Fundamentals
of
Chinese Medicine

Fundamentals of Chinese Medicine

Compiled from texts by:

Beijing College of Chinese Medicine
Nanjing College of Chinese Medicine
Shanghai College of Chinese Medicine

Translated and amended by:
Nigel Wiseman
Andrew Ellis

Consulting Editor:
Li Cheng-Yü, C.M.D.

Senior Editor:
Paul Zmiewski

East Asian Medical Studies Society

Paradigm Publications
44 Linden Street
Brookline, Massachusetts 02146

ISBN 0-912111-07-0

Copyright © 1985 East Asian Medical Studies Society

All rights reserved. No part of this publication may be reproduced, stored in a retrieval system or transmitted in any form by any means, electronic, mechanical, photocopying, recording, or otherwise, without the prior written permission of the publisher.

Consulting Editor: Li Cheng Yü
Senior Translator: Nigel Wiseman
Acumoxatherapy Translator: Andrew Ellis
Senior Editor: Paul Zmiewski

Paradigm Publications

Publisher: Robert L. Felt
Editor: Martha Lee Fielding
Chinese Character Editor: Richard Feit
Cover Design: Herb Rich, III
Editorial Assistance: Mary Kinneavy

Typesetting Software
by
Textware International: Cambridge, Massachusetts

Chinese Character Typesetting
by
Linguistic Systems: Cambridge, Massachusetts

Additional Software
and
World Distribution
provided by
Redwing Book Company: Brookline, Massachusetts

Printing
by
McNaughton & Gunn Lithographers: Ann Arbor, Michigan

Acid free, archive quality papers have been used
in the production of this text to insure longevity.

Dedication

Whenever a Great Physician treats diseases, he has to be mentally calm and his disposition firm. He should not give way to wishes and desires, but has to develop first of all a marked attitude of compassion. He should commit himself firmly to the willingness to take the effort to save every living creature.

If someone seeks help because of illness or on the grounds of another difficulty {a Great Physician} should not pay attention to status, wealth or age, neither should he question whether he is an enemy or friend, whether he is Chinese or a foreigner, or finally, whether he is uneducated or educated. He should meet everyone on equal ground; he should always act as if he were thinking of himself. He should not desire anything and should ignore all consequences; he is not to ponder over his own fortune or misfortune and should thus preserve life and have compassion for it. He should look upon those who have come to grief as if he himself had been struck, and he should sympathize with them deep in his mind. Neither dangerous mountain passes nor the time of day, neither weather conditions nor hunger, thirst nor fatigue should keep him from helping whole-heartedly. Whoever acts in this manner is a Great Physician for the living. Whoever acts contrary to these demands is a great thief for those who still have their spirits.

Sun Si-Mo, **Priceless Prescriptions** *Qiān Jīn Yào Fāng*. Quoted from Paul U. Unschuld, **Medical Ethics in Imperial China.** Berkeley: University of California Press, 1979, pp. 30-31.

Acknowledgements

This book would never have been completed without the support, encouragement, and advice of many people. We would particularly like to thank:

Hsu Fu-Su, C.M.D., for his time, patience, and expertise.

Mei Hsiang, C.M.D., Hsieh Lung-Pin, and Li Shun-Lai for valuable help concerning drug processing.

Huang Pi-Sung, C.M.D., Hsiao Chao-Hui, C.M.D., and Liu Chung-Ming, C.M.D., for their advice on terminology.

Ch'en Chun-Ch'ao and Cheng Hsiu-Lan for their help with the acupuncture sections.

Helen Seer for her careful correction of the Latin drug names.

Wang Hsun-Chih and Ting Ya-Chung for their advice on etymology and linguistics.

Michael D. McCarty for his meticulous review of the manuscript.

Sally Rimkeit, Joan Stephenson, and Kathy Denton for reading and critiquing the foreword.

Huang Sheng-Jing for her aid in compiling the glossary and bibliography.

T. Caylor Wadlington for his ideas at the inception of this project.

Stephan Schindl for his conceptual contributions, and for catching a few grievous errors.

Robert Felt and Martha Fielding for their unswerving support and encouragement.

C.D. Cheng, David Moskin, Fred Lee, and Chang Hsiu-Hsiung for their support.

Translators' Foreword

> "What is necessary is to rectify the names!"
> Confucius, *Discourses* 13:3.

> "When I use a word, it means just what I choose it to mean — neither more nor less."
> Humpty Dumpty, *Alice Through the Looking-Glass.*

The major problem facing the Western student of Chinese medicine is the dearth of literature concerning this art of healing as traditionally practiced in China. A glance at Western bookshelves shows that most of the literature categorized as "Chinese medicine" is more correctly *comment* on the subject. Much of it is comparative research in medicine and cosmology. A surprisingly large proportion of the material that has been translated into English is not from original Chinese sources, but rather from French or German. Direct translation from Chinese accounts for perhaps 10% of the available literature, and the English language usage in the greater proportion of this writing has noticeable inadequacies. Although some reliable texts on acumoxatherapy do exist, commendable works on drug therapy are scarce.

Westerners, brought up in the modern scientific tradition, often have difficulty in grasping the concepts of Chinese medicine. Preconceptions about what constitutes an effective science of healing have affected not only what is presented to the Western student, but also how it is presented. Much of English literature, including that produced in China, omits the apparently irrational, while reformulating in inexact Western medical terminology much of what is acceptable. What results is a hodgepodge presentation of Chinese medicine leading many to regard it as a morass of empirical data with few fundamental principles.

Why has this cultural barrier not been overcome? A major reason is that there is not enough literature on the bookshelves to cut through the recalcitrance of Westerners' thinking habits. Not enough effort has been put into presenting Chinese medicine faithfully as the Chinese conceive it. Translation of Chinese medicine is a formidable task, and few people are able - and even fewer willing - to do it. The complexities of translation have given rise to problems of terminology that hamper students' progress.

Translators' Foreword

It is difficult to understand and distinguish concepts unless they are clearly labelled by words.

Words and Concepts

Translation of Chinese medicine, as of any scientific discipline, requires consistent use of standardized technical terms. If different words are used by different translators to denote one concept, an unnecessary burden is placed on the student's memory. If different translators discern different concepts, the student is confused. If a translator fails to recognize a concept as such, and renders the term denoting it with a different word at each encounter, the student is completely at sea. The presentation of Chinese medicine to English-speaking readers is flawed by inconsistency both in delimitation of concepts and in the terminology that represents these concepts. This problem stems from the nature of both Chinese medicine itself and the language of the people who have devised it.

Chinese medicine deals in phenomena directly perceived by the naked human senses. Using no instruments, it focusses on quality rather than quantity. Western science, by contrast, is concerned with quantities of clearly definable substances or energies. Seeking objectivity, it is concerned with entities independent of the human mind. While Western science views perceptible qualities as the product of complex physical, chemical, physiological, and psychological processes, Chinese science focusses on the patterns of correspondences they display. What to Western science are mere appearances, to the Chinese are meaningful entities subject to clear laws. This is why Western science is said to be analytical and Chinese science synthetic or associative.

Instead of measuring quantities, the Chinese mind categorizes qualities. Yin-yang and the five phases, for example, are major systems of categorization used throughout all Chinese sciences. Both systems comprise categories of quality and relationship. All phenomena ascribed to one category are of like nature, and each stands in like relationship to a corresponding phenomenon ascribed to the other category or categories. In yin-yang theory, the relationship is one of complementarity and opposition, while in five-phase theory, the relationships are the engendering, restraining, rebelling, and overwhelming cycles. The result is a complex network of qualitative correspondences among phenomena and among relationships. Thus, yin-yang and the five phases illustrate not only the qualitative, but also the synthetic bent of Chinese thinking.

This bent pervades the whole of Chinese medicine. Physiologic processes are described as "steaming," "distilling," "bending and stretching," "flowering," etc., by dint of their similarities to processes observed in the natural environment. Relationships among organs, processes, and elements were classically expressed in the language of government, the military, and the family, as is seen in such terms as "ministerial fire," "commander of the blood," "mother of qi." In pathology, disease states are seen as being caused by, or analogous to, environmental conditions such as cold, damp, and wind.

The qualitative approach is reflected in a terminology largely comprising words that describe form, color, sound, texture, and smell, or denote qualities of motion, stasis, obstruction, and interaction. Since Chinese medicine deals in directly perceptible phenomena, it draws on the descriptive vocabulary of the layman, i.e., it uses words that need no definition other than those normally given them. It may be argued, therefore, that qualitative terms by definition are not technical terms, and do not need to be rendered with standard equivalents.

Indeed, the use of technical terms, i.e., words that are given specific meanings in a given discipline, to some extent goes against the nature of Chinese medicine, which seeks correspondences between all aspects of nature. However, when words used to describe everyday consensual reality indicate correspondences in a technical context, they assume the nature of a technical term. The word [青] qīng, for example, can mean blue or green. In the five phases, qīng corresponds to wood. English speakers naturally associate green with trees, yet they would describe as blue the complexion color denoted by qīng. If the translator only associates green with the five phases, and uses the word blue when describing complexions, his reader may not know that a connection with the five phases is intended. Although qīng is a lay word, used in a lay sense, failure to recognize its technical associations leads to loss of meaning in English. Since green cannot describe the color of complexion that qīng describes, we have chosen the word "cyan." We have done this on the grounds that the modern English word "cyan" conveys the idea of blue and green, even though cyanosis, like the original Greek root, kyanos, is associated with blue. Being an uncommon term in English, cyan can be made to convey broader associations than it normally has in a way that either green or blue cannot.

Most technical terms of Western medicine are recognizable as such by the layman largely because he is unfamiliar with the things to which they refer. He is unlikely ever to see streptococcus bacteria. Chinese medicine deals mostly in directly perceptible phenomena, so that its primary data is discussed in terms of concepts - and words - familiar to the layman. The technical nature of these concepts lies only in their significance to the physician, and is concealed by the mundaneness of the words that denote them. If such terms cannot be rendered by any existing word that can clearly convey the same technical significance, a new term must be coined, or a rarely used or archaic word must be pressed into service. The choice of comparatively rare English words highlights the technical nature of the concepts they denote.

The problem of association by no means attaches to a few words only. Although ideograms with qualitative meanings or connotations are relatively few in number, a large proportion of them are sufficiently abstract as to be able to take on a variety of concrete meanings in context. For instance, the word [淡] *dàn* describes both blandness of flavor and paleness of color, and sometimes two different doctors will give different answers as to which meaning is intended in a given context. This is because to the Chinese, there is a qualitative unity between paleness and blandness. The same is true of [膩] *nì*, which means slimy when referring to the tongue fur, and sickly when referring to the taste in the mouth. The conceptual unity in this case is underlined by the fact that both are damp signs. In such cases, the absence of a single English word to denote what the Chinese regard as a single conceptual entity may hamper the reader in forming correct associations. If only one or the other of the meanings of *dàn* and *nì* are intended in any given context they may each be rendered with two English terms. Since there is reason to believe that both of their respective meanings are intended in at least some contexts, they should ideally be treated as technical terms and rendered with single equivalents.

The relatively small corpus of ideograms expressing qualities may be used in different combinations to produce a seemingly infinite range of meanings. For example, the character [虛] *xū* means empty, insubstantial, meaningless, weak, vain, conceited, humble, etc., depending on the context in which it is found. Thus, [虛榮] *xū* (empty) plus *róng* (glory), denotes vainglory or conceit, while [謙虛] *qiān* (modest) plus *xū* (empty), means modest, in the sense of having no thought of self. English differs from Chinese in that it expresses subtle shades of meaning not by combinations, but by its much greater wealth of ready-made words. Thus, where it uses a word such as "congest," Chinese might express the notion in a form equivalent to "block-accumulate," i.e., accumulation of a substance occurring when its path is blocked. The above example of vainglory is a rare example of a combination word in English. The translator's natural bent of resorting to ready-made English equivalents to convey subtleties may deprive his readers of the associations conveyed linguistically in Chinese. While the term [淡黃] *dàn huáng*, pale yellow, can convey five-phase associations, the choice of a more expressive English term such as sallow would only provide a conceptual association. Here, *dàn* and *huáng* are technical terms in their own right.

It should be clear at this point that the problem for the translator lies in deciding whether one word represents one or more clearly definable concepts each to be rendered by technical terms, or whether it is loosely used and can therefore be translated freely according to context. If one term is seen to represent two or more clearly unrelated meanings, no harm is done by rendering these with different words. If, however, intercontextual connections are identified, a single term should be used. If, owing to limitations of his own language, the translator is forced to use different words in different contexts to convey what in Chinese is a single concept represented by a single term, he may only succeed in conveying conceptually what is clearly reflected in the language of the original. This is decidedly insufficient.

The most accurate solutions to terminological problems is to render a single Chinese term with the fewest English equivalents. We believe that it is possible to come much closer to this goal than previous writers have done. Following the principle that any Chinese term rendered by more than one English equivalent represents an act of interpretation that may cut through the associative fabric of Chinese medicine, we have sought to render terms by equivalents that will serve in as many contexts as possible. Although this approach involves the use of more abstract terms than those used by other writers, it does give the students the opportunity to discern for themselves where correspondences exist, rather than placing the onus of interpretation on the shoulders of the text writer.

Students unacquainted with Chinese should be aware that difficulties created for them by terminology are only a reflection of the difficulties translators face in rendering terms. Solutions to terminological problems vary in accordance with translators' ideas about the nature as well as the scope of a concept. In most cases, any solution is only partially correct, as every fair-minded translator would admit. Differences in terminology should be seen as providing light on concepts that are difficult to express in English. It is much more important to understand why such differences exist than to decide which solution is correct. Provided concepts are recognizable when referred to by different names, the choice of name is of secondary importance.

To give students a maximum of assistance in coping with unfamiliar terms in this text, we have included a glossary mainly comprising dictionary definitions that have been amended and expanded to permit the development of associations not inherent in English equivalents. Chinese characters accompany glossed terms not only for the benefit of those who read Chinese, but so that all students can see any connections among multiple renderings of a single Chinese term. This additional clarification should help readers to recognize familiar concepts referred to by new names. The following discussion aims to provide further insight into terminological problems and the reasons for the solutions we offer.

Technical terms

In Chinese medicine, technical terms fall into three fundamental categories: **fixed terms,** universally used by all authors throughout all ages (or over extended periods of time); **occasional terms,** used by one author; and **conditionally stipulated terms,** which, being loosely defined, are used with some degree of freedom by the writer, and are interpreted by the reader according to context. While terms of the first two categories must always be translated with standard equivalents, the latter, in theory, may be translated flexibly.

A characteristic of Chinese medicine is the unusual way in which these three categories of terms are interrelated. Owing to the reverence for classical medical works, a large number of occasional terms are used in latter-day literature to serve as allusions to a particular place in an authoritative work. Certain words used as conditionally stipulated terms are also used in some contexts as fixed terms, causing some confusion as to just when these words are being used in a strictly technical sense.

Fixed terms

Many of the basic fixed technical terms require little discussion, mainly because they represent or are derived from directly perceptible phenomena. The names of parts of the body,[1] theoretical symbols,

---

[1] The finer anatomical demarcations in ancient texts are different from those of Western medicine, but in modern texts, they are largely ignored.

and functional qualities largely belong to the realm of consensual agreement. Because of this, translation of the names of the organs, the five phases, the eight parameters, etc., is all more or less standardized. Terminological differences among writers at this level rarely give rise to confusion. If, for example, phlegm is referred to as mucus, the meaning is still clear.

This having been said, some discrepancies may still be observed in the way these fixed technical terms are rendered in English. The most obvious is the way [實] *shí* and [虛] *xū*, two of the most common words in Chinese medicine, have been rendered by different writers. "Excess" and "deficiency," coined by Bensky and others, are perhaps the most commonly used terms, and are certainly the kindest to the ears. However, it is important to understand that they are rarely suitable equivalents in contexts other than that of the eight parameters. Although it is neither possible, nor necessarily desirable, to find equivalents that cover all uses of the Chinese terms, the limited suitability of the terms deficiency and excess reflects their failure to capture fully the qualities denoted by the original terms.

Excess and deficiency denote quantitative deviations from an ideal norm. They emphasize quantity and always imply a negative value judgement. In the eight parameters, the terms *xū* and *shí* respectively denote weakness of correct qi and strength of a pathogen. Deficiency and excess are functionally adequate equivalents in this context because a relative ideal norm, health, is implied. However, they fail to reflect the essential meaning of the terms because of their quantitative and negative bias. *Shí* means having substance/force, while *xū* means not having substance/force. They are qualitative in that they stand in relation to each other, not to some predefined norm. Moreover, they have no inherent positive or negative connotations, since, for example, they imply no notion of too much or too little. When describing the root of a plant, *xū* denotes hollowness, insubstantiality, weakness, i.e., qualities analogous to those of a patient whose condition is described by the same word. Since such tangible qualities may be associated with desirable pharmacological properties, to describe such a root as "deficient" would only lead to confusion.

The ideal English equivalents should therefore be qualitative words with neither a negative nor positive value judgement. Joseph Needham uses the word "plerotic," from the Greek *plerotikos,* meaning "made full" or "filled up," and "asthenic," denoting absence of strength (having no force). Although plerotic seems to have primarily religious connotations in its rare English usage, its basic Greek meaning is more or less in keeping with the concept of *shí*. Asthenia, strictly speaking, only conveys half the meaning, the connotation of not having substance attaching to it only by association. Suggesting the idea of puniness, asthenia has clearly negative connotations. However, despite these shortcomings, these terms represent an improvement over excess and deficiency.

The words "fullness" and "emptiness" come closer to the requirements of translation. Both terms have quantitative and qualitative connotations. For example, "the bottle is half full" is a quantitative statement relating to the size of the bottle, but if we say "Jim is full of vim," the fullness referred to here is qualitative, there being no norm by which to measure it. A similar case may be made for emptiness. However, since confusion might arise with [滿] *mán,* "fullness," meaning a subjective feeling of distention, we ultimately rejected this solution.

Manfred Porkert has chosen the Latin words *repletio* and *inanitas.* These are Latin terms meaning fullness and emptiness and having a distinctly qualitative bias. *Websters New World Dictionary* defined replete as well-filled or plentifully supplied, or as stuffed with food and drink; gorged. The Chinese word *shí* means to fill, well-filled, solid, or overfilled. As with replete, its positive and negative connotations vary according to context. However, while *repletio* finds a close English derivative in "repletion," the words *inanus* (adjective) and *inanitas* (noun) took on highly specific connotations of "meaningless" and "stupidity" when they were absorbed into English as "inane" and "inanity." The Chinese word *xū* means hollow, empty, insubstantial. Only "inanition" preserves acceptable connotations. We therefore decided to use the word "repletion," but have replaced its opposite with the word "vacuity," which is more directly associated with the notion of emptiness and insubstantiality. The words repletion and vacuity are applicable in the widest variety of contexts because they convey meanings similar to the Chinese terms. Although they may seem unusual at first, our experience shows that sacrificing superficial readability for terminological precision is compensated by familiarity which comes with time and use.

Other, finer distinctions appear irrelevant to some writers and are therefore glossed over. Let us take the example of "liquid" [津] (*jīn*) and "humor" [液] (*yè*). All Chinese sources agree that liquid is the thinner fluid of the human body, while humor is the thicker one, and that the compound term [津液] *jīn-yè,* which we translate as "fluid," represents both types of fluid collectively. The differences would appear to be ignored because it is often felt that both single terms are sometimes used to denote the fluids collectively. What must be understood is that literary, and to a certain extent modern, Chinese expresses itself largely in four-character phrases, and that in some cases one character is used to represent two in order to conform with this pattern. In such cases, the ancient writers had the choice of either omitting *jīn* or *yè*. Their choice was most likely prompted by a natural emphasis on one or the other according to context, since a certain amount of regularity is observed in usage. We reflect this in our translation by adhering firmly to standardized equivalents. However, it is important to understand that the English terms "liquid," "humor," and the generic term "fluid" are more or less synonymous, although liquid tends to mean the thinner fluids, while humor tends to refer to the thicker ones.

While some writers ignore the difference between the two forms of fluid, others prefer to offer highly interpretive renderings with relatively rigid definitions. Manfred Porkert, for example, refers to them in English as "active" and "structive" (i.e., yang and yin) fluids (1974, pp. 190-191). While these terms are useful in conveying the essential significance of the Chinese words, we feel that it is not the translator's task to use words that have more precise definitions than the original terms they render. Furthermore, equating *jīn* and *yè* completely with yang and yin leaves the problem of how to translate the frequently encountered term [陰液] *yīn-yè*, rendered in this text as "yin humor." Our terms - liquid, humor, and fluid - are all more or less synonymous in conventional English usage, as are their Chinese ideograms. The advantage in using them is that they can accrete new meanings and associations, according to their context in Chinese medicine, without imposing rigid definitions. Only terms that allow for interpretation and reasonably flexible association can hope to gain currency in a discipline so fraught by differences of opinion.

Much of the terminology relating to diagnostics is oversimplified for want of clear definitions. To some extent, this problem arises out of the assumption that symptoms are perceived through the senses and that they can therefore be described in the language of consensual reality, or by merely resorting to the most likely Western medical equivalents. However, Chinese medicine uses no instruments in diagnosis, and does not rely on quantitative measurement. The Chinese physician's senses are more highly trained than those of his Western counterpart, and this is reflected in the nuances in Chinese diagnostic terminology. Distinction is made, for example, between thirst and desire for fluid; if both Chinese terms are rendered as thirst, a highly important distinction is lost.

In diagnostics, it should be remembered that distinctions indicated in Chinese texts should not be ignored simply because the reader (or translator) does not understand their significance. The translator's job is to translate all he sees, not just the part of it that suits his own conceptions or falls within his own limited experience.

Some of the problems of translating basic concepts stem from the misattribution of functions to parts of the body. For example, Chinese medical literature tells us that the term "sinews" [筋] (jīn) refers to the tendons and ligaments, although nobody seems to agree on what the precise functional correspondence is in Western medicine. The ancient Chinese perceived the existence of white sinewy tissue in the muscle (presumably through autopsy), and, for reasons which may not be wholly apparent to us, associated them with certain aspects of motor function. We felt it would be wrong to equate this concept with either tendons or ligaments, as these are precise morphological entities with clearly defined functions in Western medicine. The more neutral term, sinews, can more readily take on the functional associations its Chinese equivalent carries.

Even the names of the organs are the subject of some disagreement. Some writers have capitalized these names in order to highlight the fact that they are morphologically the same as, but functionally different from the entities referred to by the same names in Western medicine. The use of capitals in English suggests a sense of reverence, importance, or strangeness that does not exist in the original Chinese. As in Western medicine, once technical terms have been explained, they do not need to be highlighted typographically. Others treat the organs as "orbs of function" in order to underline their opinion that the organ names refer only to groups of functions. To do this constitutes altering the original information, which is not the translator's task. Rightly or wrongly, the Chinese labelled functions with terms denoting morphological entities also known in the West. Any rendering other than their simple uncapitalized English names represents an unnecessary act of interpretation.

Another example is the concept of qi, which refers to behavioral patterns seen to occur through the spatial extension of a physical medium. Qi is both activity and active substance, and to the Chinese resides firmly in the realm of consensual reality. Qi is not simply flow through the channels, as detected by pathologic changes, or reaction to needle or other stimulation along channel pathways. It occurs in terms denoting things that pervade the atmosphere, like odors [氣味] (qì wèi) and damp [溼氣] (shī qì). It describes the politeness felt to emanate from guests [客氣] (kè qì) and the physical turbulence felt in anger [生氣]

(shēng qì). In medicine, the same term is used to describe the movement of digestate through the digestive tract [濁氣] *(zhuó qì)*. Similarly, vomiting, eructation, hiccough, and facial flush are seen as counterflow rising of qi. Reluctance to recognize qi as a unique concept has caused it to be misrendered as "energy," despite the fact that it is a firmly established neologism among English-speaking students of Chinese medicine. In the entirety of Chinese medical literature there is little evidence to suggest that qi means anything like the Western concept of energy; we believe it should always be rendered by transcription until the (unlikely) discovery of a Western scientific correspondence warrants any change.

Diseases in any given system of medicine are clearly definable entities. Many Chinese medical disease categories have close, but not exact, equivalents in Western medicine. Translation of Western medical literature into Chinese provides precedents of how terms can or should be translated. In some cases, Chinese exponents of Western medicine have drawn on Chinese medical terms, while in others, they have invented new ones. The same approach can be adopted by Western exponents of Chinese medicine, provided they point out any differences of meaning if the same terms are used. Translation of disease names should always be in keeping with the definition Chinese medicine gives them.

The problem arises when Chinese and Western medicine are synthesized, i.e., when both forms of medicine are used and spoken of together, as is now often the case. We have adopted the approach of making distinctions in terminology wherever fundamental differences in the nature or conception of diseases are observed. For example, the Chinese term [氣喘] *qì chuǎn*, which is used in Western medicine to translate the notion of asthma, has been rendered in the present text as wheezing and dyspnea, since in Chinese medicine distinction is made between the two components. The term [消渴] *xiāo kě*, which frequently corresponds to one form of diabetes or another, but is not used in Western medicine, has been rendered as "diabetic disease." Here, the similarity, yet slight difference in terminology is designed to maintain the association with Western medicine, while still implying some difference. However, certain archaic terms have no equivalents in Western medicine, and in fact have so many different associations that rendering them with any single English term is impossible; in these few cases, we have had no alternative but to retain the original Chinese, defining them at length in the appended glossary. [疝] *Shàn* and [疳] *gān* are two examples of this.

Occasional terms

Occasional terms are those used by particular authors alone, or at a particular place in their writings. Where such terms occur in the ever-revered classics, they succinctly point to a particular frame of reference. For example, if the student were to see 汗出濈濈然 *hàn chū jí jí rán* (a constant stream of sweat), he would know that the author was referring to the section relating to yang ming disease in *A Treatise on Cold Damage*. Since the Chinese have a tradition of memorizing the classics, allusion suffices where a Westerner would expect an explicit reference. At present, few of the classics have been translated (and no translation is accepted as definitive), so that when these terms occur in modern writing, they are translated according to context. Even though standard translations of the classics are not available, these words should nevertheless be considered as technical terms and rendered consistently, if only to avoid confusion in identifying their sources.

Conditionally stipulated terms

The greatest problem of translation undoubtedly lies in the rendering of conditionally stipulated terms. This category mainly comprises a corpus of some two hundred ideograms describing physiopathologic activity and methods of treatment, and includes words such as those rendered in this text as "abduct," "course," "depurate," "disinhibit," "dissipate," "effuse," "percolate," "perfuse," etc. These words describe qualities of activity that are subjectively perceived by the medical community as a whole, and are therefore definable. Though they overlap in meaning and can be used with a certain degree of flexibility, they commonly occur in fixed technical terms. For example, "dissipate" [散] *(sàn)* conveys a general notion of dispersion, but in the term "dissipating cold" [散寒] *(sàn hán)*, it denotes the more specific notion of eliminating the cold pathogen in the interior.

It should be understood that qualitative terms are very often the exclusive property of one linguistic community. As such they present difficulties of translation that are often best overcome by flexible rendering according to context. However, when they function as technical terms, as they do in Chinese medicine, the necessity to render them with standard equivalents cannot be ignored.

The lack of any consistent correspondence between qualitative association of Chinese and English words means that one English word could be used to render a number of different Chinese terms, and vice-versa. For example, the words "clear," "dissipate," and "dispel" could each, by virtue of their manifold connotations, probably render at least three of the commonly used Chinese terms in some, though not all, of their contexts. However, where the use of a term is highly specific, a glut of partial equivalents is no substitute for a single equivalent that can be used consistently.

In Western sciences, technical terms are usually derived by giving an existing word a stipulated definition it did not have before, and translators will usually select equivalents by the same method. Words may be chosen on account of their analogous qualities (as "mosaic" was chosen to represent a highly specific concept in genetics), but in such cases the qualitative aspect usually serves only to aid comprehension or memory. By contrast, many words in Chinese medicine are used precisely for the qualitative value they have in nontechnical contexts. If the translator finds no ready-made equivalents, he is hard pressed to invent any. It is a linguistic fact that while words with particular qualitative associations can be given new specific meanings, they are particularly resistant to the grafting of new qualitative associations. It is for this reason that previous translators of Chinese medicine have taken the flexible approach, rendering terms with appropriate equivalents according to context. However, we believe that conditionally stipulated terms should, as far as possible, be rendered with standard equivalents. Our reasoning is as follows:

First, the flexible approach fails when words function as specific technical terms. Free translation poses the danger of blurring fine distinctions such as between the different intensities of therapeutic action denoted by "blood quickening" [活血] *(huó xuè)*, "stasis transformation" [化鬱] *(huà yù)*, and "blood breaking" [破血] *(pò xuè)*. Failure to make terminological distinctions, such as between "extinguishing wind" [熄風] *(xí fēng)*, which is a method used to treat certain forms of endogenous wind, and "dispelling wind" [祛風] *(qū fēng)*, which applies only to exogenous wind, could, if the context is not sufficiently clear, give rise to confusion. There is much evidence to suggest that up to now many fixed technical terms have not been recognized as such, and consequently have not been rendered with standard equivalents.

Second, conditionally stipulated terms often have more than one specific application. For example, [化] *huà,* rendered in this book as "transformation," describes not only the action of the spleen, but also specific methods of treating damp, static blood, phlegm, etc.. The specific application could theoretically be rendered with different words, e.g., by using "transformation" to describe splenic function and "resolution" to denote the methods of pathogen elimination. Such a solution would be justifiable were it not for the fact that it denies the unity of the concept *huà* in denoting changes of a particular nature. We feel that accurate translation should reflect the conceptual unity of the term, and so we have rendered it consistently, despite the awkwardness initially felt at having to accommodate its new connotations.

Third, only by ensuring the highest possible degree of linguistic association can students detect correspondences that are inherent in the synthetic, inductive approach characteristic of Chinese medicine, and which are crucial to its understanding. For example, the term [困] *kùn* describes the way in which damp hampers splenic function and the heaviness felt in the limbs as a result. The present text speaks of "splenic encumbrance" and "cumbersome limbs" to preserve this association. While it may be argued that this example is only a translator's nicety, the argument in favor of rendering [鬱] *yù* with "depression" as its standard equivalent carries greater force. To the Chinese, *yù* describes a repressed state of both certain physical functions and emotional activity, frequently occurring together. They see clear correspondences between the two, since they have never entertained any division between mind and body. Thus, what is referred to as a "correspondence" could be seen equally as nothing more than continuity of functional quality.

Fourth, consistent English correspondences for Chinese terms make translated literature easier reading for those conversant with Chinese and who would otherwise not wish to waste their time wading through unfamiliar English terminology. It also greatly simplifies the task of the Chinese-trained teacher of Chinese medicine attempting to teach in an unfamiliar language.

Usage of many of the conditionally stipulated terms has changed with the gradual evolution of the language. We have decided that wherever possible, a particular term should be rendered at all times by the same standard equivalent. For example, in the phrase, "depression of fire is treated by effusion" [火鬱發之] *(huǒ yù fā zhī)*, the terms "depression" and "effusion" are used to denote meanings slightly different from those they convey in modern usage. Though the basic meaning of the words has remained the same, their specific application has changed. Our decision to adhere to standard equivalent terms is designed to help those who know Chinese to recognize the classical reference. In this way, standardized terms embrace differences in usage over the history of Chinese medicine. Students should understand that the terseness of the literary style of writing, and the changes in the usage of terms, means that today's

Chinese-speaking student has to rely largely on the footnotes provided by successive generations of commentators. If the English-speaking student is confused by such phrases, he may be comforted to know that the Chinese student has no clearer idea of their meaning.

In some cases, standard equivalent terms are hard to find. On occasion we have had to resort to new coinages, e.g., "disinhibition" [利] *(lì)*, "downbearing" [降] *(jiàng)*, and "summerheat" [暑] *(shǔ)*. In view of the wordiness of English by comparison with Chinese, we have seen fit to bend English usage by introducing unconventional transitive forms, as for example in "diffusing the lung" (i.e., promoting diffusion of lung qi). Our experience over the more than two years it has taken to translate this book is that both associations and grammatical usages of words can to some extent be extended to accommodate new concepts.

Conclusion

Failure to recognize words as representing qualitatively precise technical terms reduces what in Chinese are coherent, internally consistent linguistic conventions to a conceptually impoverished jumble of words leading only to misinterpretation and confusion. What we have attempted in this present volume is to create a system of terminology paralleling that of the Chinese, thus enabling the English-speaking student to form the same series of definitions and associations as his Chinese counterpart. We feel that this is the only method by which the essential nature of Chinese medical thought can be accurately transmitted to the West, and the only way it can be understood as thoroughly, and practiced as successfully, as it is in the East. We believe that the acceptability of such a terminology depends largely on the degree of freedom left for interpretation according to context, and therefore propose standardization of terminology in a manner that presupposes no greater or lesser degree of definition than is inherent in the original Chinese.

Ideally, the work of translation should be a cooperative effort. However, because the differences of opinion about Chinese medicine are even greater in the West than in the East, gaining general agreement on a standardized terminology will be no easy task. Despite these differences (or perhaps because of them), it is of primary importance to establish a unified approach to translation. We hope that our effort will provide a first step in this direction.

Translators' Foreword

* * * *

This book is a translation of *Zhōng Yī Xué Jī Ch*, from the Shanghai College of Chinese Medicine. Certain omissions in the original text led the translators to add material from other sources. For example, acumoxatherapy was included to complete the treatment sections. Point locations were chosen through research on classical and modern texts, with the advice of experienced physicians. They therefore represent a synthesis of old and new, of clinical and theoretical methods. These additions are intended to serve as a guide for further study rather than a comprehensive exposition of the subject.

Finally, we realize that this translation will contain errors; we beg your tolerance and welcome comments and suggestions.

Introduction

Oriental Medicine: Culture, History and Transformation

The movement of Oriental medicine beyond the confines of its native languages necessarily creates more than linguistic translation. The publication of this excellent translation of a crucial, contemporary Chinese medical text is a perfect opportunity to raise some broader questions concerning cultural transmission. While the matter does continue to generate discussion, we do have some consensus as to what constitutes good literary translation. A good translation brings the sense and richness of the original to the life of a different language.

With *Fundamentals of Chinese Medicine,* the goal of translation is more than that of literary classics, which are ends of themselves. Rather, the goal is to assist in the faithful translation of an entire medical tradition. In the long run, however, the results will be the same as any cross-cultural undertaking. For instance, translating the Bible into Greek and Latin launched it on a new career. Or, closer to the material in hand, the Bodhidharma's journey East and his legendary translations, unleashed much more than a mere appreciation of Buddhism or an exact replication of its Indian style. Examples from history abound and we should not be surprised that translations of Oriental medical texts will have unimagined consequences. Perhaps, the more good translations we have, the more direct access to Oriental medicine we acquire, the faster the transmitted medicine will diverge from the presumed original.

This process is natural and occurs whether we are aware of it or not. Neither is this the first time that Oriental medicine will have changed by its travels. Yet, *Fundamentals of Chinese Medicine* comes at a time when Oriental medicine has already ceased to be a fringe phenomena and is poised to acquire a greater role in the West. Aware that change is taking place, we can begin to frame the questions Oriental medicine must answer to make the transition.

Oriental medicine will confront a series of novel and distinct situations. Viruses, diseases, work and leisure styles, diet, intra-psychic and interpersonal sensitivities, social behaviors, health care systems, economic pressures, perceptions of existential intactness, and cultural definitions of health and illness are clearly not the same. The movement of a medical system from one culture to another always necessitates an adaptation to a different cultural environment with different health requirements, divergent idioms of distress and vocabularies of discomfort. As Arthur Kleinman notes:

> Indigenous healing practices cannot be removed from their social, structural, and cultural contexts, and transferred unaltered to alien cultural settings, such as the contemporary U.S. society, as a quick way of fabricating a "holistic" system of care. Therapeutic practices and practitioners are situated in specific contexts that help determine their structure and from which they cannot be readily separated without undergoing fundamental alteration (Kleinman 1980a, 431).

All medical systems confront a changing world, even if they stay within their native culture. However, the process of moving from East to West is a particularly dramatic leap. The conservative response to this process is to resist all change with the justification that by becoming westernized, Oriental medicine is in peril of losing its initial inspiration. This underestimates its strength. Far from undermining Oriental medicine, I believe that the challenge of the new environment will attest to the validity of the Oriental medical approach. In any case, the goal is not to maintain Oriental medicine as a healing model for only those who already embrace an Eastern model of reality. To truly flourish in the West, it must treat people who have never contemplated practicing Tai Chi or thought for a moment of the nameless Tao.

As Western practitioners, students and scholars, our minimum responsibility is two fold. First, we must have access to accurate information from first-hand sources such as this translation. Concomitantly, we need to become poignantly aware of how culture and history demand from us different answers than those presently fixed in the tradition as it is variously understood in different Asian countries.

Oriental Medicine's Clinical Gaze

I would like to be explicit concerning my perception of the essential "clinical gaze" of Oriental medicine. A health care system's clinical gaze can be defined as "the conceptual structures which constitute the frame of reference within which all questions are posed and all answers offered" (Jewson 1976, 225). This method of observation, which necessarily interacts with clinical experience, is what may be formally abstracted from a medical approach, minus the specific medical demands culture and history place upon it. If such a clinical gaze can be said to exist, it seems to me that the fundamental points of departure for Oriental medicine must include the following principles:

> Change is constant. All sensations, motivations, functions, activities, and events are a manifestation of complimentary opposites. This dialectical perspective is symbolically

described by the principles yin and yang, or at other times, by the five phases or other emblematic systems. There is no sharp dichotomy between mind and body, subjective and objective. The physical, mental, emotional, behavioral, social, existential and spiritual dimensions of life interpenetrate and are "not considered mutually exclusive, to be accounted for by sharply different varieties of discourse" (Sivin 1982, 52). Health is a dynamic harmony and interaction of an inner environment with an exterior world. Sensory observation and a synthetic thought process allow us to discern and understand the qualities of being and behavior that define human reality. Human intervention can effect change. Previous clinical and theoretical understanding can guide current practice.

I think these principles encapsulate the spoken and unspoken points of agreement in the medical gaze that derives from the *Yellow Emperor's Inner Canon*, the earliest preserved text of the Oriental medical tradition. I think that the major thinkers and practitioners of Oriental medicine in China, Japan, Korea and Vietnam could live within this set of axioms and assumptions. If we accept this, or something close to it, the next question becomes: How do culture and history influence and interact with the details of this method? What are the particular pressures and constraints that modify how the clinical gaze of Oriental medicine is discussed? How is the yin and yang of Oriental medicine colored by time and place?

Cultural Perceptions of Disharmony

No human knowledge, understanding, behavior or insight is without a cultural dimension. As Malinowski (1944, 69) posited long ago,

> ". . . not even the simplest need, nor yet the physiological functions most independent of environmental influences can be regarded as completely unaffected by culture. . . . There is no human activity which we could regard as purely physiological that is "natural" or "untutored."

All activities and behaviors of people have a learned component. Even basic needs such as what to eat, who and how to mate, what to wear, how to sleep and rest, and how to eliminate bodily waste, need to be learned. All have a cultural component (Malinowski 1944).

Sociologists, anthropologists and historians have long been aware that illness is not an objective fact perceived, reacted to, and reported similarly by all cultural groups. Zola has shown this in his many dramatic studies the sociocultural determinants of perception and reaction to symptoms (Zola 1983). For example, in a study at the Massachusetts General Hospital, he demonstrated that Italian and Irish patients with a matched eye pathology had different symptoms, interpretations, and responses (Zola

1966). Zborowski has shown how Irish, Italian, and "old stock Yankee" variously experience pain, one of the most common symptoms of illness (Zborowski 1952; Zborowski 1969). Later studies extended these observations to other ethnic groups (Wolff and Langley 1964). It is even possible to find tribal peoples, the Bariba of Nigeria for example, who consistently demonstrate an absence of pain behavior (Sargent 1984). Symptoms of illness are not consistent cross-cultural variables. Individuals in any social setting learn to perceive, experience, label, express and respond to symptoms differently (Kleinman 1980b).

This has long been noticed for the more "psychological" disorders. The definition of mental and emotional abnormality is very obviously culturally determined. The frequency and patterns of symptoms in mental and affect disorders vary widely across cultures (Singer 1975). For example, some societies can accept hallucinatory experiences without anxiety. Many symptoms or syndromes exist only in specific cultures: *kuru,* "shrinking penis," in Southeast Asia (Rin 1965); *latah,* "ticklish," in Malaya; *wihitigo,* "a giant creature with a heart of ice," among the Cree Indians (Yap 1951); and *susto,* "fright," among the Mexican-Americans (Rubel 1960). We might just as well add "anorexia nervosa" in contemporary America to the list (Swartz 1985). The very notions of psychosomatic disorders (Helman 1985) and depression (Marsella 1980; Tseng and Hsu 1969), and arguably even psychology itself (Ackerknecht 1943), have cultural and ethnocentric dimensions.

Even with "purely physical" symptoms, if one can speak of purely physical problems (Leigh 1977), we need social evaluation to determine whether these are diseases. For example, some cultures consider cough, yawns, malaria, and eczema normal (Ackerknecht 1968). The very labeling and definition of bodily states as symptoms or problems is part of a social process (Zola 1976, 630). Even beyond this question, the experience, in itself, of a "physical" symptom necessarily varies between cultures. Horacio Fabrega notes:

> Although terms such as weakness or nausea may have straightforward clinical implications, it must be emphasized that they are rooted in differing phenomenological complexes. For example, what causes nausea and how it is conceptualized, experienced and reported will differ according to meanings people attribute to their body, to their food and to vomiting. . . . The influence that social and cultural patterns have in shaping the way in which subjects experience and define medical issues suggests . . . [that] altered bodily sensations fuse with their socio-moral implications and interpretations to form a culturally relevant picture that symbolizes a disarticulation of the self (Fabrega 1980, 145-146).

Most "common physical symptoms" can be semantic metaphors of psychic, social and behavioral disruption and conflict that have unique cultural components. In his studies concerning the Chinese, Kleinman sees this subtlety as so persuasive that he has called for research "to provide phenomenological accounts of common symptoms and affects in different cultural systems" to combat "biomedical and psychological reductionism [that] strips away what is most unique to these terms and the experiences they constitute and express" (Kleinman 1980b, 145).

Obviously, the observations of the social sciences have ramifications for how Oriental medicine is understood in the West. For example, "seeing ghosts," "running piglet syndrome," or "mountain-top-naked-screaming syndrome," conditions frequently cited in early Oriental medical texts, may have had a particular cultural significance not automatically understood by Westerners, or even by contemporary Chinese. There are analogous problems for "physical" symptoms. For example, the symptom of "oppression," represented by the Chinese character of a doorway enclosing a heart (*men*), is clearly uniquely Chinese and not merely a physical sensation (the gloss of this volume notes this for the first time in any English translation). The ubiquitous Chinese symptom of "spermatorrhea" in modern China has little or no relation to what a modern Westerner might think, having more to do with Chinese social-sexual conflicts than any involuntary emission of sperm (cf. Englehardt 1974; Gilbert 1975; Parsons 1977). Illness response always strongly influences the symptoms themselves (Mechanic 1972). Even "lumbago" has meanings that extend beyond simple, physical sensations of discomfort (Kleinman 1982; Nagi 1973). The unique Oriental way of experiencing disorder, limitation, impairment and inadequacy needs to be examined. Without such an inquiry we can neither expect to understand what its methods are nor sensitively apply them to real people in other cultural circumstances.

Locating Discomfort: Psyche and Soma

The clinical gaze of Oriental medicine recognizes the continuum and interaction of the psyche and soma. The methodology has always taken into account the psychosomatic truth that psychological and physiological processes are interactive and have a shared clinical significance. For example, on a very simple level, Oriental medicine can see anxiety and heart palpitations, fear and sweating, revulsion and nausea, anger and changes in metabolism, and despair and sighing, as being emotional and physical concomitants of a single yin-yang manifestation. Nevertheless, contemporary Eastern and Western people tend to experience different ends of this continuum in their lives. What may be a single "energetic" phenomena in Oriental medical theory can be a totally different experience for peoples of different culture.

Introduction

Arthur Kleinman (1980b, 135) observes that contemporary Chinese people "learn not to attend to their feelings and acquire little skill in identifying emotional states. Non-specific names lump together emotions that contemporary Westerners readily differentiate." Francis Hsu (1952, 12) saw one "fundamental contrast [between Chinese and Americans] is the prominence of emotion in the American way of life as compared to the tendency of the Chinese to underplay all matters of the heart." He saw suppression of affect as the dominant mechanism of socialization of the individual in China and Japan (Hsu 1949) and observed that Chinese people do not commonly reveal strong normal or dysphoric affects (Hsu 1971a). Cultural rules defining proper relationships prohibit "free recognition of feelings in a Western sense" (Hsu 1971b). On standard psychological tests, such as the MMPI, many responses of Chinese subjects tend to differ greatly from, or to be the opposite of, those given by American subjects (Chang 1985; Song, W. 1985). Americans tend to recognize and experience problems as derived from internal feeling states, while Chinese culture focuses on external situations of the physical (White 1982).

Illnesses that are recognized in the West as primarily affect or emotional disorders are experienced as being somatic in the East. Most cross-cultural studies seem to corroborate Tseng's conclusion (Tseng 1975, 237) that "Chinese patients tend to somatize their emotional conflicts." Kleinman (1975, 6) also comments, "Minor psychiatric problems - depression, anxiety reaction, hysteria, psychophysiological reactions, etc. - are most commonly labelled as medical (physical) illnesses. That is, the secondary physical complaints accompanying the psychological disorders are labelled as medical problems, while the psychological issues are systematically left unlabelled." Lau (1983, 114) states, "Depressive illness often passes unrecognized in domiciliary practice, because of its tendency to hide behind a facade of somatic symptoms that command the patient's as well as the doctor's attention." Once a physical or "physiomorphic label" (Ohnuki-Tierney 1984, 75) is applied, "it remains unclear to what extent the expectations alter the very nature of the symptoms, but something of this kind might well happen" (Kleinman 1980b, 143).

This process of learning to self-monitor in culturally specific ways begins in earliest childhood. A carefully matched study recorded by Caudill (1969, 16) showed that "by three to four months of age Japanese and American infants have learned in some ways to behave differently, in response to the culturally patterned behavior of their mothers." American babies were conditioned to be more verbal, assertive and expressive, while Japanese babies communicated by physical means and were conditioned to be more passive. In a follow-up study (Caudill 1977) of the same children at the age of two and a half years old, the research showed that Japanese mothers tried to monitor minor changes in the child's body in order to recognize the child's urge to eliminate; they then responded by putting the child in the right location. The American mother showed less close physical involvement and demanded that the child learn to go to the toilet by himself. The communication of bodily states was more verbal and cognitive.

Similar findings have been made in China.

> Chinese parents do not impose strict toilet training on the child when he is very young. The Chinese mother holds the baby in her arms when he wants to urinate. She learns to recognize the baby's bodily behavior and tries to respond to the baby so as to facilitate his urination. It is the mother who "trains" herself and sensitizes herself to the baby's rhythm (Tseng 1979, 7).

"The Chinese mother . . . learns to be sensitive to the minute signals and to hold her baby away from her at exactly the critical moment" (Yeh 1978, 134). The communication of changed bodily states in infancy is through physical sensation in the East, through verbal encouragement of self-consciousness in the West. A more generalized study concerning the severity of child-training practices between Chinese and American middle-class families showed that the oral, anal, and genital stages were all markedly more severe in the East, as was training around dependence and aggression issues (Scofield 1960). Even the usually culturally insensitive psychoanalytic literature could not help but observe that "the Chinese have achieved totally different solutions to the Oedipal problem" (LaBarre 1946). Caudill's study of Japanese-American children concluded that the "precursors of certain ways of behaving, thinking and feeling that are characteristic of a given culture have become part of an infant's approach to his environment well before the development of language and hence are not easily accessible to consciousness or to change" (Caudill 1969, 16).

Locating Personhood: Self and Other

Emotions and affect are not the only way in which sensitivity to states of being and behavior differs between the East and West. The sense of self, purpose and meaning of life is fundamentally different. Well-being and its accompanying sense of unhamperedness derives from different inspirations and sources (cf. Baumann 1961). This necessarily has a tremendous impact on how illness and health manifest. Francis Hsu (1971b, 29) points out that the Chinese concept of person contrasts sharply with the Western concept of personality:

> The [Western] concept of personality puts the emphasis on what goes on in the individual's psyche including his deep core of complexes and anxieties. The nature of the individual's external behavior are seen as expressions, reasons, or indicators of these forces. Since the deepest complexes and anxieties are also regarded as the prime mover of the entire psyche, the rearrangement of such complexes and anxieties are seen to hold

the key to the solution of the individual's problems. But the concept of *jen* [Chinese idea of person] puts the emphasis on interpersonal transactions. It does not consider the individual psyche's deep core of complexes and anxieties. Instead it sees the nature of the individual exterior behavior in terms of how it fits or fails to fit the interpersonal standards of society and culture.

The contemporary Western patient tends to experience selfhood as "individual-centered" and monitors his changing states in intensely personal and existential terms, while the contemporary Chinese patient tends to view selfhood as "situation-centered" and illness and health in physical terms (Hsu 1985, 12).

Godwin Chu (1985, 258) expands on Hsu's idea: "The traditional Chinese self . . . appears to be relatively more oriented towards the significant others, rather than toward the individual self." Thus a male Chinese would consider himself a son, a brother, a husband, a father, but hardly himself. It seems as if outside the relational context of the significant others, there was very little independent self for the Chinese. An old saying well illustrates this point: "One's body, hair, and skin are gifts from one's parents. One is not at liberty to do harm to them." Contrast this very physical expression with the popular attitude among some American teenagers: "This is my life, and I'll do what I want with it" (Chu 1985, 258). Margaret Lock (1978, 162) captures these differences in a valuable observation: "In Japan, the worst kind of punishment for a child is to be made to stand outside its house in the street - to be separated from its family; a striking contrast to the American child who is usually shut in. In Japan, punishment is separation from nurturance. In the U.S., it is the separation from freedom and individuality."

The Orient has a different concept of freedom, as Yeh (1978, 133) tells us:

> The word freedom is seldom used in the Confucian classics or current literature. In the traditional Chinese mind, freedom, both from external pressures and internal psychological restraints, has been entirely a matter of cultivation of the individual's moral character according to his social roles. The Chinese is free from inner conflict and feels no resentment against conformity and no compunction about behaving differently under contrasting circumstances.

In the West, Kierkegaard's question, "How does one become an individual?" and Heidegger's demand for "inward truth" or "truth as freedom," are an important undertone of people's concern, though they might not express it in these terms. Western people and patients tend to be aware that "the human being's paramount struggle is with the givens, the ultimate concerns, of existence: death, isolation, freedom, and meaninglessness" (Yalom 1985, 95). Contemporary Western patients (at least in the middle and upper classes) are acutely aware of issues such as existential doubt, emptiness, meaninglessness, estrangement, conflict, and alienation from oneself. They readily experience and acknowledge the importance to the well-being to such notions as despair, fragmented personality, anxiety of non-being, self-awareness, purpose, meaning, values, and self-realization.

Medical Implications for Oriental Medicine

The fact that the authentic self of China is more physical and interpersonal and the self of the modern West is more psychological and existential is crucial for shaping what makes a person a patient and a patient a person in each culture (cf. Shweder and Bovine 1982). Why people and patients experience or do not experience symptoms as hindering and obstructing, what converts a person to a patient and vice-versa, has much to do with multi-levels of sensitivity and self-awareness that amplify or dampen, reinforce or diffuse, the experience of wellness or sickness (Eisenberg 1980; Cassell 1982). Not to be aware of the cultural dimension of perceived wellness and illness is to assure second-rate and and inadequate medical care.

This different cultural perception and understanding is obvious to students of Chinese medicine visiting China. First-hand clinical experience frequently prompts Western observers to remark, "It seems as if all the patients have read the textbooks." Patients in China often report "neat" problems with details concerning particulars of perspiration, gradations of thirst, various tastes in the mouth and other descriptions that are routine components of health care discourse in China. People have learned to monitor themselves on this level and this is what doctors elicit. Little psychological and existential detail is involved. Western practitioners of Chinese medicine wonder why their patients never quite have these kind of simple "textbook" presentations or descriptions. It would be wrong to conclude that the Oriental medical perspective is necessarily limited to physical discussions. Rather, the situation is that the Oriental medicine of contemporary China follows the socially and culturally appropriate somatic communication of discomfort. Practitioners in the Orient "choose to focus on somatic complaints as a point of departure for therapeutic intervention. Dealing directly with psychological and social factors would destroy rapport and minimize cooperation" (Lock 1980, 221). Oriental people and their health care practitioners monitor wellness and sickness, intactness and brokenness, health and illness, in culturally unique ways.

A culture's idiom of distress not only influences clinical care and but also has a great impact on medical theory and the formalized "voice of medicine." For example, modern Chinese and Japanese medical theoreticians speak of the liver and heart as being more sensitive to emotional issues than other organs (see pages 204-211 and 232-242 of this volume). In modern China, this perspective is perfectly correct. Liver emotions such as anger and hostility or heart states of unclarity and confusion are socially inappropriate in China and very noticeable: they disrupt "face" (Hu, 1944). Yet, other emotional states that are connected with the quality of energy of other organs such as the spleen, small intestine, kidney, or lung are not part of the discourse of doctor-patient dialogue in modern China. There is no compelling theoretical or clinical reason to include their emotional presentation in books like *Essentials of Chinese Acupuncture* (Beijing 1980) or this present volume.

This is also true for the existential issues. The earliest layers of Oriental medicine are replete with existential discussion (though usually in Chinese culture-bound terms). The relation of the *hun* (non-corporal soul), *po* (corporal soul), *yi* (intention), *zhi* (intelligence), and *zhi* (will) to energetic configurations is discussed in detail throughout early medical texts, e.g., *Ling Shu,* Chapter 8, or *Nan Jing,* Chapter 34. These discussions have been systematically deleted from modern Chinese medical discourse. Given their cultural and historical needs, modern Chinese medical thinkers can legitimately talk about the kidney's relationship to hair and urination and will correctly omit its relations to will, meaning, death, fantasy, and purpose. Likewise, the spleen's relationship to muscles or digestion is amplified, but its connection with being nurtured, being "at home in the world," trustworthiness, and responsibility are glossed over. Whole areas of key questions concerning crucial areas for Western patients are not to be found in these modern texts. (In the People's Republic of China, this is reinforced by political considerations, as I will discuss later). Yet, these issues may be critical for practitioners in the developed nations. Western patients readily bring up and expect health care providers to address such well-being issues as self-abusive behavior, indecision, uncontrollable urges, shyness, feelings of inadequacy or superiority, guilt, brooding, phobias, ambivalence, anxiety, social withdrawal, distrust, jealousy, envy, resentment, failure to mourn, promiscuity, clumsiness, timidity, passivity, overactivity, obsessiveness, fastidiousness, hysteria, withdrawal, or delusions. Family relationships, work and career issues, lifestyle management, sexual problems, stress reduction, are aspects of the health care concerns of Western patients. If Western practitioners shirk these dimensions of health care, it will be impossible to understand and properly treat our patients, and the therapeutic relationship itself may become jeopardized.

The overly somatic doctor-patient dialogue of the modern East is obviously inadequate for a modern Western clinical encounter. Certainly, it would be criticized in the new "holistic" parlance that has influenced both biomedicine and alternative medicines in the West (Engel 1980; Pelletier 1979). This discrepancy poses the possibility that perhaps the "ten questions" formulated in the Ming dynasty by Zhang Jie-Bin (A.D. 1563-1640) to reflect the clinical needs of practitioners and their patients (and slightly modified in modern China, e.g., Chapter 6 of this volume), might need to be reformulated to mirror modern Western needs. Perhaps some questions similar to the following need to be formally integrated into the standard diagnostic inquiry of Oriental medical practitioners in the West:

1. How is your current relationship to the significant people in your life? How has it been in the past? What change would you like?

2. What are the significant events of your childhood? Of your adulthood? What is incompleted in your life? What is completed?

3. What is the history of and relationship to your job/career? Does it give you support? Is it a burden? Is it what you want to be doing?

4. What changes have your health problems caused in the area of job/work? family/friends? goals/plans? self-esteem/self-worth? Have there been any benefits?

5. How have these health problems confirmed or changed your ideas about who you are? Does the problem have any special meaning or special lesson for you? Is there any special dimension of pain or suffering?

6. How do you care for yourself? What other health-care providers have you consulted? How would you describe your relationship to them? How do you care for others? How do you abuse/neglect yourself and others? What do you value most in yourself? Has it changed since the illness?

7. What do you consider the major disappointments in your life? What are your major successes? Major learning experiences?

8. What are the sources of pleasure in your life? Where do you recognize sadness in yourself? How do you deal with pain? Has this approach changed because of your health problem?

9. What are your most recurrent feelings? Thoughts? Expectations? Fantasies? Dreams? Plans? Fears? Memories? Obsessions? Anxieties? How do you experience feelings?

10. For the practitioner, what response does the patient evoke from him/her? What is your emotional reaction during the clinical encounter?

Questions of this kind are not meant to deny the importance of physical signs. Nor are they appropriate at all times. Rather, they are intended to broaden the clinical dialogue and options of Oriental medicine in the West so that the yin-yang qualities of Western patients can be more accurately understood, assessed and treated. For many Westerners, the non-corporeal aspects of their being are at times more accurate indicators of their health problems. Such issues are important not merely because of the widespread incidence of psychiatric disease. Psychological issues play a significant role in the illness process for "regular" medical patients. Because of the diversity of the of measures and definitions, research in this area is very imprecise, estimates vary from between 30% to over 70% (Stoeckle, Zola, and Davidson 1964; cf Shepherd 1964). Psycho-social issues are crucial triggers for health care utilization (Mechanic 1972; Murphy 1980; Tessler, Mechanic, and Dimond 1976). Such dimensions of health care are especially important in chronic illnesses where the tendency toward chronicity has been shown to relate to psychosocial difficulties that underline or predate physical or even infectious disease (Imboden 1961a; Imboden 1961b; McQueen and Siegrist 1982). Practitioners of Oriental medicine in the West are already engaged in the dialogue just suggested because of the needs of their patients. By explicitly raising questions of this nature and seeing them as part of Oriental medicine in the West, Western clinical needs can interact more consciously and seriously with the clinical gaze of Oriental medicine.

Competition and Factionalization: A History of Transformation

Competition Among Eastern Medical Systems

The somatic preoccupation of modern Oriental medicine has historical as well as cultural roots. Psychological and existential issues can never be completely disguised and in fact have always played a prominent role in illness and health in the Far East. These issues are often raised in older texts. However, historical circumstances conspired to somatize the voice of Oriental medicine, which is the name I give the literate and formalized strata of medicine that derives from the *Yellow Emperor's Inner Canon*. In fact, the health care systems of China, Japan, and Korea were always and are still pluralistic with many competitive strata. There was never just a single traditional medicine of China, Japan, or Korea. Like health care systems anywhere in the world, there was and is now constant competition among health care providers for medical resources and patients (Unschuld 1975, 304). Huard and Wong, for instance, enumerate the following incomplete list of healers in historical and modern Chinese societies: shaman; soothsayer; geomancer; fortune-teller; eye-and-ear specialist; dentist; herbalist; masseur; itinerant doctor; bonze; Tao-shih; pharmacist, itinerant drug-peddler. Palos adds astrology, physiognomy, palmistry, pedoscopy, many other means of divination and diagnosis, charms, prayers, ritual incantations, exorcism, drawings, talismans, various local and regional folk rites, and religious ceremonies (Palos 1971).

In fact, Oriental medicine has been an "alternative" medical system for most Chinese people. Paul Unschuld (1978, 78) estimates that "the history of high medicine in China was never the medicine of 90% of the population." In the rural areas of China, where 80% of the people still live, literacy was extremely rare and health care was primarily in the hands of various magico-religious practitioners or folk herbalists. Even in the cities, during every epoch this was true. Spence comments:

> Magicians and exorcists, midwives, herbalists, apothecaries and Taoist adepts, self-taught practitioners, eminent Confucian scholars who turned to medicine out of intellectual interest or financial necessity, families of physicians jealously guarding inherited family lore, skillful practitioners with nationally known names, court specialists — all of these "practiced" during the Ch'ing Dynasty, and none can be ignored in a comprehensive study of the medical system (Spence 1975, 81).

Similarly, in the Song dynasty, "For every illness, the diagnosis and remedies varied widely according to the different schools of medicine and sick people for their part did not hesitate to try out different treatments at the same time" (Gernet 1970, 170). Even Confucius speaks of health care as being the domain of both physicians and sorcerers. (The Chinese word for sorcerer, *wu*, can also be translated as wizard, witch, medium, exorcist.) The *Inner Canon (Huang-di nei-jin su-wen* [100 B.C.] 1963) also speaks of competing medical practitioners (e.g., Chapters 11 and 13). In terms of patient population, medical systems of supernatural causation "dominated medical care among the Chinese masses" (Unschuld 1985, 224). In modern industrial Japan and Korea, traditional magic and exorcism still play a crucial but legally unsanctioned role, especially among the lower economic classes (Blacker 1975; Davis 1980; Harvey 1979; Kendall 1981). And secretly there are "spirit-mediums, diviners, priests, and other specialists [who] still perform many health care functions in Chinese culture, although they are excluded from the state system" (Leslie 1980, 192; cf. Parrish and Whyte 1978; Potter 1970).

This medical pluralism has had a great impact on the development of what the current Chinese government allows to be called traditional medicine. Intra-cultural medical tension has exerted a profound influence on the development of Oriental medicine, tending to focus discussion in certain clinical directions by a method of self-selection of patients and allowable discourse. Whenever problems affected the mind, affect, emotions, intention, will, belief, or purpose, or involved aberrant behavior, it was more likely that people brought the problem to the religious-style healers (Veith 1963). Obviously, there was no absolute distinction, e.g., during the cholera epidemic of the 1940's, prayer, healing rituals, and magical charms were an important part of health-care mobilization (Hsu 1952). Sun Si-miao, the great Tang dynasty scholar, treated demonic possession with acupuncture and herbs (Sun 1965), and later used incantations to treat physical problems (Sun 1982). Generally, however, the realms of imagination, vision, religious belief and behavior and intra-psychic conflict - what would be classed in modern terms as psychological and existential issues - were more likely directed to the practitioners of supernatural healing. The literate Oriental medicine, compared to its rivals, tended to occupy and monopolize the more sober, detached, rational, and somatic corner of health care.

The social division of labor between the scholarly physician and spiritual healer reinforced the tendency already present in the culture (especially in its more upper crust) to consider only somatic communication as proper and without moral stigma. Divided expectations themselves effected symptoms as patients tended to modify their presentation of complaints in different medical contexts (cf. Cheung and Lao 1982). Although both the religious and philosophic medicines claimed all health care issues within their expertise, the social tendencies of the Chinese people made the "psychological and existential discourse" more appropriate for the supernatural health care sector.

Interestingly, Western patients have their own cultural and historical expectations concerning Oriental medicine. Because many Western patients and practitioners see contemporary biomedicine as inordinately somatic (cf. Engels 1977), they expect Oriental medicine, correctly or not, to be particularly capable in non-somatic areas. Ironically these are precisely the areas it tended to underplay in its more recent history. Western practitioners need to be cognizant that this historical switch places new demands on the medical discourse transmitted from the East and increases our need to be adaptive and innovative.

Innovation and Debate within Chinese Medicine

In fact, innovation is nothing new to Oriental medicine. There has never been a monolithic or static medical perspective with questions and answers carved in "classical canon." Oriental medicine has always been a dynamic dialogue around a core methodology that encompassed lively and contrasting viewpoints. Though Japan, Korea, and Vietnam initially adopted the basic theories and practices of Oriental medicine from China, their national perspectives and medical requirements interpreted and developed this knowledge differently from the Chinese tradition. Any observer visiting Tokyo or Seoul cannot fail to see the great differences in how Oriental medicine is practiced there in contrast to Shanghai. Like China, Japan, Korea, and Vietnam, all had their important interpreters who adapted the Oriental medical paradigm to their circumstances and needs. In fact, such famous interpretations as those descended from the Japanese Kohoha school of Nagoya Gen (A.D. 1628-1696) (Otsuka 1977), the Korean schools based on Sa-am-do-in (fl. A.D. 1590) (Song, K. 1979), or the Vietnamese tradition based on Tue Tinh (14th Century) (Levinson 1974), are reinterpretations or simplifications of the old layers of Oriental medicine that may have been neglected in China. Westerners need to compare the interpretations of the Oriental medical tradition and critically develop a methodology of adaptation and change within Oriental medicine. Indeed, one important contribution Westerners can make to Oriental medicine's development is to carefully and critically examine these national traditions without the cultural bias that usually exists between them and help to encourage a healthy exchange for the benefit of both East and West.

China's version of Oriental medicine is rich in differing schools of thought and traditions, among them the "cooling school" of Liu Wan-Su (A.D. 1120-1200); the "purgative school" of Zhang Cong-Zheng (A.D. 1156-1228); the "gastrosplenic supplementation school" of Li Gao (A.D. 1180-1251); the "living noose" (huo tao), word therapy method of Zhu Zhen-Heng (A.D. 1281-1358); the "yang supplementation school" of Zhang Jie-Bin (A.D. 1522-1640); the "Han revivalist school" of Fang You-Zhi (A.D. 1522-1593); the "pestilence school" of Wu You-Xing (A.D. 1582-1652); and the "thermic heat disease school" of Ye Gui (A.D. 1667-1746). The list could go on for pages, depending on how tradition is defined. Arguments betweenschools wereintense and sometimes nasty. Japan's history is even more factional: "Graduates from schools representing rival factions remained competitive and aloof" (Lock 1980a, 57). In both China and Japan each tradition usually claimed authenticity by referral to the classics. These scholars and clinicians "writing for a medical audience, were able to select specific passages [of more ancient classics] for inclusion in their own works or for comment; when these same passages are considered in their historical contexts, their meaning may be quite different" (Epler 1980, 38). Scholarship too often became what one historian of another tradition called "the factory of evidence for the current faddish view" (Smith 1979, 8).

Some of these alternative approaches came from the clinical needs of different patient populations and different disease situations. Medical historians have known for a long time that the "changing pattern of epidemic infection was and remains a fundamental landmark in the human ecology" (McNeill 1985, 207). Risse (1979, 507) states, "Disease is not a 'natural' phenomenon striking man . . . according to some immutable laws. . . . Epidemiological patterns are not autonomous, but intricately linked to political, socio-economic and cultural factors." The configuration of febrile illness, symptom complex, and probable biomedical disease entities in *A Treatise on Cold Damage* by Zhang Ji (c. A.D. 220) is entirely different from that appearing in Wu Tang's *Systematized Identification of Thermic Disease* (A.D. 1798). In fact, it could not be otherwise, as China was subject to different infectious diseases throughout its long history (McNeill

1985). And even from medical texts that share the same historical epoch, social and class consideration change medical requirements. The diseases of patients in the *Inner Canon* are different from those in Zhang Ji's *Treatise on Cold Damage*. The *Inner Canon*, with its upper-class concerns, has much more room to attend to chronic ailments. Upper-class patients have different needs from poor peasants. A discussion of "lung energy" in a patient population that is overwhelmingly affected by infections and contagious disease will be very different from the refined atmosphere of the imperial court with its chronic cinnabar poisoning. The efforts of some Japanese schools to reject Chinese Yuan and Song dynasty medical revisions, and only use "Cold Damage" drug formulae or *Canon of Perplexities* style acupuncture, while making sense in terms of Japanese history, could never quite succeed. Disease patterns are different; the circumstances can never be duplicated. Cinnamon Twig Decoction (*guì-zhī tāng*) in modern Japanese herbal medicine can never be used exactly as it was in the Han dynasty. In the same way, Westerners can never duplicate what the Chinese do. "Lung energy" will necessarily be different in a post-antibiotic age where disease is predominantly rooted in social maladaptation (Burkitt 1978; Inglis 1981). Our diseases, health care options, and experience of being "healed" in sickness are just too different (cf. Blendon 1979).

Modern Discourse in China

The diverse, chaotic, but rich debate that existed within Oriental medicine has contracted within the last one hundred and fifty years. In China, Oriental medicine necessarily reacted defensively to the penetration of Western medicine in China, especially beginning with the confrontation during the First Opium War (Agren 1975). "The great diversity of individual efforts to reconcile insights from personal experience with the ancient theories of yin-yang and the five phases . . . disappeared behind the illusion of a so-called Chinese medicine" (Unschuld 1985, 250). The process that began in the Qing dynasty was tremendously accelerated by the Communist revolution, which further "reduced the internal spectrum of competing Chinese interpretations of the classics" (Unschuld 1985, 250). Japan also experienced a contraction of options, beginning with Western penetration, where "the threat posed by cosmopolitan medicine served to unite 'Kanpo' [Oriental style] doctors, who were able for the first time in several hundred years to overcome the rifts caused by professional factionalization" (Lock 1980a, 63), and organize a unity of divergent schools (Lock 1980a, 61). The post-Second World War American occupation under Douglas MacArthur forced a formal burial of conflict among Kanpo doctors. But the most severe limitation has probably occurred in contemporary China, where for political reasons debate is severely restricted.

In 1949, the newly founded People's Republic of China obviously had many conflicting ideas on how to handle what the United Nations had in the previous year declared "perhaps the greatest and most intractable public health problem of any nation in the world" (Hillier 1983, 66). While practitioners of supernatural medicine were quickly outlawed, one of the thorniest questions was what to do with practitioners of Oriental medicine. In late 1954, the Chinese government made an abrupt change of health care policy and officially recognized the Oriental medical practices of China as a " medical legacy of the motherland" as opposed to the earlier tendency to consider it "feudal medicine" (Croizier 1968, 162). This was to become the modern world's most ambitious governmental support of a non-scientific medicine (cf. Bhardwaj 1981; McCorkel 1961; Minocha 1985). But circumscribing this support was a severe restriction on allowable debate within the tradition. Oriental medicine could become "legitimate," even pretend its equality to Western medicine, but it had to groom its "appearance." Its discussions had to be consistent with the ideological and health requirements as defined by a Marxist government. While socio-political influence on health care discussions is present in every society, the orientation of medicine in modern China is an exceptionally explicit and overt political issue (Chin 1968; Lampton 1981).

With official recognition and legitimization of Oriental medicine in China came state-supported schools. By late 1955, four colleges of official traditional medicine and the Academy of Traditional Medicine were established to give the new Communist policy a strong institutional base (Lampton 1977; Neumann and Lauro 1982). The year 1955 also marked the establishment of 144 traditional medical hospitals, with 77 added the following year (Hillier 1983). In 1958, thirteen colleges of traditional medicine existed (Lampton 1977); by 1984, twenty-four were in operation (Macek 1984). The communist government had decided that the low social status to which Oriental medicine had fallen among the ruling elites of China during the late Qing and the Republic period was to be altered, at least officially. But Oriental medicine had to conform to clearly defined boundaries.

The first five schools - Beijing, Guangzhou, Shanghai, Chengdu, and later Nanjing - were assigned roles to pioneer a "modern" curriculum. The practitioners of Oriental medicine were going to learn in a fashion that resembled the training of Western medical professionals. Textbooks were needed for this type of instruction. Classical texts were rendered into the modern vernacular style and given extensive explanatory commentary that supported the official interpretation. Yet, they in themselves were insufficient; they were not written with a modern curriculum or health delivery system in mind. A more step-by-step, systematic approach was needed that would lend itself to modern examinations, study methods and acceptable medical care. Expanding a fashion that had already begun in the Qing dynasty (e.g., Chen, X. 1982), introductory books on what the public health ministry considered to be the crucial areas of Chinese medicine were written in an unprecedented blossoming of Chinese medical literature. The first of these new textbooks were compiled at the five original colleges. The parameters of development of these texts depended on the political line of the central government. "Idealist," "feudal," "incomplete," "unclear," "inaccurate," "metaphysical," and "primitive" ideas that did not fit into the acceptable dialogue were omitted. "Traditional Chinese Medicine" was to be a neat and rational set of theories and practices.

The Chinese medical textbooks of the era *prior to* the Great Leap Forward are distinct from those of the Great Leap Forward as these are distinct from the texts printed during the Cultural Revolution and during the period after this episode (cf. Agren 1975). For example, the "stems and branches" method of acupuncture (*zi-wu-liu-fa*) was included in the fifties, omitted in the seventies, and allowed back in the eighties. Very occasionally, the elegant discussion of feelings, words, and emotions from the *Jing-yue quan-shu* (Zhang Jie-Bin [1624] 1980) might be found in textbooks; but never, for example, was the presentation from *Ben-cao gang-mu* (Li Shi-Zhen [1596] 1981) on the pharmaceutical use of a hanged man's *po* (non-corporal soul) a permitted topic for investigation or even discussion. The high point of this simultaneous expansion, rationalization, and purgation was in the early 1970's, especially in Shanghai (Unschuld 1985). The Shanghai radicals of that period called for the creation of a new medicine for China and greatly stressed increased utilization of indigenous medical methods. Though heavily criticizing the theoretical basis of Oriental medicine, this period nevertheless produced some of the best and most thorough Chinese medical textbooks, such as *Fundamentals of Chinese Medicine*. The self-justification of Oriental medicine was taken outside its own methodology. By appealing to a combination of 19th century shallow positivism (i.e., "empirical practices of the masses") and 20th century watered-down dialectical materialism (i.e., "yin-yang is a rudimentary dialectic"), Oriental medicine ceased to be a coherent point of departure for illness and health and became a corpus needing rescue from modern science. The tendency that has existed for the last thirty years in China to be "interested in the empirical efficacy of traditional practice, not in the traditional theoretical framework, which supported these practices" (Kleinman 1975, 435) reached full blossom. In the post-Cultural-Revolutionary thaw, dating from the "Three Roads" policy, Oriental medicine has been given more freedom, but "Western medicine clearly dominates and controls the character of the mandated integration" (Rosenthal 1981, 611). Many classical texts reprinted in China for the first time since the fifties have appeared, but recent Oriental medical texts, while a little more independent of scientific medicine, seem to be in a quandary and are only repeating 1970s formulations minus the Mao quotes. No improvements over *Fundamentals of Chinese Medicine* have been offered, nor are any likely.

The People's Republic of China sanction of a modern version of Oriental medicine may have helped save a pre-scientific medical system from "historical oblivion and consignment to the museum of medical oddities, victim of the rising dominance of Western biomedical science" (Rosenthal 1981, 600). China's policy also had an immeasurable impact on Japan and Korea and increased the popularity of traditional practitioners (Lock 1980b). And Chinese policy certainly brought Oriental medicine to the attention of the rest of the non-Asian world. In spite of this, all practitioners of Oriental medicine in the West should be aware that the historical synthesis that has been nurtured and sanctioned by the Chinese government is only one of the many conceivable options that lie within the medical perspective of Oriental medicine. China's synthesis (which is always changing and itself has been affected by Western questions and research) is the product of complex cultural, historical, and political forces.

Questions for the West and Fundamentals of Chinese Medicine

Western practitioners of Oriental medicine have a long but exciting road ahead of them. We need to honor Oriental medicine's parentage, study its theories, and examine its long and changing practice. We need to explore the historical and cultural forces that shaped it. As more accurate information and knowledge moves West, we can begin to be selective in our adaptation. Westerners can begin to examine the Oriental tradition with our own health care needs in mind. We need to make our own choices, based on our own scholarship, research, investigation, debate, and reflection. We need to adapt the tradition to our needs. The process has already begun. By being explicit and conscious we can do a better job. The Oriental tradition needs to be examined to find earlier engagements with the type of questions Western practitioners face daily.

Our own questions may mean that we need to reprioritize the tradition. For example, is the Qing dynasty "thermic heat disease" school of Chinese medicine or the "splenic supplementation" school of the Yuan dynasty as important for the modern West as the long-forgotten Yuan dynasty "living noose" method that tried to induce different affective reactions in emotionally disturbed patients by having the practitioner embody different emotions (Chen et al. 1962; Hunan 1979; Liu 1981). Do the rationalizations of acupoint functions done in the 1950's by the Chinese medical schools need to be redone by Western scholars? Do the original pharmaceutical codifications need to be reformulated to take into account ignored Han and Tang psycho-spiritual understanding of herbs? Is the early twentieth century Japanese five-phase system of acupuncture based on the *Canon of Perplexities* exactly right for Western patients or do scholars have to reexamine the original terrain? Is the Qing dynasty "eight principles" approach to yin-yang the most appropriate? Do we need to develop Huang-fu Mi's ([282] 1979) Jin dynasty acupuncture treatments for happiness? What of Yang Ji-zhou's ([1601] 1978) Ming dynasty ideas concerning needle technique, respiration, and guided imagery? Are the "most useful" herbal prescriptions selected from the 61,739 combinations in the *Pu Ji Fang* ("Prescriptions of Universal Benefit") (A.D. 1406) the "most useful" for Western patients? For example, is the discussion of the liver's energetic relationship to the fingernails so important that it can overshadow the relationship of the liver to the *hun* (non-corporal soul) and the relationship of the liver to psychic and existential boundaries, values and virtue?

Publication of an English translation of *Fundamentals of Chinese Medicine* is an important step toward assuring that a process of serious questioning will take place and that the medical dialogue between East and West will have lasting importance and conscious direction. Only accurate information will allow the beginnings of an American or European version of Oriental medicine. A new variant of Oriental medicine must be based on careful and thoughtful study of primary sources, on reflection, and on information. Otherwise, it will be a mutant based on fantasy. Every bit of information received from the Orient must be considered a precious artifact requiring our intense examination.

Fundamentals of Chinese Medicine is an excellent example of this need and process. The translators have made an excellent choice for the commencement of their proposed series. This volume is considered by many Chinese practitioners to be the most important introductory textbook of the last two decades. It continues to be a standard work at institutes of traditional medicine throughout Asia. Western readers can finally have an accurate sense of how the Chinese are presenting the Oriental medical tradition of this era. The translators' attention to nuance and detail is impressive; each word appears to have been weighed in delicate linguistic scales. This volume is a vast improvement in translation standards and will ensure a deepened appreciation of how the Chinese have applied the methodology of Oriental medicine to the circumstances of their contemporary society.

The work and care in producing this volume is formidable. Only with this kind of effort can we in the West say we are properly appreciating the efforts of our Eastern colleagues. Many other, almost countless other, Oriental medical works need translation, as the future commitments of translators Nigel Wiseman and Andrew Ellis and senior editor Paul Zmiewski demonstrate. Yet translation must be reinforced by critical examination. Communication must mean more than imitation. Accurate information about what other cultures do is valuable experience for the understanding of possibilities in our own culture.

Hopefully, the publication of this volume will help mark the time when students in the West begin to have the self-assurance necessary to separate what of Oriental medicine is applicable in the West from what is not.

Instead of adopting wholesale an entire medical practice, we should begin, through careful analysis, to adapt it to the needs of those we treat. This effort will take decades of rigorous translation, clinical practice, scholarly research, inner reflection, collective discussion and perseverance. Only in this way can Oriental medicine in the West reflect its true methodology. Yin and yang concern the perception, understanding and encouragement of change.

Ted J. Kaptchuk
Clinical Director, Pain and Stress Clinic
Lemuel Shattuck Hospital
Boston, Massachusetts

References to the Introduction may be found on page 581.

Pronunciation Guide

The alphabetized pinyin list of Chinese sounds provided below is intended as a quick reference. In the present text, units of two or more characters are joined by a hyphen. We have deliberately strayed from standard PRC convention of writing composite terms as one word to emphasize to students the individual character entities. Composite given or adopted names are hyphenated, with the family name set apart before them (e.g., Zhang Jing-Yue, Zhang being the family name and Jing-Yue being the adopted society name).

Where Chinese transcriptions appear in Latin drug names we have used the Wade-Giles system, and in some cases pre-Wade-Giles systems, in keeping with convention, but have written the character renderings separately, again in order to empahsize character entities (e.g., Kan Sui, rather than Kansui). Compounds adjectivalized with a Latin suffix are written as one word (e.g., Szechuanensis). Finally, the apostrophe, often omitted for aesthetic reasons, has been retained to ensure greater clarity (e.g., T'ing Li Tzu instead of Tinglitzu).

Initials

b   like the unaspirated *p* in spy (not like the voiced *b* in buy)
c   a highly aspirated *ts* sound, as the *t's h* in it's hell
ch   somewhat like *tr* in *tree* or *trust*, produced by pronouncing an *r* simultaneously with the above **c** sound
d   like the *t* in *sty,* or the soft *t* in the American pronunciation of *bitter*
f   as in English usage
g   like the unaspirated *k* in sky (not like the voiced *g* in *guide*)
h   like the *ch* in *loch*, or the German *nach*
j   like the *j* in *jeep*
k   like the *k* in *kite*, but with a much stronger aspiration
l   like the English *l* in *lip* (not like the *l* in *bottle*)
m   as in English usage
n   as in English usage
p   like the *p* in *pig*, but with a much stronger aspiration
q   like the *ch* in *cheat*
r   like the *r* in *rude*, but with a slight "buzzing" sound like the *z* in *zoo*
s   like the *s* in *sit*, but with the tongue much farther forward

sh	somewhat like the *shr* in *shrine*, produced by pronouncing an *r* simultaneously with the above **s** sound
t	like the unvoiced *t* in *sty*, but highly aspirated, i.e., more like the *de h* in *wide hat* than the *te h* in *white hat*
w	as in English usage
x	a less full-bodied sound than the *sh* in *shall*, produced by saying *s* and *y* at the same time
y	as in English usage
z	like the *t's* in *it's intact*
zh	somewhat like the *dr* in *dredge*, produced by pronouncing an *r* simultaneously with the above **z** sound

Vowels

a	between the *a* in *cat* and the *a* in *father*
e	like the *e* in *bed* after *u* or *i*, and before *i* (e.g., *xue, lie, lei*), and like the *e* in *err* or the *u* in the expression *ugh* in all other positions (e.g., *she, ke, te*)
i	like the *i* in *machine*, never as in *tin*.
o	like the *aw* in *law* or the *o* in *lord*
u	like the *u* in *rule*, but with more lip-rounding and the tongue drawn further back (i.e, like German or French usage)
ü	like the *u* in the French *tu* or the German *Müller*, pronounced by forming the lips to say the above *u* sound, but trying to say the *ee* of *feet* instead; the dieresis (umlaut) is omitted when this sound follows *a, j, q, x,* or *y*.

Dipthongs

ai	like the *ie* in *lie*, but more open as in the German *Mainz* or *Heinz*
ao	like the *ow* in *cow*, but more like the *au* in the German *Haus*
ei	between the *ay* in *may* and the *e* in *bed*
ia	between the *ya* in *yap* and the *ya* in *yard*
iao	like the *yow* in *yowl*, but more like the *jau* in the German *jaulen*
ie	like the *ye* in *yet*
iou	like the *yo* in *yoke*
iu	between the *u* in *union* and the *yo* in *yoke*
ou	like the *oa* in *boat*
ua	like the *wa* in *water*
uai	like the *wi* in *wife*

üe	like the *ü* sound followed by the *e* in *bed*
ui	like the sound in *way* or *weigh*

Vowels with Final Consonants

an	between the *an* in *can* and the *an* in *khan;* after *i* or *u* this sound is more like the *en* in pen
ang	like the *a* in father (but much shorter), followed by *ng* as in *sing*
en	like the *un* in *fun,* or the *on* in *wanton*
eng	like the *ung* in *lung*
ian	like the English pronunciation of *yen*
in	like the *een* in *seen* (see **i** above)
ing	like the *ing* in *sing* (see **i** above)
iong	like the German *jung,* or a *y* plus the *u* in *put* plus the *ng* in *sing*
uan	like *wham* but with an *n* substituted for the final *m*
üan	like the Chinese *ü* sound followed by the *en* in *pen*
uang	*w* plus the above **ang** sound
un	like the sound in *won* not like the *un* in *fun*
ün	like the Chinese *ü* sound, followed by the English *in*

Tones

In English, the difference between Mother! and Mother? is one of intonation. Words and phrases are intoned in varying ways in English to express subtle differences of meaning and attitude. In Chinese, each character has its set tone (some characters may have more than one tone, or even more than one pronunciation, depending on their meaning), while much of the general work done by intonation in English is taken on by additional words, such as question particles and exclamation particles. In Mandarin, there are four basic tones. The first is a high, flat tone, the second a rising tone, the third a deep, dipping tone, and the fourth, a high falling tone. These can be schematically represented as follows:

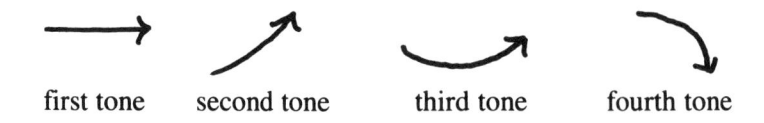

first tone   second tone   third tone   fourth tone

Thus, the sound *shi* can mean damp when pronounced in the first tone *(shī)*, stone when pronounced in the second tone *(shí)*, to cause when pronounced in the third tone *(shǐ)*, and to be when in the fourth tone *(shì)*. Each of these sounds are written with different ideograms.

Table of Contents

Part I: Basic Theories

Chapter One: Yin and Yang and the Five Phases 3
- Yin and Yang 3
- The Five Phases 10
- Tables 19
- Notes 21

Chapter Two: Qi, Blood, Essence, and Fluids 23
- Qi 23
- Blood 27
- Essence 30
- Fluids 31
- Notes 36

Chapter Three: The Channels 37
- Pathways and Theory 37
- The Twelve Regular Channels 40
- The Eight Irregular Channels 53
- Channel Distribution 58

Chapter Four: The Organs 65
- The Visceral Manifestation Theory 65
- The Heart and Pericardium 67
- The Lung 70
- The Spleen, Stomach, and Intestines 73
- The Liver and Gallbladder 79
- The Kidney, Bladder, and Associated Functions 84
- Notes 93

Chapter Five: Diseases and Their Causes 95
- Factors of Disease 95
- The Laws of Pathogenesis 104
- Struggle and Imbalance in the Development of Disease 105
- Notes 108

Part II: Pattern Identification and Treatment

Chapter Six: The Four Examinations 111

    Visual Examination 111
    Audio-Olfactive Examination 129
    Inquiry 132
    Palpation 141
    Tables of Pulses and Clinical Significance 153
    Notes 157

Chapter Seven: Eight-Parameter Pattern Identification 159

    Exterior and Interior 160
    Cold and Heat 166
    Vacuity and Repletion 170
    Yin and Yang 175
    Eight-Parameter Pattern Tables 178
    Notes 187

Chapter Eight: Qi-Blood Pattern Identification 189

    Disease Patterns of Qi 189
    Disease Patterns of the Blood 192
    Dual Disease Patterns of Qi and Blood 198
    Qi-Blood Pattern Tables 202

Chapter Nine: Organ Pattern Identification 203

    Disease Patterns of the Heart 204
    Disease Patterns of the Lung 211
    Disease Patterns of the Spleen, Stomach, and Intestines 218
    Disease Patterns of the Liver & Gallbladder 232
    Disease Patterns of the Kidney and Bladder 243
    Organ Pattern Tables 251

Chapter Ten: Pathogen Pattern Identification 265

    Wind Disease Patterns 265
    Cold Disease Patterns 274
    Heat, Fire, and Summerheat Disease Patterns 280
    Damp Disease Patterns 289
    Dryness Disease Patterns 300
    Digestate Accumulation 304
    Phlegm Disease Patterns 308
    Pathogen Pattern Tables 319
    Notes 333

Chapter Eleven: Exogenous Heat Disease 336

    Six-Channel Pattern Identification 336
    Four-Aspect Pattern Identification 348
    The Relationship Between Six-Channel
        and Four-Aspect Pattern Identification 359

    Exogenous Heat Disease Tables 361
    Notes 370

Chapter Twelve: Principles and Methods of Treatment 371
    Principles of Treatment...371
    Methods of Treatment 377
    Summary...449
    Notes 450

Glossary of Terms 453

Stroke-Order Glossary 516

Latin—Chinese Index of Chinese Drugs 541

Chinese—Latin Index of Chinese Drugs 551

English—Chinese Index of Chinese Medicinal Formulae ..561

Chinese—English Index of Chinese Medicinal Formulae ..568

Acumoxatherapy Index..571

Bibliography...579
    Works Cited in the Text..579
    Translators' References 580
    References for the Introduction 581

Concepts Index...589

Part One
Basic Theories

Chapter One
Yin and Yang and the Five Phases

The concepts of yin and yang and the five phases were devised by the ancient Chinese as a method of defining and explaining the nature of all phenomena. As such they represent the Chinese conception of Nature and were fundamental to all natural sciences; not only medicine, but astronomy, calendrical science, geography, and agriculture made extensive use of and were strongly influenced by these theories.

Chinese medicine is a vast treasury of knowledge. It is the product of millenia of practical experience in dealing with sickness. Yin and yang and the five phases have played a major role in the development of medical theory and represent the mainstay of physiology, pathology, pattern identification, and treatment.

Yin and Yang

The theory of yin and yang, derived from agelong observation of nature, describes the way phenomena naturally group in pairs of opposites — heaven and earth, sun and moon, night and day, winter and summer, male and female, up and down, inside and outside, movement and stasis. These pairs of opposites are also mutual complements. Chapter 5 of *Essential Questions*[1] states, "Yin and yang are the way of heaven and earth."

The basic principles of yin-yang theory

All phenomena in the universe may be ascribed to yin and yang (cf. Table 1-1). Each individual phenomenon possesses both a yin and a yang aspect. Yin and yang are natural complements in the sense that they depend upon and counterbalance each other. Further, they are mutually convertible, since either may change into its complement.

The following principles may be observed in the application of the theory of yin and yang to medicine:

Yin and yang as the fundamental categories of all phenomena

In medicine, the concepts of yin and yang are generally used to categorize both anatomic parts and physiologic functions. For example, the back is yang and the abdomen is yin; the six bowels are yang and the five viscera are yin; qi is yang and blood is yin; agitation is yang and moderation is yin (cf. Table 1-2). Similarly, diseases may be categorized according to yin and yang. For example, exterior, repletion,[2] and heat disorders are yang, while interior, vacuity, and cold disorders are yin.

Pulses may similarly be categorized: floating, rapid, and slippery pulses are yang, while deep, slow, and rough pulses are yin (cf. Table 1-3).

Yin and yang are divisible

Every phenomenon may be classified as yin or yang in contrast to another. Each yin or yang phenomenon itself possesses both yin and yang aspects that may be further divided in the same way. This process of division may be carried on ad infinitum. The *Inner Canon*[3] states:

> Yin and yang can be divided down to ten, and then further down to one hundred, to a thousand, to ten thousand and to a number so great as defies calculation; yet in essence all these are but one.

Medicine makes extensive use of this infinite divisibility of yin and yang not only in anatomy, physiology, and pathology, but also in pattern identification and treatment.

Yin and yang are interdependent

Interdependence is the notion that yin and yang are mutually indispensable and engendering. Yin exists by virtue of yang, and yang exists by virtue of yin. Hence it is said:

> Yang has its root in yin;
>   yin has its root in yang.
> Without yin, yang cannot arise;
>   without yang, yin cannot be born.
> Yin alone cannot arise; yang alone cannot grow.
> Yin and yang are divisible but inseparable.

In medicine, the concept of interdependence of yin and yang is widely used in physiology, pathology, and treatment. Blood and qi, two fundamental elements of the human body, provide an example: blood is yin and qi is yang. It is said that "qi engenders blood," i.e., blood formation relies on the power of qi to move and transform the digestate; "qi moves the blood," meaning that blood circulation relies on the warming and driving power of qi.[4] Furthermore, "qi contains the blood," i.e., it keeps the blood within the vessels. The functions of engendering, moving, and containing the blood are summed up in the phrase, "qi is the commander of the blood." Conversely, qi is dependent on the provision of adequate nutrition by the blood; thus it is said that "qi has its abode in the blood," and "blood is the mother of qi." Because qi has the power to engender blood, treatment of blood vacuity involves dual supplementation of qi and blood. Profuse hemorrhage, where qi deserts[5] with the blood, is first treated by boosting qi, since blood generative treatment should not be administered until qi is secured. Similarly, formulae used to treat qi vacuity often include blood-nourishing agents to enhance qi supplementation.

Another example of the interdependence of yin and yang, seen in the development of diseases, is the principle that "detriment to yin affects yang" and "detriment to yang affects yin." Since "without yang, yin cannot be born," when yang vacuity reaches a certain point, the production of yin humor is affected, and yin also becomes vacuous. Most cases of chronic nephritis indicate yang vacuity, and are characterized by water-swelling due to the inability of the kidney to transform fluids.[6] However, when the yang vacuity reaches a certain point, fluid formation is affected and a yin vacuity pattern evolves. This demonstrates the principle of "detriment to yang affects yin." Similarly, yin vacuity, when reaching a certain peak, lead to simultaneous yang vacuity, since "without yin, yang cannot arise." What is termed high blood pressure in Western medicine usually corresponds to hyperactivity of yang caused by vacuity of yin. In severe cases, this condition may develop into a dual yin-yang vacuity, illustrating the principle that "detriment to yin affects yang."

Yin and yang counterbalance each other

The yin and yang aspects of the body counterbalance each other. A deficit of one naturally leads to a surfeit[7] of the other, while a surfeit of one will weaken the other. In both cases, yin and yang no longer counterbalance each other, and disease arises as a result. In medicine, the notion of counterbalancing is widely applied in physiology, pathology, and therapy.

In physiology, for example, liver yin counterbalances liver yang, preventing it from becoming too strong. If liver yin becomes insufficient and fails to counterbalance its complement, ascendant hyperactivity of liver yang[8] develops. In the relationship of pathogens and the human body, yang pathogens invading the body will cause a surfeit of yang, which may lead to damage to yin humor and the emergence of a heat pattern. Conversely, a yin pathogen entering the body will lead to a surfeit of yin, causing damage to the body's yang qi and the emergence of a cold pattern. These processes are described in *Essential Questions* in the following way:

> If yang abounds yin ails, and if yin abounds, yang ails; when yang prevails there is heat, and when yin prevails there is cold.

In therapy, if a disease is caused by the heat pathogen, it is treated with cool or cold agents according to the principle that "cold can counteract heat," meaning yin agents combat yang pathogens. Similarly, disorders caused by cold pathogens are treated with warm or hot agents, since "heat can overcome cold," or yang agents can combat yin pathogens. This is summed up in a guiding principle of therapy, "Heat is treated with cold and cold is treated with heat."[9] It is most often applied in patterns of repletion characterized by a surfeit of either yin or yang.

In conditions caused by deficit of yin or yang, the opposing complement is no longer kept in check and becomes disproportionately strong. If yin is vacuous, yang is no longer kept in check and its strength will grow out of proportion to that of yin. Such a condition is at root a yin vacuity, manifesting itself as vacuity heat. For this reason, treatment by draining fire and clearing heat alone is not only ineffective but also detrimental to the patient's health. It is replaced by a method such as enriching yin and downbearing fire, or fostering yin and subduing yang, whereby clearing heat and draining fire are secondary to enriching yin. By supplementing yin, the yang surfeit will naturally diminish. This explains the principles, "Where cooling is to no avail, water is lacking,"[10] and "invigorate the governor of water to counteract the brilliance of yang." In the reverse situation, where yang is vacuous and fails to keep yin in check, there is exuberant yin cold in the inner body, manifesting in such forms as clear-food diarrhea, daybreak diarrhea, and water swelling. Here, treatment should aim not simply at dissipating the cold pathogen, but also at supplying the yang vacuity through such methods as reinforcing yang, boosting fire, and supplementing qi. This demonstrates the principle "where warming is to no avail, fire is lacking," and "boosting the source of fire to eliminate the entrenched surfeit of yin."

It is important to note the difference between the natural flux of yin and yang and a surfeit of one or the other complement. The natural flux of yin and yang refers to their normal relationship in the human body, which is one of constant fluctuation, rather than a rigid, immutable balance. "When yin rises, yang ebbs," and "when yang swells, yin subsides." This constant fluctuation is apparent in all the body's physiologic functions, such as fluid production and metabolism, the role of the five viscera in storing essential qi, and the role of the six bowels in conveyance and transformation of digestate. By contrast, "deficit" and "surfeit" denote the disturbance of the normal relative balance and failure to rectify the imbalance immediately. This is known as imbalance of yin and yang, which is the underlying cause of all disease.

Mutual convertability of yin and yang

In medicine, examples of yin-yang conversion are found mainly in pathology, where yang patterns can develop into yin patterns and vice versa. In practice, this means that heat patterns can either turn into or develop from cold patterns, and vacuity can give way to, or supercede, repletion.

For example, infectious hepatitis in its acute icteric phase is associated with damp-heat symptoms such as yellowing of the face and eyes, fever, nausea, vomiting, pain in the lateral costal region, oppression in the chest, dyspeptic anorexia, and a thick, slimy tongue fur. However, when the condition becomes chronic and develops into liver cirrhosis, the patient will show symptoms of vacuity such as spiritual lassitude [11] and general lack of strength, dizziness, a dull pain in the chest and lateral costal region, no enjoyment of food, and a dark, red tongue. This indicates that the condition of repletion has turned into one of vacuity. If the condition develops further, stagnation of water-damp gives rise to ascites, manifesting as distention and fullness in the chest and abdomen, showing that the condition has reverted from vacuity to repletion. However, the resultant condition of repletion is different from the original one. In the initial condition, although pathogenic qi is strong, correct qi is still relatively unaffected, whereas in the resultant condition, pathogenic qi is exuberant in a body left frail by serious damage to the correct qi.

Cold-heat and vacuity-repletion conversion are subject to specific variables such as the strength of the patient's defenses, the nature of the pathogen, and choice of treatment. For instance, wheezing dyspnea (asthma)[12] may change from the original cold pattern to a heat condition, owing to repeated contraction of exogenous pathogens. In cases of pyelonephritis, the original disorder, which in Chinese medicine is expressed as damp-heat in the lower burner, may, owing to unthorough treatment, resistance of bacteria to drugs, or repeated relapses, develop into insufficiency of kidney yin, manifesting as yin vacuity fire effulgence, a form of vacuity heat.

Medical applications of yin yang theory

The preceding explanation of the basic concept of yin and yang uses Chinese medicine as its general frame of reference. The following is a systematic analysis of the application of yin and yang in Chinese medicine.

Yin-yang analysis of anatomy

Chinese medicine sees the human body as a whole, the component parts of which may all be analyzed in terms of yin and yang. For instance, the upper part of the body is yang and the lower part is yin; the exterior of the body is yang by contrast to the interior, which is yin. The surface of the body may be further divided, the abdominal surface being yin, and the back being yang. The internal organs may be divided into the five viscera, which are yin, and the six bowels, which are yang. *Essential Questions* states:

> As to the yin and yang of the human body, the outer part is yang and the inner part is yin. As to the trunk, the back is yang and the abdomen is yin. As to the organs, the viscera are yin whereas the bowels are yang. The liver, heart, spleen, lung, and kidney[13] are yin; the gallbladder, stomach, intestines, bladder, and triple burner are yang.

Each of the organs itself has a yin and a yang aspect: there is heart yin and heart yang, kidney yin and kidney yang. The two primary elements of the human body, blood and qi, may also be thus categorized, blood being yin

Basic Theories

and qi being yang. As to the channels, those passing over the back and the outer face of the limbs are yang, while those running through the surface of the abdomen and the inner face of the limbs are yin.[14] *Essential Questions* emphasizes the importance of yin and yang when it states, "The physical manifestation of human life cannot escape the duality of yin and yang."

Yin-yang analysis of physiologic activity

Yin and yang provide a general method of analyzing the functions of the human body. These are seen in terms of four categories of movement: upbearing, downbearing, issue, and entry. Upbearing and issue are yang, while downbearing and entry are yin. These movements serve to explain the interactions between blood and qi, and the organs and channels.

Physiologic processes are explained in terms of the natural flux of yin and yang. *Essential Questions* states:

> Clear yang issues from the upper portals, while turbid yin issues from the lower portals; clear yang effuses {issues} through the striations, while turbid yin goes through {enters} the five viscera; clear yang fills the limbs, whereas turbid yin passes through the six bowels.

This explains how yang, the clear light qi of the body, ascends up to and out of the clear portals, passing outward to the surface of the skin and strengthening the limbs, and how yin, the heavy turbid qi of the body, flows in the interior, its waste products being discharged through the anus and the urethra. The four movements are considered to be interdependent and mutually supporting. Thus *Essential Questions* states, "Yin is in the inner body and protects yang; yang is in the outer body and moves yin."

Yin-yang analysis of pathologic change

In medicine, morbidity is explained in terms of yin-yang imbalance. Both pathogenic and correct qi can be analyzed in terms of yin and yang. There are both yin and yang pathogens. Yin pathogens cause a surfeit of yin, which manifests as a cold pattern; yang pathogens produce a surfeit of yang in the body characterized by repletion heat patterns. The "correct," the body's health-maintaining forces, comprise two aspects, yang qi and yin humor. Yang qi vacuity is characterized by vacuity cold patterns, whereas yin humor vacuity is characterized by vacuity heat. A vast number of diseases can be summed up in the following four phrases:

> When yin prevails, there is cold; when yang prevails, there is heat. When yang is deficient, there is cold; when yin is deficient, there is heat.

The cause of these conditions is imbalance — surfeits or deficits — of either yin or yang.

General parameters of diagnosis

Imbalance of yin and yang accounts for the emergence and development of disease. The essential nature of any disease may be analyzed in terms of yin and yang, despite the infinite number of possible clinical manifestations. Yin and yang form the basic parameters of eight parameter pattern identification: exterior, heat, and repletion disorders being yang; interior, cold, and vacuity disorders being yin. *Essential Questions* states, "Proper diagnosis involves inspecting the appearance and feeling the pulse and first differentiating yin and yang."

Treatment and drug use

Because surfeit of yin or yang is the primary cause of any disease, treatment must involve restoring the balance by reducing superabundance and supplying insufficiency.

The nature and effect of drugs may also be classified according to yin and yang. For example, cold, cool, rich, and moist agents are yin, whereas warm, hot, dry, and fierce agents are yang. Agents pungent and sweet in sapor are yang, while those that are salty, bitter, sour, or astringent in sapor are yin. Agents whose qi and sapor are bland and mild are yang, and those whose qi and sapor are strong are yin. Agents that upbear and effuse are yang in nature, and agents that contract and astringe are yin.

Therefore, in diagnosis and treatment, it is necessary to identify yin-yang surfeits and deficits among the complex array of symptoms and determine the nature of the treatment. Agents must also be selected and used to make an appropriate synthesis of their yin and yang qualities. This means that a pattern due to a surfeit of yin or yang is one of repletion, and according to the principle of reducing superabundance, is treated by the method of drainage. A pattern essentially the result of a deficit of either yin or yang is one of vacuity, and in accordance with the principle of supplying insufficiency, is treated by the method of supplementation. If yin is in surfeit, the problem is one of repletion-cold, for which warm, pungent yang agents should be used to dissipate the cold. If yang is in surfeit, the pattern is one of repletion-heat, requiring cold, bitter heat drainers, which are yin in nature. If the pattern stems from an insufficiency of yin, yin-supplementing agents with a cooling and moistening effect are prescribed to nourish blood and fluids. Conditions stemming from a yang deficit manifest themselves as vacuity-cold, and are treated with yang drugs, warm or hot agents, to warm and supplement yang qi.

The Five Phases

The theory of the five phases rests on the notion that all phenomena in the universe are the products of the movement and mutation of five qualities: wood, fire, earth, metal, and water, otherwise known as the five phases. In Chinese medicine, five-phase theory has had considerable influence in physiology, pathology, diagnosis, treatment, and pharmacology.

The basic concept of the five phases

Characteristics and categorization

The ancient Chinese gained knowledge of the nature of the five phases through long observation of nature and ascribed certain values to each. Thus:

> Wood is the bending and the straightening, having the characteristics of growth, upbearing, and effusion;
>
> Fire is the flaming upwards, having the quality of heat and upward motion;
>
> Earth is the sowing and reaping, representing the planting and harvesting of crops and the bringing forth of phenomena;
>
> Metal is the working of change, having the qualities of purification, elimination, and reform;
>
> Water is the moistening and descending to low places, having the qualities of moistening, downward movement, and coldness.

Five phase theory is based on the understanding of the nature of these qualities, attributed to all phenomena in the universe. The interaction of the five phases explains the nature of all phenomena. In medicine, the bowels and viscera, body tissues, sense organs, emotions, and even drug properties are all categorized according to these phases (cf. Table 1-4).

The four cycles

Interaction among the phases is viewed in terms of four cycles. Engendering denotes the principle whereby each of the phases nurtures, produces, and benefits another specific phase. Restraining refers to the principle by which each of the phases constrains another phase.

Arranged in cyclic form, the engendering relationships are as follows (starting with wood engendering fire):

> wood ► fire ► earth ► metal ► water ► wood

The restraining cycle (starting with wood restraining earth) is as follows: wood ▶ earth ▶ water ▶ fire ▶ metal ▶ wood

In their correspondences to the viscera, the engendering and restraining cycles appear as follows:

engendering: liver ▶ heart ▶ spleen ▶ lung ▶ kidney ▶ liver

restraining: liver ▶ spleen ▶ kidney ▶ heart ▶ lung ▶ liver

The notions of engendering and restraining posit a conception of the natural world as a united whole made up of interrelated parts. The *Illustrated Supplement to the Categorized Canon* states:

> Nature cannot be without engendering or restraining; without engendering there is no way by which things may arise, and without restraining, things may become unduly powerful and cause harm.

It also states, "in engendering, there is restraining" and "in restraining, there is utility." This belief that all movement and mutation in the phenomenal world derives from the mutually engendering and mutually restraining relationships of all phenomena has had a profound influence on the visceral manifestation theory of Chinese medicine.

The principles of overwhelming and rebellion describe disruptions of the normal cycles. In medicine, they explain pathologic manifestations. The principle of overwhelming refers to the situation where one of the five phases is weakened, causing the phase that under normal circumstances would overcome it to invade and weaken it further. For example, wood normally restrains earth, but if earth is weak, then wood overwhelms it, rendering earth even weaker. In terms of the viscera, this means that the spleen, normally only restrained by the liver, will, if weak, be completely overwhelmed, becoming even weaker. According to the original theory of the five phases, restraining and overwhelming differ in that the former denotes the normal action of a given phase in keeping another in check, while the latter refers to a disproportionately powerful influence when the normal balance has been upset. However, in Chinese convention the term restraining is often used as an alternative for overwhelming, so that the terms have become somewhat confused.

The principle of rebellion denotes the situation where one of the five phases is disproportionately strong and rebels against the phase that should normally restrain it. For example, wood is normally kept in check by metal, but if it becomes too strong it will rebel against metal. Powerless to withstand the attack, metal will succumb. In terms of the organs this means that when the liver, normally kept in check by the lung, becomes too strong, it will rebel against the lung and overcome it.

Practical application of five phases in medicine

In Chinese medicine, the five phases are used to categorize the various organs and tissues, sense organs, and drug properties. Their four cycles also explain normal physiologic activities and pathologic changes. Some examples are given later in the text. At the beginning of its development, Chinese medicine established correspondences between the five phases and the seasons, the types of weather associated with each season, and the functions of the organs of the human body.

Five-phase analysis of organ characteristics

Beginning with the liver, the physiologic characteristic of this organ is that it thrives by orderly reaching. It governs upstirring, and is like the "sprouting of trees and plants in spring." Spring corresponds to wood in the five phases, so that the liver is ascribed the attribute of wood.

The physiologic characteristic of the heart is that it governs the blood vessels. It has the function of propelling qi and blood to warm and nourish the whole body. It is likened to the heat of summer, when the whole of creation thrives. Summer corresponds to fire, and so the heart is ascribed the quality of fire.

The spleen's physiologic characteristic is that it governs movement and transformation of the essence of digestate and is the basis of the formation of blood and qi. It is associated with late summer and humid weather, when the whole of nature is at its peak. Late summer corresponds to earth, so that the spleen is ascribed the attribute of earth.

The physiologic characteristic of the lung is that it thrives by purity and governs downbearing. It is likened to the clear fresh air and purifying first frosts of autumn, when nature is withdrawing into itself. For this reason, it is ascribed the attribute of metal.

Finally, the kidney has the physiologic function of storing essence and of governing fluids. It is associated with the bitter cold of winter, when nature is dormant.

The correspondences between the five phases and organic function is clearly not without adequate foundation. However, the accumulated knowledge concerning the organs over the long history of Chinese medicine goes far beyond the confines of the five phases. For example, the liver not only governs upstirring and thrives by orderly reaching; liver yin and liver blood have a nourishing function for which the correspondence to wood cannot account. Similarly, the heart represents not only the warming function and the strength of the heart's yang qi, but also the nourishing, calming function of heart yin, which does not accord with the notion of fire. The functions of the stomach and spleen include not only formation (of blood and qi), but also upbearing effusion and free downflow, which are not entirely in keeping with the notion of earth. The lung has not only the function of depuration, but also that of diffusion, which cannot be accounted for by the notion of metal. Finally, the functions of the kidney include not only storing essence and governing water, but also warming and propulsion of fluids, which are not associated with the notion of water.

For these reasons, it is felt that the theory of the five phases is incomplete and fails to embrace all the physiologic functions of the five viscera. It is only through clinical practice and research that our understanding of the functions of the organs can be increased and new breakthroughs accomplished.

The four cycles in inter-organic relationships and prognosis

The engendering and restraining cycles each have two aspects: engendering and being engendered; restraining and being restrained. These explain the relationship of each of the phases to the remaining four. The liver, for example, is engendered by the kidney, and engenders the heart; it is restrained by the lung and restrains the spleen. The liver relies on kidney water for nourishment, a relationship known as water moistening wood. Failure of kidney water to fulfill this function is known as water failing to moisten wood. Pulmonary governance of depurative downbearing counterbalances hepatic governance of upstirring, which is known as metal constraining wood. When liver fire is effulgent and invades the lung, this is wood fire tormenting metal. Most liver disorders affect the spleen, an occurrence known as wood overcoming earth. Finally, when kidney fire and heart fire give rise to each other, it is known as water and fire sharing the same qi.

The theory of the five phases is also used in disease prognosis. If a condition spreads in the order of the engendering cycle, the prospects for a good recovery are favorable, and the disease can be considered minor. If, on the contrary, the condition spreads in the order of the restraining cycle, the prospects are unfavorable, the disease is serious. For example, a liver disease affecting the heart is considered normal, because the liver (wood) engenders the heart (fire). Should it progress in the order of the restraining cycle to the spleen, the condition is serious.

Although the preceding explanation of the physiopathologic relationships between the organs in terms of the five phases does have some definite clinical justification, current thought is that the physiologic activity of any given organ forms part of the general physiologic activity of the entire body. Morbid changes in any given organ may, under specific conditions, affect any of the other organs. For example, if kidney yin is vacuous, the liver may be deprived of its nourishing effect ("water failing to moisten wood"). Although this is accounted for by five-phase theory, unexplained is the fact that the heart or lung may be similarly affected, causing upflaming of heart fire or lung heat dry cough. Taking another example, liver fire may invade not only the lung but also the stomach, and may further affect the kidney. The inherent interrelationship among the organs cannot be explained in terms of the engendering and restraining cycles alone. To stick rigidly to the theory of the five phases in this particular area would be to go against objective reality.

As far as disease shifts and prognosis are concerned, the factors and conditions are even more complex, and are dependent on the nature of the pathogen, the strength of correct qi, and the treatment prescribed. The engendering and restraining relationships are of relatively little use in estimating a patient's progress. The errors and insufficiencies of the theory of the four relationships of the five phases in their application to medicine must be clearly identified and eliminated to salvage what is true and useful.

The engendering and restraining cycles in determining treatment

The theory of the engendering and restraining cycles can help to determine the correct method of treating disorders through a series of rules, for example:

> boosting fire to engender earth,
> banking up earth to engender metal,
> mutual engendering of metal and water,
> enriching water to moisten wood,
> banking up earth to dam water.

These rules represent practical guidelines for clinical practice. However, a critical approach should be adopted to eliminate the unreasonable elements and verify what is rational. These "rules of thumb" may be considered individually:

Boosting fire to engender earth

In practice, this means warming and supplementing kidney yang to treat disorders such as clear-food diarrhea, enduring diarrhea, or daybreak diarrhea, when caused by a splenorenal yang vacuity. In five-phase theory, the spleen corresponds to earth, and conditions such as spleen-vacuity diarrhea require that fire be supplemented to engender earth, restoring the spleen to normal functioning. Since "fire" here refers not to the heart fire (fire corresponding to the heart in the five phases) but to kidney yang (vital gate fire), this rule of thumb is not strictly in keeping with five-phase theory. The correct interpretation of the word relies on the understanding that in medicine, kidney yang is the root of the yang qi of all the organs. Warm supplementation of kidney yang indirectly strengthens splenic, cardiac, and pulmonary yang. Even assuming that fire represents kidney yang, a strict interpretation of five-phase theory would limit the effect of warm supplementation of kidney yang to mere fortification of the spleen, which is not in keeping with organ theory.

Banking up earth to engender metal

In practice, this rule denotes fortifying the spleen to treat disorders of the lung. The rule applies in cases of lung vacuity that occur in conjunction with splenogastric vacuity. Since the stomach and spleen are the source of the acquired constitution, and are the basis of blood and qi formation, supplementing these organs is generally conducive to increasing the body's resistance to disease. If we were to interpret "banking up earth to engender metal" according to five-phase theory to mean that supplementing the spleen is effective only in treating lung vacuity, the theory that the stomach and spleen are the basis of blood and qi formation would to a certain extent be invalidated.

Metal and water engender each other

This guideline is derived from the five-phase principle that metal engenders water. In practice, it refers to pulmorenal yin vacuity, where treatment is based chiefly on the method of enriching kidney yin, and complemented by that of nourishing lung yin. The disorder involves vacuity in two organs, so both are treated.

This approach is not limited to the kidney and the lung; it may also be applied to other dual vacuity patterns. For example, kidney and heart yin can be simultaneously diseased, as can kidney and heart yang. An even more common example is kidney and liver yin. All these conditions are treated by a dual approach. Because kidney yang and kidney yin are the root of the yin and yang of the whole body, treatments of dual disorders involving the kidney and another organ are primarily based on supplementing the kidney. This is an important principle of treatment in Chinese medicine.

Enriching water to moisten wood

This is taken to mean nourishing kidney yin to subdue liver yang, a principle that is applied in the treatment of ascendant hyperactivity of liver yang due to hepatorenal yin vacuity. However, five-phase theory fails to take account of the fact that kidney yin is the root of the yin of all viscera. Insufficiency of kidney yin can produce not only ascendant hyperactivity of liver yang (characterized by dizziness and upbearing fire flush), but also upflaming of heart fire (characterized by palpitations, insomnia, excessive dreaming, and erosion of the nasal and oral mucosa). Accordingly, kidney yin enrichment treats disorders stemming from both hepatorenal and cardiorenal yin vacuity.

The inherent relationships of the yin and yang aspects of the organs thus explain the supplementation of kidney yin to subdue liver yang or to clear heart fire. The axiom that the kidney is the source of all yin means that kidney yin has the definite functions of nourishing the yin aspect of all the other organs, and of counteracting the yang aspect of all the other organs. To claim that kidney yin can moisten only the liver would be erroneous. In reality, this rule of thumb falls within the scope of "invigorating the governor of water to counteract the brilliance of yang."

Banking up earth to dam water

Treatment of water swelling by fortifying the spleen and boosting qi is known as banking up earth to dam water. Here, "water" refers not to the kidney, but to water-damp pathogens in the body. According to the correspondence among the five phases and the five viscera, water can only represent the kidney and cannot refer to water-damp pathogens. Thus, banking up earth to dam water only makes sense when rephrased as fortifying the spleen to disinhibit water.

The reluctance in Chinese medical tradition to modify or discard the theories of the past means that theory is encumbered by a considerable and confusing detritus. The theories of yin and yang and the five phases are fraught with defects that should be set out clearly.

Yin and yang in Chinese medicine are abstract concepts that are used to denote different phenomena. When speaking of a condition characterized by prevalence of yin and debilitation of yang, "yin" refers to a yin pathogen, while "yang" refers to the yang qi of the body. In the phrase "yang hyperactivity due to yin vacuity," "yin" refers to yin humors, while "yang" refers to yang qi, both of which are inherent elements of the body.

Another example is seen in surfeits and deficits of yin and yang. The notion that detriment to yin or yang affects its complement can be explained in terms of interdependence. Here yin and yang refer to mutually engendering yin humor and yang qi. By contrast, a surfeit of yin or yang cannot lead to a surfeit of its complement, since yin and yang here refer to pathogenic qi, which does not stand in a relationship of mutual engendering with the body. This situation therefore cannot be explained in terms of interdependence.

In medicine, the concepts of yin and yang are always used to denote specific phenomena. Physiologic elements of the body (yin humor and yang qi) and pathogens may both be referred to by the terms yin and yang, sometimes in close proximity and without any indication as to which is intended. The problem arises because yin and yang represent a theory, rather than a natural law. Some aspects of the theory of yin and yang have only limited scope in practice and lack universal validity. Zhang Jie-Bin (Jing Yue) states:

> If yin and yang are distinguished according to heat and cold, they cannot be confused; if distinguished according to essence and qi, they cannot be separated.

In some cases, yin and yang denote cold and heat, while in other cases they refer to essence and qi. Confusion arises because different laws apply in each case.

The problem of whether the yin-yang balance is relative or absolute reveals a lack of clarity in the theory. The vague explanations found in the classical texts offer no firm conclusions. *Essential Questions* states, "When yin is calm and yang is sound, essence and spirit remain in order; if yin and yang separate, essential qi expires." This would appear to mean that yin and yang aspects of the body under normal circumstances should be in harmony and cannot be separated, but there is no indication of any absolute balance.

There is also a more metaphysical interpretation, as one author suggests:

> If yang is neither in surfeit nor deficit, and yin is not damaged nor dispersed, then the body is healthy; but if the body's yin and yang forces become mutually opposed or imbalanced, then disorders will arise, sometimes leading to death.

According to this statement, yin and yang function in perfect equilibrium.

A further example is the question of whether yin-yang conversion is subject to conditions. *Essential Questions* states:

> Double yin becomes yang; double yang becomes yin.
> Extreme cold engenders heat; extreme heat engenders cold.

"Double" and "extreme" may be said to be conditions, but this is not sufficiently clear. Thus, in later classical texts, the conversion of yin and yang was said to be cyclical, a considerably idealized interpretation.

Conspicuous shortcomings are also to be found in five-phase theory. In some areas the theory has clearly slipped into the metaphysical. It would be wrong to assume that the symbols metal, wood, water, fire, and earth are without meaning and void of practical utility in all contexts. Yet at the same time, it would be a mistake to assume the theory of the engendering and restraining cycles to be flawless without first subjecting it to due scrutiny and analysis. The five phases are used for making analogies and inferences, and sometimes broad generalizations. The functions of the organs of the human body cannot be fully explained in terms of the attributes of the five phases. Similarly, the relationships between the organs cannot be fully explained in terms of the engendering and restraining cycles, as has already been discussed. Confusion of concepts may also arise. For example, "fire" may sometimes refer to the heart and sometimes to kidney yang. "Water" may sometimes refer to the kidney and sometimes to water-damp pathogens. Clearly, explaining the functions of the organs in terms of the attributes of the five phases represents a biased approach. The engendering and restraining cycles can only be thought of as a rough guide in determining treatment, and it would be biased to regard them as universally valid laws.

In summation, today it is generally held that the yin-yang and five-phase theories derived from practical experience are based on rudimentary dialectics and have been a positive force in the development of medical theory. As a consequence of historical conditions, however, they were necessarily incomplete. Although certain aspects of these theories still provide valuable guides for clinical practice, other aspects are unclear and are therefore incompatible with modern medicine. The accurate aspects must be preserved, and the inaccurate ones eliminated. Although the terms yin and yang are still in common use, the practice of referring to the organs by their corresponding phase is dying out. It is thought that greater clarity is achieved by referring to the organs by their own names, even when discussing their interrelationships. Retaining only the theories that have practical value will do no damage to the theoretical body of Chinese medicine. Indeed, it will help to eliminate the constraints, develop it further, and raise it to the standards of a modern science. The practical aspects of the yin-yang and five-phase theories must be subject to practical analysis to separate the seed from the chaff. It would be wrong to think of these theories as entirely valid or invalid. What is required is honest analysis to select the best of past and present theory, and to use modern scientific methods in further research. Only then will China be able to develop Chinese medicine, and make its rightful contribution towards creating a new medical and pharmacological science.

Table 1-1

Yin–Yang Categorization of General Phenomena		
Phenomena	*Yang*	*Yin*
Space	Heaven	Earth
Time	Day	Night
Season	Spring Summer	Autumn Winter
Sex	Male	Female
Temperature	Hot	Cold
Weight	Light	Heavy
Brightness	Light	Dark
Motion	Upward and Outward Evident Motion	Downward and Inward Relative Stasis

Table 1-2

Yin–Yang Categorization of Body Regions, Tissues and Organs, and Physiologic Activities		
	Yang	*Yin*
Parts of the Body	Exterior back, Upper body	Interior abdomen, Lower body
Tissues and Organs	Surface skin, Body hair, Bowels	Bones, Sinews, Viscera
Activity, Function	Qi and defense, Agitation, Strength	Blood and construction, Calm, Weakness

Table 1-3

Yin—Yang Categorization of Patterns and Pulses		
	Yang	Yin
Disorder	Exterior Repletion Heat	Interior Vacuity Cold
Pulse	Rapid Floating Slippery Replete Large and surging	Slow Deep Rough Vacuous Small and fine

Table 1-4

Examples of Five Phase Categorization					
Category	*Wood*	*Fire*	*Earth*	*Metal*	*Water*
Season	Spring	Summer	Late summer	Autumn	Winter
Climate	Wind	Heat	Damp	Dryness	Cold
Direction	East	South	Center	West	North
Development	Birth	Growth	Maturity	Withdrawal	Dormancy
Color	Cyan	Red	Yellow	White	Black
Taste	Sour	Bitter	Sweet	Pungent	Salty
Viscus	Liver	Heart	Spleen	Lung	Kidney
Bowel	Gallbladder	Small Intestine	Stomach	Large Intestine	Urinary Bladder
Sense Organ	Eyes	Tongue	Mouth	Nose	Ears
Tissue	Sinews	Vessels	Flesh	Body Hair	Bones
Disposition	Anger	Joy	Preoccupation	Sorrow	Fear

Notes

[1] *Essential Questions* is the first book of *The Yellow Emperor's Inner Canon* (*circa* 200 B.C.), the earliest known treatise on Chinese medicine. The second book is the *Spiritual Axis*. The chapter titles appearing in the original *Fundamentals of Chinese Medicine* have been omitted in this text.

[2] Unusual or unfamiliar terms are defined in Appendix 1, "Glossary of Terms."

[3] *Inner Canon* is the abbreviated title of *The Yellow Emperor's Inner Canon*.

[4] The functions of qi and the blood are discussed in Chapter 2, "Qi, Blood, Essence, and Fluids."

[5] See Chapter 8, "Qi-Blood Pattern Identification," under the heading "Sequential Desertion of Blood and Qi."

[6] The functions of the kidney, as of the other organs, are dealt with in Chapter 4, "The Organs."

[7] Deviations from the natural flux of yin and yang are described in a variety of terms. A strengthening of one complement over the other is usually expressed as prevalence, while weakening is usually expressed as vacuity, or sometimes as debilitation in the case of yang. Here, the terms surfeit and deficit are synonymous with prevalence and vacuity/debilitation. Exuberance and hyperactivity describe more pronounced strengthening of yin and yang respectively, where the causal or resultant weakening of the complement is usually denoted by vacuity. Terms denoting strengthening and weakening of the body elements (qi, blood, essence, fluid) and the yin and yang (the organs) are described in the glossary under exuberance and debilitation, and under their own separate headings.

[8] Impairment of organ functions is dealt with in Chapter 4, "The Organs," and Chapter 9, "Organ Pattern Identification."

[9] Quotations such as "heat is treated with cold and cold is treated with heat" are often taken from the classics and used as general laws or principles in later texts. Traditional Chinese thinking was little concerned with absolute validity. Statements were made on the grounds of pertinence to context. The above statement adjusted to Western thought habits would read, "*Generally speaking,* heat is treated with cold and cold is treated with heat." Much of the exegetic work involved in reading classical texts stems from this need to determine the scope of statement validity.

[10] "Water is lacking": literally, "there is no water"; the meaning being "relative absence of water."

Basic Theories

[11] Lassitude of the spirit, q.v.. The spirit, in this context, is roughly synonymous with essence-spirit, i.e., that upon which mental vitality depends. Chinese medicine does not see a clear distinction between the body and the mind. States of being that Westerners would attribute to the mind or consciousness are seen by the Chinese as states of spirit, essence-spirit, spirit-disposition, spirit-affect, etc. These words are explained in Appendix 1, "Glossary of Terms."

[12] The Chinese term rendered here as "wheezing dyspnea" was chosen as the equivalent of asthma in Western medicine. In Chinese medicine, the independent nature of the two components, "wheezing" and "dyspnea," makes a single-word translation unsuitable. To reflect Chinese medical disease classification adequately, a new term has been chosen. Here, as in similar contexts throughout the book, the term added in parentheses indicates equivalence in Western medical classification.

[13] The lung and kidney are referred to in the singular (as opposed to the lungs and kidneys) to emphasize that in Chinese medicine they are regarded as functional entities rather than strictly morphological ones.

[14] Cf. Chapter 3.

Chapter Two
Qi, Blood, Essence, and Fluids

Qi, blood, essence, and fluids are the basis of all physiologic activity. Qi vitalizes the body, propels and warms, and is yang in nature. Blood and fluids are the sustenance of the body, nourishing and moistening the entire organism, and are yin in nature. Essence is the basis of physical development and reproduction. It is the stored surplus potential of the human body, and the basis of blood and fluid production. All changes that occur in the human body from birth to death result from the interaction of qi, blood, essence, and fluids.

Qi

Formation and physiologic function of qi

The ancient Chinese perceived the existence of qi and believed it to be the basic element[1] by which all movements and mutations of all phenomena in the universe arise. In the context of medicine, it is believed to be a fundamental constituent of the body. The movements and mutations of qi explain all physiologic activity. *Jing-Yue's Complete Compendium* emphatically states, "Human life depends upon this qi." The *Axioms of Medicine* posits, "When qi gathers, so the physical body is formed; when it disperses, so the body dies."

In the human body, qi appears in various forms. The basic form is original qi, which is made up of a combination of three other forms: the essential qi of the kidney; digestate qi, derived through the transformative function of the spleen; cosmic qi, the air drawn in through the lung. Original qi is highly active, flowing throughout the whole body. It is in all parts of the body at all times. The dynamic of qi is its capacity to undertake the four primary movements that occur in the organs and channels: upbearing, downbearing, issue, and entry. *Essential Questions* states, "There is no organ in which upbearing, downbearing, issue, and entry of original qi does not occur." When this movement stops, life ceases. It further states:

> Things are created by virtue of transformation; when they reach their extreme, transmutation occurs. Things evolve and dissolve by virtue of the interaction of transformation and transmutation.
>
> Evolution and dissolution are secretly reliant on the power of creation, which by its constant activity brings about transmutation.
>
> Without issue and entry, there can be no birth, growth, prime, or aging; without upbearing and downbearing, there can be no birth, growth, transformation, withdrawal, and dormancy.

These quotations all highlight the movement and mutation of qi.

Original qi flows around the whole body, manifesting as physiologic activity. Its various manifestations describe distinct aspects of this activity, each of which has been allotted its own name.

Organ qi

Original qi present in the bowels and viscera is known as organ qi. Thus each organ has its own qi, which is the basis of its physiologic activity and manifests as a major aspect of its physiologic function.

Channel qi

The original qi that flows through the channels is called the channel qi. Its movement is seen in the channels' function of transmission and conveyance. The sensation produced by needling an acupuncture point, known as "obtaining qi," demonstrates the operancy of channel qi.

Construction qi

The qi that forms the blood and flows with it in the vessels, helping to nourish the entire body, is known as construction qi. Its functions are discussed in *Essential Questions,* which says:

> It harmonizes with the viscera and is distributed among the bowels; it is thus able to enter the blood vessels, flowing up and down in them, connecting the bowels and viscera.

The *Spiritual Axis* points out:

> Construction qi secretes fluids, discharges them into the vessels, and turns them into blood, to nourish the limbs and supply the bowels and viscera.

Because the main function of construction qi is to produce blood and nourish the whole body, *Essential Questions* also states, "Construction qi is the essential qi of the digestate."

Defense qi

The qi that flows outside the vessels is known as defense qi. It is described as being fierce, bold, and uninhibited, so it cannot be contained by the vessels. Its main function in the chest and abdomen is to warm the organs. Its function on the exterior is to flow through the skin and flesh, regulate the opening and closing of the striations, protect the exterior, keep the skin lustrous and healthy, and prevent invasion of exogenous pathogens. The *Spiritual Axis* states:

> Defense qi warms the flesh and flushes the skin; it keeps the striations replenished and controls their opening and closing.
> If defense qi is in harmony, the skin is supple and the striations are kept tight and sound.

Because defense qi is "fierce and bold," flows outside the blood vessels, and provides resistance against exogenous qi, *Essential Questions* states, "Defense qi is the fierce qi of the digestate."

Ancestral qi

Ancestral qi gathers in the chest, which is also known as the "sea of qi." However, it can ascend the trachea and descend into the qi thoroughfare. The *Spiritual Axis* states:

> Ancestral qi is concentrated in the chest, and may come up through the throat to connect with the heart and produce respiration.
>
> Ancestral qi is located in the sea of qi; descending, it enters the qi thoroughfare, and ascending it goes into the respiratory tract.

The main functions of ancestral qi may be described as follows:

> Ancestral qi enters the respiratory tract and controls breathing; its health is reflected in the strength of respiration and the voice. It also causes the qi derived from the breath to descend into the qi thoroughfare. Breath control in *qi gong*[2] makes use of this function.
>
> Ancestral qi penetrates the heart and the vessels, driving the heart and regulating the pulses. Thus, the circulation of qi and blood, as well as the temperature and movement of the limbs, is largely dependent on it.

From these descriptions, qi can be seen to have five basic functions:

Activation

Qi is highly active; human growth and development, as well as all physiologic activity and metabolism, are manifestations of the activation of qi.

Warming

The temperature of the human body and the ability of the organs and tissues to perform their functional activities are dependent on the warming action of qi.

Defense

Qi is the outer defense of the body, and prevents pathogenic influences from entering. *Essential Questions* states, "Where pathogens are able to enter, qi must be vacuous." Qi, in its capacity of defending the body against pathogens, is thus known as "correct qi." When disease develops in the body, correct qi becomes active, fighting to destroy the pathogens and restore the body to health.

Qi, Blood, Essence, and Fluids

Transformation

Production of blood and fluids, distribution of fluids, and conversion of fluids into sweat and urine are all the result of the transformative action of qi. More is said about these processes in the sections specifically relating to blood and fluids.

Containment

Under normal circumstances, extravasation of blood is prevented by the containing function of qi. Hence it is said, "Qi contains the blood." This function also prevents excessive loss of fluids through oversecretion of sweat and other fluids or excessive urination.

These five aspects of the function of qi are interrelated. Basically, they are all normal functions of original qi. When original qi is in the organs it is known as organ qi. Organ qi ensures the fulfillment of the physiologic functions of each bowel and viscus. Thus, the functions of each organ are intimately related to the formation and movement of original qi. The essential qi of the kidney combines with the qi assimilated from the air by the lung and the essential qi produced from the digestate of the stomach and spleen to form original qi. Heartbeat and respiration work together in controlling the movement of original qi; the liver governs the free-coursing of qi and thus has a regulating effect on its flow.

Disorders of qi

The main pathologies of qi are qi vacuity and qi stagnation.

Qi vacuity

Qi vacuity denotes a group of diseases caused by a vacuity of original qi. The vacuity may be caused by enduring illness, old age, a weak constitution, malnutrition, or taxation fatigue. Qi vacuities are invariably characterized by general physical weakness, but affect the bowels and viscera in different ways, each according to its physiologic characteristics. Shortness of breath and a faint voice are associated with lung qi vacuity. Poor appetite and indigestion are associated with splenogastric qi vacuity. Enuresis and seminal efflux are associated with kidney qi vacuity. Aversion to wind and a tendency to catch cold are associated with defense qi vacuity.

Qi stagnation

Under normal circumstances, qi courses smoothly without impediment through the whole body. If the qi dynamic is disturbed in any part, the resultant disorder in the relevant organ or channel is known as qi stagnation. Emotional constraint, dietary irregularities, contraction of exogenous pathogens, and traumas are all potential factors of qi dynamic disturbance. Qi stagnation often occurs in the early stages of disease, which explains why it is said that "qi is implicated in the onset of disease." The main symptoms of qi stagnation are local pain, distention, feelings of oppression, or painful distention of fluctuating intensity and nonspecific location. These often occur in association with essence-spirit or emotional disturbance. If qi stagnates in the chest and lateral costal region, those areas will be painful and distended. If it stagnates in the liver channel, there may be painful swelling of the breasts and distention or prolapse in the lower abdomen. Tenesmus may also be a sign of qi stagnation.

Qi counterflow and qi fall are common disorders resulting from impairment of the normal bearing of qi. Qi counterflow denotes stagnation and counterflow upbearing of qi that normally bears downwards, and usually occurs in disorders of the lung and stomach. Impairment of the normal downbearing of lung qi presents as cough and counterflow qi ascent (cough with distressed, rapid breathing). Disturbance of gastric downbearing is characterized by such symptoms as nausea, vomiting, and hiccough. Qi fall denotes downward fall of qi from vacuity, mostly occurring in diseases of the spleen. The qi of the spleen normally bears upwards. If it falls, there may be not only dizziness and vacuity, distention or vacuity fullness in the upper abdomen, but also either enduring diarrhea efflux desertion and prolapse of the rectum, or prolapse of the uterus.

Blood

Formation and physiologic function of the blood

Blood is formed from the essential qi derived from the digestate by the stomach and spleen that becomes red blood after transformation by construction qi and the lung. The *Spiritual Axis* states, "The middle burner takes in qi, extracts the sap from it and turns it into the red substance that is blood." In another passage it states:

> From the qi that the middle burner takes in, it produces waste, and distills fluids from which it extracts the essence. This then flows into the lung channel where it is transformed into blood, which furnishes the vital needs of the body. Its preciousness is unexcelled by anything. It flows through the blood vessels and is known as construction qi.

After formation, the blood flows through the vessels, and is pumped around the whole body by the heart, whence the phrase "the heart governs the blood." The blood is stored and regulated by the liver. "When the body moves, the blood flows through the channels; when at rest, the blood returns to the liver where it is stored."[3] This explains the phrase, "The liver stores the blood." The blood is prevented from spilling out of the vessels by the containing power of the spleen. Hence it is said that "The spleen manages the blood."

The main function of the blood is to nourish the whole of the body. The skin and the body hair, the sinews and bones, the channels, the bowels and viscera, and all the other organs and tissues of the body rely on the blood for nutrition. The *Canon of Perplexities* confirms this point in stating "blood governs nutrition." *Essential Questions* states that all parts of the body rely on adequate nutrition from the blood to accomplish their functions:

> The liver receives blood, so there is sight; the legs receive blood and thus are able to walk; the hands receive blood and so are able to grip; the fingers receive blood and then are able to grasp.

Blood has the function of nourishing the body. It is produced by construction qi, and flows with the construction qi through the vessels. Consequently, blood is often referred to as construction, or in the combined form, construction-blood.

The relationship between qi and blood

Blood and qi are both basic elements indispensable to the body's physiologic activity. They are differentiable but inseparable; they complement each other and are dependent on each other.

Qi is the commander of the blood

Blood is produced by construction qi, which carries the essence assimilated from the digestate by the stomach and spleen upward into the lung, combining it with lung qi. Once formed, it then flows with qi through the vessels. The heart's function of governing the blood, the liver's function of storing the blood, and the spleen's function of keeping the blood in the vessels are all attributable to the qi of these organs. From this it can be seen that qi is indispensable for both the production and the circulation of blood. Qi engenders, moves, and contains the blood. This is why it is said that "qi is the commander of the blood."

Blood is the mother of qi

The capacity of the qi to enable all parts of the body to carry out their various activities is attributable to the adequate supply of nutrition from the blood. This is why it is said that "blood is the mother of qi." Qi and blood are interdependent, together forming the basis for the life and activity of the body. Further, as the *Canon of Perplexities* states, "Qi invigorates, and blood nourishes." As mutually complementary elements, they flow endlessly around the whole body, enabling it to grow, develop, and fulfill its metabolic activities. *Essential Questions* states, "If blood and qi fall into disharmony, a hundred diseases may arise."

Disorders of the blood

The main disorders of the blood are blood vacuity, blood stasis, and blood heat.

Blood vacuity

Blood vacuity is the manifestation both of insufficiency of the blood caused by heavy blood loss or diminished blood production, and of local impairment of the blood's nourishing function. It can occur when the blood is not immediately replenished after heavy blood loss or when blood formation diminishes as a result of splenogastric transformation failure. It may also be result from failure to eliminate static blood and produce new blood. Blood vacuity characteristically displays such symptoms as dizziness, palpitations, a lusterless or withered, yellow, drawn complexion, colorless lips and tongue, a thin pulse, insomnia, flowery vision, hypertonicity, dry skin, or dry, lifeless hair.

Blood stasis

Blood stasis refers to generalized impairment of the smooth flow of blood, local stagnation of blood in the vessels, or local accumulation of extravasated blood. Among the causes are: stagnation or vacuity of qi, impairing the free flow of blood; blood cold, causing congealing and stagnation of the blood; blood heat that "boils" the blood; and impact trauma that causes extravasation of the blood (internal hemorrhage and contusion). Blood stasis is characterized by general signs such as a dark, dull complexion, cyan-purple lips and tongue, stasis macules on the margins of the tongue, and a thin or rough pulse. Local stagnation is characterized by painful swelling and stabbing pain of specific location. In serious cases there may be palpable internal masses attended by general signs such as a soot black complexion and cyan-purple lips and tongue. Bleeding, which arises when blood vessels can no longer withstand the pressure created by static blood obstruction, is usually recurrent, while the blood is purple-black and clotted. Bleeding due to the presence of static blood is most common in gynecological disorders. Bruises resulting from impact trauma are one type of stasis macule. If blood stagnation affects the heart, essence-spirit disturbances such as raving and delirium may be observed.

Blood heat

Blood heat is a disorder resulting from heat toxin entering the blood. It is usually characterized by frenetic blood movement, hemorrhage (with bright red blood), or maculopapular eruptions. If blood heat harasses the heart spirit, symptoms include restlessness, a crimson tongue, a rapid pulse, or even delirium or coma.

Essence

Essence is a primary element responsible for determining physical growth and development and maintaining life activity and metabolism in the body. It may be considered the substantial (yin) counterpart of the active (yang) spirit. The combination essence-spirit is used to denote "vitality," in both its physical and mental senses. There are two basic forms of essence: the part forming a constituent part of the body is termed congenital essence, while the part maintaining life activity is referred to as acquired essence, from which reproductive essence and essential qi are both derived.

Essence is the basis of life. If it is abundant, the life force is strong, facilitating adaptation to environmental changes and helping to prevent sickness. If it is insufficient or vacuous, the life force is weak, reducing adaptability to the environment and resistance to disease. As such, essence serves as the body's reserve potential used to compensate in emergency situations.

Congenital essence

Congenital (or prenatal) essence is inherited from both parents, and determines the individual's constitution, physical development, and to some extent, eventual lifespan. Congenital essence is a fixed quantum at birth; it is nonrenewable, and when it is eventually exhausted life ceases.

Congenital essence is responsible for effecting the transformative action of middle burner qi, activating the stomach and spleen which are then able to assimilate and transform the digestate into both blood and acquired essence. It is thus said that "essence and blood proceed from the same source." Considered together, the strength of the essence-blood is a good indicator of the health of a person. Because the kidney stores essence and the liver stores blood, in clinical practice vacuities of essence-blood are often treated by strengthening the liver and the kidney.

Acquired essence

Acquired (or postnatal) essence is produced from food and air, and is responsible for the continuing healthy function of the organs. As such, it serves to supplement and reinforce the congenital essence. Acquired essence is constantly being used and replenished from the essence of digestate.

Reproductive essence

The kidney is considered the basis of essence formation. When the acquired essence of the organs is abundant, it returns to the kidney to be stored. When the reproductive function becomes fully developed, the kidney is able to transform this stored essence into reproductive essence, and the individual is able to produce offspring. The reproductive essence of the mother and father combine in the womb, creating new life and determining the eventual congenital essence of the newborn.

Essential qi

Essence that has been mobilized to maintain the functional activity of the organs is often referred to as essential qi. In this sense, it also includes the qi of construction and defense derived from food, and is indispensable for maintaining life activity. However, it cannot be considered separate from the acquired essence stored in the kidney, which may also be mobilized for reproduction. Only when the essential qi of the organs is abundant can there be plentiful supplies of stored essence in the kidney.

It can be seen from an understanding of the function of essence that weakness or depletion of essence in any of its forms would be a major cause of congenital defects, late or improper maturation, premature senility, or sexual and reproductive dysfunctions.

Fluids

Formation and physiologic function of fluids

The term "fluids" embraces all the normal fluid substances of the human body. It refers to fluids actually flowing within the human body, and to sweat, saliva, digestive juices, urine, and other fluids secreted by or discharged from the body. The main functions of fluids are to keep the organs, muscles, skin, mucous membranes, and portals adequately moistened, lubricate the joints, and nourish the brain marrow and bones.

Though referring to a single entity, the term fluids is often differentiated into two component aspects, liquid and humor, to highlight specific characteristics. Liquid refers to fluid that is relatively thin, mobile, and yang in quality, whereas humor denotes thicker, less mobile yin fluid. Liquid is mostly found in the surface of the flesh and in the mucous membranes, moisturizing the flesh, skin, and hair, and keeping the eyes, ears, mouth, nose, and other portals moistened. Sweat and urine are both produced from fluids. Humor is located primarily in the bowels and viscera, the brain, and the bones, and is responsible for lubricating the joints, and also partially responsible for moistening the skin. It must not be forgotten, however, that liquid and humor form a single entity and are mutually convertible. Distinction is most often made in pathology, as in cases of damage to liquid or humor desertion.

The term yin humor is sometimes used synonymously with humor, emphasizing its yin nature (thick, heavy, and relatively immobile). It may also loosely denote all the nutritious fluids of the body, and as such, is used in contradistinction to yang qi.

The formation, distribution, and discharge of fluids involve complex processes in which the lung, spleen, kidney, stomach, small intestine, large intestine, bladder, and other organs play major roles. *Essential Questions* gives the following description:

> Ingested fluids enter the stomach. Here, they are churned and their essential qi is strained off. This is then carried to the spleen and further distributed by spleen qi. It passes up to the lung which ensures regular flow through the waterways down to the bladder. In this way, water essence is distributed throughout the five channels and the four parts of the body.

Fluid processing begins in the stomach, where the essential qi (the useful part) of the fluids is absorbed. The spleen then carries this essential qi up to the lung and distributes it among the other organs. The statement appearing elsewhere in *Essential Questions,* that the spleen "moves the fluids of the stomach," highlights the active role of the spleen in assimilation of fluids. The lung, by governing diffusion and depurative downbearing, ensures the regular flow of water through the waterways. The kidney's function is to "distill" fluid, bearing the clear up and the turbid down. It plays a part in distributing fluids around the entire body, and is responsible for transforming surplus and waste fluid into urine, which is discharged through the bladder. The intestines are also involved in the absorption of fluids; the small intestine separates the clear from the turbid, and the large intestine conveys the waste material downward while further absorbing fluid. The *Spiritual Axis* comments, "The small intestine governs humor" and "the large intestine governs liquid."

Thus, assimilation and initial conveyance of fluids are dependent on gastric ingestion and splenic movement and transformation. The distribution of fluids around the body, including moisturization of the muscle and skin, and surface skin and body hair, is dependent on the lung's function of ensuring diffusion and depurative downbearing. The transformation of fluids into sweat is also dependent on this function. For these reasons, the lung is said to be the "upper source of water" and to ensure regular flow through the waterways. The kidney plays the most important role in the formation and replacement of fluids, since the roles of the stomach, the spleen, and the lung are dependent on the warming and activating function of kidney qi. More importantly, the production and discharge of urine and normal replacement of fluids in the body is intimately related to the transformative action of kidney qi. This is why it is said, "The kidney governs the water of the whole body."

Finally, because the lung, spleen, stomach, and kidney are located in all three burners, the term "triple burner" is often used to denote the waterways; and the formation, movement, and discharge of fluids is attributed to the transformative action of triple burner qi. *Essential Questions* states, "The triple burner holds the office of the sluices; it manifests as the waterways."

Relationship of the fluids to blood and qi

The main source of fluids, blood, and qi is the essential qi of the digestate. As three fundamental elements of the human body, they are closely interrelated.

Relationship between the fluids and qi

The production, distribution, and discharge of fluids relies on the upbearing, downbearing, issue, and entry of qi. It is intimately related to the transformative action of the triple burner qi, and to the qi dynamic of the relevant organs. If the qi dynamic of any of these is disturbed, the transformative action of triple burner qi will be invariably affected, leading to fluid disorders such as "insufficiency of the basis of fluid formation," and abnormal accumulations of fluid forming water qi. Where qi is vacuous and thus unable to perform its containing function, heavy fluid loss may result. Examples of this are profuse sweating from yang qi vacuity desertion, or long micturition with clear urine due to kidney qi vacuity. Conversely, cases of major damage to the fluids invariably culminate in desertion of original qi, and abnormal fluid accumulations may cause local impairment of the transformative action of qi.

Relationship between fluids and blood

Fluid is an important constituent of the blood. Its richest elements flow into the vessels and combine with construction qi, flow into the vessels of the lung, and are there transformed into blood. The *Canon of the Golden Coffer and Jade Sheath* states, "Water enters the channels and becomes blood." This implies that the quantity of fluids and the quantity of blood are interrelated. For example, in cases of massive bleeding, there may be thirst, dry skin, scant urine, and other signs of fluid depletion. Fluid depletion may also lead to insufficiency of the basis of blood formation, which is known as exhaustion of liquid and blood. The *Spiritual Axis* states, "Blood retrenchment diminishes sweat, and sweat retrenchment diminishes blood." *A Treatise on Cold Damage* warns, "Patients suffering from nosebleed may not be given diaphoretic treatment," and "patients suffering from blood collapse may not be given diaphoretic treatment."

Disorders of the fluids

Disorders of the fluids fall into two categories: damage and abnormal accumulations. Damage to the fluids can manifest as damage to liquid or humor desertion. Abnormal fluid accumulations can appear as water swelling or phlegm-rheum.

Damage to liquid and humor desertion

Minor depletion of fluids is known as damage to liquid; major depletion is known as humor desertion. Among the causes are great fever, enduring fever, profuse sweating, heavy urination, vomiting, and diarrhea. The most common pathomechanisms are scorching of the fluids by pathogenic heat or wearing of the fluids through enduring sickness. Iatrogenic causes include inappropriate or excessive use of diaphoretics, urine disinhibitors (diuretics), draining precipitants (purgatives), or warm, dry agents.

Damage to liquid denotes temporary depletion of the body's fluids. The main signs are: thirst; dry, rough tongue fur; dry throat, lips, tongue, nose, and skin; dry, bound stool; and short micturition with scant urine.

Humor desertion generally refers to serious depletion of the body's yin humor. Thus, symptoms are more pronounced than those of damage to liquid, and treatment is generally slower. Humor desertion mostly occurs as a result of prolonged sickness or in the latter stages of exogenous heat diseases. In addition to pronounced signs of damage to liquid, symptoms include extremely poor general health and a dry mouth with a strong desire for fluids; the tongue may be dry, red or crimson in color, and peeled clean of fur.

Water swelling and phlegm-rheum

Water swelling and phlegm-rheum refer to abnormal accumulations of fluid in the body, mainly resulting from impairment of the transformative action of qi in the lung, spleen, and kidney, affecting the distribution or discharge of fluids. Water swelling may occur when impairment of pulmonary diffusion and depuration or of splenic movement and transformation affects the flow of fluid and leads to accumulations. However, a far more common cause is impairment of the transformative action of kidney qi, affecting upbearing of the clear and downbearing of the turbid, and the production and discharge of urine.

Phlegm-rheum denotes accumulations of fluid for reasons similar to those that cause water swelling. Therefore, in some cases water swelling and phlegm-rheum are interrelated. Phlegm-rheum arises when fluid distribution is disturbed owing to impairment of pulmonary diffusion and depuration or splenic movement and transformation; fluids then accumulate and form phlegm, giving rise to cough and expectoration of copious, white, foaming mucus. The statements, "the spleen is the basis of phlegm formation" and "the lung is the collecting place of phlegm" essentially refer to phlegm-rheum. Impairment of the transformative action of kidney qi can also cause a surplus of water, which ascends, transforms into phlegm, and enters the heart or lung. These conditions are known as water-rheum intimidating the heart and water-rheum shooting into the lung. Signs such as palpitation, rapid breathing, cough, and expectoration of large quantities of white, foaming phlegm, which occur in what Western medicine terms cardiac failure and pulmonary edema, are mostly attributable to this type of pathology.

A disturbance of the transformative action of lung, spleen, or kidney qi may affect the other two organs. For example, disturbance of fluid distribution due to impairment of splenic movement and transformation may affect the pulmonary regulation of the waterways, causing dyspnea and fullness with phlegm cough. It may also affect the kidney's distilling function, causing swellings in the groin and lower limbs, and short micturition with scant urine. Impaired regulation of the waterways may affect splenic governance of fluid distribution. This either gives rise to accumulations of damp, which may transform into phlegm, or it may affect the transformative action of kidney qi, causing water qi to flood and transform into phlegm. Impaired transformation of water qi due to debilitation of kidney yang may place an added burden on other viscera. If it affects pulmonary diffusion and depuration, the result will be dyspnea and cough with expectoration of copious amounts of phlegm. If splenic movement and transformation is affected, inhibited urination, water swelling, and abdominal fullness may be observed.

Notes

[1] The Chinese text uses the word "substance" to explain qi, blood, essence, and fluids. Since the translators cannot accept qi as a single form of matter capable of being isolated, the term "element," in the sense of a component part or quality, has been chosen instead.

[2] Qi cultivation exercises using special breathing and meditative techniques.

[3] From Wang Bing's annotated *Inner Canon*, A.D. 762.

Chapter 3
The Channels

Pathways and Theory

The channels are pathways that carry qi, blood, and fluids around the body. They are the communication lines between all parts of the organism. The *Canon of Perplexities* states, "The channels move blood and qi and ensure the free flow of yin and yang, so that the body is properly nourished." The organs, portals, surface skin and body hair, sinews and flesh, bones, and other tissues all rely on communication through the channels, forming an integrated, unified organism.

Channel theory, derived to some extent from human anatomy, is an important element of Chinese medicine. The *Spiritual Axis* states:

> Regard the body of an eight cubit man; when alive, take his measurement, feel his pulses; when dead, dissect his body and regard the strength of his viscera, the size of his bowels, the volume of the trunk cavity and the organs within it, the length of the channels, the clarity of the blood and the state of the qi. . . . All are shown to conform to a standard.

This quotation provides evidence that by the time of the Warring States Period, knowledge about the channels was gained from human anatomy. However, channel theory was largely derived from clinical practice and the subjective experiences of patients undergoing acupuncture treatment. Thus, this theory represents a synthesis of anatomical and clinical findings with subjective sensory experience. It is applied in the clinical practice of all branches of medicine, particularly in acupuncture and moxibustion, and has led to major medical developments such as acu-analgesia.

The channels are described in two main categories: major channels, having clearly defined pathways that penetrate deep into the body, and connecting channels, which are their branches. *The Gateway to Medicine* states, "The major channels represent the main pathways, and their ramifications are the connecting channels." There are two types of major channels: the twelve regular channels and the eight irregular channels. Concerning the difference between the regular channels and the irregular channels, *The Savior General Compendium* states:

> There are regular and irregular major channels. The twelve {organ-related} channels are the regular channels. The eight irregular channels are so named because they do not conform to the norm. Qi and blood constantly flow through the twelve regular channels and, when abundant, overflow into the irregular channels.

The connecting channels are described in three categories: the large ones, of which there are fifteen, are called collateral connecting channels, and serve to connect interior (yin) and exterior (yang) major channels; those that run through the exterior of the body are called superficial connecting channels; their finer ramifications are known as the reticular connecting channels. Twelve divergent channels enhance communication between organs and the major channels, and between the channels themselves. Finally, twelve sinew channels and twelve cutaneous regions divide the body's musculature and integument into twelve distinct regions corresponding to the twelve regular channels.

Channel theory is of significance in physiology, pathology, pattern identification, and treatment. In physiology, the channels represent the principal pathways by which qi, blood, and the fluids are distributed around the body, providing nourishment and warmth. They also serve as vital links among the organs and other parts of the body. The *Spiritual Axis* explains:

> The channels are the routes by which blood and qi circulate, regulating yin and yang, keeping the bones and sinews moistened and the joints lubricated.

The blood and fluids are carried through the channels by qi, and in acupuncture the sensation produced when obtaining qi shows that the channel is live, or has abundant qi. The channels are the transmission lines between the various parts of the body, making the organism a unified whole.

In pathology, exogenous pathogens invade the body through the exterior and penetrate into the interior, affecting the organs. *Essential Questions* states:

> A pathogen settling in the body must first abide in the surface skin and body hair. If it resists expulsion, it will enter the reticular connecting channels. If it continues to resist, it will enter the larger connecting channels. If it persists, it will enter the major channels that communicate with the organs in the inner body. When the pathogen spreads to the stomach and intestines, yin and yang are both affected and all the organs suffer damage. This is the sequence by which pathogens penetrating the body through the surface skin and body hair eventually affect the five viscera.

Similarly, organic pathologies may spread to other parts of the body through the channels. A disorder in a given organ may be transmitted through the relevant channel, manifesting as morbidity in regions along the channel's course. An example of this is seen in upflaming of liver fire which may be characterized not only by ocular rubor and pain in the center of the chest, but also by pain in the related channel along the inner face of the arm. Disease in one organ can also spread to other organs through the channels. Examples include heart fire, which can spread to the small intestine, and kidney vacuity water-flood, which intimidates the heart or shoots into the lung. Through channel transference, morbidity in the organs may also be reflected in areas of palpatory tenderness, swellings, indentations, nodules, and hyperemia. These signs are often helpful in diagnosis.

The main significance of channel theory in pattern identification and treatment is found in a series of methods based on the laws governing the flow of channel qi, interorganic connections, physiopathologic characteristics of the channels, and channel interrelationships. There are three most common uses of these methods. Determining channel relevance based on pathology location involves determining the channels relevant to a disorder based on its location. Pattern identification by channels involves analyzing symptoms based on the physiopathologic features of the channels. Acupoint and drug prescription by channels denote methods of determining treatment through the physiopathologic features of the channels.

For example, the forehead, cheeks, teeth, lips, and throat are all located on the foot yang ming stomach channel and the hand yang ming large intestine channel. Therefore, disorders such as frontal headache, wind-fire toothache, and sore throat may be treated as yang ming channel disorders. In acumoxatherapy, they are treated by needling the points ST-6, ST-7, ST-36, ST-44 on the foot yang ming stomach channel; or LI-4 and LI-1 on the hand yang ming large intestine channel may be chosen. If drug treatment is indicated, agents that dissipate yang ming wind-fire may be used:

Agents that dissipate yang ming wind-fire	
Radix Puerariae	*gé gēn*
Rhizoma Cimicifugae	*shēng má*
Radix Angelicae	*bái zhǐ*
Radix Ledebouriellae	*fáng fēng*

Agents that clear yang ming repletion-heat may also be employed:

Agents that clear yang ming repletion-heat	
Gypsum	*shí gāo*
Rhizoma Anemarrhenae	*zhī mǔ*
Rhizoma Phragmitis	*lú gēn*

Since the hand and foot yang ming channels are linked to the intestines and stomach, agents that flush gastrointestinal heat-bind may also be employed:

Agents that flush gastrointestinal heat-bind	
Rhizoma Rhei	dà huáng
Mirabilitum	máng xiāo

In summation, channel theory represents an important part of the body of medical theory, and is widely applied in pattern identification and treatment in the clinical practice of all branches of medicine. It is of greatest importance in organ pattern identification and six-channel pattern identification; in external medicine, where attention is paid to the proximity of lesions to channels; and in the regulation of the penetrating and conception vessels in gynecology. Recent research has led to major advances in acu-analgesia, as well as facial and scalp acupuncture.

The Twelve Regular Channels

Distribution of channels throughout the body

The twelve channels (listed in Table 3-1) are duplicated on both sides of the body. They are identified according to the limb along which they flow and according to yin and yang. The yin channels run along the inner surface of the limbs, and across the chest and abdomen. Each is also associated with a viscera. The yang channels run along the outer surfaces of the limbs and over the back and buttocks, and are each associated with a bowel. Yin and yang are each further divided into three subdivisions. In the normal standing position, the tai yin channels run along the forward inner edge of the limbs; the shao yin channels run along the rear inner edge, and the jue yin channels run along the midline of the limbs' inner surface. Similarly, the yang ming channels run along the forward outer edge of the limbs; the tai yang channels run along the rear outer edge of the limbs, and the shao yang channels run along the midline of their outer surface (cf. Table 3-2).

Directions of the twelve channels

Specific laws govern the direction of the twelve regular channels. The three yin channels of the hands all start in the chest and run outward to the hands, where they each join a hand yang channel. The three yang channels of the hands all start from the hands and ascend to the head and face, where they each meet with the foot channel of the same yang subdivision. The three yang channels of the feet all start from the head and face and descend to the feet, linking with the three yin channels of the feet at the toes. The three yin channels of the feet start at the toes and ascend to the chest, meeting the three yin channels of the hands, to complete the cycle. Thus, all the channels are linked together, enabling qi and blood to circulate throughout the body.

Interior-exterior relationships of the twelve channels

The twelve channels have two forms of interior-exterior relationships. First, each yang channel is joined to its corresponding yin channel, "interior" being yin and "exterior" being yang. Second, each channel "connects" with the organ that stands in interior-exterior relationship with the organ to which it belongs, or "homes."

The homing and connecting relationships between the channels and organs are as follows:

Channel Relationships		
Channel	**Homing Organ**	**Connecting Organ**
hand tai yin	lung	large intestine
hand yang ming	large intestine	lung
hand jue yin	pericardium	triple burner
hand shao yang	triple burner	pericardium
hand shao yin	heart	small intestine
hand tai yang	small intestine	heart
foot tai yin	spleen	stomach
foot yang ming	stomach	spleen
foot jue yin	liver	gallbladder
foot shao yang	gallbladder	liver
foot shao yin	kidney	bladder
foot tai yang	bladder	kidney

In this way, each channel links both a bowel (exterior) and a viscera (interior), and each yang channel is connected to a yin channel, forming a twofold link between the exterior and the interior.

Exterior — Interior Linkage of Channels	
Interior Channel	**Exterior Channel**
Lung	Large Intestine
Pericardium	Triple Burner
Heart	Small Intestine
Spleen	Stomach
Liver	Gallbladder
Kidney	Bladder

Interlinkage is further enhanced by the divergent channels and the connecting channels.

The interior-exterior pairing of channels is significant in acupuncture treatment, since the points on one channel may be needled to remedy a disorder associated with the corresponding exterior or interior channel. For instance, the points on the lung channel may be used to treat disorders of the large intestine or those associated with the large intestine channel. The same significance also applies to drug treatment; for example, liver coursers and bile disinhibitors may be combined to great effect, as may spleen fortifiers and stomach harmonizers. The interior-exterior interrelationships of the channels are utilized in ear point diagnosis and in auricular acupuncture. For example, diseases of the heart are reflected in the small intestine acupoints, and pyelonephritis is reflected in the bladder acupoints.

Although the organs are all paired in interior-exterior correspondences, the closeness of the relationships varies. The relationships between the stomach and the spleen, the liver and the gallbladder, and the kidney and the bladder are closest, while the relationships between the heart and the small intestine and the lung and the large intestine are relatively less so. Although the triple burner and pericardium are linked together through the channels, they have little bearing on each other functionally.

Channel communication

The hand and foot channels of the same name are said to "communicate" with each other. These relationships are as follows:

Channel Communications	
Channel	**Communicates with**
hand tai yin lung	foot tai yin spleen
hand jue yin pericardium	foot jue yin liver
hand shao yin heart	foot shao yin kidney
hand yang ming large intestine	foot yang ming stomach
hand shao yang triple burner	foot shao yang gallbladder
hand tai yang small intestine	foot tai yang bladder

In acupuncture, a disorder of a particular organ or its associated channel can be treated by needling points on its communicating channel. For example, disorders of the large intestine may be treated by needling points on the foot yang ming stomach channel. The principle of channel communication is reflected in physiology, pathology, pattern identification, and treatment. For example, the lung and the spleen function in close cooperation in the formation of qi and blood, and the method of strengthening the spleen can be used to transform phlegm-damp in the lung. Disorders of the pericardium are invariably seen in conjunction with liver wind symptoms, and in treatment, the methods of opening the cardiac portals and extinguishing liver wind are often used together. Zhang Ji (Zhong Jing) of the Han Dynasty, who classified exogenous heat diseases according to the channels they affected (as tai yang, shao yang, yang ming, tai yin, shao yin, and jue yin disorders) wrote of the significance of the communicating channels. He points out that shao yin disorders include heart and kidney affections, and that yang ming disorders include hand and foot yang ming exuberant heat disease, constipation, diarrhea, and abdominal pain and distention caused by gastrointestinal heat-bind. He also points out that shao yang disorders include gallbladder patterns (vomiting, pain and fullness in the chest and lateral costal region), as well as combined gallbladder and triple burner patterns such as pain in the lateral costal region, deafness, visual dizziness, and headache.

Channel pathways and their pathologic signs

Hand tai yin lung channel

Pathway:

The hand tai yin lung channel starts in the region of the stomach in the middle burner and descends to connect with the large intestine. It then returns upward through the cardiac orifice, passes through the diaphragm, and homes to the lung. Continuing its ascendant path, it passes through the respiratory tract into the throat, then veers downward, following the clavicle to enter the axilla. From here it runs down the anterior aspect of the upper arm, lateral to the heart and pericardium channels, traverses the cubital fossa, and continues along the anterior aspect of the forearm to the radial styloid process of the wrist. It crosses the radial pulse, traverses the thenar eminence, and travels along the radial side of the thumb to its tip.

A ramification leaves the main pathway proximal to the wrist, passes round to the dorsum of the hand, and then runs down the inside of the index finger to its tip.

Main pathologic signs:

Symptoms associated with the external course of the channel are: fever and aversion to cold (with or without sweating), nasal congestion, headache, pain in the supraclavicular fossa, chest, shoulders, and back, and cold pain along the channel on the arm.

Symptoms associated with the internal course of the channel are: cough, wheezing, and dyspnea, rapid breathing, fullness and oppression in the chest, expectoration of phlegm-drool, dry throat, change in urine color, restlessness, spitting of blood, heat in the palms. Other possible symptoms include fullness and distention in the abdomen and thin stool diarrhea.

Hand yang ming large intestine channel

Pathway:

The hand yang ming large intestine channel begins at the radial side of the tip of the index finger and proceeds upward between the first and second metacarpal bones of the hand and between the tendons of the extensor pollicis longus and brevis muscles at the wrist. It continues along the radial margin of the forearm to the radial margin of the lateral aspect of the elbow, then up the lateral aspect of the upper arm and over the shoulder joint. After intersecting the hand tai yang channel at SI-12, it rises to just below the spinous process of the seventh cervical vertebra, and intersects with the governing vessel at GV-14, where all six yang regular channels meet. It then travels straight into the supraclavicular fossa to ST-12, from where it connects through to the lung, passes through the diaphragm, and homes to the large intestine.

A branch separates from the main channel at ST-12 in the supraclavicular fossa, passes up the neck, and traverses the cheek before entering the lower gum. From here it skirts around the lips, passes the foot yang ming channel at ST-4, and then meets the same channel coming from the other side of the body at the philtrum. It then continues around the nostril of the opposite side to terminate at the side of the nose. In other words, the right and left channels cross over at the philtrum and run for the last short stretch on the opposite side of the body from which they originated.

The *Spiritual Axis* describes yet another branch that separates from the main channel at ST-12, descends past ST-13 and penetrates the lung, passes through the diaphragm, homes to the large intestine, and descends to the lower limb to emerge at ST-37, which is the lower uniting point of the large intestine.

Main pathologic signs:

Symptoms associated with the external course of the channel are: fever, parched, dry mouth and thirst, sore throat, nosebleed, toothache, ocular rubor and pain, swelling of the neck, palpable red swelling and inhibited bending and stretching of the fingers. There may also be pain, sensation of cold, or painful and palpably hot, red swelling in the region of the shoulder and upper arm.

Symptoms associated with the internal course of the channel are: lower abdominal pain, migratory abdominal pain, borborygmi, thin stool, and excretion of thick, slimy yellow matter. There may also be rapid breathing and dyspnea.

Foot yang ming stomach channel

Pathway:

The foot yang ming stomach channel starts at the side of the nose, and then ascends to the inner canthus of the eye to intersect the foot tai yang bladder channel at BL-1. It then descends parallel to the nose, penetrates the maxilla into the upper gum and joins the governing vessel at GV-24 in the philtrum. It skirts back along the upper and lower lips to join the conception vessel at CV-24 in the mentolabial groove on the chin. From this point, it runs along the mandible to the point ST-5 and rounds the angle of the mandible to ST-6. It proceeds upward in front of the ear, intersects with the foot shao yang gallbladder channel at GB-3, and continues along the hairline, intersecting the foot shao yang channel again at GB-6, from where it crosses to the middle of the forehead to intersect with the governing vessel at GV-24.

A branch separates at ST-5, runs down the throat to the point ST-9, and then continues down to in the supraclavicular fossa. From here it crosses through to the back to intersect the governing vessel at GV-14, and then descends internally, crossing the diaphragm and intersecting with the conception vessel internally at CV-13 and CV-12 before homing to the stomach and connecting with the spleen.

Another branch separates at ST-12, runs down the surface of the trunk along the mammillary line, and continues downward, passing beside the umbilicus to enter the qi thoroughfare (the inguinal region) at ST-30.

Yet another branch starts in the area of the pylorus, descending internally to join the branch just described at ST-30 in the inguinal region. It emerges here and runs down to ST-31 on the anterior aspect of the thigh. It travels down the thigh to the high point above the knee at ST-32, and on down to the patella, then proceeds downward along the lateral side of the tibia to ST-42 on the dorsum of the foot, finally terminating at the lateral side of the tip of the second toe.

A branch separates at ST-36, three body-inches below the knee, and runs down lateral and parallel to the main branch, terminating on the lateral side of the middle toe.

Still another branch breaks off from the main branch on the dorsum of the foot at ST-42, terminating on the medial side of the great toe, where it connects with the spleen channel at SP-1.

Main pathologic signs:

Symptoms along the external course of the channel are: high fever or malaria, flushed face, sweating, clouding of the spirit and delirium, manic agitation, and aversion to cold; pain in the eyes, dry nose and nosebleed, lesions of the lips and in the mouth, sore larynx, swelling in the neck; wry mouth; chest pain; cold or pain, redness, and swelling in the lower limbs.

Symptoms along the internal course of the channel are: pronounced abdominal distention, fullness, and edema; restlessness and discomfort while active or recumbent; or mania and withdrawal. There may also be hyperpepsia and rapid hungering, and yellow urine.

Foot tai yin spleen channel

Pathway:

The foot tai yin spleen channel starts on the medial tip of the great toe and runs up the medial aspect of the foot along the border of the light and dark skin. It then passes in front of the medial malleolus and up the posterior side of the leg along the posterior margin of the tibia. Here it crosses and runs anterior to the foot jue yin liver channel, passing medial to the knee and running up the anteromedial aspect of the thigh. It penetrates the abdomen and intersects with the conception vessel at CV-3 and CV-4 before homing to the spleen and connecting with the stomach. It continues upward, passes through the diaphragm to intersect with the foot shao yang gallbladder channel at GB-24 and the foot jue yin liver channel at LV-14, ascends to the side of the esophagus, crosses the hand tai yin lung channel at LU-1, and finally proceeds up to the root of the tongue to disperse over its lower surface.

A branch breaks off in the area of the stomach, crossing the diaphragm to transport qi to the heart.

Main pathologic signs:

Symptoms associated with the exterior course of the channel are: heaviness in the head or body, fatigue and weakness of the limbs, and general fever; pain in the posterior mandibular region and the lower cheek, and motor impairment of the tongue; wasting and atony of the muscles of the limbs; cold along the inside of the thigh and knee, or edematous swelling of the legs and feet.

Symptoms associated with the internal course of the channel are: ventral pain and thin diarrhea or stool containing undigested food, borborygmi, retching and nausea, abdominal lump glomus, reduced food intake, jaundice, and inhibited urination.

Hand shao yin heart channel

Pathway:

The hand shao yin heart channel starts in the heart, emerging through the blood vessels surrounding this organ. Traveling downward, it passes through the diaphragm to connect to the small intestine.

Another branch separates from the heart, traveling upward along the side of the esophagus to meet the tissues surrounding the eye.

A further channel separates from the heart and travels directly up into the lung, and then veers downwards to emerge below the axilla. It travels down the medial aspect of the upper arm, medial to the hand tai yin lung and hand jue yin pericardium channels, and passes over the antecubital fossa. It continues down the anteromedial margin of the forearm to the capitate bone on the wrist, travelling along the radial side of the fifth metacarpal bone to terminate at the tip of the little finger.

Main pathologic signs:

Symptoms associated with the external course of the channel are: general fever, headache, pain in the eyes, pain in the chest and back muscles, dry throat, thirst with the urge to drink, and hot or painful palms; inversion frigidity of the limbs; or pain in the scapular region and/or the medial aspect of the forearm.

Symptoms associated with the internal course of the channel are: cardialgia, fullness and pain in the chest and lateral costal region, pain in the hypochondriac region; restlessness; rapid breathing, discomfort when recumbent, dizziness with fainting spells; and essence-spirit disorders.

Hand tai yang small intestine channel

Pathway:

The hand tai yang small intestine channel starts on the outside edge of the little finger tip, and travels along the ulnar side of the hand to the wrist, emerging at the ulnar styloid process. Continuing up the posterior aspect of the ulna, it passes between the olecranon of the ulna and the medial epicondyle of the humerus on the medial side of the elbow. It then runs on up the posteromedial side of the upper arm, emerging behind the shoulder joint and circling around the superior and inferior fossae of the scapula. At the top of the shoulder it intersects the foot tai yang bladder channel at BL-36 and BL-11, connecting with the governing vessel at GV-14 before turning downward into the supraclavicular fossa. Here it submerges at ST-12, connects with the heart, and follows the esophagus down through the diaphragm to the stomach. It then intersects with the conception vessel internally at CV-13 and CV-12 before homing to the small intestine.

A branch separates from the channel at ST-12 and runs up the neck to the cheek. It then travels to the outer canthus of the eye where it meets the foot shao yang gallbladder channel at GB-1, and then turns back across the temple to enter the ear at SI-1.

Another branch breaks off from the former on the mandible, rises to the infraorbital region, and continues to the inner canthus where it meets the foot tai yang bladder channel at BL-1, then crosses horizontally to the zygomatic region.

The *Spiritual Axis* claims that another branch descends internally from the small intestine to emerge at SI-9, the lower uniting point of the small intestine.

Main pathologic signs:

Symptoms associated with the external course of the channel are: erosion of the glossal and oral mucosa, pain in the cheeks, sore pharynx, lachrymation, stiffness of the neck, pain on the lateral aspect of the shoulder and upper arm.

Symptoms associated with the internal course of the channel are: lower abdominal pain and distention with the pain stretching around to the lumbar region; lower abdominal pain radiating into the testicles; diarrhea; pain in the stomach with dry feces, and constipation.

Foot tai yang bladder channel

Pathway:

The foot tai yang bladder channel starts at the inner canthus of the eye, travels upwards over the forehead, intersecting the governing vessel at GV-24 and the leg shao yin gallbladder channel at GB-15. It travels on up to the vertex and again meets the governing vessel at GV-20.

A branch separates at the vertex and goes down to the area just above the ear, meeting the foot shao yang gallbladder channel at GB-7, GB-8, GB-10, GB-11, and GB-12.

A vertical branch enters the brain from the vertex to meet the governing vessel at GV-17, and reemerges to run down the nape of the neck and the muscles of the medial aspect of the scapula, meeting the governing vessel again at GV-14 and GV-13. It continues downward, parallel to the spine, to the lumbar region. Here, the channel submerges, following the paravertebral muscles, and connects with the kidney before homing to the bladder.

A branch separates in the lumbar region and runs down the buttocks and the posterior midline of the thighs to the popliteal fossa behind the knee.

A further branch separates from the main channel at the nape of the neck, descending lateral to the paravertebral branch mentioned above along the medial border of the scapula and down to the gluteal region, where it crosses the buttocks and intersects with the gallbladder channel at GB-30. It then passes down the posterolateral aspect of the thigh to meet the other branch of the same channel in the popliteal fossa. The channel continues downward through the gastrocnemius muscle, emerges posterior to the lateral malleolus, and then runs along the lateral margin of the fifth metatarsal bone, crossing its tuberosity, to the lateral tip of the little toe at BL-67.

Main pathologic signs:

Symptoms associated with the exterior course of the channel are: chills and fever, headache, stiff neck, pain in the lumbar region and along the spine, nasal congestion, ocular pain and lachrymation; pain in the posterior thigh, popliteal region, gastrocnemius, and foot.

Symptoms associated with the internal course of the channel are: pain and distention in the lower abdomen, inhibited micturition, urinary block and enuresis; mental disorders; and opisthotonos.

Foot shao yin kidney channel

Pathway:

The foot shao yin kidney channel starts on the underside of the little toe, crosses the sole of the foot obliquely to emerge out of the arch of the foot under the navicular tuberosity at KI-2. It then proceeds posterior to the medial malleolus and continues into the heel. From here, it travels up the rear medial aspect of the lower leg to intersect with the foot tai yin spleen channel at SP-6. Traveling up through the gastrocnemius muscle, it ascends across the medial aspect of the popliteal fossa and the posteromedial aspect of the thigh to the base of the spine, where it meets the governing vessel at GV-1. It continues up the interior of the spinal column to home to the kidney, after which it turns downwards to connect with the bladder and intersect with the conception vessel at CV-4 and CV-3.

A branch ascends from the kidney, goes directly to the liver, crosses the diaphragm, enters the lung, and follows the throat up to the root of the tongue.

A further branch separates in the lung, links through to the heart and disperses in the chest.

Main pathologic signs:

Symptoms associated with the external course of the channel are: low back pain, counterflow frigidity of the legs, atony of the legs, dry mouth, sore pharynx, and pain in the lateral gluteal region and in the posterior aspect of the thigh; there may also be pain in the soles of the feet.

Symptoms associated with the internal course of the channel are: dizziness, facial edema, bleary eyes, ashen complexion, shortness of breath, short rapid breathing, somnolence or restlessness, enduring diarrhea, thin stool, or dry stool evacuated with difficulty; there may also be abdominal distention, nausea and vomiting, or impotence.

Foot jue yin pericardium channel

Pathway:

The foot jue yin pericardium channel starts in the chest, where it homes to the pericardium. Descending through the diaphragm into the abdomen, it connects successively to the upper, middle, and lower burners.

A branch runs out horizontally from the center of the chest, emerges at the flank three body-inches below the anterior axillary fold, and then skirts around the axilla to the upper arm. It runs down the medial midline of the upper arm between the hand tai yin lung channel and the hand shao yin heart channel, crosses the center of the cubital fossa and then proceeds down the forearm between the tendons of the palmaris longus and flexor carpi radialis muscles. It travels through the palm and along the ulnar aspect of the middle finger until it reaches the tip.

Another branch separates in the palm and proceeds along the lateral aspect of the fourth finger to its tip.

Main pathologic signs:

Symptoms associated with the external course of the channel are: stiffness of the neck, spasm in the limbs, red facial complexion, pain in the eyes, subaxillary swelling, hypertonicity of the elbow and arm inhibiting movement, and hot palms.

Symptoms associated with the internal course of the channel are: delirious speech, clouding inversion, restlessness, fullness and oppression in the chest and lateral costal region, aphasia, palpitations, cardialgia, constant laughter and other essence-spirit disorders.

Hand shao yang triple burner channel

Pathway:

The hand shao yang triple burner channel starts at the ulnar side of the tip of the fourth finger and travels up between the fourth and fifth metacarpal bones on the dorsum of the hand to the outside of the wrist. Proceeding up the posterior midline of the forearm between the radius and the ulna, it runs over the olecranon process of the elbow, and then travels up the posterior midline of the upper arm to the shoulder. Here it meets the hand tai yang small intestine channel at SI-12 and then runs over to the back to meet the governing vessel at GV-14. It crosses back over the shoulder to intersect the foot shao yang gallbladder channel at GB-21 before running into the supraclavicular fossa, penetrating internally at ST-12 and traveling into the mid-chest region to meet the conception vessel at CV-17, where it links with the pericardium. It then descends internally, homing through each of the three burners successively.

A branch breaks off from the mid-chest region at CV-17, rises to emerge in the supraclavicular fossa, then runs up the neck and behind the ear to intersect with the foot shao yang gallbladder channel at GB-6 and GB-14 on the forehead, before winding down around the cheek to return to the infraorbital region where it meets the hand tai yang small intestine channel at SI-18.

Another branch separates behind the ear, enters the ear to reemerge in front of it, and intersects with the hand tai yang small intestine channel at SI-19. It then crosses in front of the foot shao yang gallbladder channel at GB-3 and runs along the zygoma to terminate at the outer canthus at TB-23.

The *Spiritual Axis* adds that an internal branch descends from the triple burner to emerge at its lower uniting point, BL-53.

Main pathologic signs:

Symptoms associated with the external course of the channel are: sore throat, pain in the cheeks, ocular rubor and pain, deafness; pain behind the ears and on the posterior aspect of the shoulder and upper arm.

Symptoms associated with the internal course of the channel are: abdominal distention and fullness, or hardness and fullness in the lower abdomen; urinary frequency and distress, vacuity edema of the skin, water swelling, and enuresis.

Foot shao yang gallbladder channel

Pathway:

The foot shao yang gallbladder channel starts from the outer canthus of the eye, traverses the temple to TB-22, then rises to the corner of the forehead where it intersects with the foot yang ming stomach channel at ST-8. Descending behind the ear, it passes down the neck in front of the hand shao yang triple burner channel and meets the hand tai yang small intestine channel at SI-17. After reaching the shoulder it turns back and runs behind the triple burner channel to intersect the governing vessel at GV-14. It then moves parallel with the shoulderline outwards to intersect with the hand tai yang small intestine channel at SI-12, before crossing over to ST-12 in the supraclavicular fossa.

A branch separates from the main channel behind the ear, and passes the hand shao yang triple burner channel at TB-17 before entering the ear. It emerges in front of the ear, meeting SI-19 on the hand tai yang small intestine channel and ST-7 on the foot yang ming stomach channel before terminating at the outer canthus of the eye.

Another branch separates from the outer canthus and runs downwards to ST-5 on the mandible. Turning upwards, it crosses the hand shao yang triple burner channel and ascends to the infraorbital region before travelling down the cheek into the neck where it joins the main channel again at ST-12 in the supraclavicular fossa. From here it submerges in the chest, meets PC-1 of the hand jue yin pericardium channel, and passes through the diaphragm before connecting with the liver and homing to the gallbladder. It then follows the inside of the false ribs to emerge in the qi thoroughfare in the inguinal region, where it skirts round the genitals and submerges into the hip at GB-30.

Yet another branch separates from the main channel at the supraclavicular fossa at ST-12, descending into the axilla and running down the lateral aspect of the thorax. It intersects the foot jue yin liver channel at LV-13 before turning back to the sacral region to cross the foot tai yang bladder channel at BL-31 and BL-34. From here it passes laterally over to GB-30 on the hip joint, descending down the lateral aspect of the thigh and knee, and passing along the anterior aspect of the fibula to its lower extremity. It crosses in front of the lateral malleolus, and runs over the dorsum of the foot, travelling between the fourth and fifth metatarsal bones before terminating at the lateral side of the tip of the fourth toe at GB-44.

Another branch separates on the dorsum of the foot at GB-41 and runs between the first and second metatarsal bones to the end of the great toe, crossing under the toenail to join with the foot jue yin liver channel at LV-1.

Main pathologic signs:

Symptoms associated with the external course of the channel are: alternating fever and chills, headache, malaria, ashen complexion, ocular pain, pain under the chin, subaxillary swelling, scrofulous swellings, deafness, and pain in the lateral aspect of the buttocks and in the thigh, knee and fibula.

Symptoms associated with the internal course of the channel are: pain in the lateral costal area, vomiting, bitter taste in the mouth, and pain in the chest.

Foot jue yin liver channel

Pathway:

The foot jue yin liver channel starts on the dorsum of the great toe and runs up the foot between the first and second metatarsal bones to a point one body-inch in front of the medial malleolus. It then proceeds upward to SP-6, where it intersects with the foot tai yin spleen channel. Continuing on up the medial aspect of the leg, it recrosses the foot tai yin spleen channel eight body-inches above the medial malleolus, thereafter running posterior to that channel over the knee and thigh. Once again it crosses the foot tai yin spleen channel at SP-12 and SP-13, and then skirts around the genitals and penetrates the lower abdomen where it meets the conception vessel at CV-2, CV-3, and CV-4. It ascends, moving toward the lateral aspect of the trunk to home to the liver and connect with the gallbladder. Continuing its upward course through the diaphragm and the lateral costal region, it runs up to the neck posterior to the pharynx, enters the nasopharynx, and meets the tissues surrounding the eyes. The channel finally runs up the forehead to meet the governing vessel at the vertex.

A branch breaks off below the eye and runs through the cheeks to contour the inside of the lips.

Another branch separates from the liver, passes through the diaphragm, and enters the lung.

Main pathologic signs:

Symptoms associated with the external course of the channel are: headache, dizziness, blurred vision, tinnitus, fever, spasm of the limbs.

Symptoms associated with the internal course of the channel are: fullness, distention and pain in the costal region with lump glomus, fullness and oppression in the chest and venter, abdominal pain, vomiting, jaundice, swill diarrhea, lower abdominal pain, shan qi, enuresis, urinary block, or yellow urine.

The Eight Irregular Channels

The eight irregular channels are the governing vessel, the conception vessel, the penetrating vessel, the girdling vessel, the yin linking vessel, the yang linking vessel, the yin motility vessel, and the yang motility vessel. They are thus named because they do not fit the pattern of the other major channels: they have neither a continuous, interlinking pattern of circulation, nor are they each associated with a specific major organ. Rather, they serve as compensating reservoirs, filling and emptying in response to the varying conditions of the major channels and exerting a regulating effect on them; hence the appellation as "vessels."

The functions of the eight irregular channels are as follows:

> They provide additional interconnections among the twelve regular channels.
>
> They regulate the flow of qi and blood in the twelve regular channels. Surplus blood and qi is taken up from the twelve regular channels, and is released when qi and blood in the regular channels is vacuous.
>
> They are closely related to the liver, the kidney, and some of the minor organs. "The eight irregular channels serve the liver and the kidney."

They are directly related to the womb, the brain, and other anatomic structures discussed below.

The governing vessel

Pathway:

The governing vessel has four courses. According to the *Spiritual Axis,* the main course of this channel originates in the pelvic cavity. Emerging in the perineum at CV-1, it then passes posteriorly to GV-1 at the tip of the coccyx. From this point, it ascends along the spine to GV-16 in the nape of the neck. It enters the brain and ascends to the vertex, emerging at GV-20, continuing forward along the midline to the forehead, running down the nose and across the philtrum to terminate in the upper gum.

The second channel starts in the lower abdomen, and runs down through the genitals into the perineal region. From here it passes through the tip of the coccyx, where it diverts into the gluteal region. Here it intersects both the leg shao yin kidney channel and the leg tai yang bladder channel before returning to the spinal column. It then travels up the spine and links through to the kidney.

A third path starts at the same two bilateral points as the foot tai yang bladder channel at the inner canthi of the eyes. The branches rise up over the forehead to meet at the vertex. The channel then enters the brain and splits into two channels that descend along opposite sides of the spine to the waist, to join with the kidney.

The fourth path starts in the lower abdomen, travels up past the navel, continues upward to join with the heart, then enters the throat, crosses the cheek, splits into two and rounds the lips, and runs up the cheek to the center of the infraorbital region.

Basic functions:

The governing vessel is the sea of the yang channels. All six yang channels converge at the point GV-14. The governing vessel has a regulating effect on the yang channels, so it is said that it governs all the yang channels of the body.

The governing vessel homes to the brain and connects to the kidney. The kidney engenders marrow, and the brain is known as the "sea of marrow." Therefore, the governing vessel reflects the physiology and pathology of the brain and the spinal fluid, and their relationship with the reproductive organs.

Main pathologic signs:

Opisthotonos, malaria, pain and stiffness in the back, child fright-wind, heavy sensation in the head, hemorrhoids, sterility, essence-spirit disorders.

The conception vessel

Pathway:

The conception vessel originates in the pelvic cavity, connects with the internal genitourinary organs, and emerges in the perineum at CV-1. It ascends through the region of the pubic hair and then runs up the midline of the abdomen, chest, and neck to the mentolabial groove beneath the lower lip. Here it splits into two branches that contour the mouth and ascend to the infraorbital region.

A second course arises in the pelvic cavity, enters the spine and ascends up the back.

Basic functions:

The conception vessel is the sea of the yin channels. The three yin channels of the foot all join the conception vessel, allowing their bilateral courses to communicate. In this way, the conception vessel has a regulating effect on the yin channels, for which reason it is said that it regulates all the yin channels of the body.

The conception vessel regulates menstruation and nurtures the fetus. Thus it is said, "The conception vessel governs the fetus."

Main pathologic signs:

Menstrual irregularities, menstrual block, white vaginal discharge, miscarriage, sterility, shan qi, enuresis, and abdominal masses.

Penetrating vessel

Pathway:

The penetrating vessel has a total of five paths. The first path starts in the lower abdomen and emerges in the qi thoroughfare, traveling up with the foot shao yin kidney channel and passing the navel to the chest area, where it disperses in the intercostal spaces.

The second path begins where the channel disperses in the chest. It runs up the throat and face, running around the lips and terminating in the nasal cavity.

The third path emerges from the qi thoroughfare in the lower abdomen at KI-11, then descends along the medial aspect of the thigh to the popliteal fossa. Continuing down along the medial margin of the tibia, it passes behind the medial malleolus before dispersing in the sole of the foot.

The fourth branch diverges from ST-30 and descends obliquely down the lower extremity to the medial malleolus. It enters the heel, crosses the tarsal bones of the foot and finally reaches the great toe.

The fifth channel separates from the main course in the pelvic cavity and runs to the spine, which it then ascends.

Basic functions:

The penetrating vessel is the sea of the major channels. It has a regulating effect on all twelve regular channels, and its main function is to regulate menstruation, for which reason it is also said, "The penetrating vessel is the sea of blood."

Main pathologic signs:

In women: gynecologic disorders, including metrorrhagia, miscarriage, menstrual block, irregular menses, scant breast milk, lower abdominal pain; and hematemesis. In men: prostatitis, urethritis, orchitis, seminal emission, impotence.

Girdling vessel

Pathway:

Starting below the lateral tip of the tenth rib, this channel encircles the trunk like a belt, dipping down into the lower abdominal region anteriorly, and running across the lumbar region posteriorly. It intersects with three points on the foot shao yang gallbladder channel, GB-26, GB-27, and GB-28.

Basic functions:

This channel serves to bind up all the channels running up and down the trunk, thus regulating the balance between upward and downward flow of qi in the body.

Main pathologic signs:

(White) vaginal discharge, prolapse of the uterus, fullness and distention in the abdomen, limpness of the lumbar region.

Yin and yang motility vessels

Pathways:

The yin motility vessel originates at KI-6 below the medial malleolus, runs up the medial aspect of the leg, penetrates the genital region and then continues internally up the abdomen and chest to emerge in the supraclavicular fossa at ST-12. It proceeds up the throat, passing in front of ST-9, then continues up the medial aspect of the cheek to the inner canthus, where it joins the foot tai yang bladder and yang motility channels to ascend over the head and enter the brain.

The yang motility vessel starts below the lateral malleolus at BL-62 and runs up the lateral aspect of the trunk, gradually curving around posteriorly to the lateral aspect of the shoulder. It crosses over the shoulder to the front of the body, then runs up the neck, over the jaw, past the corners of the mouth to the inner canthus of the eye. From here it joins with the yin motility vessel and the foot tai yang bladder channel to run up the forehead and over the lateral aspect of the head to GB-20 posterior to the mastoid process, before entering the brain at GV-16.

Basic functions:

The main physiologic functions of both the yin and yang motility channels are to control the opening and closing of the eyes, control the ascent of fluids and the descent of qi, and to regulate muscular activity in general.

Main pathologic signs:

Yang motility vessel: eye diseases, dry and itching eyes, insomnia, lack of agility, pain in the lumbar region, and spasm along the lateral aspect of the lower extremity, with corresponding flaccidity along its medial aspect.

Yin motility vessel: eye diseases, heavy sensation of the eyelids or inability to open the eyes, hypersomnia, watery eyes, lower abdominal pain, pain along the waist extending into the genitals, hernia, leukorrhagia, tightness and spasms along the medial aspect of the lower limb, with corresponding flaccidity along its lateral aspect.

Regarding these latter symptoms, the "Twenty-Ninth Perplexity" of the *Canon of Perplexities* states, "When the yin motility vessel is diseased, the yang vessel is relaxed and the yin vessel is tense; when the yang motility vessel is diseased, the yin vessel is relaxed and the yang vessel is tense."

Yin and yang linking vessels

Pathways:

The yin linking vessel starts at the point KI-9 of the foot shao yin kidney channel, then runs up the medial aspect of the leg, and up the abdomen and across the chest to the throat, where it meets the conception vessel. Along its course, it intersects the foot tai yin spleen channel at SP-12, SP-13, SP-15, and SP-16. It intersects the foot jue yin liver channel at LV-14, and the conception vessel at CV-22 and CV-23.

The yang linking vessel starts below the lateral malleolus at the point BL-63 of the foot tai yang bladder channel, and runs up the leg along the path of the foot shao yang gallbladder channel. It proceeds up the posterolateral aspect of the trunk, running past the axilla, behind the shoulder, ascending the neck and crossing behind the ear to the forehead. After doubling back over the top of the head, it ends at GV-16 at the nape of the neck. Along its course, it intersects the foot shao yang gallbladder channel at GB-39, GB-21, GB-20, GB-19, GB-18, GB-17, GB-16, GB-15, GB-14, and GB-13. It intersects the hand shao yang triple burner channel at TB-15, the hand tai yang small intestine channel at SI-10, the governing vessel at GV-15 and GV-16, and the foot yang ming stomach channel at ST-8.

Basic functions:

The yin linking vessel serves to connect the flows of the yin major channels, reinforcing and balancing their respective flows, and generally regulating their activity.

The yang linking vessel serves to unite all the yang major channels, strengthening their respective flows, compensating for superabundance or insufficiency in channel circulation, and generally regulating yang channel activity.

Main pathologic signs:

Yin linking vessel: cardialgia, circulatory problems, pain in the center of the chest, and emotional disorders such as timidity and fear, apprehension, nervous laughter, delirium, nightmares, and emotional depression.

Yang linking vessel: chills and fever, dizziness, muscular fatigue, stiffness, and pain; arthritis and articular pain; lateral headache; pain and distention in the waist.

Channel Distribution

There are channels passing through all parts of the body. The physiologic functions and pathologic changes of each part of the body have specific relationships to the channels and organs with which they are associated.

The head

"The head is the confluence of yang." This phrase refers to the fact that all the yang channels of the body pass through the head: the governing vessel, the three yang channels of the hand, and the three yang channels of the foot. The governing vessel ascends the nape of the neck and the back of the head to pass over the vertex. The foot tai yang bladder channel runs parallel to the governing vessel on either side. The foot yang ming stomach channel passes over the temple, in front of the ear, and around the mandible, then circles the lips, passes through the upper gum, and passes along the side of the nose. The foot shao yang gallbladder channel runs over the temporal bone, passes through and around the ear and extends to the outer canthus of the eye. The hand tai yang small intestine channel passes the posterior margin of the mandible, in front of and through the ear, the cheek, and both the inner and outer canthi of the eye. The hand yang ming large intestine channel passes through the lower gum, the lips, the nostrils, and the nasal alae. The hand shao yang triple burner channel passes through and around the ear and over the cheek.

Most of the yin channels also pass through the head, usually at a deeper level. The foot jue yin liver channel travels through the area of the nose and throat, extends into the tissues surrounding the eye, travels around the inside of the lips, and reaches the vertex. The foot tai yin spleen channel rises as far as the root of the tongue, dispersing over its inferior surface. The foot shao yin kidney channel reaches both sides of the root of the tongue. The hand shao yin heart channel links through to the eyes. The conception vessel travels over the face to the infraorbital region.

The yin and yang motility channels converge at the inner canthus of the eye, and the yang linking channel runs from the forehead over the head to the nape of the neck. Although the other channels do not reach the head directly, they nevertheless have an indirect relationship with the head and face. For this reason, the Tang Dynasty physician Sun Si-Mo stated, "The three hundred sixty-five connecting channels all rise to the head."

The vertex

The left and right foot tai yang bladder channels join at the vertex; the governing vessel, running over the midline, passes over the vertex; the foot jue yin liver channel and the governing vessel meet at the vertex; the divergent channels of the hand shao yang triple burner channel and the foot shao yang gallbladder channel pass through the vertex.

The brain

The governing vessel homes to the brain; the foot tai yang bladder channel connects with the brain; the divergent channel of the foot yang ming stomach channel passes through the eyes and enters the brain.

The eyes

The liver opens at the eyes, and the channels that join at the eyes are the divergent channels of the foot jue yin liver channel, the hand shao yin heart channel, the foot yang ming stomach channel, and the foot shao yang gallbladder channel. Reaching the area surrounding the eyes are the yin and yang motility vessels, the foot tai yang bladder channel, the foot shao yang gallbladder channel, the hand tai yang small intestine channel, and the hand shao yang triple burner channel, as well as the conception vessel.

The ear

The kidney opens at the ear, and the channels reaching the surrounding area of the ear or entering the ear itself are the foot tai yang bladder channel (at the apex of the ear) and the foot yang ming stomach channel (anterior to the ear). There is also a divergent channel of the hand yang ming large intestine channel; and the divergent channels of the six yin channels all link with the ear. Thus, "the ear is the area of confluence of the main channels" and "the twelve regular channels all connect with the ear." This helps to explain the significance of ear acupuncture.

The nose

The lung opens at the nose, and the channels that reach the nose and its surrounding region are the hand yang ming large intestine channel, the foot yang ming stomach channel, and the hand tai yang small intestine channel. The foot jue yin liver channel reaches the nasopharyngial cavity.

The lips

"The spleen opens at the mouth, and its health is reflected in the condition of the lips." Of the irregular channels, the governing and penetrating vessels both skirt around the lips, the conception vessel reaches the lower lip, and the yang motility vessel runs up through the corners of the mouth. Of the regular channels, the foot yang ming stomach channel and the hand yang ming large intestine channel both encircle the lips, and the foot jue yin liver channel flows through the inner lips.

The tongue

The heart opens at the tongue, and the channels that pass through the tongue region are the divergent channel of the foot shao yin kidney channel, the foot tai yin spleen channel, and the hand shao yin heart channel.

The teeth

The hand yang ming large intestine channel spreads through the lower teeth, and the foot yang ming stomach channel enters the upper teeth.

The eyes, ears, nose, lips, tongue, and other sense organs are not only the external portals of the five solid organs, but are also intimately related with the channels. The *Spiritual Axis* states:

> The blood and qi of the twelve regular channels and the three hundred sixty-five connecting channels rise to the face and the portals. The pure yang qi rises to the eyes, giving sight. . . . Qi goes into the ears, giving the power of hearing, and ancestral qi rises into the nose, bestowing the sense of smell. The turbid qi rises from the stomach and goes to the lips and tongue giving the sense of taste, and the fluid of their qi rises to nourish the face.

Clinical practice in facial, nasal, and auricular acupuncture over recent years has verified many of these theories.

The neck

The governing vessel runs along the midline of the nape of the neck, while the conception vessel runs along the midline of the throat. The six yang channels also pass through the neck region. The foot yang ming stomach channel runs up the front of the neck through the region of the common carotid artery; the hand yang ming large intestine channel passes over the lateral anterior aspect of the neck roughly at the point of the external maxillary artery. The hand tai yang small intestine channel runs up the side of the neck on a line parallel to the angle of the mandible. These three channels all run in front of the ear. Running behind the ear are the hand shao yang triple burner channel, which travels up the mastoid bone along a line roughly parallel to the edge of the lobe and the helix, and the foot shao yang gallbladder channel, which travels along the edge of the mastoid process. The gallbladder and triple burner channels meet at the neck, and the foot tai yang bladder channel runs down the nape of the neck, roughly along the outer margin of the trapezius muscle.

A number of channels pass through the throat. The conception and penetrating channels meet in the throat, the foot yang ming stomach channel and the foot shao yin kidney channel both run through the throat; the foot jue yin liver channel runs up the back of the throat to the nasopharyngeal cavity. The hand shao yin heart channel and the foot tai yin spleen channels both run up the trachea to the pharynx; and the divergent channels of the hand tai yin lung channel, the hand yang ming large intestine channel, and the foot jue yin pericardium channel all pass through the throat region.

The trunk

All the channels running through the anterior aspect of the trunk, with the exception of the foot yang ming stomach channel, are yin channels. All the channels running through the back, with the exception of an internal branch of the foot shao yin kidney channel, are yang channels.

Anterior aspect

The conception vessel runs up the midline of the abdomen and chest; the foot shao yin kidney channel runs parallel to it at a distance of one-half body-inch on either side. At two body-inches from the midline (roughly bisecting the supraclavicular fossa) is the foot yang ming stomach channel, and at a further distance of a two body-inches is the foot tai yin spleen channel.

Posterior aspect

The governing vessel runs up the midline of the back, with its collateral connecting channels and the foot tai yang bladder channel running closely parallel at both sides. In the lumbar region there is also an internal branch of the foot shao yin kidney channel.

The lateral aspects

The foot shao yang gallbladder channel and the foot jue yin liver channel run along the sides of the trunk, and the foot tai yin spleen channel's main connecting channels run through the lateral costal region.

The genitals

Running through the external reproductive organs and directly related to the internal reproductive organs are the penetrating vessel, the conception vessel, the governing vessel, the foot jue yin liver channel, the foot shao yang gallbladder channel, and the yin motility channel.

The major organs

The lung

The hand tai yin lung channel homes to the lung, and the hand yang ming large intestine channel connects with the lung. The hand shao yin heart channel rises to the lung, the foot shao yin kidney channel enters the lung, and the foot jue yin liver channel flows upward into the lung.

The spleen

The foot tai yin spleen channel homes to the spleen and the foot yang ming stomach channel connects with the spleen.

The heart

The hand shao yin heart channel starts in the heart, and the hand tai yang small intestine channel connects with the heart. The foot tai yin spleen channel flows into the heart, the foot shao yin kidney channel connects with the heart, and a branch of the governing vessel passes through the heart. Apart from this, the divergent channels of the foot tai yang bladder channel, the foot shao yang gallbladder channel, and the foot yang ming stomach channel, as well as the connecting channels of the hand jue yin pericardium channel, are all linked to the heart.

The kidney

The foot shao yang kidney channel homes to the kidney, and the foot tai yang bladder channel connects with the kidney. The governing and conception vessels also connect with the kidney.

The liver

The foot jue yin liver channel homes to the liver, and the foot shao yang gallbladder channel connects with it as well. The foot shao yin kidney channel also connects with the liver.

The stomach

The foot yang ming stomach channel homes to the stomach, and the foot tai yin spleen channel connects with it. The foot jue yin liver channel passes around the outside of the stomach and the hand tai yin lung channel passes through the cardiac orifice. The hand yang ming large intestine channel and the hand tai yang small intestine channel both connect with the stomach.

These are the most important channel connections with the major organs.

Table 3-1

Channel Distribution — Body	
Hand Channels	
Yin	*Yang*
hand tai yin lung	hand yang ming large intestine
hand jue yin pericardium	hand shao yang triple burner
hand shao yin heart	hand tai yang small intestine
Foot Channels	
Yin	*Yang*
foot tai yin spleen	foot yang ming stomach
foot jue yin liver	foot shao yang gallbladder
foot shao yin kidney	foot tai yang bladder

Table 3-2

Channel Distribution — Limbs		
Upper Limb	**Yin Channels**	**Yang Channels**
	Inner Face	Outer Face
	Hand Channels	
Front	hand tai yin lung	hand yang ming large intestine
Midline	hand jue yin pericardium	hand shao yang triple burner
Rear	hand shao yin heart	hand tai yang small intestine
Lower Limb	**Yin Channels**	**Yang Channels**
	Inner Face	Outer Face
	Foot Channels	
Front	foot tai yin spleen	foot yang ming stomach
Midline	foot jue yin liver	foot shao yang gallbladder
Rear	foot shao yin kidney	foot tai yang bladder

Chapter 4
The Organs

The Visceral Manifestation Theory

All knowledge concerning the organs is embodied in visceral manifestation theory, which includes not only their anatomy, physiology, and pathology, but also the identification of organic disease patterns and their treatment. The heart, lung, spleen, liver, and kidney are the five viscera. The stomach, small intestine, large intestine, gallbladder, and triple burner are the bowels. These are referred to collectively as the major organs. In addition, there are the curious organs: the brain, bones, marrow, blood vessels, and the womb. The gallbladder is considered both a bowel and a curious organ. Since all other parts of the body are seen as being subordinate to, or governed by, the viscera, the major organs as a whole can be said to govern all physiologic activity. Thus, the major organs represent not only their morphologic counterparts in Western medicine, but also spheres of influence jointly governing the whole body. The broad scope of visceral manifestation theory makes it of paramount significance in clinical practice.

In view of their preeminent position in physiology, the major organs are often simply referred to as "the organs." The term minor organs denotes all organs that do not fall in this category.

This chapter outlines the physiologic functions of the organs together with the various morbid changes they may undergo. The identification of organ patterns and their treatment are discussed in Chapter 9. Before discussing the individual characteristics and functions of each organ, some introductory remarks concerning visceral manifestation theory are pertinent.

Holistic approach

Visceral manifestation theory does not confine itself to discussing the functional characteristics of each organ in isolation; rather, it places considerable emphasis on relationship to the other organs. Taking the spleen and stomach as an example, visceral manifestation theory states that the spleen governs movement and transformation, while the stomach governs ingestion; and spleen qi governs upbearing while stomach qi governs downbearing. Here, emphasis is given to splenic governance of movement and transformation and gastric governance of ingestion as two mutually indispensable facets of the digestion process, and upbearing and downbearing as mutually counterbalancing and complementary movements. According to visceral manifestation theory, the various tissues of the body such as the hair, skin, muscles, blood vessels, sinews, and bones, as well as the minor organs such as the eyes, ears, nose, mouth, tongue, anus, and genitals are related to the major organs in specific ways. For example, the lung opens into the nose and moves essence to the surface skin and body hair; the heart opens into the tongue and has its unfoldment in the blood vessels; the kidney opens into the ears and the two yins, the anus and genitals, and has its unfoldment in the bones. Account is also taken of the interdependence of mind and body. Perturbation of normal essence-spirit and emotional activity may affect the functioning of one or more of the organs, causing physical illness; similarly, organic disease may affect normal essence-spirit and emotional activity. Thus, the holistic approach represents an important facet of Chinese medicine.

Differentiation between the viscera and bowels; preeminence of the viscera

Functional distinction is made between the bowels and viscera: the function of the viscera is to produce and store essence; that of the bowels is to decompose food and convey waste. Thus, *Essential Questions* states:

> The so-called five viscera store essential qi and do not discharge waste. Thus they are full, but cannot be filled. The six bowels process and convey matter, and do not store. Thus they are filled, yet are not full.

This is the physiologic difference between the five viscera and the six bowels.

In addition, there are also the "curious organs": the brain, the marrow, the bones, the vessels, the womb, and the gallbladder. Their generic name derives from their functions, which distinguish them from both the viscera and the bowels. For instance, the gallbladder is considered as a bowel because it plays a part in the processing and conveyance of digestate, and is in an interior-exterior relationship with its paired viscus, the liver. But the bile that it produces is considered as a "clear fluid" rather than waste. Hence it is also classed among the curious organs.

Visceral manifestation theory provides more detail about the viscera than about the bowels. The viscera are considered interior, while the bowels are considered exterior. Each viscus is linked by channels to a bowel, thus forming pairs of interior-exterior correspondences. Because there are six bowels and only five viscera, channel theory considers the pericardium as a viscus separate from the heart, corresponding to the triple burner and associated with the pericardium channel. However, for all purposes other than acupuncture, the pericardium is to some extent considered as part of the heart, which it surrounds.

Finally, it should be mentioned that in Chinese medicine, the lung, spleen, liver, kidney, stomach, small intestine, large intestine, gallbladder, and bladder are morphologically equivalent to the organs of the same name in Western anatomy. However, the explanation of their physiologic functions and pathologic disorders differs widely from those of Western physiology and pathology.

The Heart and Pericardium

The heart is located in the chest, and is surrounded by the pericardium. The heart governs the blood vessels, stores the spirit, and opens into the tongue. Its associated channel connects with the small intestine, which is its corresponding exterior organ. The heart's principal functions are pumping the blood through the vessels and governing consciousness and mental activity. The importance of the heart is emphasized in the *Spiritual Axis*, where it states, "The heart is governor of the five viscera and the six bowels, and is the abode of the spirit." In clinical practice, cardiovascular disorders, many nervous and mental disorders, and conditions involving erosion of the tip of the tongue, are all treated as heart diseases.

Physiology and pathology of the heart

The heart governs the blood vessels

By the phrase, "The heart governs the blood vessels of the body," *Essential Questions* emphasizes that all the blood vessels of the body are subordinate to the heart. Although blood is produced from the essence of digestate assimilated by the stomach and spleen, it is the heart that ensures its constant circulation, maintaining the supply of nourishment to the whole body. Thus *Essential Questions* also states, "All blood is subordinate to the heart," and "the vessels are the dwelling place of the blood."

The heart stores the spirit

"The heart stores the spirit" is the same in meaning as "the heart governs the spirit." Here, spirit refers to the strength of essence-spirit and clarity of consciousness. In Western physiology, both consciousness and mental activity are considered functions of the brain, but in Chinese medicine their different aspects are variously attributed to the organs. The heart is considered particularly important in this context. If the heart fulfills its functions normally and blood and qi are abundant, the spirit-disposition is lucid, making the individual alert and responsive to the environment. If, however, the heart is diseased, the heart spirit may be disquieted, precipitating such symptoms as restlessness, susceptibility to fright and palpitations, diminished sleep, or excessive dreaming. In serious cases there may be signs either of loss of sensibility, such as hypersomnia or coma, or of essence-spirit disorders, feeblemindedness, raving delirium, or manic agitation.

Heart qi, heart blood, heart yin, and heart yang

Heart qi and heart blood form part of the blood and qi of the whole body and represent the basis for the physiologic activity of the heart. When heart qi and heart blood are abundant, the heartbeat is regular, the pulse is moderate and forceful, and the complexion is healthy and lustrous. Insufficiency of heart qi and depletion of heart blood are characterized by a lusterless complexion, palpitation, and slow, rapid, or interrupted pulses. Insufficiency of heart qi may lead to blood stagnation characterized by a cyan-purple complexion and pronounced lack of warmth in the extremities. Heart blood depletion leads to impairment of the blood's nourishing function. It may also deprive heart qi of support, giving rise to dizziness, spiritual fatigue, shortness of breath, and copious perspiration. Heart blood and heart qi are very much interdependent.

Heart yin and heart yang refer to the complementary aspects of the heart's functions. Heart yang refers to a strong heartbeat, smooth blood flow, and the lively, expansive aspect of essence-spirit activity. Heart yin refers to a regular, moderate heartbeat and the calm, passive aspect of essence-spirit activity. Yin and yang complement and counterbalance each other, ensuring that the heart beats forcefully and regularly, and performs all its normal functions. An essential prerequisite of normal function is an abundance of heart blood and exuberance of heart qi. Insufficiency of heart blood or heart qi may lead to debilitation of heart yin or yang. Since "when yang is vacuous there is cold," and "when yin is vacuous there is heat," such cases present with signs not only of qi or blood vacuity, but also of vacuity cold and vacuity heat.

The heart opens into the tongue

"The heart opens into the tongue" is identical in meaning to "the tongue is the sprout of the heart." This implies that disturbances of the heart are invariably reflected in the tongue. For example, in cases of heart yin vacuity or effulgence of heart fire, the tip (or the whole body) of the tongue is red, prickly, or eroded. In heart qi vacuity and insufficiency of heart qi or blood, the tongue is either pale or dark. Stagnation of the heart blood is characterized by a purple tongue with dark blood stasis speckles. When a pathogen enters the heart, the tongue becomes stiff and speech is impeded.

Despite the special relationship between the heart and tongue, the condition of all the other organs, particularly the spleen, is reflected in the state of the tongue and its fur.

The relationship of the heart to other organs

The heart stands in interior-exterior relationship with the small intestine

The heart and small intestine are connected by channels. The two organs are also related in pathology. If, in a condition of heart fire effulgence, heat spreads to the small intestine, there may be such signs as erosion and lesions in the oral cavity. In addition, urine may be scant and dark in color, with a burning sensation during urination.

The heart governs the blood and the spleen manages the blood

Physiologically, the heart governs the blood, while the spleen represents the basis of qi and blood formation, and also manages the blood. Thus, we can see that the relationship between these two organs is very close. Pathologically, essence-spirit disturbances may not only cause excessive wear on the blood, but may also affect splenic movement and transformation. Conversely, impairment of splenic movement may reduce the supply of essence of digestate to the heart, while hemorrhage due to failure of splenic management of the blood can result in insufficiency of heart blood. Such conditions are known as cardiosplenic vacuity, manifesting as dizziness, palpitations, poor memory, insomnia, lusterless complexion, and little thought of food.

The heart and kidney interact

The heart is located in the upper burner and the kidney in the lower burner. Physiologically, the heart connects with the lower burner through the kidney and the kidney connects with the upper burner through the heart. The two organs are interdependent and counterbalance each other. If this relationship is upset, the resulting condition is known as breakdown of cardiorenal interaction, characterized by insomnia, excessive dreaming, pain in the lumbar region, and dream emissions.

The pericardium

The pericardium is the outer casing of the heart. It was believed in ancient China that pathogens invading the heart would first affect the pericardium, so that conditions such as spiritual clouding and delirious mania due to high fever were termed heat entering the pericardium, while essence-spirit derangement due to phlegm-damp was termed phlegm-turbidity clouding the pericardium. Both these conditions are in reality heart disorders.

The Lung

The lung is located in the chest, connects with the throat, and opens into the nose. *Essential Questions* states, "The lung is the panoply of the viscera." Hence the appellation "florid panoply," that was coined later. The lung is interior and is connected by its channel down to the large intestine, which is the corresponding exterior organ. The main functions of the lung are governing qi and controlling respiration. Lung qi faces the hundred channels, ensures regular flow through the waterways, conveys essence to the surface skin and body hair, and governs the defensive exterior of the whole body.

According to visceral manifestation theory, the lung is associated with the respiratory function, and also with fluid regulation, the movement of qi and blood, and the capacity of the skin and the striations to resist the invasion of exogenous pathogens. Hence, in clinical practice, most disorders of the respiratory system, as well as some fluid metabolism and circulatory disorders, exterior patterns of exogenous diseases, and certain skin diseases, can be treated through the lung.

The physiology and pathology of the lung
The lung governs qi

"The lung governs qi" denotes the respiratory function and role played by the lung in the production of true qi.

The lung is the point of exchange between the gases within and outside the body. It takes in clear, natural qi and expels turbid qi. Lung qi has the functions of ensuring diffusion and depurative downbearing. If these two functions are fulfilled, air can pass in and out of the lung freely, the respiratory channels are kept free, and breathing is even. Non-diffusion of lung qi or impairment of depurative downbearing are characterized by cough, rapid or distressed breathing, as well as distention and fullness in the chest and lateral costal region. *Essential Questions* states, "Qi patterns characterized by respiratory distress and thoracic depression are associated with the lung."

The respiratory function of the lung is also related to the production of true qi. Inhaled air becomes a main constituent of true qi. The *Spiritual Axis* states, "True qi is derived from air and from the digestate qi, and fills the body." Inhaled air and digestate qi are combined with the essential qi of the kidney to form the true qi that vitalizes the human body. This is why it is said in *Essential Questions*, "The lung governs the qi of the whole body" and "all qi is subordinate to the lung." In addition to impairing respiration, insufficiency of lung qi may also affect the formation of true qi and thereby precipitate generalized qi vacuity, characterized by fatigue and weakness, shortness of breath, and spontaneous sweating.

The lung ensures regular flow through the waterways

The spleen, lung, kidney, intestines, and bladder are jointly responsible for regulating water metabolism. The specific role of the lung is called "ensuring regular flow through the waterways," and represents a combination of the two functions of diffusion and depurative downbearing. Diffusion means distributing fluids throughout the body, particularly to the skin, where they leave the body in the form of sweat. Depurative downbearing refers to the downward conveyance of water to the bladder. For this reason it is said, "The lung is the upper source of water." If diffusion is impaired, then the striations will close up, preventing perspiration. If depurative downbearing is impaired, there may be water swelling, inhibited urination, and oliguria.

The lung governs the surface skin and body hair

The surface skin and body hair represent the surface of the body, including the skin, sweat glands, and body hair, and have the function of secreting sweat and resisting exogenous pathogens. These functions of the skin and hair depend on the supply of defense qi. Defense qi also ensures that the surface skin and body hair are adequately moistened. The *Spiritual Axis* states, "Defense qi warms the flesh and flushes the skin; it replenishes the striations and controls their opening and closing." Defense qi's capacity to fulfill these functions is mainly attributable to pulmonary diffusion. This is discussed in *Spiritual Axis* in the following way:

> The upper burner opens, diffuses the five sapors, nourishes the skin, fills the body, and moistens the hair, just as the dew waters the earth. Such is the action of qi.

Because of the close relationship between the lung and the surface skin and body hair, *Essential Questions* states, "The lung is connected with the surface skin, and its health is reflected in the body hair." Exogenous pathogens entering the body through the exterior usually affect the lung first. Failure of lung qi to ensure diffusion of defense qi and conveyance of essence to the skin and hair not only produces such signs as dry and lifeless skin and hair, heavy sweating, or absence of sweating, but also increases vulnerability to exogenous pathogens. Thus, diseases caused by exogenous pathogens may be cured by treating the lung, and some skin diseases may also be successfully treated. Evidence of the intimate relationship between the lung and the skin and body hair may be seen in the treatment of neurodermatitis by needling the lung points of the ears.

The lung opens at the nose

Since the lung governs respiration and the nose is the outer extremity of the respiratory tract, the nose may be referred to as the portal of the lung. The sense of smell can function normally only if lung qi is in harmony and respiration is smooth. Thus the *Spiritual Axis* states, "Lung qi flows to the nose, enabling it to sense fetor and fragrance." Many lung disorders are the result of the contraction of exogenous pathogens through the nose and mouth, and may be detected by their condition. For example, counterflow ascent of lung qi caused by lung heat frequently leads to flaring of the nostrils. Such conditions as congested and running nose, or impaired sense of smell are usually treated by pungent dissipating lung diffusion.[1] Recent treatment of nasal polyps and chronic rhinitis by needling pulmonary acupoints on the ear also demonstrates the principle that the lung opens at the nose.

In addition, the throat is the gate of respiration; it contains the vocal organs and is located on the path of the lung channel. Vacuity or repletion of the lung may lead to hoarseness of voice and other throat disorders.

The relationship of the lung to other organs

The lung stands in interior-exterior relationship with the large intestine

The lung and the large intestine are functionally interconnected. Since lung qi ensures regular flow through the waterways, and the large intestine governs liquid, they are closely linked relative to water metabolism. Thus, the two organs are said to stand in interior-exterior relationship. In the treatment of pulmonary phlegm-heat congestion, bowel purgation can therefore sometimes drain lung heat and precipitate phlegm, while some cases of constipation can be treated with formulae containing agents that enhance pulmonary diffusion and depuration.

The lung governs qi and the heart governs blood

The relationship between the lung and the heart is principally seen in the relationship between qi and blood. The blood in all the channels of the body must pass through the lungs. Only after being combined with and diffused by lung qi can blood nourish the organs and convey essence to the surface skin and body hair. *Essential Questions* states:

> Alimentary qi goes into the stomach; turbid qi goes to the heart. Pure essence goes into the vessels, and the qi of the vessels flows into the channels. The lung, to which channel qi is subordinate, faces the hundred vessels and carries essence to the surface skin and body hair. The blood vessels and the skin share of one same essence...

Furthermore, ancestral qi, which gathers in the chest, connects with the heart and powers respiration. The physiologic relationship between the lung and heart is extremely close, and for this reason, congestion of lung qi can affect the cardiac governance of the blood vessels, causing inhibited blood flow and, in severe cases, produce blood stagnation, which is characterized by palpitations, oppression in the chest, and cyan-purple lips and tongue. Similarly, impairment of the smooth flow of blood associated with insufficiency of heart qi may affect pulmonary diffusion and depuration, giving rise to cough or dyspnea.

The lung is the collecting place of phlegm and the spleen is the basis of phlegm formation

The lung's relationship to the spleen centers on the distribution of fluids. The spleen governs movement and transformation of fluids and the lung ensures their regular flow through the waterways. Fluids are passed to the lung by the spleen; then, by pulmonary diffusion and depuration, they are distributed throughout the body and down to the bladder. If splenic movement and transformation is impaired, water may accumulate and turn into damp or phlegm. In severe cases it can effect swelling or invade the lung, causing dyspnea. Thus it is said, "The spleen is the basis of phlegm formation and the lung is the collecting place of phlegm." In accordance with this principle, coughs due to phlegm-rheum are often treated by the method of fortifying the spleen and drying damp, combined with the promotion of pulmonary depuration and transformation of phlegm.

The lung is the governor of qi and the kidney is the root of qi

The lung controls respiration and governs the qi of the whole body. However, lung qi must combine with the essential qi of the kidney to produce true qi. Thus, it is said in *Jing Yue's Complete Compendium*, "The lung is the governor of qi and the kidney is the root of qi." Although respiration is the function of the lung, it is nevertheless in one aspect dependent on the kidney. Only when kidney qi is sufficient can respiratory qi be constrained. Hence it is said, "The kidney governs the absorption of qi." If kidney essential qi is insufficient, it is incapable of ensuring the absorption of qi through the lung. This results in respiratory insufficiency characterized by shortness of breath and rapid breathing at the slightest exertion. Such conditions are termed kidney failing to absorb qi (qi absorption failure) and qi not descending to the root. Sun Si-Mo's *Priceless Prescriptions* states, "Kidney disease. . . will result in weakness of qi and respiratory qi shortage." The only effective treatment for such cases is the method of supplementing the kidney to improve qi absorption.

Spleen, Stomach, and Intestines

The spleen, stomach, and intestines are the main organs in the digestive system. The most important of these are the spleen and stomach, which are interconnected by channels and stand in interior-exterior relationship. The spleen governs movement and transformation, while the stomach governs ingestion. The spleen governs upbearing while the stomach governs downbearing. The formation of qi, blood, and fluids relies on the splenogastric function of moving and transforming the essence of digestate. This is why it is said that the spleen and stomach are the basis of formation and the root of the acquired constitution. The small and large intestines are connected by channels to the heart and the lung, with which they stand in interior-exterior relationship. However, the small intestine's function of separating the clear and the turbid and the large intestine's function of transforming and conveying waste are part of the digestive process. In clinical practice, intestinal pathology pattern identification and treatment are closely related to the spleen and stomach. Early recognition of the functional relationship of the intestines to the stomach and spleen is found in *Essential Questions,* which states:

> The spleen, stomach, small and large intestines. . . manage the granaries and are the seat of construction; they are called receptacles, having the ability to transform the five sapors entering, and the waste leaving, the body.

In clinical practice, most disorders of the digestive system are treated as disorders of the stomach and spleen. Other disorders such as water-damp, phlegm-rheum and failure of qi to contain the blood frequently stem from impairment of splenic movement and transformation and thus are also treated as disorders of the spleen.

Physiology and pathology of the spleen, stomach, and intestines

The spleen governs movement and transformation of the digestate

Initial decomposition of the digestate is carried out by the stomach. The spleen then extracts the essence of digestate (nutrients) and dispatches it to the other organs. Ultimately, it reaches all parts of the body. Thus, it is said that the spleen moves the fluids of the stomach, and governs movement and formation of the essence of digestate. Modern writers explain this function as comprising digestion, assimilation, and distribution of nutrients. *Essential Questions* explains this in the following terms:

> Ingested fluids enter the stomach. Here, they are churned and their essential qi is strained off. The essential qi is then carried to the spleen and further distributed by spleen qi. It passes up to the lung, which ensures regular flow through the waterways down to the bladder. In this way, water essence is distributed throughout the five channels and the four parts of the body.

Because of its importance in providing nutrients for the production of blood and qi that maintain the life and health of the organism, the spleen is described as the basis of qi and blood formation and the root of the acquired constitution.

Impairment of splenic movement and transformation can lead to a variety of disorders. Deficient digestion and assimilation may cause abdominal distention, diarrhea, or nutritional disturbances. If the distributive function is impaired, improper movement of fluids may give rise to endogenous damp, phlegm, rheum, or water swelling. For this reason it is said that the spleen ails by damp and is the basis of phlegm formation. Disorders resulting from impaired movement and transformation are commonly denoted by the term splenic vacuity (splenic vacuity damp, splenic vacuity phlegm, splenic vacuity diarrhea, and splenic vacuity water-swelling). According to *Essential Questions*, "Damp, swelling, and fullness are associated with the spleen." For example, splenic vacuity cold, characterized by duck stool or diarrhea, would, according to Western medical classification, be a disorder of the small intestine. Finally, it should be noted that some disorders of the spleen are attributed to other organs in Western medicine.

The spleen manages the blood

This statement refers to the role of the spleen in blood production, and also to its function of preventing extravasation of blood. The spleen is the basis of blood and qi formation, and when healthy it ensures plentiful supplies of qi and blood in the body. Thus, blood is both engendered and kept within the vessels. The two phrases "the spleen manages the blood" and "qi contains the blood" are therefore essentially synonymous.

Pathologically, hemorrhage occurring in qi and blood vacuity patterns stemming from impairment of splenic movement and transformation is explained as the spleen failing to manage the blood. Considered strictly from the point of view of bleeding, such conditions could also be described as failure of qi to contain the blood. Metrorrhagia due to cardiosplenic vacuity and qi vacuity hemafecia are conventionally attributed to blood management failure.

The spleen governs the muscles and limbs, and opens into the mouth

Because the spleen is the basis of blood and qi formation, all the muscles of the body rely for their nourishment on the capacity of the stomach and spleen to move and transform the essence of digestate. Only when the stomach and spleen are functioning properly are the muscles full and sound and the limbs powerful. Impairment of splenic function may therefore lead to wasting of the muscles, loss of limb power, and in severe cases atony and paralysis.

"The spleen opens into the mouth" refers to the relationship of the splenic movement and transformation to appetite and taste in the mouth. If the stomach and the spleen are functioning normally, the individual has a good appetite and normal taste in the mouth. The *Spiritual Axis* states, "Spleen qi passes through to the mouth; if the spleen is functioning harmoniously, then the mouth can taste the five sapors." Disorders of the spleen and stomach are often reflected in changes in appetite and changes in taste in the mouth (a bland, sweet, or sickly taste).

The stomach governs ingestion and decomposition of digestate

The function of the stomach is to receive ingested foods and perform the initial stage of digestion. Normal performance of this function is dependent on "free downflow" of the digestate to the small intestine. The spleen's role in the digestive process is nevertheless preeminent, since it moves and transforms the essence of digestate and moves the fluids of the stomach.

Impairment of stomach function may take the form of gastric qi disharmony, characterized by distention and fullness in the upper abdomen, dyspeptic anorexia, stomachache, or counterflow ascent of stomach qi, presenting signs of nausea, vomiting, eructation, or hiccoughing. Gastric repletion heat characterized by constipation and halitosis is attributed in Western medicine to the intestines.

The small intestine governs separation of the clear and the turbid; the large intestine governs transformation and conveyance of waste

The small intestine's function of further transforming the digestate already decomposed by the stomach is referred to as separation of the clear and the turbid. The clear refers to what is useful to the body, while the turbid denotes waste. In the small intestine, the essence of digestate is assimilated into the body by the action of the spleen. Waste water is absorbed and, by the transformative action of kidney qi, is conveyed to the bladder. Hence, "The small intestine governs liquid." Solid waste is passed to the large intestine where it is formed into stool before being discharged from the body. Thus, the large intestine is said to govern transformation and conveyance of waste. Since it absorbs further fluid from the waste, it is also said to govern humor.

Disorders of the small intestine are attributable to failure to separate the clear and the turbid. These disorders manifest as stool and urinary disturbances. Common symptoms are abdominal pain, diarrhea, and scant urine. Disorders of the large intestine most commonly manifest as diarrhea (including intestinal vacuity efflux desertion), dry stool, or constipation.

Relationships among the stomach, spleen, intestines, and the other organs

The spleen and stomach stand in interior-exterior relationship

The spleen and stomach are interconnected by channels, forming an interior-exterior correspondence. Physiologically, the spleen governs movement and transformation, while the stomach governs ingestion. The spleen governs upbearing, while the stomach governs downbearing. The stomach and the spleen thus complement and counterbalance each other. Together the spleen and stomach perform the major part of digestion and assimilation.

The stomach governs ingestion and decomposition, thus preparing for movement and transformation. The spleen moves the fluids of the stomach, adapting to the stomach's continuing capacity for food intake. Both organs function in close cooperation in performing digestive activity. If the stomach's ingestive function is impaired, the spleen is left with fewer raw materials from which to form blood and qi; therefore a good appetite with indigestion is a pathologic state. *Referenced Medical Remedies* states:

> The stomach governs ingestion, and the spleen governs digestion, so if the patient can ingest food but cannot digest it, the disorder is attributable to the spleen.

A clear distinction is made between the gastric governance of ingestion and the splenic governance of movement and transformation. In clinical practice, loss of appetite or clamoring stomach with rapid hungering is attributable to the stomach. If, however, the patient suffers from indigestion, has a bloated stomach after eating, and has thin stools, then the disorder is attributable to the spleen. In the first instance, treatment should be directed toward increasing the appetite and harmonizing the stomach, while in the second case, therapeutic efforts should aim at fortifying the spleen.

The spleen's governance of upbearing and the stomach's governance of downbearing again show the complementarity of the two organs. The spleen not only moves and transforms the essence of digestate, but also carries it up to the heart and lung. This is why it is said, "The spleen governs upbearing." Failure of splenic upbearing can lead to center-qi fall, characterized by distention and prolapse in the upper abdomen, diarrhea, and prolapse of the rectum. Gastric governance of downbearing refers to conveyance of the digestate to the small intestine and, in a broader sense, to downflow throughout the whole of the digestive tract. "The stomach functions properly when there is free downflow" highlights the advantage to the stomach of unimpaired downbearing. However, should stomach qi bear upward instead of downward, such symptoms as nausea, vomiting, eructation, and hiccoughing are observed. Ye Tian-Shi of the Qing Dynasty wrote:

> Ingestion of food is the primary function of the stomach while movement and transformation constitute the primary functions of the spleen; spleen qi normally bears upward, while stomach qi normally bears downward.

Upbearing and downbearing are mutually complementary. The spleen upbears clear qi (the essential qi extracted from the digestate), while the stomach downbears turbid qi (the remaining digestate). Failure of the clear qi to bear upward may impair the downbearing of turbid qi. Similarly, failure of the turbid qi to bear downward may affect the bearing of the clear qi; signs such as poor appetite, bloating in the upper abdomen, nausea, eructation, indigestion, diarrhea, and thick, slimy tongue fur often occur simultaneously. *Essential Questions* says, "Downbearing movement of clear qi causes swill diarrhea; upbearing movement of turbid qi causes distention." In clinical practice, such conditions are treated by fortifying the spleen (upbearing the clear) and harmonizing the stomach (downbearing the turbid).

Furthermore, the spleen thrives by dryness and ails by dampness while the stomach thrives by dampness and ails by dryness. In clinical practice there is a difference in nature between disorders of the spleen and those of the stomach. The spleen is particularly susceptible to invasion by the damp pathogen that disrupts movement and transformation, and if this function is already disrupted owing to other causes, it may easily produce damp. When damp affects movement and transformation, the spleen is said to be encumbered by damp. This condition is treated with warm, bitter agents that dry damp and fortify the spleen. The stomach, by contrast, is vulnerable to heat pathogens that "scorch" the stomach juices. Frequent vomiting due to counterflow ascent causes detriment to the stomach juices characterized by signs of dryness. Such patterns are treated by moistening dryness and nourishing the stomach.

Physiologically, the stomach and the spleen are closely related and the complementary nature of splenic upbearing and gastric downbearing are of particular importance in the digestive process. Disruption of this balance constitutes a primary cause of digestive disturbances, and its restoration figures frequently in the treatment of splenogastric disorders.

The influence of liver qi over splenogastric movement and transformation

The normal functioning of the stomach and spleen is to some extent dependent on the liver's governance of free-coursing. Depression of liver qi, which results from impairment of free-coursing, invariably portends digestive disturbances characterized by painful distention in the upper abdomen, dyspeptic anorexia, eructation, nausea, vomiting, and diarrhea.

The *Spiritual Axis* states, "Disorders to which the liver gives rise include fullness in the chest, eructation, and swill diarrhea." Such conditions are termed hepatosplenic disharmony.

The influence of kidney yang over splenogastric movement and transformation

Kidney yang, also known as "fire of the vital gate," represents a motive force in the digestive process. Insufficiency of kidney yang (debilitation of vital gate fire) leads to impairment of the digestive function. This disorder is known as splenorenal yang vacuity and is characterized by cold and pain in the abdomen, persistent diarrhea, daybreak diarrhea, incomplete digestion, and water swelling.

The Liver and Gallbladder

The liver is located on the right side beneath the diaphragm, and the gallbladder is located on the undersurface of the right hepatic lobe. The liver is an interior organ and is connected by channels to the gallbladder, which is its corresponding exterior organ.

The liver governs free coursing, stores blood, and governs the sinews. Governance of free coursing is seen in the regulating effect the liver has over the movement of qi, essence-spirit and emotional activity, and the secretion and discharge of bile. "The liver stores blood" implies that the liver can retain blood and regulate the amount of blood flowing throughout the body. "The liver governs the sinews" means that the liver maintains the proper movement of the sinews, the muscles, and the joints. Its associated channel starts from the great toe, passes up the leg, passes through the genitals and lower abdomen, crosses the lateral costal region and the throat, connects through to the eyes and then continues on to the vertex of the head. Diseases that occur in parts of the body traversed by the liver channel are often treated as liver disorders.

The functions of the gallbladder are included among those of the liver listed below. According to visceral manifestation theory, only the gallbladder's function of secreting and discharging bile is the same as that of Western medical physiology. All its other functions differ from those attributed to it by Western medicine.

The physiology and pathology of the liver and gallbladder

The liver governs free coursing

This phrase refers to the liver qi's function of ensuring smooth, uninterrupted flow, which can be seen in the following areas.

Ensuring unimpeded qi dynamic

The liver's governance of free-coursing is reflected in the regularity and smoothness of qi dynamic. When this function is normal, qi dynamic is smooth and regular, so that qi and blood remain in harmony, the channels are kept free, and the organs all function normally. When it is impaired, qi dynamic is disturbed and a whole variety of disorders may arise as a result. If liver qi is depressed in the liver itself and its associated channel, pain and distention develops in the chest and lateral costal region or lower abdomen, or the breasts become painfully swollen. If liver qi invades the stomach, such signs as attacks of pain in the upper abdomen, nausea, vomiting, and eructation appear; if liver qi invades the spleen, there may be painful distention in the chest, lateral costal region, and abdomen; borborygmi; and diarrhea. In a further stage of development, qi stagnation may lead to blood stasis and the development of concretions, accumulations, or lump glomi. Transformation of depressed qi into fire may cause wearing of the blood or frenetic blood movement, affecting the liver's blood-storing function.

Secretion and discharge of bile

The gallbladder is located behind the right lobe of the liver and stores bile. It stands in interior-exterior relationship with the liver, to which it is connected by channels. Production and secretion of bile depends on surplus qi from the liver being channelled into the gallbladder, where it then accumulates and forms into bile. This means that bile secretion and discharge represents an important aspect of the liver's function of governing free coursing. Disruption of free coursing may thus lead to irregularities in bile secretion and discharge, characterized by jaundice, bitter taste in the mouth, vomiting of yellow fluid, painful distention in the lateral costal region, flatulence, and diminished food intake.

Emotional disturbance

Impairment of hepatic governance of free-coursing may cause and be caused by emotional disturbance. Joy, anger, anxiety, preoccupation, sorrow, fear, and fright are the seven affects. Under normal circumstances, these are the individual's natural responses to the environment. Overintensity of one or more of these affects can lead to endogenous damage (disturbance of organ functioning). Hepatic governance of free coursing is among the physiologic functions most vulnerable to endogenous damage. Moreover, impairment of this function may lead not only to disturbance of qi dynamic and regular secretion and discharge of bile, but also to emotional disturbances such as essence-spirit depression, rashness, impatience, and irascibility.

These three aspects of free coursing are clearly interrelated. Impairment of qi dynamic may affect either emotional activity or the secretion and discharge of bile. Emotional disturbance may similarly affect qi dynamic. Disorders of bile secretion and discharge can cause gastric, splenic, or intestinal dysfunction and thereby upset qi dynamic, which in turn may affect normal emotional activity. The three different aspects of free-coursing cannot, therefore, be looked at in isolation. Only by a comprehensive approach can this aspect of the liver be fully understood in clinical practice.

The liver stores blood

The liver is capable of retaining blood and regulating the amount of blood in the body. The amount of blood in the various parts of the body varies in accordance with physiologic needs. During physical exertion, the blood is distributed throughout the body, meeting the increased need for nutrients. When the body is at rest or asleep, blood flows back to the liver to be stored. Therefore it is said, "When the body moves, blood flows through the channels, and when the body is at rest, the blood flows back to the liver where it is stored"; and "the legs receive blood and walk, the hands receive blood and grip." When the liver's blood-storing function is disrupted, two possible disorders may arise. In the first case, the storage capacity of the liver is reduced so that there is not enough blood in the body to supply all needs; if the blood does not nourish the eyes, such disorders as flowery vision, dry eyes, and night blindness may occur; if the blood fails to nourish the sinews, sinew-vascular hypertonicity gives rise to inhibited bending and stretching; in women, blood may fail to flow into the penetrating and conception vessels, causing reduced menstrual flow or amenorrhea. In the second case, the blood-storing function of the liver is impaired, giving rise to a tendency toward bleeding, such as menorrhagia, metrorrhagia, and other forms of bleeding, such conditions being known as failure of the liver to store blood (or blood storage failure).

Liver qi, liver yang, liver blood, and liver yin

Liver qi and liver yang, physiologically speaking, form a single entity, but the term liver yin is considerably broader in meaning, including the "essence" referred to in *Essential Questions,* which states, "Alimentary qi enters the stomach and sends essence to the liver." The liver's yang and qi and its yin and blood under normal circumstances are interdependent and mutually counterbalancing. Liver yin and liver blood nourish liver yang qi, and also prevent it from upstirring excessively. At the same time, they are dependent on the liver qi's function of governing free-coursing to be able to nourish the limbs, the sinews and vessels, the eyes, and the penetrating and conception vessels.

The liver is said to thrive by orderly reaching and is prone to upstirring; consequently it is known as the unyielding organ. This is seen most clearly in pathologic conditions, such as free-coursing failure. This condition is known as binding depression of liver qi, which can lead to liver blood stagnation. Depressed qi can also form fire, damaging liver yin and liver blood. If liver yin or liver blood are insufficient, the yang qi of the liver is no longer kept in check and bears upward. This condition is known as ascending hyperactivity of liver yang. All these conditions are due to disruption of the balance between the liver's yin and yang aspects, or liver blood and liver qi.

Liver qi depression and ascending hyperactivity of liver yang are both disorders of yang qi. The liver is unique in that morbidity of its yang qi is usually attributable to superabundance, while yang qi of other organs is prone to insufficiency. Similarly, liver yin and liver blood are prone to insufficiency, which again represents a deviation from the norm. This is summed up in the axiom, "liver qi and liver yang tend toward superabundance, while liver blood and liver yin tend toward insufficiency."

The liver governs the sinews; its efflorescence is in the nails

"The liver governs the sinews" means that sinew movement throughout the body is associated with the liver. Only when liver blood is abundant can replete qi reach the sinews, enabling them to move normally. If liver blood is insufficient, the resulting failure of the blood to nourish the sinews adequately brings on hypertonicity or numbness in the limbs, with difficulty in bending and stretching. When endogenous liver wind stirs, tremors, convulsive spasms, and opisthotonos are observed. "The nails are the surplus of the sinews" means that when liver blood is abundant, the nails are red, lustrous, and healthy. When liver blood is insufficient, the nails are pale in color and brittle. This explains the phrase, "The liver's efflorescence is in the nails."

The liver opens at the eyes

The eyes are intimately related with the liver. The *Inner Canon* states, "The liver receives blood, so there is sight," and "Liver qi connects through to the eyes; if the liver is in harmony, then the five colors may be distinguished." These lines emphasize that the eyes are dependent on the nourishing action of liver blood. In clinical practice, there are a considerable number of eye disorders that may be treated as liver conditions. Insufficiency may provoke such conditions as night blindness, dry eyes, and blurred vision; upflaming of liver fire may occasion ocular rubor and painful swelling of the eyes; ascendant hyperactivity of liver yang may express itself as visual dizziness; and endogenous liver wind may cause a sideways or upward squint.

Although the eyes are the specific opening of the liver, the essential qi of all the organs is reflected in them. The *Spiritual Axis* states, "The essential qi of the five viscera and the six bowels flows up into the eyes and becomes essence." Thus to some degree the eyes are associated with all the organs, and apart from their special relationship with the liver, the heart and the kidney are perhaps next most closely related. Heart fire effulgence, for instance, is associated with ocular rubor, and diminished visual acuity is associated with vacuous kidney yin.

The relationship of the liver to other organs

The liver stores the blood, the heart moves the blood

The spleen is the basis of blood formation, the liver stores the blood, and the heart pumps the blood around the body. The Tang Dynasty version of the *Inner Canon* annotated by Wang Bing states, "The blood is stored by the liver and is moved by the heart." If the yin blood of the whole body is abundant, the liver has its object of storage and the heart has its object of governance. Thus the blood can circulate and nourish the whole body. Abundance of yin blood also prevents heart and liver yang from becoming hyperactive. Insufficiency of yin blood not only deprives the liver of its object of storage and the heart of its object of governance, but also leaves liver and heart yang unchecked and precipitates simultaneous effulgence of heart and liver fire. Thus, heart and liver vacuities are closely interrelated.

The liver stores the blood and the kidney stores essence; the liver governs free coursing; the kidney governs storage

The liver and the kidney are intimately related. The two organs have manifold connections through the channels, and physiologically they are mutually engendering and counterbalancing. Clinically, the kidney and the liver are often treated together. The relationship between them may be divided into two broad aspects: the liver stores blood and the kidney stores essence. Kidney essence and liver blood are mutually engendering, for which reason it is said, "The liver and kidney are of the same source." Depletion of kidney essence and insufficiency of liver blood may both lead to what is known as dual vacuity of liver and kidney yin. Conversely, hyperactivity of liver yang and liver fire are not only detrimental to liver blood, but may also, at a further stage of development, damage kidney essence. Hence, in therapy, liver nourishment and kidney enrichment are often used in combination.

Governance of free coursing and governance of storage are interdependent, mutually counterbalancing functions of the liver and kidney. Their disruption may bring on such disorders as premature menstruation, menorrhagia, menstrual block, and seminal loss, which are frequently eliminated by combined treatment of the two viscera.

The liver governs upbearing and the lung governs downbearing

The liver is the unyielding organ and governs the upbearing of qi. The lung is the body's uppermost organ and governs downbearing of qi. These complementary movements represent a major factor in the upward and downward bearing of qi in the body. Pathologically, if hepatic upbearing is stronger than pulmonary downbearing, liver fire may invade the lung, provoking such symptoms as irritability, pain in the chest and lateral costal region, counterflow qi cough, or expectoration of blood.

The Kidney, Bladder, and Associated Functions

The kidney is located in the small of the back, on either side of the spinal column.[2] It opens at the ears and the "two yins" (the anus and genitals); its condition is reflected in the hair of the head. The kidney is an interior organ, and its corresponding exterior organ is the bladder, with which it is connected by channels. The main function of the kidney is storing essential qi that is the basis for growth, development, reproduction, and maintenance of the normal functioning of the organs. The kidney is also said to govern water and the bones, and produce bone marrow, although properly all these are functions of kidney essential qi. Its important role in human physiology has caused it to be referred to as the root of the congenital constitution. The functions of the kidney according to Chinese medical theory differ somewhat from those ascribed to it in Western medicine. Its functions correspond to urinary metabolism, reproduction, secretion, and part of the function of the brain in Western medicine. By contrast, the bladder, according to both Chinese and Western medicine, has the function of storing and discharging urine.

The physiology and pathology of the kidney and bladder

The kidney stores essential qi, and is responsible for growth, development, and reproduction

Growth, development, and reproduction are reliant on the essential qi stored by the kidney. Kidney essential qi is derived from the reproductive essence of the parents (congenital essence), out of which the embryo develops. After birth, it is gradually nurtured by the essence of digestate (acquired essence) and reaches fullness in puberty; men are able to produce sperm and women ovulate according to the monthly cycle. Thus the reproductive function comes to maturity. In old age, the kidney essential qi weakens, so that the reproductive function gradually fades away, and the body degenerates. *Essential Questions* states:

> {In the male} at the age of sixteen, kidney qi is exuberant, the reproductive function matures, essential qi flows forth, yin and yang are in harmony, and he can beget offspring. . . . At the age of fifty-six, the reproductive function ceases, essence

diminishes, the kidney grows weak, and the body loses its tone; at sixty-four the teeth and hair fall out.

{In the female} at the age of fourteen, the reproductive function matures, the conception vessel flows, the penetrating vessel fills, the menses come according to their times, and she can bear offspring. . . . At forty-two, the conception vessel empties, the penetrating vessel weakens, fertility wanes, the passages of the Earth are cut, the body deteriorates, and she can no longer bear children.

The kidney governs the bones and engenders marrow

Governance of the bones and engendering of marrow account for a large part of the function of the kidney essential qi to stimulate growth and development. The kidney stores essence, essence engenders marrow, and marrow nourishes the bones. Hence it is said, "The kidney engenders bone and marrow," "the health of the kidney is reflected in the solidity of the bones," and "the kidney governs the bones." The growth, development, and healing of the bones depends on the nourishment and propelling force provided by kidney essential qi. Insufficiency of kidney essential qi may result in retarded closure of the fontanels and soft bones. It may also lead to marrow vacuity characterized by atony of the legs preventing the patient from walking, or pain or stiffness of the lower lumbar spine preventing him from lying either prone or supine. Many kidney-supplementing agents can accelerate bone healing, providing further evidence of the connection between the kidney and the bones.

Furthermore, the teeth are the surplus of the bones. In clinical practice, slow growth of teeth in children and the premature loosening and loss of teeth in adults are found to be due to vacuity of kidney essential qi. Hence, some dental disorders are vacuity patterns that can be treated through the kidney.

Because the kidney governs the bones and engenders marrow, and the brain is known as the "sea of marrow," a close link can be seen between the kidney and the brain. Insufficiency of kidney essential qi may lead to vacuity of the sea of marrow, manifesting as dizziness, sluggish mentation, or impaired memory, all of which can by treated as kidney complaints.

The kidney governs water

The kidney distills fluids, regulates their distribution, and discharges waste water, thereby maintaining normal water metabolism in the body. For this reason, the kidney is said to govern water. Body fluids are derived from fluid ingested by the stomach and transformed by the spleen. Through splenic movement and pulmonary regulation of the waterways, they are distributed throughout the body, and waste water is carried down to the bladder before being discharged. The transformative action of kidney qi plays a vital role in this. Impairment of this action as a result of kidney yang vacuity can either cause disorders of fluid metabolism such as oliguria or water swelling, or lead to water containment failure characterized by long micturition with clear urine, and nocturia.

The function of the bladder is to store and discharge urine and is closely related to the kidney. Storage is reliant on the retentive power of kidney qi, while discharge is reliant on the power of the kidney to permit flow. This is known as the "opening and closing" function of the kidney that controls the flow of urine down to the bladder, and enables the bladder to store up to a certain amount of urine before permitting its discharge. *Essential Questions* says, "The bladder. . .stores fluid, and by the transformative function of qi ejects it." In reality, the transformative function here referred to is properly that of the kidney. Disruption of the opening and closing function of the kidney may lead to a blocked, distended bladder, with dribbling discharge of urine. Disorders of the bladder are characterized by such symptoms as urine retention, dribbling incontinence, frequency and urgency of urination, dysuria, polyuria, enuresis, and incontinence, which in the absence of intrinsic bladder disease are generally attributable to renal morbidity.

The kidney opens into the ears and the two yins and its health is reflected in the hair of the head

Since only when kidney qi is abundant is hearing acute, the kidney is said to open into the ears. The *Spiritual Axis* states, "The kidney qi connects to the ears, and if the kidney is in order, the ears can perceive the five sounds." Insufficiency of kidney essential qi gives rise to tinnitus and diminished hearing. Debilitation of essential qi in old age often leads to deafness.

The kidney opens at the "two yins," the "posterior yin," which refers to the anus, and the "anterior yin," which refers to the genital organs. These organs are located in the lower burner, and their functioning is associated with kidney qi, so that they are referred to as the outer portals of the kidney. This relationship is also reflected in various pathologies. For example, kidney vacuity may lead to changes in micturition and evacuation such as oliguria, anuria, long micturition with clear urine, incontinence and enduring diarrhea, or fecal incontinence. The reproductive system may also be affected, causing sexual impotence, premature ejaculation, or seminal efflux.

Essential Questions states, "The health of the kidney. . . is reflected in the hair," meaning that the general condition of the hair, hair growth, and hair loss are all associated with the strength of the kidney essential qi. Loss of hair in old age is one sign of debilitation of essential qi. However, the hair is also reliant on the nourishing action of the blood, so it is also said, "The hair of the head is the surplus of the blood."

Kidney yin and kidney yang are the root of the yin and yang of all the organs

The physiopathology of the kidney can be explained in terms of kidney yin and kidney yang, both of which are rooted in kidney essential qi. Kidney yin has a moistening and nourishing effect on all the organs, and when it is vacuous, such general signs as interior heat, dizziness, tinnitus, atony of the knees and lower back, seminal emission, red tongue, and dry mouth are likely to appear. Owing to the loss of the nourishing effect of the kidney yin, a whole variety of disorders, such as ascendant hyperactivity of liver yang, endogenous liver wind, upflaming of heart fire, or breakdown of cardiorenal interaction, may develop in the other organs. If the lung is affected, such signs as dry cough, tidal fever, upbearing fire, and dry pharynx are observed. Kidney yang warms and activates the other organs. Vacuity of kidney yang may therefore lead to disturbances of water metabolism and the reproductive function, and may as well diminish the activity of the other organs. If kidney yang fails to perform its activating function, signs of cardiorenal yang vacuity such as palpitations, slow pulse, sweating, shortness of breath, and frigidity of the limbs may be observed. Impairment of renal governance of qi absorption affects the lung, provoking rapid breathing at the slightest exertion. If the spleen is deprived of the warming action of kidney yang, there may be daybreak diarrhea or incomplete digestion. Conversely, yin or yang vacuities in other organs may affect kidney yin or yang. For example, liver yin vacuity, hyperactivity of liver yang, heart yin vacuity, or effulgence of heart fire may eventually damage kidney yin. Such conditions are known as sapping of kidney yin. Often, lung yin vacuity also affects kidney yin, and diarrhea caused by splenic yang vacuity may eventually affect kidney yang, this condition being known as splenorenal yang vacuity. Since kidney yin and kidney yang are the root of the yin and yang of all the organs of the body, they may also be referred to as "true yin" or "original yin," and "true yang" or "original yang."

The relationship between kidney yin and kidney yang

Kidney yin and kidney yang are basically two opposing, yet complementary aspects of kidney essential qi. They are interdependent and mutually counterbalancing, each being indispensable to the other. Imbalance of kidney yin and kidney yang, where one or other complement becomes vacuous, is fundamentally attributable to insufficiency of kidney essential qi. When kidney yin or yang vacuity reaches a certain point, it may affect its complement, so that the condition becomes one of dual vacuity of kidney yin and yang. Here, we see in operation the principle that detriment of yin or yang affects its complement.

The vital gate

Reference to a "vital gate" as part of the body first appears in the *Canon of Perplexities,* which states, "On the left is the kidney, and on the right is ming men {the vital gate}." Since that time there has been a continuous debate concerning the location and function of the vital gate. Some support the view posited by the *Canon of Perplexities,* while others claim that ming men is an independent organ separate from the kidney. Regarding function, some claim that the "vital gate fire" is synonymous with kidney yang, while others maintain that it is distinct from kidney yang. Zhang Jie-Bin states:

> The vital gate is the root of qi and is the dwelling place of fire and water. But for it, the yin qi of the five viscera would fail to have its nourishing effect, and the yang qi of the five viscera would be left unmobilized.

This clearly implies that the vital gate fire refers to kidney yin and kidney yang. In clinical practice, agents that supplement the fire of the vital gate are kidney yang warming agents. We believe that the concept of the kidney is broad and includes many functions of internal secretion. Other sources also suggest that the vital gate is the source of life, which in women manifests in the form of the uterus and the ovaries, and in the male as the testicles and the prostate. The fire of the vital gate (ministerial fire) is also said to correspond to the "fatty membrane" located in the sacral and lumbar region, that rises up the outside of the spinal column and passes into the chest and abdomen, where it controls the activity of the organs. In Western medicine, this fatty membrane corresponds to the sympathetic nerve of the lumbar region and the parasympathetic nerve of the sacral region.

The brain

The brain is located in the skull and is continuous with the spinal cord. The *Inner Canon* classifies the brain as a "curious organ," and states that it "stores yet does not discharge." The governing vessel "follows the spine up to the point *feng-fu* {GV-16}, whence it enters the brain." The foot tai yang bladder channel "connects through to the brain from the top of the head."

Chinese medicine ascribes the spirit, consciousness, and thought to the heart, and to some extent to the liver and kidney. According to tradition, "the brain is the sea of marrow; all marrow belongs to the brain, flowing up to the brain and down to the coccyx. This is the path of the upward flow of essential marrow." In later times, Li Shi-Zhen, Jin Zheng-Xi, and others explicitly stated, "The brain is the seat of the original spirit," explaining that memory, consciousness, and mental activity were functions of the brain. They also believed that the senses and control of physical movement were related to the brain. The *Spiritual Axis* states, "If the sea of marrow is insufficient, the brain turns and the ears ring, there is aching in the neck, dizziness, visual blackouts, and lethargy."

According to visceral manifestation theory, the main functions of the brain as perceived by Western medicine are ascribed to the heart, liver, kidney, and other organs. "The heart stores the spirit" refers basically to the brain's function of mental activity and thought. Such conditions as heat entering the pericardium and phlegm confounding the cardiac portals correspond to what Western medicine describes as disorders of the central nervous system. Imbalance of heart yin and heart yang, and heart qi and heart blood, are explained in Western medicine as disturbance of the brain function. Blood-nourishing spirit quietants, portal openers, phlegm transformers, heart yin nourishers, and heart yang warmers have been found to act on the nervous system. "The liver governs free-coursing" and "the liver governs the sinews" corresponds to what in Western medicine are brain functions. Disorders such as liver qi depression and ascendant hyperactivity of liver yang may be partially explained in Western medicine as being associated with the nervous system. Liver coursers, liver calmatives, yang subduers, and wind extinguishers all act on the nervous system. Since the kidney stores essence and produces bone marrow, and the brain is the sea of marrow, there is a close relationship between the kidney and the brain. Insufficiency of kidney essence can cause diminished cerebral function in adults and the elderly. Practice shows that some kidney-supplementing agents have a beneficial effect on cerebral function.

The uterus

The uterus is considered as another of the "curious organs." It is the organ of childbearing and the menstrual cycle. However, the menstrual cycle and reproductive function are also related to the three following factors:

Kidney essential qi

Only when there is abundant essential qi can the female reproductive organs develop to maturity, ensuring proper menstruation and adequate conditions for conception and childbearing. In old age, the kidney essential qi grows weak and menstruation ceases; the reproductive function is then lost. *Essential Questions* states:

> At the age of seven, the kidney qi of the female is strong, the teeth are replaced, and the hair is long. At the age of fourteen, the reproductive function matures, the conception vessel flows, and the penetrating vessel fills, the menses come according to

their times, and she can bear offspring.... At forty-two, the conception vessel empties, the penetrating vessel weakens, fertility wanes, the passages of the Earth are cut, the body deteriorates, and she can no longer bear children.

This highlights the key role of the kidney essential qi in maintaining normal menstruation and the conditions for childbearing.

The conception and penetrating vessels

Both these vessels start from the uterus. The conception vessel joins with the three yin channels of the foot in the abdomen and regulates all the yin channels of the body. Thus it is sometimes referred to as "the sea of the yin channels." When there is an abundance of blood and qi in the twelve channels, it flows into the conception and penetrating vessels, which control the flow into the womb, permitting menstruation. Menstruation begins during puberty, when the kidney essential qi comes to fullness and the uterus develops. It was traditionally held that before the opening of the conception vessel and the full development of the penetrating vessel, the menses would not start. At the age of about fifty, the penetrating and conception vessels become vacuous as a result of the weakening of essential qi, causing menstrual irregularity, and finally, menopause. This represents the normal, natural course of development, but disruption of menstruation may occur at other times, owing to disorders of the penetrating and conception vessels.

The heart, liver, and spleen

The blood is governed by the heart, stored by the liver, and commanded by the spleen, indicating that all three of these organs have some bearing on menstruation. If the liver fails to store blood or the spleen fails to command the blood, conditions such as menorrhagia, shortening of the menstrual cycle, prolonged menstrual periods, or metrorrhagia may occur. Such conditions are known as the liver and spleen failing to store and command the blood. Underproduction of blood resulting from diminished assimilation of the essence of digestate in splenic vacuity conditions, or heart blood vacuity caused by mental and emotional disturbances, may lead to reduced menstrual flow, prolongation of the menstrual cycle, or even menstrual blockage, all of which fall under the general term of dual vacuity of heart and spleen. Essence-spirit depression may affect hepatic governance of free-coursing, giving rise to liver qi depression, which may also disrupt menstruation.

To sum up, menstruation is not a process that can be dealt with in isolation; it is closely connected to the general physical and mental condition of the individual. Normal menstruation and the conditions for childbearing are especially dependent on kidney essential qi, hepatic free-coursing, and the proper regulation of the penetrating and conception vessels.

The triple burner

The triple burner is the collective term for the upper, middle, and lower burners, and is classified as a hollow organ according to visceral manifestation theory. The hand shao yang triple burner channel passes through all three burners, linking up with many of the organs. The triple burner is an exterior organ, and its corresponding interior organ (for the purposes of acupuncture only) is the pericardium, to which it is connected by the hand jue yin pericardium channel.

The nature of the triple burner has always been the subject of disagreement. The following three points, however, seem to be well established:

The triple burner refers to specific body areas

According to this view, the organs of the human body are divided among three segments, referred to as the upper, middle, and lower burners. The upper burner includes the head and chest, the heart and the lung. The middle burner corresponds to the upper abdomen (the area above the umbilicus) and includes the stomach and the spleen. The lower burner corresponds to the lower abdomen (inferior to the umbilicus) but includes the liver and kidney.

The triple burner represents the waterways

Essential Questions explains, "The triple burner holds the office of the sluices; it manifests as the waterways." This suggests that the main functions of the triple burner are the processing of fluids by the transformative action of qi and ensuring free flow through the waterways, and that as such the transformative action of triple burner qi is a global expression for the roles played by the lung, spleen, kidney, stomach, small intestine, large intestine, and bladder in regulating the body's water metabolism. The *Spiritual Axis* states, "When the triple burner is open and permits effusion, it causes the five sapors of the digestate to diffuse, nourishes the skin, makes the body firm, and keeps the body hair moistened, like the sprinkling of mist and dew. Such is the action of qi." This corroborates with the saying, "the upper burner is like mist," which in practice refers to the diffusion of defense qi and distribution of fluids by the lung. The *Spiritual Axis* states:

> The middle burner . . . strains off the waste and distills the fluids out of which the essence of digestate is formed. This then flows upward into the lung channel where it is transformed into blood.

This supports the phrase, "The middle burner is like foam," which refers to the movement and formation of the essence of digestate by the stomach and spleen, the basis of blood formation.

> In the middle burner, the small intestine connects through to the bladder. . . . It transforms waste that is then sent down to the large intestine. . .and distills the juices, sending them down to the bladder.

Hence, "The lower burner is like a sluice." In actual practice this refers to the small intestine's governance of liquid, the large intestine's governance of humor, and the role of the kidney and bladder in controlling the movement of fluids and discharging urine.

The triple burner is a concept in pattern identification

Triple burner pattern identification represents one method of diagnosing exogenous heat diseases. Diseases of the upper burner include invasion of the lung by exogenous pathogens, construction-aspect pathogen patterns, and anticipated pathogen penetration to the pericardium, which for the most part correspond to first-stage exogenous heat diseases. Diseases of the middle burner include gastrointestinal heat-bind and splenogastric damp-heat, which usually correspond to mid-stage exogenous heat diseases. Diseases of the lower burner include such conditions as deep penetration of pathogens, wearing of kidney yin, insufficiency of liver blood, and yin vacuity wind, which correspond to the advanced stages of exogenous heat diseases. The concept of the three burners and the triple burner method of pattern identification are also used in diagnosing endogenous damage and miscellaneous disorders, but to a much lesser degree and in a less systematized way than that of exogenous heat diseases.

Notes

[1] "Pungent-dissipating lung diffusion" refers to the promotion of lung qi diffusion with pungent, dissipating agents.

[2] Although morphologically there are two kidneys, Chinese medicine regards them as a single unit of function, and as such are they referred in this text.

Chapter 5
Diseases and Their Causes

Under normal circumstances, yin and yang, blood and qi, and the organs and channels complement, support, and counterbalance each other, so that a harmonious balance between all these elements is maintained. This is described in *Essential Questions* in the following way: "When yin is calm and yang is sound, the spirit is undisturbed." Furthermore, there is constant interaction between the human body and the environment, and normally, the relationship between these two is one of balance. Disruption of the physiologic or physio-environmental balances is the starting point of all disease. The *Inner Canon* therefore maintains, "If blood and qi fall into disharmony, a hundred diseases may arise." *Essential Questions* states:

> Yin and yang and the four seasons are the beginning and end of all things, the root of life and death. To go against them is injurious to life; to go with them prevents serious diseases from arising.

Imbalance is attributable to exogenous, endogenous, and independent factors, known collectively as the three disease factor categories. Exogenous factors are causes originating outside the body and include the six environmental excesses and pestilential qi. Endogenous factors are causes originating in the inner body, i.e., affective disturbances. Independent factors are causes resulting from of lack of restraint in daily life, and include dietary irregularities, taxation fatigue (fatigue from mental or physical overexertion), and sexual intemperance. Traumas and parasites are also included in this latter category. In addition, pathologic products such as static blood and phlegm are secondary causes that may be attributed to one or more of these factors.

The balance between yin and yang and the struggle between correct and pathogenic qi are an important aspect of the development of diseases. This subject and the laws of pathogenesis are dealt with below in the section subsequent to disease factors.

Factors of Disease

Exogenous factors

The term "exogenous factors" refers to pathogens that assail the body from outside. They include the six environmental excesses and pestilential qi. These factors represent two major systems of analysis and treatment of exogenous diseases.

The six environmental excesses

The ancient Chinese observed how changes in the environment could directly or indirectly influence the human body, affecting the balance of yin and yang, blood and qi, and channels and the organs. According to the *Spiritual Axis:*

> If thick clothing is worn in hot weather, the striations open and the body perspires.
>
> In cold weather the striations close, qi contracts and becomes less mobile, and water flows down to the bladder, becoming urine.

These quotations illustrate how in spring and summer yang qi effuses and both qi and blood tend to move towards the exterior of the body. At this time, the skin is relaxed and the pores open easily to permit perspiration. Conversely, in the fall and winter, yang qi withdraws and becomes dormant, the skin contracts, the pores open less easily, and sweating is reduced. Such physiologic changes are the body's adaptive response to changes in the natural environment. If this adaptive function is weak, excessively severe or abrupt environmental changes, such as exceptionally hot summers or cold winters, or unseasonable warm or cold spells, may become a factor of disease. Observation of the interaction between the human body and the environment, together with clinical analysis, is the basis of the theory of environmental excess diseases.

The ancient Chinese observed six different environmental conditions: wind, cold, summerheat, damp, dryness, and fire, generally referred to as the six environmental qi's. Only when they cause sickness are they referred to as the six environmental excesses. The diseases caused by these excesses are to some degree seasonal in nature, e.g., summerheat diseases are particularly common in summer, while cold diseases are most prevalent in winter. However, owing to the complexity of environmental changes and the variability of personal factors (such as the individual's particular living environment, psychological makeup, resistance, and constitution), different exogenous pathogens may cause sickness in any season. Furthermore, a given pathogen may cause various disorders. Under the historical conditions of ancient China, it was only possible to discuss causes of these different diseases on the basis of clinical signs. They were therefore classified as wind, cold, summerheat, damp, dryness, and fire pathogens, and the diseases that these engendered were known collectively as exogenous diseases.

The concept of environmental excess diseases and clinical procedures for dealing with them were developed and refined over a long period of practical experience in the art of healing. To identify the offending pathogen, each exogenous disease is analyzed on the basis of clinical signs. Wind dispelling, cold dissipation, damp transformation, heat clearage, dryness moistening, and fire drainage are then prescribed accordingly. This process is known as identifying the pattern, determining the disease factor, and prescribing the appropriate treatment.

Modern clinical research has shown that conditions classified as bacterial and viral infections in Western medicine correspond to the category of environmental excess diseases, and that Chinese medical methods of pattern identification and treatment are effective.

Finally, some diseases attributable to organ dysfunction present signs similar to those of exogenous diseases. These are denoted by the term "endogenous," e.g., endogenous wind. Although arising in the inner body, they are not necessarily attributable to endogenous factors (affective disturbance). Since in many cases these diseases are interrelated with exogenous diseases, they are included in the discussion of the six environmental excesses.

Wind

The nature of wind as a pathogen and its clinical manifestations are similar to those of the meteorological phenomenon from which it derives its name: it comes and goes quickly, moves swiftly, blows intermittently, and sways the branches of the trees. The clinical manifestations of wind as a pathogen bear the following characteristics:

> Rapid onset and swift changes in condition; thus it is said, "Wind is swift and changeable."
> Convulsive spasm, tremor, shaking of the head, dizziness, and migratory pain and itching.
> Invasion of the upper part of the body and the exterior, e.g., the head (the uppermost part of the body), the lung (the uppermost of the major organs), and the surface skin and body hair.

If these signs are present, the disease may be ascribed to a wind pathogen. The ancient Chinese believed that such disorders were caused by the meteorologic phenomenon of wind. However, a subsequent theory posited that an upstirring of yang qi could also give rise to signs similar to those of wind. Liver yang and liver fire can transform to wind, presenting signs of dizziness, tremor, and convulsive spasm. Such conditions are known as liver wind. Furthermore, extreme heat may also engender wind, such conditions being characterized by high fever, spasms, and stiffness of the neck. This is termed extreme heat-stirring wind. Such conditions, occurring during the development of diseases, are clearly not attributable to meteorological phenomenon, and are thus termed endogenous wind. It is thus important to note the difference between endogenous and exogenous wind. It should also be noted that although wind is associated with movement, by giving rise to stiffness and trismus, it can also be seen to have the power to check normal movement.

Cold

The nature of cold as a pathogen and its clinical manifestations are similar to those of cold in the natural environment, e.g., low temperature, deceleration of activity, and congealing. It bears the following features:

> Generalized or local symptoms of cold, such as aversion to cold, desire for warmth, pronounced lack of warmth in the extremities, and cold and pain in the lower abdomen.
>
> Frigid, thin, clear excreta; for example, a running nose with clear mucus, clear phlegm, watery vomitus, long micturition with clear urine, or clear watery diarrhea. *Essential Questions* states, "Any disease characterized by frigid, thin, clear fluids is associated with cold."
>
> Tendency to develop qi stagnation and blood stasis, characterized by severe pain. It has been said, "When cold prevails, there is pain."
>
> Contracture and sinew-vascular hypertonicity, denoting invasion of the channels by cold pathogens; hence it is said, "Cold is associated with contracture and tautness."

Diseases characterized by these signs may be attributed to the cold pathogen, if they occur as a result of severe or sudden exposure to cold, e.g., catching chills, excessive consumption of cold fluids, or exposure to frost. They are also commonly caused by debilitation of the yang qi that keeps the body warm. Such cases are said to be a result of "cold arising from within," and are termed endogenous cold. Exogenous cold and endogenous cold are to some degree mutually conducive. For example, individuals whose yang qi is weak are especially vulnerable to the exogenous cold pathogen; and damage to the body's yang qi by cold can give rise to endogenous cold.

Fire

The characteristic of the fire pathogen is heat. The fire pathogen is basically a heat pathogen. It symptoms are as follows:

> Pronounced generalized or local signs of heat, such as high fever, aversion to heat, desire for coolness, flushed complexion, ocular rubor, dark-colored urine, red tongue, yellow fur, rapid pulse, pain, heat, swelling, and red lesions.
>
> Thick, sticky excreta, such as: thick nasal mucus, thick, yellow phlegm, sour, watery vomitus, murky urine, blood and pus in the stool, acute abdominal diarrhea, or foul-smelling stools, often with a burning sensation on discharge. For this reason *Essential Questions* states, "Turbid water is associated with heat," and "vomiting of sour matter, fulminant downpour, and lower body distress are associated with heat."

Damage to the fluids characterized by dry tongue with little liquid, thirst with desire for cold fluids, and dry, hard stools.

Hemorrhage, and maculopapular eruptions that occur when the fire pathogen scorches the blood and causes frenetic blood movement.

Disturbances of the spirit, such as clouding of spirit-disposition and deranged vision, or manic agitation, confirming the sayings from *Essential Questions:* "Heat patterns characterized by deranged vision are associated with fire," and "excessive agitation and mania are associated with fire."

Distinction is made between repletion fire and vacuity fire. Most of the conditions just described would be classified as repletion fire, the result of either direct contraction of the fire pathogen or the transformation of other pathogens into fire. Wind, cold, damp, and dryness pathogens may, once contracted, transform into fire (heat patterns), so that fire symptoms may appear in the heat stage of most exogenous heat diseases. Vacuity fire is endogenous heat from yin vacuity, and in the main differs from repletion heat in the following ways:

Signs of yin vacuity are present.

The fire and heat symptoms are generally less pronounced than in repletion heat, the most common being restlessness and a red, dry, or mirror tongue.

Generally, there is no high fever.

Thirst, if present, is generally not severe.

The pulse is generally rapid but feeble.

Distinction is also made between endogenous and exogenous fire. Intense fire patterns occurring in exogenous heat diseases are attributable to exogenous fire. Conditions caused by yin-yang imbalance and excesses of the five dispositions are referred to as endogenous fire (or heat). Exogenous fire conditions are repletion fire patterns, while endogenous fire conditions may be either vacuity or repletion fire patterns.

Damp

Damp as a pathogen occurs as damp in the natural environment. It is associated with persistent high humidity from meteorologic or climatic factors and from stagnant water in places where ground drainage is poor. To some extent, it is seasonal in nature, tending to occur when the weather is wet or damp. Sitting and lying in wet places, living in damp conditions, working in a damp or wet environment, or wearing sweat-soaked clothing may cause damp disorders out of damp seasons. The characteristics of damp disorders and their clinical manifestations are as follows:

Damp is clammy, viscous, and persistent. Diseases involving damp are persistent and difficult to cure.

Damp tends to stagnate. When a damp pathogen invades the exterior, the patient may complain of physical fatigue, heavy, cumbersome limbs, and a heavy head. If it invades the channels and the joints, the patient may complain of aching joints and inhibited bending and stretching.

The spleen is particularly vulnerable to damp pathogens. Associated symptoms are: loss of appetite, indigestion, oppression in the chest, heartburn, abdominal distention, thin stool, short micturition with scant urine, thick and slimy tongue fur, and a soggy, moderate pulse.

There may be generalized or local stagnation or accumulation of water-damp, such as water swelling, foot qi disease, vaginal discharge, or exudating lesions such as eczema.

Distinction is made between exogenous and endogenous damp. Endogenous damp patterns occur when the spleen is vacuous and fails to move and transform fluids. These two forms of damp are interrelated and mutually conducive: a vacuous spleen not only makes the body vulnerable to exogenous damp but also may spontaneously give rise to endogenous damp. Exogenous damp entering the body may easily damage the spleen, giving rise to endogenous damp.

Summerheat

Summerheat[1] as a pathogen is seasonal in nature. There are basically two forms: one form is categorically due to summerheat diseases, e.g., sunstroke and heatstroke. The second form is exogenous diseases occurring during hot weather, such as infectious encephalitis B. Conventionally regarded as due to the summerheat pathogen, these are also termed summerheat thermia diseases. Because summerheat as a meteorologic phenomenon is characterized not only by heat but also by humidity (in China), there are two forms:

Summerheat-heat — conditions characterized by high fever, thirst, restlessness, absence of sweating, and a surging pulse. High fever can easily damage qi and fluids, engendering weakness, short, distressed, rapid breathing, and dry tongue fur.

Summerheat-damp — conditions characterized by remittent generalized fever, fatigued limbs, loss of appetite, oppression in the chest, nausea and vomiting, abnormal stool, short micturition with dark-colored urine, soggy pulse, and thick, slimy tongue fur.

Summerheat-heat patterns are essentially heat patterns, while summerheat-damp is heat with damp complications.

Dryness

Dryness as a pathogen has characteristics of the environmental phenomenon of dryness. Dryness that invades the body from the outside is known as exogenous dryness, and normally occurs in dry regions or in dry weather. Symptoms include dry nostrils, nosebleed, dry mouth, dry cracked lips, dry, "tickly" or sore throat, dry cough with little or no phlegm, rough dry skin, and dry tongue with relatively little liquid. Because depletion of the bodily fluids and yin blood presents similar symptoms to those of dryness, it may be regarded as endogenous dryness. Such conditions are not caused by any pathogen, either exogenous or endogenous, but by an insufficiency of blood and fluids. These conditions are usually called damage to fluids, damaged yin, or exhaustion of the blood and fluids.

Pestilential qi

Pestilential qi is a type of disease factor posited by the Ming Dynasty physician Wu You-Ke. His theory concerns widely contagious diseases, which he claimed were due not to wind, cold, summerheat, damp, dryness, or fire, but to pestilential qi transmitted through the nose and mouth. His theory also explicitly states that under certain circumstances, for example, during epidemics, there are numerous kinds of "miscellaneous qi" that enter the body causing sickness. Wu You-Ke maintained that there were far more types of miscellaneous qi than the traditionally recognized pathogens, which numbered only six. He further claimed that the nature of diseases was determined by the nature of the pathogen. This theory is summed in the phrase, "One disease, one qi." This is a remarkably parallel to the concept of viruses in Western medicine.

Endogenous factors

The seven affects — joy, anger, anxiety, preoccupation, sorrow, fear, and fright — are an individual's normal emotional response to their environment. When excessively intense or persistent, the affects may disturb the yin-yang and qi-blood balance and give rise to organ dysfunction. This is known as endogenous damage.

Endogenous damage to the heart and spirit is characterized by palpitation or racing of the heart, poor memory, and insomnia; or abstraction, sorrow or anxiety with tendency to weep, and visceral agitation with frequent stretching and yawning. It may also take the form of fulminant exuberance of heart fire, characterized by manic agitation or essence-spirit derangement. Endogenous damage to the liver may take the form of binding depression of liver qi characterized by essence-spirit depression, irascibility, pain in the lateral costal region, eructation, and globus hystericus.

In women, this condition may give rise to breast lumps, painful distention in the lower abdomen, and menstrual irregularities. Affective disturbance that damages both the heart and spleen takes the form of disquieting of the heart spirit and impairment of splenogastric movement and transformation. This is characterized by attacks of abdominal pain, together with retching and nausea; or borborygmi and diarrhea. Other patterns include glomus and oppression in the chest and venter, little thought of food, and menstrual block. If splenic management of the blood is also impaired, metrorrhagia may also occur.

Emotional factors have a distinct bearing on physical health. In treating endogenous damage conditions, a dual approach is necessary. Patients must be encouraged to deal with their emotional problems, while a proper physical analysis should be made of the state of yin and yang, blood and qi, and the organs. Only in this way is it possible to provide adequate treatment and break the vicious cycle of depression causing sickness and sickness causing depression.

Independent causes

Dietary irregularities

There are three forms of dietary irregularity:

Ingestion of raw, cold, or unclean foodstuffs.[2]
Voracious eating, and overindulgence in fatty and sweet foods.
Habitual consumption of alcohol and hot, spicy foods.

Dietary irregularities may not only affect the spleen and the stomach, causing digestive disruptions, digestate accumulation, stomachache, diarrhea, etc., but in cases of excessive alcohol consumption and overindulgence in sweet and fatty foods, dietary irregularity may create heat, phlegm, and damp. In addition, improper diet may combine with the six environmental excesses to cause disease.

Excessive sexual activity

Excessive sexual activity refers not only to overindulgence in sex, but also to giving birth to too many children. Both may wear kidney essence, thereby weakening the health and increasing vulnerability to disease. Commonly observed signs include pain in the lumbar region, seminal emission, spiritual fatigue and general lack of strength, lassitude, and dizziness. Excessive childbirth may damage the penetrating and conception vessels. This is characterized by menstrual disruptions, menstrual block, and vaginal discharge.

Taxation fatigue

"Taxation" refers to any harmful form of overexertion. *Essential Questions* states:

> Prolonged vision damages the blood; prolonged recumbency damages qi; prolonged sitting damages the flesh; prolonged standing damages the bones; and prolonged walking damages the sinews. These are the five forms of taxation damage.

Taxation fatigue frequently damages the spleen, causing debilitation of original qi characterized by fatigue and weakness, lassitude of essence-spirit, yellow complexion, and emaciation.

Trauma

Traumas include: impact trauma, incised wounds, burns and scalds, and snake bites. Most traumas involve damage to the skin and flesh, the sinews and bone, and the qi and blood. Impact traumas include most bone fractures and sinew damage. Incised wounds primarily lead to loss of blood; burns and scalds cause damage to the skin and flesh and damage to yin. Chinese medicine has had long experience with traumas and has accumulated vast experience, particularly in bone-setting. There is also considerable experience in the use of heat-clearing detoxicants in the treatment of snake bites. In recent years, efforts have been made to restore and improve these methods of treatment.

Parasites

A basic understanding of parasites was gained early in the development of Chinese medicine. Treatment was devised for water poison and tympanic distention, diseases that are now known to be caused by blood flukes. Diseases caused by roundworm, hookworm, pinworm, and tapeworm were even more clearly understood as caused by the parasites lodging in the body, and were known to be connected with unclean food. *The Origin and Outcome of Diseases* by Chao Yuan-Fang of the Sui Dynasty (A.D. 610) clearly states that "whiteworm" (tapeworm) is a result of eating improperly cooked beef. The theory that damp and heat give rise to parasites is attributable to the fact that some intestinal parasitic infestations are associated with splenogastric damp-heat conditions.

Miscellaneous factors

Phlegm

In Chinese medicine, phlegm denotes the viscid mucus secreted in the respiratory channels and pathologic products in the body that are secondary causes of a wide variety of diseases. Phlegm arises as a result of either the impaired fluid movement and transformation associated with morbidity of the lung, spleen, and kidney, or the "boiling" of the fluids by depressed fire. Since disease of the spleen is the most important single cause of phlegm patterns, this organ is said to be the basis of phlegm formation. Phlegm appears in many shapes and forms, for example, phlegm congesting the lung, characterized by expectoration of large amounts of phlegm; phlegm lodging in the stomach, characterized by nausea and vomiting; phlegm lodging in the channels, possibly leading to subcutaneous phlegm nodules; and phlegm confounding the cardiac portals, disturbances of the spirit-disposition, or coma.

Static blood

Blood stasis refers to generalized impairment of the smooth flow of blood, local stagnation of blood in the vessels, or local accumulation of extravasated blood. Static blood, or blood affected by stasis, is a pathologic product. Since it impairs physiologic functions, it is also regarded as a pathogen. Static blood and the morbid changes to which it gives rise are identified by localized pain, stasis macules, and masses, indicating the presence of concretions and gatherings. When blood vessels are blocked by static blood and can no longer withstand, hemorrhage may occur. This is most commonly seen in gynecologic disorders. Generalized signs of blood stasis include a dull complexion, cyan-purple lips and tongue, and stasis macules on the edge of the tongue. The pulse is fine or rough.

The Laws of Pathogenesis

According to Chinese medicine, the various physiologic activities of the human body, the natural flux of yin and yang, the production of blood and qi, and the flow of construction and defense, all have an inherent resistance to disease. This resistance is termed correct qi, or simply "the correct." Pathogenic influences (the six environmental excesses, phlegm, digestate accumulations, static blood, etc.) stand in opposition to this resistance. The relationship between health and disease is a struggle between pathogenic and correct qi; the former is only able to cause disease when the latter is disrupted. When the correct qi is strong or the pathogen is relatively weak, the correct can fend off pathogens and prevent sickness. The *Spiritual Axis* states:

> Though there may be wind, rain, cold, or heat, without vacuity, pathogens alone cannot harm the body. The ability to stand up to raging wind and sudden storms without becoming ill indicates that there is no vacuity allowing harm to the health.

Essential Questions states, "When the correct qi dwells within the body, pathogens cannot enter." Conversely, when the body's correct qi is weak, or the pathogen is relatively strong, the correct fails to ward off pathogens and sickness arises. In another passage, *Essential Questions* states, "For pathogens to enter the body, its qi must be vacuous."

In the concept of the struggle between pathogens and correct qi, emphasis is placed on the notion that disease is not essentially caused by exogenous pathogens, but by imbalance within the body. The subsequent development of disease is seen in terms of changes due to yin-yang and qi-blood imbalance, and disequilibrium among channels and organs. Chinese medicine stresses the resistance factor without neglecting the disease factor.

Chinese medicine looks at the body holistically. It not only sees diseases affecting the whole body as an imbalance of forces, but also takes into account how localized disorders may affect the whole body, and how originally generalized disorders can manifest themselves in localized disorders. For example, erosion of the mouth and tongue, abscesses and gangrenous disease, and clove lesions are all related to general yin-yang and qi-blood imbalance.

Struggle and Imbalance in the Development of Disease

The fundamental cause of disease is the disruption of the natural flux of yin and yang. Pathogens are precipitating factors that can only affect the organism when weakness is present. The pathogen thus stands in opposition to the correct.

The struggle between pathogenic and correct qi and yin-yang imbalance are the common denominators of all disease. Generally speaking, in exogenous heat diseases the struggle between pathogenic and correct qi is more prominent, while in endogenous damage and miscellaneous diseases yin-yang imbalance is the more prominent factor, but the relative importance of these two factors is not immutable.

The struggle between correct qi and the pathogen

Exogenous diseases all involve an exogenous pathogen such as wind, cold, summerheat, damp, dryness, or fire. When an exogenous pathogen enters the body, it meets with the opposition of the correct. The ensuing fight for supremacy between these two forces is the essential characteristic of exogenous diseases. Symptoms of aversion to cold, fever, shivering, and sweating, such as occur during the development of exogenous diseases, are all the manifestations of the organism's fight against the invading pathogen. Under normal circumstances, correct qi gradually gains ascendancy, and the patient eventually recovers. However, under some circumstances, the correct is unable to withstand the attack, and the patient's condition steadily deteriorates, resulting in death. Thus, the patient's fate rests on the relative strength of the two opposing forces. If the correct is stronger, the pathogen weakens and the patient will recover; if the pathogen is stronger and correct qi weakens, the patient's condition will deteriorate.

Prevalence of correct qi and abatement of the pathogen

When correct qi gradually gains prevalence over the pathogen, the disease is eventually eliminated. Although there may be a period when the correct is left weak after the pathogen has abated, the patient then enters the recovery stage in which the damage to qi and blood is repaired and the organs and channels are restored to health.

Exuberance of the pathogen and debilitation of correct qi

If the correct is too weak or the pathogen too strong for the balance between the two forces to be reestablished, the patient's condition will continue to deteriorate. Such a trend culminates in collapse of either yin or yang, when the patient's condition becomes critical. At this point, death follows if treatment fails to eliminate the pathogen and restore correct qi.

Some diseases are not resolved so decisively. The pathogen and the correct may come to a deadlock, or the pathogen may be eliminated leaving correct qi severely damaged. For instance, an acute disease may change into a chronic disease, or sickness may leave the patient with aftereffects, preventing the swift recovery of qi, blood, and the organs. The prevention and treatment of such eventualities require special care.

Clinical experience shows that when the chief imbalance is between the pathogen and the correct, the most effective method of treatment is "attack." Attack, sometimes referred to as offensive treatment, is the use of potent drugs to eliminate the pathogen. Exterior resolution, heat clearage, detoxification, draining-precipitation (purgation), phlegm dispersion, damp transformation, water disinhibition, and stasis breaking are examples of attack. Support may be given to the correct, but only as it enhances attack or braces the interior in the face of imminent penetration of pathogens from the exterior. This dual approach is exemplified by such methods as dispelling the pathogen and preserving the correct, and supporting the correct and outthrusting the pathogen, specific forms of which include enriching yin and resolving the exterior, and boosting qi and disinhibiting water. In some cases, a two-stage approach is adopted. In supplementation followed by attack, for example, correct qi is first strengthened to minimize the damaging effects of the offensive treatment that follows. Only after the struggle between the correct and pathogenic qi has ceased, when the pathogen has been eliminated but correct qi is weak, can supplementation be used as the principal approach.

Imbalance between yin and yang

Yin and yang describe all mutually complementary and counterbalancing forces in the human body. When the natural flux of yin and yang is maintained, the body is healthy. When a surfeit or deficit of either complement develops, the balance is disrupted and disease arises.

Although imbalance between yin and yang can be said to be at the root of all diseases from incipience to resolution, in the case of exogenous diseases, the struggle between the correct and the pathogen is always the more pronounced characteristic and the decisive factor determining the outcome. An imbalance between yin and yang is always present, though it is of relatively less importance. However, in endogenous damage and miscellaneous diseases, though a struggle between resistance and pathogen is not entirely absent, the imbalance between yin and yang is of relatively greater importance. For instance, breakdown of cardiorenal interaction and hyperactivity of yang due to yin vacuity are both characterized by a predominance of the imbalance between yin and yang.

It should be understood that a different method of treatment must be used for each different condition. Conditions essentially characterized by a struggle between the correct and a pathogen should be treated by eliminating the pathogen and restoring correct qi (as discussed above). Diseases primarily involving a yin or yang imbalance are treated by restoring that balance, by eliminating surfeits and supplying deficits. Because imbalances essentially caused by surfeits of either yin or yang occur mostly in exogenous diseases, the imbalance is restored by the method of dispelling the pathogen and supporting the correct. Imbalances resulting from deficit of either complement, as mostly found in endogenous diseases, require determining which complement is in deficit. If yang is vacuous, it must be strengthened; if yin is vacuous, it must be nourished. Blood vacuities are treated by nourishing the blood, and qi vacuities by boosting qi.

The relative importance of the struggle between correct qi and the pathogen on one hand, and the yin-yang imbalance on the other, is not immutably fixed. Predominance may shift from one factor to another. The struggle between the correct and the pathogen, normally the predominant factor in exogenous disease, may cause such serious damage to yang qi or yin humor that the yin-yang factor becomes predominant. The dual yin and yang vacuity seen in the final stages of exogenous diseases is an example of this. Shifts are also seen in endogenous damage and miscellaneous diseases. For example, splenic vacuity, a yin-yang disorder, may engender damp and lead to the development of phlegm-rheum. The resulting condition is characterized by predominance of the body's struggle against the pathogen. A similar example is seen in insufficiency of kidney yang, where failure of qi to transform water leads to gathering of water in the form of edema.

Notes

[1] We write "summerheat" as a single word to ensure greater clarity when occurring in combinations, such as "summerheat-heat."

[2] Traditional texts frequently refer to raw food as a cause of disease owing largely to poor water purification.

Part II
Pattern Identification and Treatment

Chapter 6
The Four Examinations

Visual examination, audio-olfactive examination, inquiry, and palpation are referred to as the four examinations. Together, they are the basic method of learning about a patient's condition. Visual examination involves observing the patient's spirit, tongue, complexion, and overall appearance, as well as his excreta. Audio-olfactive examination involves observing the quality of voice, enunciation, and verbal expression, listening to respiration and coughing sounds, and smelling the body and excreta. Inquiry mainly involves questioning the patient about the development of the illness, the present symptoms, and any previous treatment. Palpation comprises taking the pulse and palpating relevant parts of the body. In practice, visual tongue examination and pulse palpation represent the most important sources of the information required for diagnosis. Strictly speaking, however, accurate diagnosis can be made only by synthesizing data from all four examinations.

Data obtained through the four examinations is correlated to physiological and pathological theory (i.e., visceral manifestation theory, channel theory, pathogen theory), to create a comprehensive picture of the patient's condition. Under certain circumstances, Western methods may be used to provide additional information for diagnosis.

Visual Examination

In visual examination, the physician observes the patient's general physical appearance, paying special attention to any part relevant to the presenting condition. Apart from observing the patient's spirit, overall appearance, and complexion, the physician also carefully examines the tongue, which can provide invaluable information about the state of the bowels and viscera.

Observing the spirit

"Spirit" in this context refers to a combination of the patient's facial expression, complexion, bearing, quality of voice, enunciation and verbal expression, and consciousness. It is said, "If the patient is spirited, he is fundamentally healthy; if he is spiritless, he is doomed." Conditions of the spirit may be arranged in three fundamental categories: spiritedness, spiritlessness, and false-spiritedness. The spirit sheds useful light on the severity of a given complaint.

Spiritedness

If the patient has bright eyes, normal bearing, clear speech, and responds coherently to inquiry, the condition is said to be spirited, indicating that correct qi is undamaged and the complaint is relatively minor. Although certain aspects of the patient's health may be seriously affected, swift improvement may be expected.

Spiritlessness

Essence-spirit debilitation, apathy, abnormal bearing, torpid expression, dark complexion and dull eyes, low voice, slow, halting speech, and incoherent response to inquiry are signs of a spiritless condition. They indicate a relatively serious condition in which correct qi has suffered damage. Although no critical signs may be present, extreme care is necessary. Where a spiritless condition is particularly marked, there may be signs of deranged speech, stupor of the spirit-disposition, carphologia, and a general feeling of heaviness preventing the patient from turning over in bed.

False-spiritedness

False-spiritedness generally occurs in enduring or severe illness and extremely severe cases of essence-spirit debilitation. If, suddenly, during a disease characterized by taciturnity, a low voice, halting speech, and an extremely dark complexion, the patient becomes strangely garrulous and his cheeks are flushed and unusually rosy, this new condition is said to be one of false-spiritedness. Such conditions are extremely serious and should not be mistaken for improvement. False-spiritedness implies a superficial improvement in certain aspects of the patient's mental state, which does not fit in with other aspects of the condition. It is a sign that the patient's condition will soon deteriorate dramatically, and therefore demands special attention.

Observing general physical appearance

This part of the examination involves inspecting the patient's body to see whether it is thin or fat, strong or weak, and observing the patient's movements.

Observing the body

A well-developed, strong, firm body indicates a strong constitution. Poor development and emaciation indicate a weak constitution.

Obesity with soft muscles, white, lusterless skin, diminished qi, lack of strength, and lack of essence-spirit vitality indicate what is known as a full form with vacuous qi, implying a physical constitution characterized by a yang qi vacuity. Such conditions are often seen in diseases described by Western medicine as endocrine disturbances, hypothyroidism, and some forms of hypertension.

Thinness and pallor, emaciation, and dry skin indicate insufficiency of yin-blood, generally seen in constitutional yin vacuity. Such conditions occur often in cases of tuberculosis, which has lead to the maxim, "The thin are prone to taxation coughs."

Observing the bearing

Flailing of the limbs, agitation and talkativeness, or manic agitation and dislike of restricting clothing or bedclothes usually indicates a yang disorder, i.e., one due to heat or repletion.

A patient who sleeps curled up, is uncommunicative, suffers from a general feeling of heaviness and difficulty in movement, and who keeps his body well wrapped, is usually suffering from a yin disorder, i.e., one of cold or vacuity.

"Groping in the air and pulling at invisible strings" and carphologia indicate that the illness has reached its most advanced stage and that the condition is serious.

Wry eyes and mouth, convulsive spasm of the limbs, shaking of the head, and twitching of the lips or cheeks are conditions mostly attributable to endogenous liver wind. Pronounced forceful spasm is usually seen in repletion heat patterns while milder forms are usually indicative of vacuity wind.

Rigidity of the neck, opisthotonos, and trismus indicate tetanic diseases.

Hypertonicity in the limbs inhibiting normal bending and stretching, and rigidity, distention, and deformation of the joints usually indicate obturation.

Limp, powerless limbs, or reduced prehensile and locomotive ability, indicate atony patterns.

If the patient suffers from rapid breathing while recumbent, and is thus forced to sit up, an exuberant pathogen is present and correct qi is vacuous. Dizziness experienced when sitting up, confining the patient to a recumbent posture, usually indicates either a vacuity pattern or phlegm turbidity harassing the upper body, depending on the other symptoms.

Observing the complexion

The state of blood and qi is intimately related to the facial complexion. The *Spiritual Axis* states, "The qi and blood of the twelve primary channels and the 365 connecting channels {all the channels of the body} rise to the face." It can be inferred from this that the facial complexion is of particular importance when observing the general bodily complexion of a patient.

The color of the complexion is analyzed in terms of the colors corresponding to the five phases. The five colors — cyan, red, yellow, white, and black — are primary colors from which the infinite gamut of hues is derived. When applied to the human complexion, they take on a relative significance. Thus, two people who have vastly different complexions when healthy, may be described as having an equally "white" complexion when suffering from a certain disease, even though the actual color is different. "White" here refers to a relative paling by comparison with the normal complexion. A healthy Chinese complexion is of a pale ochre hue with a slight reddish luster, though it may darken markedly when exposed to wind and sun. The five colors may therefore be similarly applied to the skins of all races.

Observing the complexion of the entire body also involves paying attention to the presence of maculopapular eruptions and miliaria.

Observing the facial complexion

White complexion

White (or pale) complexions usually indicate cold or vacuity. A drained white complexion with facial vacuity edema generally indicates yang qi vacuity and occurs after massive bleeding, in chronic nephritis, or in wheezing dyspnea patterns. A pale white, lusterless complexion, together with general and facial emaciation, normally points to blood vacuity. The *Spiritual Axis* states, "Blood desertion is characterized by a white, perished, and sheenless complexion." The sudden appearance of a somber white complexion in acute diseases is usually attributable to fulminant yang qi desertion and is seen in various forms of shock. However, somber white may also be observed in cases of exogenous wind-cold diseases characterized by aversion to cold, shivering, and severe abdominal pain due to interior cold.

In addition, there are grayish white macules that occur in infantile ringworm, known as ringworm patches.

Cyan complexion

Cyan or bluish complexions are principally associated with wind-cold, blood stasis, pain, and qi-block patterns. Infantile fright-wind and epilepsy are characterized by a dark, cyan complexion. A grayish cyan complexion with cyan-purple lips is associated with inner body blood stasis and impaired flow of qi and blood, and occurs in diseases classified in Western medicine as cirrhosis of the liver and cardiac failure. In severe wind-cold headaches and abdominal pain due to interior cold, impeded flow of yang qi may be reflected in a bluish somber white complexion. In cases of blocked lung qi, a dark, cyan-purple complexion may result from obstructed flow of blood and qi. This corresponds to conditions such as pulmogenic heart disorders and asphyxia in Western medicine.

Red complexion

Red complexions generally occur in heat patterns, with distinction being made between vacuity heat and repletion heat. Exogenous wind-heat diseases are characterized by a red face and ocular rubor. Interior repletion heat patterns are characterized by tidal flushing of the face, heavy sweating, thirst, constipation, and other signs of repletion heat. A somber white complexion with tidal flushing of the cheeks in the afternoon indicates yin vacuity fire effulgence. In severe illnesses characterized by cold sweats, inversion frigidity in the limbs, etc., a sober white complexion with flushed, unusually rosy cheeks indicates *dai yang,* or overfloating of vacuity yang, critical signs of imminent outward desertion of yang qi. In addition, in some severe or enduring illnesses, signs such as those described in the *Spiritual Axis* may appear: "If red, thumb-sized flushes appear on the cheeks, although there may be slight improvement, death will ensue promptly."

Yellow complexion

Yellow is associated with dampness and vacuity. Yellowing of the sclerae and generalized yellowing of the skin indicate jaundice. A vivid yellow indicates damp-heat and is known as yang yellow. A dark yellow color points to cold-damp, and is known as yin yellow. Yang yellow is seen mostly in cases described in Western medicine as acute icteric infectious hepatitis, acute cholecystitis, cholelithiasis, and toxic hepatitis; yin yellow occurs in cirrhosis of the liver and cancer of the head of the pancreas. A pale yellow skin that is dry and puffy, accompanied by pale lips but no yellowing of the sclerae, is referred to as withered yellow, a vacuity yellow. The condition characterized by this complexion is sometimes called yellow swelling, and is normally caused by excessive loss of blood or depletion of blood and qi after major illnesses, or by splenogastric damage resulting from intestinal parasites. It may thus be seen in diseases known in Western medicine as ankylostomiasis (hookworm disease), anemia, and malnutrition due to poor assimilation.

Black complexion

Black is associated with kidney vacuity and blood stasis. A soot-black complexion, dark gray complexion, or purple-black complexion may occur in enduring diseases, patterns characterized by kidney essence depletion, or in static blood accumulation patterns. In Western medicine, a soot-black complexion may be seen in chronic hyperadrenocorticalism, or in the final stages of cirrhosis of the liver. A dark gray complexion may be seen in chronic kidney dysfunction; and a purple-black complexion may occur in chronic cardiopulmonary dysfunctions.

A black complexion indicates intractable or severe illness. *Essential Prescriptions of the Golden Coffer* states that "black jaundice" is associated with kidney vacuity and blood stasis, and usually indicates that the condition is hard to cure.

Maculopapular eruptions

Macules and papules are symptoms of many diseases. Their appearance and disappearance, form and color, and distribution can provide valuable information about a patient's condition.

The appearance of maculopapular eruptions in exogenous heat diseases indicates heat-penetrating blood-construction. Macules are not raised above the surface of the skin and vary in size. Papules are like grains of millet in shape and size, and are raised above the surface of the skin. Provided that they are not too dense or widespread, maculopapular eruptions indicate that correct qi is capable of expelling pathogenic qi from the body. Thus it is said, "The appearance of macules and papules is a favorable sign, provided they are not in excess." The absence of such lesions may indicate a pathogen blockage. In excess, they indicate that the pathogen is strong. Macules reflect more serious conditions than papules; for example, intense toxic heat in the blood aspect. Therefore, careful attention should be paid to them.

Maculopapular eruptions are a favorable sign when red in color, and an unfavorable sign when dark. Deep red indicates intense heat, while purplish black indicates intense toxic heat in the blood aspect, a sign that the condition is extremely serious. A dark, blackish color indicates that correct qi is seriously debilitated, and the condition is critical. However, the significance of lesions can only be judged in correlation with other symptoms. *A Treatise on Thermic Heat Diseases* states, "They {macules and papules} must be viewed together with other external signs before a diagnosis can be made."

Maculopapular eruptions may also occur in endogenous damage and miscellaneous diseases, usually indicating blood heat. If they continually appear and disappear, are purplish red in color, and if signs of blood heat are absent, maculopapular eruptions indicate the failure of the qi to contain the blood. Qi vacuity with a blood stasis complication may also be indicated. If the eruptions are deep-seated and well-defined, the condition is serious. Deep-seated eruptions do not blanch when pressure is applied. Well-defined eruptions have clear edges or are characterized by localized tissue necrosis. If the edges are not well-defined, and the color fades under pressure, the condition is mild.

Miliaria

Miliaria alba appears as small white vesicles and often occurs in damp thermic diseases. It is usually located on the neck, but may spread down the upper arms and abdomen. It only occurs when there is sweating. Although its appearance usually indicates that the damp-heat is able to escape from the body, it also shows that the damp pathogen is viscous and resists transformation. For this reason there is recurrent outthrust. When miliaria takes the form of clear, plump vesicles, it is known as miliaria crystallina (sudamina) and is a positive sign. If it is a dull white, containing no fluid, it is known as dry miliaria, and indicates exhaustion of liquid qi.[1]

Maculopapular eruptions and miliaria are not considered negative signs if, once having appeared, they gradually disappear. But if, having developed erratically, they suddenly disappear, they indicate a critical condition where correct qi is debilitated and a pathogenic toxin has penetrated the interior.

When conducting the visual examination, the physician must also look for the presence of dilated abdominal veins (caput medusae) and spider nevi. Spider nevi are categorized as "red marks" in Chinese medicine. They are the result of blood amassment.

Other skin lesions belong to the field of external medicine and are beyond the scope of this book.

Digital venule examination

Digital venule examination involves observing the appearance of the venules just below the surface of the skin on the radial palmar aspect of the index finger. It is only applicable to infants under three years of age. Subsequent natural thickening of the skin makes the venules increasingly indistinct. Digital venule examination provides supplementary diagnostic data that is particularly useful in judging the severity of disease. It also helps to compensate for difficulties of pulse examination that are due to the infant's very short radial pulse, which must be taken with only one finger, and to disturbances of the pulse that result from the distress commonly experienced by children in unfamiliar surroundings.

The finger is divided into three segments, known as barriers. The first segment, from the metacarpophalangeal joint to the proximal interphalangeal joint, is known as the wind barrier. The second segment, from the proximal interphalangeal joint to the distal interphalangeal joint, is known as the qi barrier. The final segment, from the distal interphalangeal joint to the fingertip, is called the vital barrier.

The examination should be conducted in good light. Using thumb and index finger, the physician holds the child's fingertip. Then, using the other thumb, the child's finger is gently rubbed from the tip downwards several times. This makes the veins more distinct.

In healthy children, the veins appear as dimly visible, pale purple to reddish brown lines. Generally, they are visible in the wind barrier only. When the child is sick, the color and degree of fullness of the venules may change. Venules that are particularly distinct and close to the surface indicate an exterior pattern. If the venules are bright red they indicate contraction of an exogenous pathogen. If they are located at a deeper level, a pathogen is present in the interior. Purplish red venules indicate heat; cyan venules indicate wind-cold, fright-wind, a pain pattern, ingesta damage, or ascendant counterflow of phlegm and qi. Black generally indicates blood stasis. A visually discernible impairment of blood flow through the venules is associated with repletion patterns such as phlegm-damp, digestate stagnation, or binding depression of pathogenic heat.

If the venules are distinct only in the wind barrier, the condition is relatively mild. If they are also distinct in the qi barrier, the condition is more serious. Extension of visible venules through all the barriers to the fingertip indicates a critical condition.

To sum up simply, the depth of the venules indicates the depth of penetration into the interior. Red indicates heat, cyan indicates cold; pale indicates vacuity, and a stagnant appearance indicates repletion. The degree of penetration through the barriers indicates the severity of the condition.

Tongue examination

The significance of the tongue examination

Tongue examination provides some of the most important data for pattern identification. The tongue objectively reflects the state of qi and blood, progression and regression of disease, the degree of heat and cold, and the depth of pathogen penetration. Changes in the appearance of the tongue are particularly pronounced in exogenous heat diseases and disorders of the stomach and spleen. The ancient Chinese said, "The tongue is the shoot of the heart," and "the tongue is the external indicator of the stomach and spleen."

However, in clinical practice, serious illnesses are not necessarily reflected in major changes in the appearance of the tongue. Furthermore, normal healthy individuals may show abnormal changes in the appearance of the tongue. Therefore, the data provided by the tongue examination must be carefully weighed against other signs and symptoms, the pulse, and the patient's history, before an accurate diagnosis can be made.

The method of tongue examination

Distinction is made between the body of the tongue and the tongue fur. Examination of the body of the tongue involves observing color, form, and movement. Examination of the tongue fur involves observing color and nature.

When examining the tongue, the following four points should be kept in mind:

Light

The tongue examination should be conducted in adequately lit surroundings, with light shining directly into the mouth. Inadequate lighting may blur color differences, such as the difference between yellow and white, or red and purple.

Stained fur

Some foods and medicines affect the color of the fur, and potentially the diagnosis. Milk and soya bean milk stain the tongue fur white; coffee, tea, and tobacco leave brown stains; egg yolk, oranges, Rhizoma Coptidis *(huáng lián)*, and Gelatinum Corii Asini *(lǘ pí jiāo)* leave yellow stains. Staining normally affects only the surface of the fur, and is washed away by saliva. If in doubt, the physician should ask the patient if anything that may have caused staining has been eaten.

The bearing of the tongue on extension

The patient should ensure that the tongue is relaxed and flat when extended. Forced or tense protraction may deepen the color of the tongue.

Miscellaneous factors

Consumption of rough foodstuffs or chewing gum may remove the tongue fur and deepen the color of the tongue body. Patients with missing teeth may tend to chew food on one side of the mouth, which may cause irregularities in fur distribution. In windstrike patients, motor impairment of the tongue may cause an increase in tongue fur. In patients tending to breathe through the mouth owing to nasal congestion or other factors, the surface of the tongue may be abnormally dry. Such changes in the tongue and tongue fur should not be mistaken as reflecting internal morbidity.

Observing the form of the tongue

Enlargement

A swollen tongue, with dental impressions on the margin, is known as an enlarged tongue, and indicates qi vacuity or the presence of water-damp. An enlarged tongue that is pale in color, with a white, glossy fur, indicates qi vacuity. With a slimy tongue fur, enlargement generally indicates damp or damp-heat. In Western medicine, tongue enlargement may be seen in myxedema, chronic nephritis, and chronic gastritis, and is thought to be due to hyperplasia of the connective tissue, tissue edema, or blood and lymphatic drainage disturbances. Enlargement is markedly different from a painful, swollen, red tongue, which characterizes an intense heat pathogen or upflaming of heart fire.

Shrinkage

A thin, shrunken tongue indicates a yin liquid vacuity or a dual vacuity of yin and qi. A shrunken tongue due to damage to yin humor by exuberant heat is crimson in color and dry. In dual yin and qi vacuities, the tongue is pale in color. Modern clinical observation shows that shrinkage generally occurs in the latter stages of exogenous heat diseases, and in conditions described in Western medicine as pulmonary tuberculosis, and in advanced-stage carcinoma. It is explained as atrophy of the lingual muscle and epithelium due to malnutrition.

Red speckles and prickles

Red speckles and prickles appear on the tip or margins of the tongue and indicate exuberant heat. They occur in various exogenous heat diseases, particularly yang ming repletion heat patterns, and in conjunction with maculopapular eruptions. Speckles, prickles, and pain in the tongue may also occur in patients suffering from insomnia or constipation or those working late at night. According to Western medicine, speckles and prickles are due to an increase in the size or number of fungiform papillae.

Fissures

Fissures vary in depth and position. Occurring in conjunction with a dry tongue, they indicate fluid vacuity. They may also occur in exuberant heat patterns, in conjunction with a crimson tongue. Fissures are seen by Western medicine to be the result of mucosal atrophy, chiefly associated with chronic glossitis, and in 0.5% of cases to causes wholly unrelated to disease.

Mirror tongue

A completely smooth tongue, free of liquid and fur, is sometimes referred to as a mirror tongue and indicates severe yin humor depletion. A smooth, red or deep red tongue indicates damage to yin by intense heat. If pale in color, a smooth tongue indicates damage to both qi and yin. According to recent clinical observation, the mirror tongue mostly occurs in the latter stages of glossitis, but may also be seen in vitamin B deficiencies, anemia, and the latter stages of certain diseases. It is attributable to shrinkage of the filiform and fungiform papillae.

Observing the bearing of the tongue

Stiffness

If the tongue moves sluggishly, inhibiting speech, it is called a stiff tongue. This occurs in a number of serious diseases, such as heat entering the pericardium, phlegm confounding the cardiac portals, phlegm obstructing the connecting channels, and liver wind stirring in the inner body. Other signs are therefore decisive in determining the nature of the disease. In Western medicine, a stiff tongue generally indicates diseases of the central nervous system.

Limpness

A tongue that is soft and floppy, moves with difficulty, and cannot be extended, is known as a limp tongue. When limpness is due to intense heat or to yin humor depletion, the tongue is also red or deep red, and dry. In qi and blood depletion, it is limp and pale. In Western medicine, a limp tongue is seen as a sign of neurologic disorders or lesions affecting the lingual muscle.

Trembling

If the tongue trembles when it moves, the cause is ascendant hyperactivity of liver yang, endogenous wind stirred by exuberant heat, or qi vacuity. In the first two cases, the tongue is red or deep red, while in qi vacuity the tongue is pale. Synthesized Western and Chinese clinical observation shows that trembling of the tongue occurs in high fever, hyperthyroidism, hypertension, and a number of neurologic disorders.

Wry tongue

In cases of windstrike due to endogenous liver wind or phlegm obstructing the connecting channels, the tongue often inclines to one side. Synthesized clinical observation associates a wry tongue with disorders of the hypoglossal nerve or intracranial lesions.

Contraction

Contraction of the tongue preventing extension is a critical sign in most cases. The cause is either damage to yin by extreme heat or fulminant yang qi desertion. A short frenulum due to congenital factors may also prevent extension.

Worrying

Habitual extension of the tongue and licking of the lips is known as a worrying tongue. It is a sign of cardiosplenic heat, and heralds the stirring of wind. It also occurs in mentally retarded children.

Observing the color of the tongue

The normal color of the tongue is a pale red. In tongue diagnosis, the term "pale" denotes any color paler than normal, while "red" denotes a color deeper than normal. If considerably deeper in color, the term "crimson" is used. A "cyan-purple" tongue is a red tongue with a blue, or in pronounced cases, indigo hue. Changes in the color of the body of the tongue reflect the state of blood and qi and the severity of disease. In Western medicine, changes in the tongue color are explained by changes in blood chemistry, in the viscosity of the blood, and by hyperplasia or atrophy of the epithelial cells of the glossal mucosa.

Pale Tongue

A pale tongue indicates vacuity qi and blood. A pale, enlarged, well-moistened tongue accompanying cold signs indicates yang qi vacuity. In Western medicine, a pale tongue is associated with the latter stages of schistosomiasis, chronic nephritis, carcinoma, and various forms of anemia, and is seen as the result of a reduction of red corpuscles, disruption of protein metabolism, and tissue edema.

Red Tongue

A red tongue indicates heat, due to either vacuity or repletion.

Crimson Tongue

A crimson tongue is also associated with heat, but the added depth of color indicates that the heat is located in the construction or blood aspect.

Red and crimson coloring of the tongue, according to synthesized clinical observation, is associated with fever due to infection, burns, postoperative conditions, advanced carcinoma, hyperthyroidism, cirrhotic ascites, and tuberculosis. It is thought to be due to inflammation of the tongue causing dilation of the capillary vessels of the glossal mucosa.

Purple Tongue

Purple coloration indicates an impaired flow of blood and qi leading to congealing blood stasis. This is a part of either heat or cold patterns. A generalized cyan-purple coloration indicates severe blood stasis. Purple macules indicate less severe or localized blood stasis. A glossy cyan-purple tongue characterizes cold patterns caused by failure of yang qi to warm and move the blood. A reddish purple, dry tongue indicates binding blood stasis due to penetration of heat to the blood aspect. Purple coloration is seen in diseases classified in Western medicine as cirrhosis of the liver, heart diseases, asthma, cholecystitis, ulcerations, and gynecologic disorders. It is associated with hemostasis of the blood in the portal vein and superior vena cava.

Observing the tongue fur

Healthy people have a thin layer of fur on their tongue, which is due to upward steaming of stomach qi. Tongue furs are categorized as glossy, dry, thick, thin, clean, slimy, unclean, and peeling.

Moistness

A healthy tongue is kept moist naturally by saliva. A tongue covered with a transparent or semitransparent film of fluid is described as having a glossy fur, and indicates damp-phlegm or cold-damp. Exuberant damp due to splenic vacuity is characterized by a slimy, glossy fur in association with splenogastric signs of oppression in the chest, nausea, and diarrhea. Yang vacuity water-flood is characterized by white, glossy tongue fur, as well as symptoms of frigidity of the limbs and edematous swelling. A dry fur is generally indicative of heat. A tongue that is so dry that it looks rough, and feels dry or even prickly to the touch, is described as being "rough." It is mainly seen in exogenous heat diseases and indicates damage to humor by exuberant heat. However, failure of fluids to reach the upper body in patients suffering from center phlegm-damp obstruction may also cause a dry fur. In such cases, the dryness is less severe; some degree of sliminess is present and the patient experiences thirst without any urge to drink. Western medical research shows that the moistness of the tongue depends on saliva secretion, viscosity, and evaporation speed. Dryness of the surface of the tongue is the most pronounced sign of dehydration.

Thickness

The tongue fur is regarded as thin if the underlying tongue surface shows through faintly, whereas a thick fur is one that blots out the tongue surface completely. The thickness of the tongue fur is an index of pathogen exuberance, progression, and regression. A thick fur indicates a strong pathogen, while a thin fur indicates a weak pathogen. If the fur thickens the condition is advancing; if the fur thins, it is said to be transforming, and the condition is improving. Synthesized research shows that the thickness of the tongue fur is associated with the length of the filiform papillae. If the papillae are long, the tongue fur is thick; if short, the fur is thin.

Clean, slimy, and unclean furs

An extremely fine fur with a grainy appearance is described as clean fur, and is a normal healthy fur. If the fur is thicker, appears as a layer of mucus covering the tongue, and no longer has its normal grainy appearance, it is described as slimy fur. If the mucus layer looks dirty, the terms unclean fur, slimy fur, or turbid slimy fur are used. A slimy fur indicates damp, phlegm, and digestate accumulations (q.v. Chapter 5). These pathogens are said to be extremely strong when the slimy coating is "generalized," that is, covering the entire tongue. A slimy fur that covers only the center or the root of the tongue indicates a chronic condition, and does not transform (i.e., disappear) easily. An unclean slimy fur indicates, on the one hand, the presence of turbid pathogens such as turbid damp and turbid phlegm, and on the other, stomach qi vacuity. In stomach qi vacuity attention must be paid to safeguarding stomach qi when dispelling the pathogen. Synthesized research attributes slimy tongue furs to an increase in the number of filiform papillae and their branches, and the collection of mucus, putrid matter, and sloughed epithelial cells between the papillae.

Peeling

A patchy fur interspersed with mirror-like, furless areas is known as peeling fur. This generally indicates insufficiency of yin humor and vacuous stomach qi. A peeling fur in conjunction with a non-transforming slimy fur indicates non-transformed phlegm-damp, damage to yin humor and stomach qi, and suggests that the pattern is complex. A thick, slimy fur that suddenly completely peels away indicates major damage to correct qi.

Observing the fur color

White fur

The clinical significance of a white tongue fur is fourfold. Thin, white, clean, moist fur is normal and healthy, but may also appear at the onset of sickness indicating that the pathogen has not yet entered the interior and correct qi remains undamaged. Glossy white fur indicates cold; thin, glossy white fur indicates exogenous wind-cold or endogenous cold. Thick, glossy white fur indicates cold-damp or cold-phlegm. Dry white fur indicates transformation of the cold pathogen into heat. Thin, extremely dry white fur indicates insufficiency of fluids; thick, dry fur indicates transformation of damp into dryness. White, floury fur with a red tongue body indicates impeded damp and deep-lying heat, which is treated by first transforming the damp to allow the heat to escape rather than with excessive use of cool agents. Thick, slimy white fur indicates phlegm damp, and is usually accompanied by a sickly taste in the mouth, oppression in the chest, and dyspeptic anorexia.

White fur occurs in a variety of disorders. Synthesized research views it as an essentially normal phenomenon. Thick white fur is mainly associated with hypertrophy of the corneal layer of the filiform papillae for unknown reasons.

A white, mold-like coating covering the tongue and the whole of the surface of the oral cavity, or small patches of mucosal erosion known as erosion spots, are termed oral putrefaction. A cottage cheese fur is a lumpy, easily removable fur classically compared to crumbs of beancurd. These symptoms indicate the development of sweltering damp-heat in patterns of damage to yin by gastric vacuity. This generally occurs in enduring or serious illnesses and indicates complex patterns that are difficult to treat.

Yellow fur

A yellow fur usually signifies heat. Because heat patterns vary in severity and may involve different pathogens, different forms of yellow fur are distinguished. Thin, dry, yellow fur indicates damage to liquid by the heat pathogen, posing the need to safeguard liquid. Slimy yellow fur usually indicates damp-heat. Old yellow fur (dark yellow) and burnt yellow fur (blackish yellow) indicate binding of repletion heat. Mixed white and yellow fur indicates the initial stages of the transformation of cold into heat that is associated with pathogen interiorization.

Synthesized research suggests that yellow fur is associated with the infectious stage of inflammatory conditions and is mainly attributable to hypoplasia of the filiform papillae, coloring by bacteria, and localized manifestation of an inflammatory disease.

Black fur

Black fur may occur in cold, heat, repletion, and vacuity patterns, but most commonly indicates an exuberant pathogen. A rough, dry, black fur, somewhat parched in appearance, together with a red or deep red tongue body, indicates damp-heat transforming into dryness or damage to yin by intense heat. Usually, a thick, slimy black fur indicates a phlegm-damp complication. A glossy black fur signifies either gastric or renal vacuity. A slimy yellow fur with a grayish black coating is generally indicative of an exuberant damp-heat pathogen. A mixed gray and white fur or a gray, thin, slimy, glossy fur is generally indicative of cold-damp.

Synthesized research shows that black fur is most often seen in acute pyogenic infections, such as toxemia, gangrenous appendicitis, peritonitis, and cholecystitis. However, it may also occur in disorders such as chronic bronchitis and uremia. It mostly corresponds to what Western medicine calls a black, hairy fur. Opinions differ as to the exact causes of black fur. Explanations include: growth of bacteria after long administration of antibiotics, absorption by the tongue fur of iron present in blood from minor bleeding in the oral cavity, and high fever and loss of fluid.

Organ correspondences in tongue examination

Though subject to argument, some correspondence between parts of the tongue surface and the viscera is accepted. It is generally thought that the root of the tongue is related to the kidney, which in a sense is the root of the body. The center of the tongue's surface is said to reflect the condition of the spleen and stomach, which are at the body's center. The tip of the tongue reveals the condition of the heart. Agreement ends here. Some texts state that the condition of the liver and gallbladder is reflected on the sides of the tongue, and that the lung is reflected at the tip. In other sources, the left side of the tongue is assigned to the lung, and the right side to the liver. A few other variations may also be found. In view of these inconsistencies, organ correspondences should always be correlated with data from the other examinations.

The tongue examination is ascribed an important place in the four examinations. The body of the tongue is of greatest significance in judging the strength of correct qi. It may also provide an indication of the severity of the condition, as in the case of a pale tongue, which indicates blood and qi vacuity, or a deep red tongue, which indicates yin vacuity or penetration of pathogenic heat to the construction aspect. The tongue fur, though primarily an indicator of the severity of a disorder, is sometimes a useful measure of the strength of correct qi. This is true in the case of a thick, slimy fur, which indicates exuberant damp turbidity, or a peeling fur, which indicates stomach qi vacuity or damage to yin humor. The moistness of the tongue sheds light on the state of the fluids. For these reasons, the tongue examination is of special importance in exogenous heat diseases.

Observing the color and shape of the various parts of the head and face

Infants

In infants, a head that is unusually small or large generally indicates depletion of kidney essence or an insufficiency of the congenital constitution that may be accompanied by water-rheum. Depressed fontanels indicate yin humor depletion, while bulging fontanels indicate acute or chronic fright-wind. Failure of the cranial sutures to close and the inability to keep the head upright indicate an insufficiency of kidney essence and bone marrow vacuity. An uncontrollable shaking of the head indicates a wind disorder.

Hair

Scant, dry hair indicates insufficiency of kidney qi or qi-blood vacuity. After middle age, the hair naturally grays and becomes scant. Graying may occur in young people, usually due to non-pathologic constitutional factors.

Eyes

Observing the eyes most often involves observing the spirit. Since the "essence of the bowels and viscera flows up into the eyes," the eyes reflect the state of the organs to some extent. Furthermore, the eyes connect through to the brain, which is referred to as the sea of marrow, and "the essence of marrow is in the pupils." Therefore, when the pupils are normal in enduring or severe illnesses, the disease is still curable. Conversely, if a patient has lusterless eyes, and tends to keep the eyes shut, taking no interest in the world, or if the spirit of his eyes has an abnormal appearance, the condition is critical. If the eyes are turned upwards or sideways, or look fixedly ahead, the condition is one of endogenous liver wind. Dilation of the pupils may, in serious illness, be a sign of approaching death.

Conjunctival injection or reddening of the eyes, often with copious discharge that occurs as part of a broader pattern, usually indicates exogenous wind-heat, heart fire, or liver fire. Lusterless conjuctivae indicates a dual vacuity of blood and qi. Swollen and painful corneae are generally associated with liver fire. Yellowing of the sclerae indicates jaundice, which in most often signifies damp-heat, and in rare cases, cold-damp.

Dark rings around the eyes indicate renal vacuity, while cyan-purple rings indicate intraorbital bleeding. Sunken eyes indicate a serious condition of damage to liquid and humor desertion. Slight puffiness around the eyes indicates incipient water swelling. However, senile debilitation of kidney qi may be characterized by slackening and puffiness of the lower lids, though in most cases this does not constitute a sign of disease. Bulging of the eyes is usually caused by binding phlegm-fire depression.

Nose

Flaring nostrils are associated with rapid breathing due to lung heat. Dry nostrils indicate lung heat or contraction of the dryness pathogen. A dry, parched-black nose indicates intense heat toxin. Prominent blood vessels at the root of the nose in infants are a sign of a weak constitution or weakness of the organs. When this occurs during the course of an illness it indicates fright-wind. In patients suffering from measles, extremely scant papules at the sides of the nostrils indicate non-diffusion of lung qi and the incomplete outthrust of pathogenic heat. Treatment should aim to prevent the inward fall of the pathogen.

Lips, teeth, and throat

Pale lips indicate a dual vacuity of blood and qi. Cyan-purple lips are seen in both blood stasis and cold patterns and indicate impaired flow of blood and qi. Parched lips indicate damage to liquid. Gaping corners of the mouth and shrinking of the philtrum signify imminent desertion of correct qi. Drooling from the corners of the mouth during sleep generally indicates splenic vacuity or gastric heat. In infants this may be a sign of intestinal parasites. Drooling from one side of the mouth is associated with wryness of the mouth and facial paralysis. Trismus is seen mostly in tetanic diseases. When accompanied by foaming at the mouth, trismus is generally symptomatic of epilepsy. When associated with a phlegm rattle in the throat, and wryness of the eyes or mouth, it indicates windstrike.

Dry teeth indicate damage to liquid by intense heat. "Teeth as dry as old bones" indicate exsiccation of kidney yin. Red, swollen, hot and painful gums, putrifying, cracked gums, or bleeding gums generally indicate stomach fire. Gingival vacuity edema and loose teeth point to renal vacuity. Since "the teeth are the surplus of the kidney" and "the stomach is connected to the gums," gingival morbidity is connected mainly with gastric heat and renal vacuity. Bruxism during sleep by children is generally indicative of gastric heat, intestinal parasites, or gan accumulation. Red, swollen, hot and sore throat or tonsils are indicative of upflaming stomach or lung heat. When yellowish white putrefaction speckles are also present, intense toxic heat is indicated. A dry, slightly swollen, sore, red throat generally indicates yin vacuity fire effulgence. A sore, pale red throat, without the presence of heat or swelling, may indicate upfloating of vacuity fire. A sore, slightly red and swollen throat, with grayish white putrefaction speckles or patches that are not easily removed, may indicate diphtheria. It is attributable to scorching of pulmogastric yin liquid by dryness-heat.

Ear

The ear is the meeting place of all the channels of the body, and is also the outer portal of the kidney. Withering of the auricles and shrinking of the lobes in the course of enduring or serious illness is a sign of qi and blood depletion and impending expiry of kidney qi.

In recent years, extensive research into ear acupuncture has shown that some organic diseases are reflected by changes in ear point reactivity.

Neck

Morbid changes in the neck include struma, scrofulous swellings, and phlegm nodules. If these are soft to the touch, the pattern is generally one of binding depression of phlegm and qi. If the nodules are hard to the touch and static, the pattern is one of congealing stagnation of qi and blood. Conspicuous throbbing of the *ren-ying* pulse (at the common carotid artery) accompanied by cough, dyspnea, or water swelling, is generally indicative of cardiopulmonary qi vacuity or cardiorenal yang vacuity.

Visual examination of excreta

Phlegm

Thin, clear phlegm indicates cold, while yellow or thick white phlegm indicates heat. Scant phlegm expectorated with difficulty signifies either heat or dryness. Copious, easily expectorated phlegm indicates damp. Coughing of fishy-smelling pus and phlegm generally indicates lung abscesses in a pattern of toxic heat brewing in the lung. Expectoration of phlegm containing blood, or coughing of pure blood, are due either to vacuity fire or lung heat damaging the connecting vessels. The distinction is dependent on the general signs. In these patterns, expectoration of purplish black blood may indicate a blood stasis complication.

Nasal mucus and tears

Nasal congestion and runny nose with clear nasal mucus is a sign of non-diffusion of lung qi, and usually occurs in the initial stages of colds and influenza, but may also appear at the onset of some acute infectious diseases. Recovery from colds or influenza can be expected when the thin, clear nasal mucus thickens and becomes yellow. Turbid yellow, foul-smelling nasal mucus accompanied by recurrent headaches generally indicates paranasal sinusitis, which is a lingering wind-heat pattern. The presence or absence of lachrymation in children is important: crying without tearing is a sign of a relatively serious condition.

Vomitus

Vomiting of phlegm and water indicates gastric phlegm-rheum, and generally forms part of a cold pattern. Vomitus containing digestate without sour taste or bad odor indicates vacuity cold or invasion of the stomach by liver qi. Vomitus with a sour taste and bad odor indicates digestate accumulation, stomach heat, or hepatocystic damp-heat. Bitter, yellow vomitus is generally indicative of hepatocystic damp-heat. Vomiting of purplish black blood can only be diagnosed by taking account of other symptoms.

Stool

Malodorous, yellow, thin stool is associated with damp-heat. Frequent evacuation of small amounts of sticky stool containing blood is a sign of dysentery. Watery stool containing improperly digested food may be symptomatic of cold-damp, as may duck stool. Stool with bright red blood indicates heavy bleeding, usually in the anus or rectum, and is known as precipitation of blood due to intestinal wind. Thin, glossy, blackish duck stool is generally associated with bleeding in the digestive tract. However, identification of this pattern requires the correlation of other signs. Dry, hard stool, bearing the appearance of sheep droppings, and accompanied by evacuative difficulty, is due to intestinal heat-bind and is generally associated with gastric reflux and esophageal constriction (cf. diarrhea, Glossary of Terms).

Urine

Long micturition with clear urine is most frequently associated with cold. Short micturition with dark-colored urine is generally associated with heat; when accompanied by painful urination, urinary urgency, and frequency, it indicates damp-heat in the lower burner. Turbid urine that clears when left to stand, or clear urine that turns murky when left to cool does not usually indicate morbidity. Urine that is turbid upon urination and remains turbid when left to stand is indicative of unctuous strangury. This may involve either damp-heat in the lower burner or renal vacuity. Hematuria is attributable to various causes, including damp-heat in the lower burner, yin vacuity fire-effulgence, calculous strangury, or tumors. Accurate diagnosis must be made based on the accompanying signs.

Audio-Olfactive Examination

Sounds

The "listening" of audio-olfactive examination involves listening to the sound of the patient's voice, respiration, cough (if present), and the sounds that express pain and discomfort. Changes in enunciation and respiration are a direct reflection of disease changes in the lung and the state of original qi. Verbal expression and response to questions reflect the state of the spirit.

Quality of voice and enunciation

A faint, frail voice with faltering speech, which in serious cases hampers comprehension, indicates a vacuity of lung or original qi. *Essential Questions* states, "If the patient has a faint voice and takes a long time to get his words out, his qi is depleted." This condition is most often seen in damage to the lungs by enduring cough, pneumonia affecting the kidney, or vacuous original qi. A rough, turbid voice generally indicates a repletion pattern where the lung has been invaded by an exogenous pathogen, preventing diffusion of lung qi. This may occur in diseases classified in Western medicine as bronchitis and laryngitis. A hoarse voice or aphonia indicates lung-block when it is associated with repletion signs. It indicates pulmonary detriment when accompanied by vacuity signs. Diagnosis is made based on accompanying signs. Groaning, outcries, etc., indicate distention, pain, or oppressive sensations. Their significance must be determined by thorough questioning. *Essential Prescriptions of the Golden Coffer* states:

> If the patient tends to keep still and frequently emits cries, he has pain in the joints. If his voice is weak and indistinct, the pain is in the center of the chest and diaphragm. If he can talk clearly without interruption, but keeps his voice low, the pain is in the head.

In other words, when the disorder is in the joints, movement causes pain. Thus, the patient tends to keep as still as possible, and may utter sounds of pain and discomfort when he moves. When the disorder is in the center of the chest and diaphragm, the respiratory tract is constricted, so that the patient's voice is faint and broken. Any attempt to talk only aggravates the pain. In those suffering from headaches, raising the voice causes cranial vibrations that increase pain; however, since the respiratory tract is not affected, the voice is clear and undistorted.

Verbal expression

Incoherent expression and response to inquiry indicate disorders of the heart. *Essential Questions* states:

> Failure to keep apparel and bedclothes adjusted, loss of all sense of propriety in speech, and inability to recognize relatives indicate derangement of the spirit.

The pattern may be repletion or vacuity, the former characterized by a vigorous or strident voice, the latter by a low, weak voice. Confused, strident speech in exogenous heat diseases is known as delirious speech and most commonly occurs in repletion patterns. Mussitation, where the patient talks to himself in a low voice with frequent repetitions, is usually seen in vacuity patterns.

Respiration

Weak, short, distressed breathing indicates insufficiency of lung qi or original qi. Rough breathing generally occurs in repletion patterns where the lung has been invaded by an exogenous pathogen. Dyspnea occurs in replete and vacuous forms; the difference is succinctly elucidated in *Jing Yue's Complete Compendium* as follows:

> In repletion dyspnea, breathing is deep, inhalation seeming to be never-ending. In vacuity dyspnea, breaths are short, with a slight pause between inhalation and exhalation. In repletion dyspnea, the chest feels distended and breathing rough, and the voice is high and strident; the chest swells as if to burst, unable to contain all the breath it draws in, and relief from discomfort only comes with exhalation. In vacuity dyspnea, the patient is distressed and anxious, and his voice is low and faint; he is panicky, feeling as if he is about to stop breathing; he is unable to catch his breath and feels as though the air is not being absorbed by the lungs; the short, rapid breaths give the impression of panting, and relief is felt only when a long breath can be drawn.

In Western medicine, classical repletion dyspnea is seen in acute attacks of bronchial asthma, while vacuity dyspnea occurs in pulmonary emphysema or dyspnea due to cardiac failure.

Cough

Cough and dyspnea with qi ascent, accompanied by a frog rattle in the throat, is caused by phlegm in the respiratory tract obstructing the smooth flow of air. This condition is a commonly observed cold-rheum cough and dyspnea pattern. A heavy, turbid cough with a gurgling sound of phlegm is indicative of phlegm-turbidity congesting the lung. A dry cough indicates pulmonary dryness or yin vacuity. A faint, feeble cough indicates lung qi or lung yin vacuity. Long bouts of continuous coughing that are finished with a sonorous crow and accompanied by pronounced flushing of the face (which may even turn purple in serious cases) indicate pertussis, or whooping cough.

Hiccoughing

Although occasional bouts of hiccoughing are not abnormal, when occurring in enduring or serious illness they must be given special attention. Short, relatively high-pitched, forceful hiccoughs indicate repletion heat. Protracted, low-pitched, weak hiccoughs indicate counterflow ascent of stomach qi.

Odors

The smell of the patient's breath and excreta can give some indication of their condition. *Major Thermic Pestilences,* by Dai Bei-Shan, mentions "identification of odors" as one of five main diagnostic methods, emphasizing that special attention should be paid to unusual smells.

Breath and body smells

Halitosis is generally attributable to stomach heat. In some cases, however, it is due to stagnation of digestate in the stomach and intestines or indigestion; in other cases, it is due to oral gan, periodontal gan, caries, or throat diseases. Belching of sour, foul-smelling gas is due to ingesta damage.

The unusual fetid smell given off by patients suffering from hepatic coma, known as the hepatic odor (and which may be synonymous with the "cadaverine odor" referred to in *Major Thermic Pestilences*) is due to exuberant toxic heat in the inner body.

Excreta odors

The putrid smell of phlegm, pus, urine, or stool that is thick and turbid indicates damp-heat or toxic heat. The "fishy" smell of thin excreta is usually due to vacuity cold.

Inquiry

Inquiry represents an important way of gaining information about the patient's condition, and considerable emphasis has always been placed on it. *Essential Questions* states:

> If, in conducting the examination, the physician neither inquires as to how and when the condition arose, nor asks about the nature of the patient's complaint, about dietary irregularities, excesses of sleeping and waking, and poisoning, but instead proceeds straightway to take the pulse, he will not succeed in identifying the disease.

Through inquiry, which Zhang Jie-Bin of the Ming Dynasty believed to be "the essential element of examination, and the most indispensable of all aspects of clinical practice," the practitioner may learn of the origin and development of the present condition, as well as of pre-existing and previous complaints and drug reactions. Physicians today hold to the principle that inquiry should precede physical examination.

Important though it may be, inquiry nevertheless poses the problem of subjectivity. While the visual and audio-olfactive examinations and palpation are relatively objective, the information provided by the patient in response to the physician's questions is not fully reliable, since it frequently tends to be clouded by his own fears and misjudgement. Traditionally, it was recognized that although the patient must be questioned in detail regarding his condition, the information he provides must be set against the picture presented by the other examinations. The patient's conception of his condition may be confused. Accurate diagnosis depends on thoroughness. Standard practice dictates the synthesis of information from all four examinations.

Zhang Jie-Bin summarizes diagnosis in ten steps:

Inquire about:

1. Cold and heat
2. Perspiration
3. Head and body
4. Stool and micturition
5. Diet
6. Chest
7. Hearing
8. Thirst

Then:

9. Identify yin and yang from the pulse and complexion.
10. Note any strong odors and abnormalities of the spirit.

Since only the first eight rules properly belong to inquiry, in the interests of completion, the last two steps were later changed to asking about previous illness and any previous prescriptions. Han Fei-Xia proposed an eight-point inquiry:

1. Location of pain and discomfort
2. Possible cause
3. Onset of present condition
4. Time of greatest discomfort (day or night)
5. Predominance of hot or cold symptoms
6. Patient's preferences
7. Previous medication
8. Places visited

These lines summarize well the scope of the inquiry examination. Today, we would add only "working conditions." In the following sections, each of the aspects of inquiry is discussed in detail.

Cold and heat

The practitioner should inquire whether the patient suffers from sensations of cold or heat. Exogenous diseases classically present with fever and aversion to cold at the onset. The prominence of aversion to cold indicates the presence of exogenous wind-cold. A more pronounced fever with milder aversion to cold suggests exogenous wind-heat. Alternation of fever and chills is usually seen in mid-stage penetration patterns, such as malarial disease.

An unabating high fever without aversion to cold indicates that the disease has already interiorized, i.e., penetrated the interior. A persistent but remittent high fever, unabated by sweating, with intermittent aversion to cold, indicates that the pathogen is intense and the condition is relatively serious. Late afternoon tidal fever, principally associated with gastrointestinal heat-bind, is a persistent high fever that peaks from about 3 to 5 p.m. Persistent fever accompanied by signs of the damp pathogen indicate lingering damp-heat. A low fever (often little more than hot palms and soles and flushed cheeks) that occurs in the afternoon or evening, and is abated by night or morning sweating, is known as steaming bone tidal fever. It is attributable to yin vacuity. A fever that is present during the day and rises at night indicates a relatively serious condition. If the patient feels hot and restless, but has a normal or slightly high body temperature, the condition is generally found to be organic heat (heat in the organs). An irregularly intermittent fever with lassitude and weakness is usually indicative of qi vacuity.

Aversion to cold and aversion to wind are essentially the same; the latter is merely a milder form. Aversion to cold with shivering is usually simply referred to as shivering. It frequently occurs in conjunction with fever. Aversion to cold without fever is principally associated with yang vacuities. Often occurring as a result of a sudden drop in body temperature, such a condition demands special attention since it may indicate vacuity desertion due to collapse of yang.

Perspiration

Sweat is produced from the fluids and blood, and normal secretion is regulated by construction and particularly defense. Abnormal secretion, therefore, reflects the state of the fluids and blood, as well as that of construction and defense.

Excessive sweating during the daytime or sweating at the slightest physical exertion is termed spontaneous sweating. This most often occurs in patients suffering from qi or yang vacuities and is an indication of vacuous defense qi and a slackening of the striations. Sweating during the night is termed night sweating and generally occurs in patients suffering from yin vacuities. It indicates yin vacuity endogenous heat and insecurity of construction qi.

Fever with dry skin and absence of perspiration may occur either in depletion of blood and fluids, or in exogenous disease when the exterior is assailed by a pathogen, depressing defense qi and blocking the striations. Correlation with other symptoms is necessary to ensure a correct diagnosis.

Perspiration provides a valuable indicator of the patient's condition. Oily sweat streaming constantly from the skin indicates yang collapse vacuity desertion, and is a serious condition. If, as a result of sweating, the body temperature drops and the pulse stabilizes, correct qi is dispelling the pathogen from the body. A much less common sign of pathogen expulsion is shiver-sweating. This refers to a shivering bout followed by sweating which reduces a persistent high fever. Sweating fails to abate fever in two cases: in construction-defense disharmony, where continuing, intermittent, but not severe fever, and spontaneous sweating accompanied by aversion to cold, indicate that the body is incapable of expelling an exterior pathogen; and in great qi-aspect heat patterns where high fever and profuse sweating are accompanied by aversion to heat and great thirst and restlessness.

Head and body

The head contains the brain marrow and is an area of high channel concentration. Most of the regular and irregular channels, in particular the yang channels, pass through the head. Headaches and dizziness are among the most common symptoms of disease, occurring in both exogenous diseases and endogenous damage.

The nature, severity, and duration of headaches are all important factors in diagnosis. Headaches of recent onset usually indicate exogenous disease. Enduring headaches indicate endogenous damage. Severe headaches usually form part of repletion patterns, while dull headaches are generally associated with vacuity. If the pain is exacerbated by exposure to wind and cold, the patient is likely to be suffering from a wind-cold disorder. Exacerbation by warmth generally indicates ascendant hyperactivity of liver yang. A headache accompanied by heavy-headedness, known as a "bag-over-the-head" sensation, is generally attributable to phlegm-damp clouding the upper body. Frontal headaches are often associated with the yang ming channel. Pain in the temporal area is generally associated with the shao yang channel. Pain in the back of the head and neck is associated with the tai yang channel; and pain at the vertex is generally associated with the jue yin channel.

Dizziness may be associated with liver yang, wind-phlegm, and vacuity disorders. The exact nature of the sensation should be ascertained.

Where there is a pronounced feeling of imbalance (such as felt on a boat), ascendant hyperactivity of liver yang is the most probable cause. Visual whirling suggests wind-phlegm harassing the upper body. Flowery vision and tinnitus, when accompanied by pale white complexion, indicate insufficiency of blood and qi.

Inquiry about the body involves asking the patient about pain, discomfort, lumps, or similar irregular phenomena in the trunk or limbs. Generalized aching accompanied by fever and aversion to cold generally occurs in exterior patterns. Pain of specific location, or migratory pain in the joints, is generally indicative of an obturation pattern. Qi and blood vacuities, where the blood fails to nourish the sinews, may give rise to a relatively mild aching and numbness in the sinews and bones. Heaviness and fatigue in the body and limbs are generally attributable to damp-encumbrance.

Micturition and stool

Inquiring about the patient's micturition and stool is an indispensable part of the inquiry examination. It provides a valuable indicator of repletion, vacuity, cold, and heat.

Urine is produced from fluids, and normal secretion and voiding depend on the transformative action of qi. This means that micturition can provide useful information about the state of the fluids and the transformative action of qi.

Polyuria and in particular nocturia indicate vacuous kidney yang failing to perform its containing function. Short micturition with scant urine and anuria occur in three cases: fulminant fluid desertion exhausting the source of urine; insufficiency of kidney yang causing impaired transformation and thus reduced urine production; or a vesicular qi-block, whereby urine is produced but cannot be voided and is thus retained in the bladder. Short, scant voidings are normal in hot weather when the fluids lost in sweating are not replaced by adequate fluid intake. Occurring in pregnancy, frequent short micturition with scant urine indicates fetal pressure and is attributable to qi vacuity. Frequency, small voidings, dark-colored urine, and stinging pain during urination are symptoms associated with vesicular damp-heat. Dribbling incontinence refers to a constant dribbling discharge of urine and inability to achieve a full stream of urine, and is due to a vacuity of either center qi or of kidney qi. Enuresis is generally attributable to a vacuous kidney failing to secure.

Stool

Stool changes are largely attributable to morbidity of the spleen, stomach, and intestines, but may also be associated with hepatic and renal dysfunction.

Constipation and hard, dry stool are mainly attributable to heat and repletion, although cold and vacuity are not uncommon causes. Constipation with fullness, distention, and pain in the abdomen occurring in exogenous heat disease as a result of gastrointestinal heat-bind is termed heat constipation. This is a repletion pattern. Vacuity constipation is a pattern of insufficiency of intestinal humor due to blood and fluid depletion that produces dry, hard stools without pronounced abdominal distention. This pattern includes cold constipation, referring to the evacuative difficulty experienced by the elderly as a result of yang vacuity affecting movement and transformation of digestate.

Diarrhea and thin stool occur in vacuity, repletion, cold, and heat patterns. Fulminant diarrhea usually indicates repletion. Enduring diarrhea generally indicates vacuity, or a vacuity-repletion complex. Diarrhea characterized by frequent evacuation of small amounts of stool with tenesmus and a burning sensation indicates damp-heat in the large intestine. Abdominal pain followed, and relieved, by diarrhea is most often attributable to digestate accumulations. Bouts of diarrhea with abdominal pain that is unrelieved by evacuation are brought on by emotional stimulae. The root cause is to be found in hepatosplenic disharmony. Diarrhea occurring shortly after eating indicates splenogastric qi vacuity. Diarrhea each day before dawn is known as daybreak diarrhea and is attributable to splenorenal yang vacuity. Diarrhea with loss of the voluntary control over bowel movements, sometimes accompanied by prolapse of the rectum, is known as intestinal vacuity efflux desertion, and is attributed to vacuity cold or to center-qi fall.

Diet

Dietary considerations are categorized in three parts: thirst and fluid intake; food intake and digestion; and taste in the mouth.

Thirst and fluid intake

Inquiry about thirst and fluid intake provides a valuable indicator of heat and cold. Absence of thirst, or intake of warm fluids in small amounts, indicates a cold pattern. Thirst with little or no urge to drink, or immediate vomiting of ingested fluids, indicates water-damp collecting in the inner body and impaired upbearing of fluids. Thirst with a preference for cold fluids and severe thirst with high fluid intake are signs of heat. Thirst unallayed by a large fluid intake, together with a high increase in urine volume, indicates diabetic disease.

Food intake and digestion

Information concerning the patient's intake of solid foods is particularly valuable in prognosis. Maintenance of a good appetite and digestion in spite of long or serious illness shows that the stomach qi has not expired and the patient's prospects for recovery are good. Hence it is said, "If sustenance is taken, the body thrives." Persistent loss of appetite may affect the prospects for recovery. Most illnesses characterized by a reduced food intake, distention, and oppression after eating are traceable to splenogastric vacuity or inner body damp-heat obstruction. A normal appetite with indigestion signifies a strong stomach and a weak spleen. High food intake with rapid hungering and clamoring stomach after eating indicates stomach heat. Stomachache slightly relieved by eating signals a vacuity. Predilection for rich and fatty foods increases susceptibility to phlegm-damp. A perverted appetite indicates parasitic accumulations.

Taste in the mouth

Changes in the taste in the mouth are of corroborative value in pattern identification. If the taste in the mouth is unaffected by illness, the mouth is said to be in harmony. This indicates that there is no heat in the interior. A bitter taste in the mouth is a sign of heat, and usually indicates stomach heat, liver heat, or hepatocystic damp-heat. A sweet, sickly, or bland taste in the mouth indicates damp obstruction or splenic vacuity with damp. A sour, putrid taste is usually attributable to digestate stagnation. Intermittent acid upflow is usually indicative of stomach heat, or invasion of the stomach by liver fire.

Chest and abdomen

All the major organs, with the exception of the brain, are located within the chest and abdomen. Most organic disorders are therefore reflected by pain or discomfort in this region. Inquiry thus involves identifying possible glomus, fullness, distention, and pain, and determining their parametric nature.[2]

Glomus with fullness and occasional pain, accompanied by coughing and copious phlegm, indicates thoracic obturation or a cold-rheum pattern. If the same symptoms are accompanied by restlessness and fever, thirst, and slimy tongue fur, the pattern is one of phlegm-heat. A feeling of oppression in the chest with weak respiration is symptomatic of vacuity. Painful distention in the lateral costal region indicates either binding depression of liver qi, or hepatocystic damp-heat. Both of these are readily identifiable by the correlation of other symptoms. Lancinating pain and oppression around the heart, with ashen complexion, and profuse cold sweating, is termed cardialgia and is a critical condition.

Abdominal pain relieved by pressure is associated with vacuity; pain exacerbated by pressure is attributable to repletion. Pain soothed by application of heat is attributable to cold. Stabbing or lancinating pain of specific location indicates accumulation of static blood forming an internal abscess. Remittent scurrying pain of non-specific location is usually qi pain. Intermittent scurrying pain in the umbilical region may indicate parasites.

Abdominal distention relieved by passing flatus or belching is usually related to qi stagnation or digestate accumulation; it is often further characterized by dyspeptic anorexia. Continued distention without relief, together with hard stools, indicates repletion. Periodically abating vacuity distention combined with thin stool form a vacuity pattern. *Essential Prescriptions of the Golden Coffer* describes the former as "abdominal fullness with little or no relief," and the latter as "abdominal fullness recurring after periods of relief."

Hearing and vision

The ears are the portals of the kidney, and vacuity of kidney essential qi may give rise to tinnitus and hearing loss. Because the ears are located on the path of the shao yang channel, disease affecting the shao yang may lead to deafness. Loss of hearing may also occur in warm disease repletion patterns where pathogenic qi clouds the clear portals. Loss of hearing acuity and deafness, occurring in some chronic diseases, generally are part of qi or kidney vacuity patterns. Gradual loss of hearing in old age is due to vacuity. Tinnitus and deafness are fundamentally of identical significance in pattern identification.

The eyes are the portals of the liver. Visual dizziness and flowery vision are generally associated with liver fire or ascendant hyperactivity of liver yang, and hepatorenal essence-blood depletion. Loss of visual acuity and dry eyes are usually attributable to hepatorenal insufficiency.

Sleep

Insomnia characterized by reduced and restless sleep, excessive dreaming, palpitations, and susceptibility to fright and fear, is largely attributable to insufficiency of heart blood, disquieting of the heart spirit, or liver blood insufficiency. When characterized by restlessness and interior heat, initial insomnia, or in serious cases, nightlong sleeplessness, it is attributable to yin vacuity fire effulgence. Persistent, severe insomnia with signs of both heart fire and kidney vacuity indicate breakdown of cardiorenal interaction. Insomnia due to phlegm-fire harassing the upper body, splenogastric vacuity, or indigestion, is loosely termed "troubled sleep due to gastric disharmony."

Somnolence, denoting extended periods of sleep interspersed with drowsy consciousness, occurs most notably in exogenous diseases such as heat entering the pericardium or phlegm clouding the cardiac portals. It may also be a sign of debilitation of yang qi, which is referred to in *A Treatise on Cold Damage* where it states, "When the shao yin is affected by disease... there is desire only for sleep." Patients suffering from yang vacuity may fall asleep almost instantly, but readily waken. This condition is distinguished from the former by the absence of heat symptoms.

History

Information about the patient's history of illness is important when judging new conditions. The following points should be noted:

Presence of perduring ailments

The physician should ask patients whether they were already suffering from any perduring complaint when the present condition arose. The regular presence of liver fire and liver yang disease is a predisposing factor for stirring of endogenous wind and sudden wind strokes. Enduring diarrhea or water swelling frequently indicates splenorenal yang vacuity. The regular presence of phlegm-rheum may be due to insufficiency of the transformative action of the lung, spleen, and kidney qi.

Previous treatment and its implications for medication

Patients should be questioned about previous treatment and its effects. If, for example, a condition was previously identified as a heat pattern, yet treatment with cold or cool agents produced no marked effect, either the pattern was wrongly identified, or the diagnosis was correct but the formula chosen was inappropriate. Possibly, the formula was simply not strong enough. Reappraisal in the light of presenting symptoms should pinpoint the error.

Attitudes, emotions, lifestyle, and working environment

People who are taciturn and melancholy by nature are more prone than others to binding depression of liver qi. Impulsiveness, rashness, and impatience are predisposing factors for upflaming of liver fire and upstirring of liver yang. Predilection for cold, raw, and fatty foods, and smoking tobacco, may cause phlegm-damp. Attention should be paid to the diseases commonly associated with the patient's occupation; for example, the occupational diseases of outdoor manual laborers include low back pain and aching legs, and cold-damp obturation.

Gynecologic considerations

Menstruation and childbearing are associated not only with the uterus, but also the heart, the liver, the spleen, and kidney, as well as the penetrating and conception vessels. Information concerning menstruation, pregnancy, and childbirth is therefore relevant in many non-gynecologic disorders. The physician should ask about menstruation, history of pregnancy and childbirth, and future plans with regard to having children.

When inquiring about menstrual history, attention should be paid to the length of the menstrual period (premature or delayed arrival of periods), flow, color (light red, red, purple), and the consistency (thin, thick, clotted) of the discharge. Premature arrival of periods, with a heavy flow and a thick red discharge, generally indicates blood heat. Delayed arrival of the period, with reduced flow and a light-colored discharge generally implies blood vacuity. A heavy flow with a thin, light-colored discharge indicates qi vacuity. Purple discharge with clots is symptomatic of blood stasis. Irregularity of menstrual periods and flow is generally associated with disorders of the penetrating vessel. Excessive childbearing frequently leads to depletion of the penetrating and conception vessels. Women with histories of miscarriage and difficult deliveries may be suffering from non-gynecologic disorders such as insufficiency of qi and blood or hepatorenal depletion.

Information concerning menstruation and pregnancy is of vital importance in selecting medication for non-gynecologic disorders. Zhang Zi-He states:

> Female patients should always be questioned about possible pregnancy. If the slightest suspicion of pregnancy exists, qi breakers and blood quickeners should not be prescribed.

The following acupoints are also proscribed during pregnancy: LI-4, SP-6, GB-21, and any points on the lower abdomen. Mild stimulation may be used on other points.

Children

For infants and children, general inquiry about their development is important for assessing the state of their kidney essential qi and splenogastric function. When infants are breast-fed, inquiry about lactation may be pertinent.

Palpation

Palpation is the process of examining the surface of the body by touch to detect the presence of disease. Pulse taking, an essential part of routine examination, is the most common form of palpation.

Pulse examination

"The blood vessels are the dwelling place of qi and blood." That is, they are the pathways of qi and blood. By palpating the blood vessels in specific parts of the body, it is possible to judge the state of the qi and the blood, and to thereby assess whether the patient's condition is improving or deteriorating, and determine the ultimate prospects for recovery. *Essential Questions* comments:

A long pulse indicates that qi is in order; a short pulse indicates a disorder of qi; a regularly interrupted pulse indicates debilitation of qi; a large pulse indicates that the condition is advancing.

The length, size, rate, and rhythm of the pulse provide information not only about the state of correct qi, but also about the location and nature of the disease. For example, a floating pulse is associated with the exterior and a deep pulse is associated with the interior. A rapid pulse indicates heat and a slow pulse indicates cold.

Pulse examination method

Pulse examination involves feeling the pulsation of the blood vessels by placing the fingertips on the surface of the body. The following considerations should be noted:

Time

Essential Questions states, "The pulse should be taken in the early morning." This is the time when the body is least subject to external influences. Usually, the best the physician can do is to ensure that the pulse is taken in as quiet and relaxed an atmosphere as is possible, so that external and emotional factors will cause minimum distortion of the patient's pulse. The pulse should be felt for at least one or two minutes in order to ensure maximum accuracy.

Position

Up to the Han Dynasty, the pulse was commonly taken at three positions: the *ren-ying* (common carotid artery), the *cun-kou* (radial styloid pulse), and the *fu-yang* (dorsalis pedis artery). Today, the first and third positions are rarely used.

The radial pulse is divided into three points: the inch, the barrier, and the cubit. The barrier point is located on the anterior face of the radial styloid process. The inch point is located on its distal side, and the cubit point on its proximal side. Since the pulse is taken on both wrists, there are six points in all, known as the six pulses.

According to classical literature, the condition of each of the various bowels and viscera is reflected in the six pulses: the right inch pulse is associated with the lung, and the right barrier pulse is associated with the stomach and spleen. The left inch pulse is associated with the heart, and the left barrier pulse is associated with the liver and gallbladder. The kidney and the bladder are reflected in both cubit pulses. Through the centuries, other theories of organ correspondence have also been postulated.

Posture

The patient should be either seated upright or lying supine. His forearm should be in a horizontal position level with the heart. The palm of the hand should be facing upward, and the wrist, which should be resting on a soft pad, is kept straight and relaxed. Incorrect posture may affect the flow of qi and blood, and thus falsify the pulse.

Normal breathing

To ensure maximum accuracy when taking a patient's pulse, physicians should make sure that their own respiration is natural and even. The mind should be fully collected and thus able to detect even the slightest changes.

The method of feeling the pulse

Normally, the physician places the index finger on the inch point. The middle and fourth fingers rest on the barrier and cubit points respectively. When taking the pulse, the following considerations should be noted:

The spacing of the three fingers used in taking the pulse should depend on the height of the patient. For a tall patient, the fingers should be spaced apart, whereas with short patients, they should be kept close together. For infants, the use of only one finger may be necessary. To ensure the greatest accuracy in pulse reading, it is important to use only the very tips of the fingers, and to apply even pressure with all three fingers. The practitioner should note the difference in the pulse at the various levels of pressure applied. There are three basic pressure levels: the superficial level is found by placing the fingertips lightly on the skin. The deep level is felt by pressing firmly. Between these two is the mid-level. The practitioner feels for the different levels by moving the fingers slightly across the skin and by applying different amounts of pressure. Simultaneous palpation is the normal method of pulse-taking, involving the application of all three fingers at the same time. However, sometimes a clearer picture of the patient's condition can be gained by applying the fingers individually to the three points.

The nature of the pulse

The practitioner is said to have "found" the pulse when the pulsation is distinctly felt. Then the physician concentrates on the different aspects of the pulse. The rate is measured by counting the number of beats to one complete respiration (one inhalation and one exhalation). The quality is judged by the size, thickness, and length, the smoothness of the flow, and the regularity of the beat. Taking the pulse involves counting the number of beats, and identifying a form and pattern. Later in this text the most common pulse types and their clinical significance, and a comparative analysis of similar pulses where confusion easily arises, will be presented. Some of the rarer pulses are mentioned in the comparative analysis, although they are not described in detail under separate headings. It should be borne in mind that each of the types represents only one aspect of a given pulse. For example, floating and deep describe the depth; slow and rapid describe the rate, while surging and thin describe the size of the pulse. In actual practice, these qualities occur in combinations. In most cases a patient's pulse is described with a composite term such as floating, slippery, and rapid, or deep, wiry, and thin.

Normal pulse

With approximately four beats per respiration, the normal pulse is steady and even, providing a threefold significance. Its smoothness and strength indicate the presence of spirit. It is neither deep nor floating, and the beat rises and falls evenly and effortlessly, indicating the presence of stomach qi. Strength at the deep level indicates the presence of foundation.

The pulse may be affected by such factors as age, sex, build, and constitution. The pulse of a child tends to be soft and rapid; that of a woman is softer and slightly faster than a man's. Corpulent people tend to have fine and deep pulses, while thin people have large pulses. Athletes have moderate pulses, and pregnant women usually have slippery, slightly rapid pulses. These variations are all within the bounds of normal health. Some people display congenital irregularities, such as a particularly narrow artery, which makes the pulse comparatively fine, or a dorsal styloid pulse, where the artery runs around the posterior face of the styloid process of the radius. These irregularities have no significance in pattern identification.

Floating pulse

The floating pulse is pronounced at the superficial level, but vacuous at the deep level. Described as being "like a cork floating on water," it is felt as soon as the fingers touch the skin, but becomes markedly less perceptible when further pressure is applied.

Although classically associated with exterior patterns, the floating pulse may be indistinct in patients of heavy build, with weak constitutions, or suffering from severe water-swelling, even when an exterior pattern is present. A floating pulse may also occur in enduring illnesses or after a major loss of blood, indicating a severe insufficiency of correct qi rather than an exterior pattern. It is said, "A floating pulse seen in enduring illness is cause for great concern." In these cases it differs slightly from the floating pulse occurring in exogenous disease. It is slightly less pronounced at the superficial level, and markedly less pronounced at the deep level; thus it is sometimes referred to as a vacuous floating pulse.

A floating, large pulse without foundation is known as a scattered pulse. This pulse is large at the superficial level, but because of its lack of force, ceases to be felt as soon as the slightest pressure is applied. It indicates the dissipation of qi and blood, and the impending expiry of the essential qi of the organs. It is usually attended by other critical signs.

A floating pulse that is empty in the middle is known as a scallion-stalk pulse. It is a sign of heavy blood loss and usually occurs in cases of major hemorrhage.

Deep pulse

A deep pulse is one that is distinct only at the deep level. A deep pulse is associated with interior disease. However, the exterior patterns of exogenous diseases may temporarily present with a deep, tight pulse when the body's yang qi is obstructed.

The hidden pulse is even deeper than the deep pulse and considerable pressure has to be applied in order to feel it. The *Bin Hu Sphygmology* states, "The hidden pulse is found by pressing through the sinews right to the bone." It is associated with fulminant desertion of yang qi and deep-lying cold, and generally appears in conjunction with severe vomiting, diarrhea, and pain.

The weak pulse is deep and without force, and is associated with vacuity of qi and blood.

The confined pulse is deep and strong and feels as though "tied to the bone," hence its name. It is associated with cold pain.[3] In clinical practice, this term is no longer in popular use. The pulse is described as a deep wiry pulse or a deep full pulse.

Slow pulse

A slow pulse is one that has three or less beats per respiration. The slow pulse is principally associated with cold and yang vacuity. It may occur in any disease involving insufficiency of yang qi or obstruction of qi dynamic, such as cold, phlegm turbidity, and static blood. Occurring during pregnancy, this pulse signifies uterine vacuity cold or insecurity of fetal qi.

Like the slow pulse, the moderate pulse is also slower than the standard pulse, although usually it has more than three beats per respiration, and is not an indication of morbidity.

Rapid pulse

A rapid pulse has six beats per respiration and is distinct from a pulse having between five and six beats, which is termed a slightly rapid pulse. The rapid pulse is usually quite smooth-flowing, so it is often confused with a slippery pulse. However, the term "rapid" refers exclusively to the pace, while "slippery" denotes a quality. The *Bin Hu Sphygmology* clearly points out, "Rapid and slippery should not be considered as being the same; rapid refers to the pace only."

The rapid pulse is associated with heat, but may sometimes be an indication of vacuity. A strong, rapid pulse indicates repletion heat and is most commonly seen in exogenous heat disease. A fine, weak, rapid pulse is indicative of yin vacuity fire effulgence and is generally seen in depletion patterns, such as are described in Western medicine as pulmonary tuberculosis. A large, weak, rapid pulse generally indicates qi vacuity. Most healthy infants have rapid pulses, and a slippery, rapid pulse is a normal sign in pregnancy.

A pulse having seven or more beats per respiration is known as a racing pulse. Its significance is basically the same as that of the rapid pulse, but more thought should be given to the possibility of vacuity.

Slippery pulse

The slippery pulse is very smooth-flowing, and is classically described as "pearls rolling in a dish" or "small fish swimming." A slippery pulse is commonly seen in pregnancy, particularly in the early stages where extra blood is needed to nourish the fetus. It is also sometimes seen in healthy people, indicating an abundance of qi and blood. Phlegm-rheum patterns and digestate accumulation may also be characterized by a slippery pulse.

The animated pulse is a combination of the rapid, short, and slippery pulses. Smooth-flowing, short, small, and rapid, it is seen in tachycardia, high fevers associated with exogenous diseases, and in pregnancy.

Rough pulse

A rough pulse is the opposite of a slippery pulse, and does not flow smoothly. Sometimes termed a choppy or dry pulse, it is classically described as "a knife scraping bamboo." It tends to be somewhat fine, is generally slightly slower than the normal pulse, and has been described as being "fine, slow, short, dry, and beating with difficulty."

The rough pulse is often seen in blood stasis patterns and dual vacuity of blood and qi.

Wiry pulse

The wiry pulse is long and taut and feels like a guitar or violin string to the touch. The wiry pulse is associated with diseases of the liver and gallbladder, and in particular with ascendant hyperactivity of liver yang. It is also associated with pain and with phlegm-rheum patterns. It may be commonly seen in diseases classified by Western medicine as hypertension, arteriosclerosis, chronic bronchitis, and in diseases characterized by severe pain. The wiry pulse is generally strong; if weak, it is termed a vacuous wiry pulse, indicating vacuity of yin and hyperactivity of yang.

A tight pulse is a wiry pulse that has marked forcefulness. "Wiry" denotes a quality, whereas "tight" denotes a quality and forcefulness. A tight pulse is always wiry, while a wiry pulse is not necessarily tight. A tight pulse is associated with cold and pain. A drumskin pulse is wiry and empty in the middle. Its significance is the same as that of the scallion-stalk pulse, the name by which it is more commonly denoted.

Soggy pulse

"Soggy" signifies softness and relative lack of force. A soggy pulse is thin, though less distinctly so than a thin pulse, and tends to float. The soggy pulse is associated with dual vacuity of blood and qi and with damp encumbrance.

A faint pulse is extremely fine and weak, indistinct, and almost imperceptible. It indicates qi and blood vacuity desertion.

Like the soggy pulse, the empty pulse is weak, but differs as it is large rather than thin. The term is also generally used to connote weakness, particularly in combinations such as vacuous rapid pulse, vacuous wiry pulse, etc.

Surging pulse

This pulse is broad and large, and is forceful at all levels, especially the superficial. The onset is longer and more forceful than the falling away, which accounts for the description, "Forceful in rising and feeble in falling." It is thought of as waves beating against the rocks, an initial strong swell followed by a sharp but calm ebbing away.

A surging pulse indicates exuberant heat, and is usually a sign of repletion. Observed in enduring diseases (such as tuberculosis) or in vacuity patterns due to profuse hemorrhage, it indicates that correct qi is extremely weak and that the condition is deteriorating.

A full pulse is similar to a surging pulse, although it is as forceful when it falls as when it rises. It indicates that the body is afflicted by an exuberant pathogen, but that correct qi is still holding firm.

A large pulse in clinical practice has roughly the same significance as the surging pulse. However, it should be noted that "large" refers only to the breadth of the blood vessel as it feels to the touch. It bears no connotations of strength.

Fine pulse

The fine pulse, sometimes called a small pulse, feels like a well-defined thread under the fingers. The fine pulse indicates dual vacuity of qi and blood or of yin and yang, and in particular points to blood and yin vacuities.

Interrupted pulses

There are three interrupted pulses. The slow irregularly interrupted pulse, sometimes referred to as a bound pulse, is slow with pauses at irregular intervals. The rapid irregularly interrupted pulse, or skipping pulse, is also broken by irregular pauses, but is relatively fast. A pulse interspersed with more relatively regular pauses is called a regularly interrupted pulse. These three are referred to under the collective name of interrupted pulses.

The interrupted pulses indicate debilitation of visceral qi, and in particular insufficiency of heart qi. They may also indicate blood stasis or phlegm turbidity obstructing yang qi in the chest, and can be seen in cardiac obturation patterns. Interrupted pulses may also occur in healthy individuals and in patients suffering from emotional depression.

Long pulse

A long pulse is one that can be felt beyond the inch and cubit positions. The long pulse is not usually a sign of morbidity. However, a long wiry pulse frequently occurs in patients suffering from what Western medicine terms arteriosclerosis.

Short pulse

A short pulse is one that is felt only at the barrier point. The short pulse signifies dual vacuity of blood and qi, or impaired flow of blood and qi. (see Table 6-1, "Comparative Table of 29 Pulses".)

Precedence of pulse or symptoms

Pulse examination represents only one method of gathering information for the purpose of diagnosis. The pulse reflects different conditions to different degrees and with varying accuracy. Its value is therefore relative rather than absolute. A rapid pulse, for instance, generally signifies heat, but it may also occur in vacuity patterns. Some conditions are reflected indistinctly or even falsely in the pulse, while in others, the pulse may be the only truthful indicator among unpronounced or misleading symptoms. When there is incongruity between pulse and symptoms, a synthesis of data from all four examinations reveals the order of precedence.

Two possibilities exist: of the two factors (signs and pulse), either one factor may be the true reflection of the patient's condition, while the other is false or misleading; or both factors may be the true reflection of different elements of a vacuity—repletion complex.

An example of the first case is a condition with signs of palpatory tenderness in the abdomen, constipation, and a thick, yellow, parched tongue fur, with a slow and thin pulse. The signs faithfully reflect gastrointestinal heat-bind, while the pulse reflects only its false or misleading side effects, in this case heat binding the interior, impairing qi dynamic and thereby inhibiting the smooth flow of blood through the vessels. Here, the signs should be given precedence over the pulse, and the condition treated by emergency precipitation of the repletion. Giving precedence to the symptoms accords with the principle applied in pattern identification of distinguishing true and false.

Another example of the first case is an inner-body heat block, where the pulse is deep and rapid and the symptoms are inversion frigidity of the limbs. Here, the pulse faithfully represents the true condition. The symptoms only reflect the misleading presence of cold due to the confinement of heat in the interior. The pulse thus overrides the signs and the proper treatment is to outthrust the interior heat.

An example of the second case would be when ascites is accompanied by a weak, faint pulse, where the signs reflect the repletion of pathogenic qi, while the pulse reflects the vacuous state of correct qi. Both truly reflect different aspects of the condition. In such cases, the information derived from all four examinations must be carefully synthesized, and the relative predominance of repletion or vacuity determined.

If the repletion of the pathogenic qi is found to be more pronounced than the vacuity of correct qi, the symptoms override the pulse and the principle of attack followed by supplementation (q.v. Chapter 12) is applied. If the correct qi vacuity is more pronounced than the repletion of pathogenic qi, the pulse overrides the symptoms and the principle of supplementation followed by attack applies. Most often, the principle of simultaneous supplementation and attack is used. Generally speaking, where a vacuity-repletion complex accounts for incongruity between pulse and symptoms, it is readily identifiable. Greater difficulty lies in evaluating the relative severity of vacuity and repletion and deciding whether the pulse or the symptoms should govern treatment. Where incongruity involves a false factor, the true factor is usually readily identifiable, whereas the false factor tends to cause confusion. The solution in both cases lies in thorough examination and careful analysis. In the example of gastrointestinal heat-bind, careful observation reveals the pulse to be slow, thin, and forceful, distinguished from the slow, thin, feeble pulse that would otherwise indicate a vacuity pattern.

In an inner-body heat block with inversion frigidity of the limbs, all the other symptoms point to the presence of heat. No signs of heat accompany inversion cold in the legs, when the cause is yang collapse vacuity desertion. Extremely careful diagnosis is therefore required to avoid the mistake of strengthening repletion or exacerbating vacuity. Li Shi-Zhen (sobriquet Bin Hu) states in his *Bin Hu Sphygmology:*

> The pulse ranks last among the four examinations... and must be placed against the background of all the information gathered. All four examinations must be carried out.

General palpation

General palpation involves feeling the surface of the body with the hand to determine the presence of heat, cold, moistness, distention, and pain, and to observe the patient's reaction to pressure. General palpation may be divided into five parts: palpation of the skin, the limbs, the chest, the abdomen, and the acupoints. When conducting the examination, the physician should ensure that his hands are warm and that he applies pressure gently and evenly. In winter, the patient should be prevented from catching cold if required to undress.

Palpation of the skin

The principal goal of skin palpation is to assess the temperature and degree of moistness of the skin. The skin provides a reasonably faithful reflection of the body temperature; however, since the surface temperature varies from place to place, accuracy of judgment depends on a comprehensive examination. For instance, in the case of an inner-body pathogenic heat block, the chest and abdomen are palpably hot, while the limbs may not show any marked rise in temperature or may even be slightly lacking in warmth. The degree of moistness of the skin may reflect the amount of sweating, but provides considerably more information when combined with the temperature information. For example, a skin that is dry and palpably hot, such as is encountered at the onset of acute diseases, indicates fever due to exterior repletion. A hot, moist skin generally indicates heat in the qi aspect, and in some cases qi vacuity fever. It may also indicate sweating prior to the abatement of a fever. A cold, clammy skin may indicate yang-collapse vacuity desertion, or a fever-reducing sweat; the correct diagnosis becomes clear when correlated to other symptoms. A dry, shrivelled skin indicates damage to liquid, humor desertion, or major damage to qi and yin. A condition of extreme dryness and roughness of the skin in enduring illness, known as cutaneous cornification, indicates insufficiency of qi and blood or static blood binding in the inner body. Temporary depression of the skin after applying pressure indicates water swelling. Grossness of the limbs where the flesh feels soft like cottonwool and rebounds immediately on release of pressure is qi swelling or vacuity corpulence.[4]

Palpation of the limbs

Temperature assessment is the most important aspect of palpation of the limbs. A lack of warmth in the extremities is a sign of yang vacuity. Inversion frigidity indicates yang collapse or the presence of a heat pathogen causing an inner-body block. Generalized fever with coldness at the tips of the fingers and toes may portend yang-collapse vacuity desertion, or heat block tetanic inversion. This sign should be accorded special attention if it occurs in children. Heat in the palms and the soles together with a subjective feeling of feverish oppression in the chest, known as "fever in the five hearts," is a sign of yin vacuity fever. Palpation of the limbs also involves identification of deformity and paralysis.

Palpation of the chest

Palpation of the *xu-li* pulsation constitutes the main aspect of chest palpation. The point *xu-li* is located below the left nipple. Described as being "the source of all blood vessels," it is the point where the heart is closest to the surface, corresponding to the apical pulse in Western medicine. Too strong or too weak a pulsation indicates insufficiency of heart qi; excessive strength of the pulsation is known by a special term, "outward draining of ancestral qi." The *xu-li* pulse is relatively indistinct in corpulent people and more pronounced in thin people. This is not an indication of disease.

Palpation of the abdomen

Through palpation of the abdomen, the physician is able to locate disorders, determine the nature of any pain or distention, or identify any concretions and gatherings.

Location of disorders

The correspondences between location of pathologic symptoms and the relevant diseased organ are as follows: the lateral costal region corresponds to the liver and gallbladder; the lumbar region to the kidney; the umbilical region to the stomach and intestines; and the lower abdomen to the liver, the bladder, or the kidney. The results of palpation should be correlated with other symptoms, with special attention paid to the relationship between the location of symptoms and the channels.

Determining the nature of pain

Pain relieved by pressure is cold pain, vacuity pain, or qi pain. Palpatory tenderness indicates heat or repletion pain.

Identification of concretions and gatherings

Masses of specific location that are hard and resist dispersion under pressure are either concretions or accumulations. Concretions and accumulations generally occur when repletion pathogens such as static blood or phlegm-rheum gather and bind. Abdominal masses that are soft or that disperse under pressure are conglomerations or gatherings. Conglomerations and gatherings are generally attributable to qi stagnation. These four forms are referred to collectively as concretions and gatherings.

Palpation of acupoints

Organic morbidity may be reflected in palpatory tenderness or sensitivity at certain acupoints. For example, hepatitis is reflected in palpatory tenderness at LV-14 and BL-18. Diseases of the gallbladder are reflected by palpatory tenderness at BL-19 or *dan-nang-xue* (M-LE-23). Gastric or duodenal ulcers are reflected in palpatory tenderness in the region of ST-36. Acute appendicitis is reflected in palpatory pain at *lan-wei-xue* (M-LE-13). Diseases are not only reflected at these points, but may also be treated by acupuncture or massotherapy at the sensitive spots.

Table 6-1
Comparative table of 29 pulses, page 1

Pulses and Their Clinical Significance

Pulse	Beats (per resp.)	Strength	Form	Clinical Significance	Notes
Floating		Superabundant at the superficial level and insufficient at the deep level.		Exterior exogenous contraction pattern	Floating pulse in enduring disease or hemorrhage is a negative sign
Deep		Not felt until heavy pressure is applied		Interior pattern	
Slow	3 or less			Cold pattern, yang vacuity	
Rapid	6 or more			Heat pattern or yin vacuity	
Vacuous		Very weak	Relatively small	Vacuity, especially of yang	General term for all forceless pulses
Replete		Very strong	Relatively large	Repletion patterns	General term for all forceful pulses
Slippery			Rises and falls smoothly, like pearls rolling in a dish	Pregnancy, phlegm patterns, digestate accumulation	

Table 6-1
Comparative table of 29 pulses, page 2

Pulses and Their Clinical Significance

Pulse	Beats (per resp.)	Strength	Form	Clinical Significance	Notes
Rough		Relatively weak	Rises disfluently, like a knife scraping bamboo	Blood vacuity or stasis	
Wiry		Usually forceful	Long and straight, like a guitar string	Hepatocystic disease, phlegm-rheum, pain	
Soggy		Relatively weak	Slightly floating and fine	Insufficiency of blood and qi, damp encumbrance	Also called a soft pulse
Surging		Strong	Broad and large, falls away weakly after an exuberant onset	Heat, pathogen exuberance, advancing condition	
Faint		Very weak	Fine, faint, and indistinct, sometimes felt and sometimes not	Vacuity desertion of qi and blood	
Fine		Generally very weak	Thin and threadlike	Insufficiency of qi and blood, and especially of qi and yin	Also called a small pulse

Table 6-1
Comparative table of 29 pulses, page 3

Pulses and Their Clinical Significance

Pulse	Beats (per resp.)	Strength	Form	Clinical Significance	Notes
Weak		Deep and forceless	Fine and small	Insufficiency of blood and qi	
Large			Broad and large		Refers to pulse size, no connotation of strength
Scattered		Very weak	Floating and forceless, large and without root	Dissipation of qi and blood, impending expiry of essential qi	
Tight		Strong	Wiry and markedly forceful	Cold and pain	
Scallion Stalk		Weak (forceless when heavy pressure is applied)	Floating and empty in the middle, like a scallion stalk	Blood collapse, seminal loss, commonly occurs in massive bleeding	
Drumskin		Weak (forceless when heavy pressure is applied)	Occurs with wiry pulse	Blood collapse, seminal loss, commonly occurs in massive bleeding	
Confined		Deep and forceful		Cold pain, inner body exuberance of yin cold	Commonly referred to as a deep wiry pulse or a deep replete pulse

The Four Examinations

Table 6-1
Comparative table of 29 pulses, page 4

Pulses and Their Clinical Significance

Pulse	Beats (per resp.)	Strength	Form	Clinical Significance	Notes
Racing	7 or more		Soft, slippery, rapid, bouncing like beans	Basically the same as a rapid pulse, but suggests vacuity	
Animated	6 or more			High fever, palpitations, pregnancy	
Hidden			Deeper than a deep pulse	Inner body pathogen block, fulminant desertion of yang qi	
Moderate	3 - 4			Normal	
Rapid irregularly interrupted	6 or more		Pausing irregularly	Debilitation of organ qi, obstruction of heart blood or heart qi flow	Sometimes seen in healthy persons
Slow irregularly interrupted	4 or less		Pausing irregularly	Debilitation of organ qi, obstruction of heart blood or heart qi flow	Sometimes seen in healthy persons
Regularly interrupted			Relatively regular pauses		
Long			Extending beyond barrier and cubit positions		
Short			Felt only at barrier		

156

Notes

[1] "Liquid qi" denotes liquid, but emphasizes its active aspect. See the glossary entry for qi.

[2] Parametric nature signifies cold or heat, vacuity or repletion (q.v Chapter 7).

[3] Q.v. Chapter 10, the discussion of cold pain, under Cold Disease Patterns.

[4] See the glossary entry for water.

Chapter 7
Eight-Parameter Pattern Identification

Pattern identification is the process of determining the significance of symptoms and assembling them into a coherent picture. The first and most important stage of this process is eight-parameter pattern identification. The fundamental nature and location of the disease is determined according to eight parameters: exterior and interior; cold and heat; vacuity and repletion; yin and yang. In subsequent stages, investigation focuses on specific aspects of the organism to reveal a more detailed picture of the patient's condition. For instance, if by eight-parameter pattern identification a heat pattern is detected, qi-blood pattern identification will show whether the heat is located in the blood or qi; organ pattern identification will determine what organ or organs are affected, and pathogen pattern identification will identify any pathogen present.

The eight parameters may be divided into four pairs: exterior and interior; cold and heat; vacuity and repletion; and yin and yang. These pairs are of unequal value and vary in significance according to types of disease. Yin and yang are general parameters that embrace the other six, since exterior, heat, and repletion are yang, and interior, vacuity, and cold are yin. However, because disease represents a complex state of imbalance in the body, yin and yang alone are too vague to be the only parameters of analysis. Interior and exterior, the parameters measuring the depth of disease, are of great importance for identifying exogenous diseases. Pathogens rarely invade the interior without first passing through the exterior. Interior-exterior are, however, of negligible significance in endogenous damage and in miscellaneous diseases, which almost invariably manifest as interior patterns. Cold and heat describe the nature of disease, and provide the criteria for selection of cool or warm agents in drug therapy, and the use of moxibustion in acumoxatherapy. Finally, vacuity and repletion indicate the relative strength of correct and pathogenic qi. Thus, vacuity-repletion determines whether treatment should focus on restoring the correct or dispelling the pathogen. For these reasons, the more specific parameters, especially cold, heat, vacuity, and repletion, are of greater importance in clinical practice.

The eight parameters are not mutually exclusive and unrelated; combinations, conversions, and complexes commonly occur. The term "combination" denotes the simultaneous occurrence of symptoms in two or more parameters. For example, initial stage exogenous heat diseases appear as exterior patterns, which must be further differentiated as exterior cold or exterior heat. Enduring diseases presenting as vacuity patterns must be further differentiated into vacuity cold and vacuity heat. Clearly the parameters follow a strict order of importance. Exterior cold and exterior heat patterns are primarily exterior patterns, and secondarily cold or heat patterns. Vacuity cold and vacuity heat patterns are primarily vacuity patterns and secondarily cold or heat patterns. In interior-exterior combinations, parameter precedence varies from case to case.

"Conversion" denotes the displacement of symptoms of one parameter by symptoms of the opposing parameter of the pair. Any pattern's parameter may, under given circumstances, convert into its opposite. An example of this can be seen in exogenous heat diseases. These are characterized in the initial stages by symptoms such as headache, generalized pain, aversion to cold, and fever. If in such cases the pathogen interiorizes, as a result of either its own strength, vacuity of correct qi, or inappropriate treatment, the original exterior pattern converts into an interior pattern. Patterns of all the other parameters may similarly convert in specific circumstances. The aim of treatment is therefore to foster favorable and prevent unfavorable conversion.

The term "complex" denotes the simultaneous appearance of symptoms of paired parameters, such as cold and heat, or vacuity and repletion. The simultaneous appearance of interior and exterior signs, which is referred to as a combination rather than a complex, is an exception.

Finally, some conditions may be characterized by false signs, such as extreme heat simulating cold, extreme cold simulating heat, repletion falsely presenting as vacuity, and vacuity falsely presenting as repletion. In pattern identification, care is required to not be misled by false signs, since this may lead to incorrect diagnosis and inappropriate treatment.

Exterior and Interior

"Exterior" and "interior" refer to parts of the body. The surface skin and the body hair, the muscle and skin, and the superficial channels are exterior. The bone marrow, the bowels and viscera, etc., are considered as interior. Exterior-interior pattern identification involves determining the depth of penetration of exogenous pathogens. Pathogens invariably pass through the exterior before penetrating the interior. This is much less significant in endogenous damage and miscellaneous diseases that arise in the inner body and generally manifest as interior patterns.

Exterior patterns

In exterior patterns only the exterior is affected by disease. They generally indicate that the disease is in its initial stages and relatively mild. *Jing Yue's Complete Compendium* states, "In exterior patterns, pathogenic qi enters the body from the outside," and "a pathogen settling in the body must first abide in the surface skin and body hair."

Pattern identification

Disease caused by any of the six environmental excesses entering the body is characterized in the initial stages by aversion to cold, aversion to wind, fever, headache, pain in the joints and limbs, and a floating pulse. These are the classical exterior pattern signs. What in Western medicine are termed upper respiratory tract infections and other acute infectious diseases appear in their initial stages as exterior patterns.

Exterior patterns are seen when exogenous pathogens depress the muscle striations and impede the diffusion of defense qi, producing aversion to cold or wind. When defense qi, which is the body's outer resistance to disease, is impeded by an invading pathogen, the ensuing fight to repel the invader gives rise to fever. Disease in the exterior is characterized by a floating pulse. The forcefulness at the superficial level reflects the exuberant exterior pathogen. Thus, aversion to cold, fever, and a floating pulse represent basic exterior pattern symptoms. Headache and pain in the limbs and joints are attributable to pathogenic qi in the channels impairing the smooth flow of blood and qi. Although diffusion of lung qi may be impaired, giving rise to such symptoms as nasal congestion and cough, the interior and all organs other than the lung remain unaffected, and the appearance of the tongue, with a thin, white fur, is relatively normal.[1]

Exterior patterns vary according to the nature of the offending pathogen and strength of the correct. Distinction is made between patterns of exterior cold, exterior heat, exterior vacuity, and exterior repletion.

Exterior cold patterns

Exterior cold patterns are characterized by pronounced cold signs with a distinct aversion to cold. The pulse is tight and floating, and the tongue fur is thin, white, and moist. When cold prevails there is pain, hence headache, and generalized pain and heaviness may also be felt. Running nose with clear nasal mucus, and expectoration of thin, clear phlegm are common symptoms. Exterior cold patterns are generally caused by contraction of the wind-cold pathogen.

Exterior heat patterns

Exterior heat patterns are characterized by pronounced heat signs, such as a red, sore pharynx and a relatively red tongue with dry fur. In addition to the regular external signs, the pulse is floating and rapid. Other symptoms include cough and production of thick white or yellow phlegm. Most exterior heat patterns are attributable to contraction of the wind-heat pathogen.

Identification of exterior cold and heat patterns is based on assessment of heat and cold "signs" rather than the actual body temperature. Fever as a symptom does not necessarily correspond to heat in the sense of the eight parameters. Depressed wind-cold may transform into heat, so that the exterior cold pattern converts into an exterior heat pattern (or interior heat pattern).

Exterior repletion patterns

Adiaphoretic exterior patterns, those characterized by the absence of sweating, are referred to as exterior repletion patterns. In most cases, these are cold exterior patterns brought about by contraction of a strong cold pathogen that obstructs defense qi and blocks the striations. Such patterns are reflected in a tight, floating pulse.

Exterior vacuity patterns

Exterior patterns with persistent sweating and fever are referred to as exterior vacuity patterns. They occur as a result of construction-defense disharmony where resistance to exogenous pathogens is lowered. When a pathogen is contracted, it cannot be expelled from the body even though there may be sweating. Such conditions are reflected in a moderate, floating pulse (moderate here is used in contradistinction to tight) (cf. Table 7-1).

Treatment

Drug therapy

Exterior patterns are treated by diaphoresis to expel the pathogen from the body. Cold exterior patterns are treated with warm, pungent exterior resolvents. The most commonly used are:

Warm, Pungent Exterior Resolvents	
Herba Ephedrae	má huáng
Ramulus Cinnamomi	guì zhī
Rhizoma et Radix Notopterygii	qiāng huó
Folium Perillae	sū yè
Herba Schizonepetae	jīng jiè
Radix Ledebouriellae	fáng fēng

Formulae include:[2]

Warm Exterior Resolvent Formulae	
Ephedra Decoction	má-huáng tāng
Schizonepeta and Ledebouriella Detoxifying Powder	jīng fáng bài dú sǎn

Exterior heat patterns are treated with cool, pungent exterior resolvents such as:

Cool, Pungent Exterior Resolvents	
Herba Menthae	bò hé
Fructus Arctii	niú bàng zǐ
Semen Sojae Praeparatum	dòu shǐ
Folium Mori	sāng yè

Formulae include:

Cool Exterior Resolvent Formulae	
Lonicera and Forsythia Powder	yín qiào sǎn
Mulberry and Chrysanthemum Cool Decoction	sāng jú yǐn

Exterior patterns without perspiration (exterior repletion patterns), where strong diaphoretic action is needed, are treated with warm, pungent exterior resolvents. Exterior patterns with sweating should be treated with formulae having a milder diaphoretic effect. A persistent exterior pattern with sweating characterized by pronounced exterior vacuity signs such as a moderate, floating pulse and a thin moist tongue fur should be treated with Cinnamon-Twig Decoction *(guì-zhī tāng)*. This formula harmonizes construction and defense.

Acumoxatherapy

Exterior cold patterns can be treated with such points as LI-4, SP-6‡,[3] GB-20‡, GB-15, SI-3‡, BL-12‡, BL-13‡, and KI-7. Exterior heat patterns can be treated with points such as the following: LU-10, LI-4, LI-11, GV-14, KI-7, and BL-13. Where vacuity is present, such points as LU-9, ST-36‡, LI-4‡, and GB-20 can be used to supplement the exterior. LI-4 and KI-7 may be used to stop vacuity sweating. Exterior repletion patterns are commonly treated with such points as LU-5, LU-7, LU-11, and GV-l4 in addition to previously mentioned points such as LI-4 and KI-7.

Interior patterns

The term "interior pattern" stands in opposition to "'exterior pattern," and indicates that the disease is located in the interior. *Jing Yue's Complete Compendium* states, "In interior patterns, the disease is in the inner body, in the viscera." In exogenous heat diseases, a pathogen in the exterior that is not expelled by the body will in most cases interiorize (i.e., enter the interior). *Essential Questions* states:

> A pathogen settling in the body must first abide in the surface skin and body hair. If it resists expulsion, it will enter the reticular connecting channels. If it continues to resist, it will

enter the larger connecting channels. If it persists, it will enter the major channels that communicate with the organs in the inner body. When the pathogen spreads to the stomach and intestines, yin and yang are both affected and all the organs suffer damage. This is the sequence by which pathogens penetrating the body through the surface skin and body hair eventually affect the five viscera.

Interior patterns may therefore emerge as a result of environmental excesses passing from the exterior to the interior, as described in the above quotation, or directly, which is known as "direct strike." However, these patterns may also be caused by affect damage, taxation fatigue, or dietary irregularities that directly affect the bowels and viscera, blood, qi, and fluids.

Pattern identification

Interior patterns occurring in endogenous damage and miscellaneous diseases may be characterized by a wide variety of symptoms (these are discussed in the relevant following chapters). In interior patterns occurring in exogenous heat diseases, distinction must be made between heat, repletion, cold, and vacuity, the first two being the most common.

Interior heat and repletion patterns

If an exterior pathogen interiorizes and transforms to heat, the original exterior pattern gives way to one of fever without aversion to cold, a red tongue with yellow fur, a rapid pulse, and short micturition with dark-colored urine. All these indicate pronounced heat. In severe cases, there may be tidal flushing of the face, aversion to heat, restlessness, a rapid, surging pulse, profuse sweating, and thirst, each of which indicates intense interior heat. Exterior pathogens penetrating the interior may also produce pain, distention, and fullness in the chest and abdomen, hard stool, a deep, full pulse, and thick, slimy, yellow tongue fur. These signs are indicative of gastrointestinal heat-bind (interior repletion).

Developing a stage further, interior heat and repletion may be characterized by a crimson tongue, clouding of the spirit, tetanic inversion, and convulsive spasms, as well as maculopapular eruptions. These symptoms are indicative of pathogenic heat penetrating construction-blood or the pericardium, or of extreme heat stirring wind. All are serious conditions.

Interior cold and vacuity patterns

Pathogen interiorization may produce cold or vacuity, characterized by the absence of fever, an aversion to cold, vomiting, thoracic pain, diarrhea, and absence of thirst. The tongue fur is white and moist, while the pulse is moderate and soggy. These signs indicate devitalization of splenic yang. In severe cases, there may be somber white complexion, sweating and frigidity of the limbs, spiritual lassitude and somnolence, and a fine, faint pulse. These signs collectively indicate cardiorenal yang debilitation.

This is only a simple analysis of interior patterns. When interior patterns occur in exogenous heat diseases, it is also necessary to identify six-channel, four-aspect, and pathogen patterns. In endogenous damage and miscellaneous diseases, the wide range of patterns associated with the various organs and the variety of diseases and pathogens are such that eight-parameter pattern identification must be followed by organ and qi-blood pattern identification before treatment can be prescribed.

Interior patterns are presented schematically in Table 7-2.

Treatment

Since distinctions are made between cold, heat, vacuity, repletion, and their various combinations, a broad variety of interior patterns exists. Accordingly, treatment may take the form of warming, clearage, supplementation, or attack. Diseases affecting specific organs, channels, and functional aspects all require particular methods of treatment. For elaboration, see the relevant sections on pathogen, organ, and exogenous heat disease pattern identification.

Midstage and dual exterior-interior patterns

Midstage patterns

Midstage patterns are exogenous heat disease patterns that neither fit the category of exterior patterns nor the category of interior patterns. They are chiefly characterized by alternating fever and chills, bitter fullness in the chest and lateral costal region, restlessness, no desire for food and drink, bitter taste in the mouth, dry pharynx, visual dizziness, and wiry pulse. The etiology of midstage patterns is considered in detail in Chapter 11, "Exogenous Heat Disease Pattern Identification." Since these are not exterior patterns, they cannot be treated by diaphoresis. Because the pathogen has not completely penetrated the interior, the normal procedures for treatment of interior patterns are also excluded. Instead, the method of harmonization and resolution is applied. The basic formula is Minor Bupleurum Decoction *(xiǎo chái-hú tāng)*, which outthrusts exterior pathogens and clears the interior.

Dual Exterior-Interior Patterns

Conditions characterized by the simultaneous presence of both exterior and interior patterns are known as dual exterior-interior patterns. These patterns occur when a cold pathogen simultaneously invades the exterior and interior, creating exterior symptoms such as aversion to cold, fever, headache, and aching bones, and interior signs such as abdominal pain and diarrhea. Dual exterior-interior patterns also occur when a pathogen that initially produces an exterior pattern subsequently interiorizes creating an interior pattern before the exterior pattern is resolved.

The term "dual exterior-interior pattern" generally does not include superimposure of an exterior pattern resulting from contraction of an environmental excess on a pre-existing interior pattern. Rather, such an exterior pattern is simply referred to as a complicating contraction. Similarly, it does not include ingesta damage patterns superimposed on pre-existing exterior exogenous disease patterns. These are known as ingesta damage complications.

Cold and Heat

Cold and heat are terms denoting the nature of a disease. Identification of cold and heat symptoms is of crucial importance for the selection of warm and cool agents in treatment.

Cold and heat pattern identification involves using clinically observable signs to determine whether the pathogen is yin or yang in nature, or whether the yin-yang imbalance is attributable to vacuity of yin or yang. The chapter entitled "Cold and Heat" of the *Jing Yue's Complete Compendium* states, "Cold and heat are mutations of yin and yang." The author continues:

> When yang is exuberant, there is heat; when yin is exuberant there is cold; when yang is vacuous, there is cold; when yin is vacuous there is heat.

Cold patterns

Cold patterns may be caused by either yin pathogens entering the body ("when yin is exuberant there is cold") or by an insufficiency of the body's yang qi ("when yang is vacuous there is cold").

Pattern identification

Cold patterns are generally characterized by aversion to cold, somber white or cyan complexion, desire for quiet, curled-up recumbent posture, and counterflow frigidity of the limbs. The mouth is moist, and there is either no thirst, or thirst with desire for warm fluids. There may be fulminant pain in the abdomen, fulminant vomiting, or fulminant diarrhea. Since cold is associated with thin, cold, clear excreta, micturition is long with clear urine, and the tongue fur is moist and white. The pulse is slow or tight.

Pronounced cold signs such as pain in the abdomen, fulminant vomiting, fulminant diarrhea, cyan complexion, and tight pulse are associated with prevalence of yin, i.e., an exuberant yin pathogen. Symptoms such as desire for quiet, curled-up recumbent posture, long micturition with clear urine, clear-food diarrhea, inversion frigidity of the limbs, and slow pulse are chiefly attributable to yang vacuity. However, since cold pathogens may damage yang, and yang vacuity may engender cold, the two forms of cold are interrelated. Cold form and frigid limbs, and somber white complexion, which are commonly observed cold signs, are attributed to the debilitation of yang qi and the presence of an exuberant cold pathogen.

Treatment

Drug therapy

Since "cold is treated with heat," warming is the chief form of treatment for cold patterns. Patterns in which invasion by an exogenous pathogen is the primary element are treated by dissipation of the cold pathogen with warm agents. Those patterns primarily characterized by debilitation of yang qi are treated by warming yang and boosting qi. Commonly used agents that dissipate the cold pathogen include:

Warming Agents	
Radix Aconiti Fu Tzu	fù zǐ
Cortex Cinnamomi	ròu guì
Rhizoma Zingiberis Recens	shēng jiāng
Rhizoma Zingiberis Exsiccatum	gān jiāng
Fructus Evodiae	wú zhū yú
Rhizoma Alpiniae Officinaris	gāo liáng jiāng

Radix Aconiti Fu Tzu *(fù zǐ)* and Cortex Cinnamomi *(ròu guì)* also possess a yang-warming effect. Radix Ginseng *(rén shēn)* or Radix Codonopsis Pilosulae *(dǎng shēn)*, Radix Glycyrrhizae *(gān cǎo)*, Rhizoma Atractylodis Macrocephalae *(bái zhú)*, and other qi fortifiers may be added to boost qi. Cold-dissipating formulae include:

Cold-Dissipating Formulae	
Alpinia and Cyperus Pills	liáng fù wán
Ginseng and Aconite Decoction	shēn fù tāng
Counterfow Cold Decoction with Ginseng	sì nì jiā rén-shēn tāng
Center-Rectifying Pills	lǐ zhōng wán

These are commonly used yang-warming, qi-boosting formulae. Alpinia and Cyperus Pills help to relieve pain.

Acumoxatherapy

The use of moxibustion is important in treating cold patterns and conditions characterized by yang debilitation. Commonly used points include the following: CV-6‡, CV-4‡, ST-36‡, SP-6‡, BL-20‡, and GV-4‡.

Heat patterns

Heat patterns are the result of either an invasion of a yang pathogen ("when yang prevails there is heat") or of insufficiency of yin humor ("when yin is vacuous, there is heat"). Yang prevalence and yin vacuity thus represent the two essential factors for the emergence of heat patterns.

Pattern identification

Heat patterns due to prevalence of yang are termed repletion heat patterns. These patterns are characterized by red complexion, ocular rubor, vigorous fever, agitation, thirst, and desire for cold fluids. The stool is hard and micturition is short with dark-colored urine. The tongue is red or deep red with yellow fur, while the pulse is rapid or large, surging, and rapid. Heat due to insufficiency of yin humor (see following section, "Yin and Yang") is termed vacuity heat, and is characterized by fever in the five hearts, steaming bone tidal fever, dry throat and mouth, red, mirror tongue, and a thin, rapid pulse.

Treatment

Drug therapy

Vacuity heat and repletion heat are treated differently. Repletion heat is treated by clearage, according to the principle that heat is treated with cold. Heat-clearing, fire-draining agents such as these are commonly used:

Heat-Clearing, Fire-Draining Agents	
Gypsum	*shí gāo*
Rhizoma Anemarrhenae	*zhī mǔ*
Radix Scutellariae	*huáng qín*
Rhizoma Coptidis	*huáng lián*
Rhizoma Rhei	*dà huáng*

Heat-clearing toxin-resolving agents are useful in specific cases. Formulae frequently used to treat repletion heat patterns include White Tiger Decoction *(bái hǔ tāng)* and Heart-Draining Decoction *(xiè xīn tāng).*[3]

In treating vacuity heat, nourishing yin is of greater importance than clearing heat. For details about yin-nourishing agents, see "Vacuity and Repletion" in this chapter. Drugs frequently used for clearing vacuity heat include:

Vacuity Heat Clearers	
Herba Artemisiae Apiaceae	qīng hāo
Radix Cynanchi Atrati	bái wéi
Radix Stellariae Dichotomae	yín chái hú
Cortex Radicis Lycii	dì gǔ pí
Rhizoma Anemarrhenae	zhī mǔ
Cortex Phellodendri	huáng bó

Two-A Decoction *(qīng-hāo biē-jiǎ tāng)* is a formula commonly used for clearing vacuity heat.

Acumoxatherapy

General points for repletion heat include ST-25, ST-41, and LI-4. Where there is constipation ST-25 is especially important, along with TB-6 and LI-6. Vacuity heat may be treated with some of the above-points together with HT-5, KI-3, LV-3, and SP-6. The selection of points is dependent on the organ systems involved. Severe repletion heat may be treated by bleeding such points as BL-54 and GV-14.

Combinations of heat and cold with repletion and vacuity

Most cold patterns are vacuity cold patterns. However, there are repletion cold patterns that are characterized by pain and distention in the abdomen, constipation, and dyspnea with fullness in the chest. In severe cases, there is cyan complexion, frigid limbs, trismus, and block-clouding inversion. These signs are explained either by gastrointestinal obstruction due to the presence of a cold pathogen and digestate accumulation, or to cold blocking lung qi. Most heat patterns are replete, though vacuity heat patterns are not rare. Table 7-3 shows the basic differences between vacuity and repletion cold, and vacuity and repletion heat.

Cold—heat complexes

Cold-heat complexes, which are patterns including both cold and heat signs, are commonly seen in clinical practice. Signs such as a sensation of heat and feverishness in the chest, pain in the venter, clamoring stomach, and vomiting of sour and bitter matter, occurring at the same time as abdominal pain relieved by warmth and pressure, borborygmi, and diarrhea with undigested food in the stool, indicate upper-body heat and lower-body cold, one example of a cold-heat complex. In such cases, the relative prominence of heat and cold must be determined before treatment can be prescribed.

False heat and cold

"Extreme heat simulates cold and extreme cold simulates heat." This describes the situation where heat or cold, on reaching its extreme, gives rise to some symptoms that conflict with the existing original pattern. For instance, tidal flushing of the face is a heat symptom, and appearing in a pronounced cold pattern, is at variance with the other signs. This situation is described as cold falsely presenting as heat. Similarly, if inversion frigidity of the limbs appears side by side with pronounced heat signs, the pattern should be rightly identified as one of heat falsely presenting as cold. Since false symptoms occur only in relatively severe diseases, it is of vital importance to distinguish true signs from false signs.

Heat falsely presenting as cold

If symptoms such as unsurfaced heat, inversion frigidity of the limbs, and even aversion to wind, occur in combination with dry mouth, dry throat, thirst with desire for cold fluids, short micturition with dark-colored urine, hard stool, red tongue with slimy, yellow fur, and a strong, rapid pulse, the latter signs govern. The inversion frigidity of the limbs and aversion to cold are due to depressed heat in the interior preventing yang qi from reaching peripheral regions. They are therefore false signs of cold and the pattern should be correctly identified as one of heat.

Cold falsely presenting as heat

When inversion frigidity of the limbs, diarrhea with undigested food in the stool, or faint pulse verging on expiry, occur simultaneously with agitation, no aversion to cold, thirst with desire for warm fluids, upbearing fire flush, or sore pharynx, the pattern is one of cold falsely presenting as heat. Here, the cold signs are caused by exuberant yin cold in the inner body while the false heat signs (agitation, upbearing fire flush, and sore pharynx) are attributable to overfloating of vacuous yang. This is a critical condition treated by salvaging yang and checking desertion.

In general, where the presence of false signs is difficult to determine, the tongue, pulse, thirst, and type of fluids desired provide the most reliable indication of the true pattern.

Vacuity and Repletion

"Where pathogenic qi is exuberant there is repletion, and where essential qi is retrenched there is vacuity." These words sum up the laws underlying the emergence of vacuity and repletion patterns. The parameters of vacuity and repletion reflect the strength of correct qi and pathogens. Their identification also provides the basis for determining whether offensive or supplementing treatment should be prescribed.

Vacuity patterns

Vacuity patterns may be due to such causes as a weak constitution, damage to correct qi either through enduring illness, loss of blood, seminal loss, and profuse sweating, or by invasion of an exogenous pathogen (yang pathogens readily damaging yin humor and yin pathogens readily damaging yang qi). These causes are succinctly summed up in the phrase, "Where essential qi is retrenched, there is vacuity."

Pattern identification

Distinction is made between general insufficiencies of qi, blood, yin, and yang. Since these frequently affect specific organs, further distinction is made between such forms as heart yin vacuity, liver blood vacuity, kidney yang vacuity, and lung qi vacuity. This section deals with the major distinctions only, while the organ-related forms are dealt with in Chapter 9.

Qi and yang vacuity are both forms of yang qi insufficiency, hence their clinical manifestations are similar. Signs include drained or somber complexion, spiritual fatigue, weakness, spontaneous sweating, and low voice. Yang vacuity is characterized by pronounced cold signs. Blood vacuity denotes depletion of the blood and often occurs in conjunction with qi vacuity (dual vacuity of qi and blood) or with yin vacuity (dual vacuity of yin and blood). Yin vacuity refers to insufficiency of the yin humor, and is invariably characterized by signs of heat and dryness. (See Table 7-4.)

Treatment

Drug therapy

"Vacuity is treated by supplementation." Thus, supplementation is the principal method of treating vacuity patterns. Qi boosting, blood supplementation, yang warming, and yin enrichment are the methods used for treating the four basic forms of vacuity. However, since qi and blood are mutually dependent and engendering, vacuity of either qi or blood is generally treated by providing support for its complement. Qi boosters include:

Qi Boosters	
Radix Astragali	*huáng qí*
Radix Codonopsis Pilosulae	*dǎng shēn*
Radix Glycyrrhizae	*gān cǎo*

Yang warmers include:

Yang Warmers	
Radix Aconiti Fu Tzu	fù zǐ
Cortex Cinnamomi	ròu guì
Cornu Cervi	lù jiǎo

Blood supplementers include:

Blood Supplementers	
Radix Angelicae Sinensis	dāng guī
Radix Rehmanniae Conquita	shóu dì

Yin enrichers include:

Yin Enrichers	
Radix Rehmanniae Cruda	shēng dì
Herba Dendrobii	shí hú
Radix Scrophulariae	xuán shēn
Tuber Ophiopogonis	mài dōng
Carapax Amydae	biē jiǎ
Plastrum Testudinis	guī bǎn

As to formulae, Four Nobles Decoction *(sì jūn zǐ tāng)* is commonly used to fortify qi; Aconite and Cinnamon Eight Pills *(fù guì bā wèi wán)* are used to warm yang; Four Agents Decoction *(sì wù tāng)* is used to supplement the blood; and Rehmannia Six Pills *(liù wèi dì-huáng wán)* are frequently used to enrich yin.

Acumoxatherapy

Qi-boosting points include GV-14‡, LI-4‡, CV-6‡, CV-4‡, BL-38‡, and ST-36‡. Blood-nourishing points include SP-1O, SP-6‡, KI-3‡, and BL-2O‡. To warm yang, points such as GV-4‡, GV-2O‡, LI-4‡, and BL-23‡ may be used. Finally, yin enrichment can be achieved by needling KI-3, PC-7, TB-2, and LV-3.

Repletion patterns

Repletion may be due to such factors as an invading pathogen, phlegm-rheum, water-damp, static blood, parasitic accumulations, and digestate accumulations. For this reason it is said, "Where pathogenic qi is exuberant, there is repletion."

Pattern identification

Repletion patterns vary according to the nature of the pathogen and the organ affected. Specific patterns are dealt with in the chapters on pathogen and organ pattern identification. However, a common feature of repletion patterns is that they are associated with exuberant pathogenic qi. Thus, when a heat pathogen is exuberant, a repletion heat pattern emerges; the presence of an exuberant cold pathogen gives rise to a repletion cold pattern; and exuberant phlegm gives rise to phlegm and drool congesting the upper body. Table 7-5 provides a comparison of vacuity and repletion patterns.

It should be pointed out that repletion may reflect not only the exuberance of a pathogen but also the strength of the body's reaction to it. This explains why rapid, surging pulses, slippery, wiry pulses, and large, replete pulses, which are all strong at the deep level, are associated with repletion patterns.

Treatment

Drug therapy

Since repletion is treated by drainage, attack is the chief method of treating repletion patterns. In practice, this embraces a wide range of treatment methods, including heat clearage and detoxification, fire drainage, restoration of stool flow, water expulsion, offensive elimination of phlegm, expulsion of static blood, qi breaking, abductive dispersion, and parasite expulsion. For further details, see the chapters relating to exogenous heat disease, pathogen, qi-blood, and organ pattern identification.

Acumoxatherapy

The draining method in acupuncture generally involves the use of a strong stimulus. The choice of points is dependent on the nature and location of the repletion.

Complexes, conversions, and false signs of vacuity and repletion

Vacuity-repletion complexes

Vacuity of correct qi and pathogen exuberance occurring simultaneously is known as a vacuity-repletion complex. For example, if a patient suffering from a cough expectorates thick, sticky phlegm and has a yellow tongue fur, his condition is described as pulmonary phlegm-heat congestion, which is a repletion pattern. If, at the same time, his breathing is short and shallow, and becomes rapid at the slightest exertion, he is said to be suffering from insufficiency of lung qi, which is a vacuity pattern. The two sets of symptoms together form a vacuity-repletion complex.

A further example is inner-body static blood obstruction, manifesting as abdominal lump glomi. If this repletion pattern occurs with signs of dual vacuity of yin and blood, characterized by emaciation, cutaneous cornification, and dark rings around the eyes, the patient is said to be suffering from a vacuity-repletion complex. Such patterns may be due to contraction of an exogenous pathogen by patients suffering from regular vacuity of the correct, or may be caused by an invading pathogen at once causing repletion and damaging the correct.

Conversion of vacuity and repletion

Under certain conditions, vacuity of correct qi and pathogen exuberance are mutually convertible. In their initial stages, exogenous diseases are usually characterized by repletion. However, if the pathogen disappears, leaving the correct damaged, or if the correct is damaged before the pathogen disappears, a vacuity pattern evolves. Vacuity of the correct is fundamentally a vacuity pattern, but by affecting the flow of blood or movement of fluids, it may give rise to phlegm-rheum, water-damp, and static blood, or lead to further pathogen contraction. In this event, the original qi, blood, yin, or yang vacuity converts into a repletion pattern. Vacuous constitutions, exuberant pathogens, repeated contraction of pathogens, as well as inappropriate or unthorough treatment, may all give rise to the conversion of vacuity or repletion into its opposite.

False vacuity and repletion

Vacuity and repletion may simulate each other. For this reason it is said, "Severe repletion presents signs of weakness, and extreme vacuity presents symptoms of strength." False signs occurring in diseases with a complex array of symptoms easily cause confusion. When damp-heat obstruction in the initial stage of non-icteric hepatitis presents such signs as fatigue and lack of strength, limpness and pain in the limbs, little thought for food, and a soft, soggy pulse, the condition may be wrongly identified as one of vacuity. Although there may be a splenogastric vacuity complication, the pattern of damp-heat obstruction is one of repletion. Careful examination will point to the correct diagnosis. Exhaustion and weak limbs, together with oppression in the chest, abdominal distention, and a slimy tongue fur indicate encumbering damp rather than vacuity of original qi. If the tongue fur is yellow and slimy, and micturition is short with dark-colored urine, the condition may be identified as one of damp-heat. Treatment should therefore involve draining the repletion rather than supplying the vacuity. The classics state, "Where the symptoms may be false, the pulse should govern, and where the pulse may be false, the tongue should govern." This provides a useful guide in correct identification of vacuity and repletion.

False repletion signs may also occur. For example, vacuity dyspnea occurring in failure of renal governance of qi absorption may be characterized by exuberant phlegm, dyspnea and fullness, rapid breathing and inability to lie flat, as well as a slippery, wiry pulse, and a slimy tongue fur.

These signs may easily be misinterpreted as repletion dyspnea. Although there is lower body vacuity and upper body repletion, the pattern is, at root, one of vacuity. The exuberant phlegm congesting the upper body represents only the branches. Careful examination leads to the correct diagnosis. Respiration is short, rapid, and distressed, hence different from the rough breathing and strident voice typifying repletion dyspnea; the slippery, wiry pulse has no strength when firm pressure is applied; and finally, although the tongue fur is slimy, the body of the tongue usually has a slightly cyan-purple hue. These symptoms all indicate vacuity falsely presenting as repletion, and the additional presence of frigid limbs and cold sweating on the head provide further confirmation that vacuity dyspnea is the correct diagnosis. Treatment should therefore center on restoration of qi absorption. Generally speaking, when faced with a confusing array of symptoms, all the information derived from the four examinations should be carefully synthesized, paying special attention to such factors as age, constitution, and duration of the disease. Misidentifying vacuity or repletion as its opposite or as a vacuity-repletion complex may lead to grave errors in treatment.

Yin and Yang

Yin and yang pattern identification may be discussed under two rubrics: identifying yin and yang patterns; and identifying vacuity and collapse of yin and yang.

Yin and yang patterns

Since yin and yang are categories by which all disease may be classified, they form the basic parameters of pattern identification. The remaining pairs of parameters may also be classified according to yin and yang: exterior patterns are yang while interior patterns are yin; cold patterns are yin, while heat patterns are yang; and vacuity patterns are yin, while repletion patterns are yang. In clinical practice, however, yin and yang have little significance other than in describing classical patterns such as vacuity cold and repletion heat, which are termed yin and yang patterns respectively. By convention, vacuity cold is described as a yin pattern. All other patterns are now rarely qualified by these terms. (See Table 7-6.)

Vacuity and collapse of yin and yang

Yin and yang are used to identify vacuity and debilitation of yin humor and yang qi. Yin vacuity therefore denotes insufficiency of yin humor, while yin collapse refers to fulminant desertion of yin humor. Similarly, yang vacuity denotes insufficiency of yang qi, while yang collapse refers to fulminant desertion of yang qi. Although all four conditions are essentially vacuities, distinction is made between cold and heat: yin vacuity and collapse are characterized by heat signs, whereas yang vacuity and collapse are characterized by cold signs.

Pattern identification

Yin vacuity and yang vacuity

Refer to "Vacuity and Repletion" earlier in this chapter.

Yin collapse

The chief signs are copious perspiration, palpably hot skin, and warm limbs. There is agitation, or in serious cases clouding of spirit-affect. There is thirst with desire for cool fluids. Respiration is short, rapid, and distressed, with difficulty in catching the breath. The tongue is dry and red, while the pulse is weak and rapid.

Yang collapse

Signs include sweating and cold skin and inversion frigidity of the limbs. The patient is apathetic or (rarely) agitated, and in serious cases his spirit-affect is clouded. There is either no thirst, or else desire for warm fluids. The pulse is either hidden, deep, fine and faint, or agitated and racing. The tongue is pale.

Collapse here refers to acute, critical forms of vacuity. High fever, profuse sweating, fulminant vomiting, fulminant diarrhea, and heavy bleeding may all lead to serious depletion of yang qi and yin blood. In such cases, both yang qi and yin humors are damaged. Since yin and yang are interdependent, when yin collapses yang has no support and scatters, and when yang collapses, yin humor is no longer produced and is gradually depleted. Thus, yin collapse may swiftly give rise to yang collapse, and yang collapse invariably causes damage to yin.

Treatment

Methods for treating yin and yang vacuity have been discussed. Yin and yang collapse are treated by restoring the correct and securing against collapse. Yin collapse is treated by boosting qi and constraining yin, and by heavy supplementation of original qi. This engenders yin humor and prevents collapse of yang. Although this method involves qi boosting, the use of potent warm and hot agents is nevertheless avoided.

Drug therapy

Pulse-Engendering Powder *(shēng mài sǎn)* is a formula commonly used to treat yin collapse. Yang collapse is treated by salvaging yang, boosting qi, and securing against desertion. The most commonly used drugs are Radix Ginseng *(rén shēn)* and Radix Aconiti Fu Tzu *(fù zǐ)*. Yin-constraining anti-desertives such as Os Draconis *(lóng gǔ)* and Concha Ostreae *(mǔ lì)* may be added. Thus, two formulae that may be used are

Ginseng and Aconite Decoction *(shēn fù tāng)* and Ginseng, Aconite, Dragon Bone, and Oystershell Decoction *(shēn fù lóng mǔ tāng)*. Where there are signs of damage to yin, formulae including Radix Rehmanniae *(dì huáng)*, Radix Paeoniae *(sháo yào)*, and Gelatinum Corii Asini *(ē jiāo)* may be used.

Acumoxatherapy

Yin collapse is often treated by needling such points as GV-14, CV-4, CV-12, KI-3, and KI-7. Moxibustion is indicated for the treatment of yang collapse, provided the fluids have not been severely damaged, the commonly used points being GV-26, GV-20‡, KI-1, LI-4, ST-36‡, BL-38‡, and GV-4‡.

Yin and yang lesions

Finally, in external medicine, distinction is made between yin and yang lesions. Generally, lesions white in color, characterized by diffuse swelling, absence of heat, and clear, thin pus, or accompanied by generalized physical weakness, are classified as yin lesions, whereas those characterized by pronounced redness, swelling, heat, pain, and thick pus, and associated with generalized repletion heat patterns, are classified as yang lesions.

Table 7-1

	Exterior Cold, Heat, Vacuity, and Repletion Patterns	
Pattern	*Principal Signs*	*Method of Treatment*
Exterior Cold	Marked aversion to cold Headache Pronounced general pain Thin, moist tongue fur Tight, floating pulse	Warm, pungent Exterior resolution
Exterior Heat	Mild aversion to cold Sore throat Thin, dry tongue fur Red tongue Rapid, floating pulse	Cool, pungent exterior resolution
Exterior Vacuity	Sweating Moderate, floating pulse	Construction-defense harmonization
Exterior Repletion	No sweating Tight, floating pulse	Warm, pungent exterior resolution

Table 7-2 page one

Pattern	Principal Signs	Method of Treatment
Interior Cold and Heat Patterns		

Interior Cold	Somber white complexion
	Aversion to cold
	  and frigidity of the limbs
	  no thirst
	  or desire for warm beverages
	Abdominal pain
	  relieved by warmth
	Long micturition
	  with clear urine
	Thin or clear stool
	Pale or white glossy tongue
	Deep, hidden pulse
	  or deep, slow pulse
		Warming

Interior Heat	Red complexion or tidal flushing
	Fever
	Aversion to heat
	Agitation
	Desire for warm beverages
	Short micturition
	  with dark-colored urine
	Hard, bound stool or diarrhea
	  with foul-smelling stool
	  or blood in stool
	Red or crimson tongue
	  with yellow fur
	Rapid pulse
		Clearage

Table 7-2 page 2

Interior Vacuity and Repletion Patterns		
Pattern	*Principal Signs*	*Method of Treatment*
Interior Vacuity	Fatigue and lack of strength Shortness of breath Low voice Dizziness Flowery vision Palpitations Mental distraction Reduced appetite Thin stool Fine, weak pulse	Supplementation
Interior Repletion	Abdominal fullness, distention with discomfort exacerbated by pressure Constipation Delirious mania Thick, slimy, yellow tongue fur Deep, replete pulse	Attack

Table 7-3 page 1

Combinations of Cold with Vacuity and Repletion

Pattern Type	Pathomechanism	Principal Signs	Method of Treatment
Vacuity Cold	Debilitation of yang qi	Aversion to cold Inversion frigidity of the limbs Drained white complexion Torpor of essence spirit Clear-food diarrhea Long micturition with clear urine Pale, enlarged tongue with thin, moist tongue fur Thin, slow, weak pulse	Warming Yang & Restoring the Correct
Repletion Cold	Cold pathogen congestion	Aversion to cold Cold limbs Cold and pain in the abdomen White, slimy tongue fur Deep, hidden pulse (or) tight, wiry pulse	Warming & Freeing Repletion Cold

181

Table 7-3 page 2

Combinations of Heat with Vacuity and Repletion

Pattern Type	Pathomechanism	Principal Signs	Method of Treatment
Vacuity Heat	Yin humor depletion	Tidal fever Night sweating Emaciation Lack of strength Fever in the five hearts Dry throat and mouth Red tongue with little fur Fine, rapid pulse	Nourishing Yin & Clearing Heat
Repletion Heat	Intense heat pathogen	Vigorous fever Restlessness and thirst Clouding of the spirit Delirious mania Abdominal fullness and distention with pain exacerbated by pressure Red tongue with yellow fur Fast, surging, slippery and replete pulse	Heat Clearage & Fire Drainage

Table 7-4 page 1

Qi and Yang Vacuities

Pattern	Common Signs	Distinguishing Signs	Method of Treatment
Qi Vacuity	Drained white or somber white complexion Spiritual fatigue and lack of strength Spontaneous sweating No energy to speak Low voice Non-transformation of ingested food Pale, enlarged tongue	Shortness of breath Lack of strength Rapid breathing at the slightest movement (all of these relatively pronounced) Thin stool Dribbling incontinence Soggy pulse	Boosting Qi
Yang Vacuity		Aversion to cold Inversion frigidity of the limbs Dark or cyan-purple complexion Long micturition with clear urine Clear food diarrhea Cyan-purple tongue Slow pulse	Warming Yang

Table 7-4 page 2

Blood and Yin Vacuities

Pattern	Common Signs	Distinguishing Signs	Method of Treatment
Blood Vacuity	Emaciation Dizziness Flowery vision Insomnia Palpitations Little tongue fur Fine pulse	Pale white (or sallow) complexion White nails Numbness of the limbs Pale tongue	Supplementing the Blood
Yin Vacuity		Rising fire flush Fever in the five hearts Dry throat and pharynx Night sweating Seminal emission Red or crimson tongue Peeling tongue or completely furless tongue Fine, rapid pulse	Enriching Yin

Table 7-5

	Vacuity and Repletion Patterns	
Aspect	*Pattern Type*	
	Vacuity	*Repletion*
Essence-spirit	Lethargy	Agitation
Bearing	Curled posture Desire for quiet	Flailing limbs
Complexion	Somber white, drained white, or withered yellow	Tidal flushing
Enunciation	Low	Strident
Speech	Little desire to speak (or) mussitation	Restlessness and talkativeness Delirious speech
Breathing	Shortness of breath	Rough
Chest and abdomen	Vacuity softness or pain and distention with intermittent relief	Hard, distended glomus with pain exacerbated by pressure
Pulse	Forceless	Forceful
Tongue Fur	Little or none	Thick and slimy

Table 7-6

Aspect	Yin and Yang Patterns	
	Pattern Type	
	Yang Patterns *Repletion Heat*	*Yin Patterns* *Vacuity Cold*
Essence-Spirit	Manic agitation	Lethargy
Complexion	Tidal flushing	Drained white or somber white
Cold & Heat	Vigorous fever (or) no aversion to cold	No fever Frigidity of limbs Aversion to cold
Stool & Urine	Constipation and dark-colored urine	Clear urine and stool
Voice & Breathing	Rough breathing and strident voice	Shortness of breath Low voice
Thirst & Drinking	Thirst Desire for cold beverages	No thirst Desire for warm beverages
Tongue	Red or crimson with yellow fur	Pale with white fur
Pulse	Rapid Slippery Replete Surging	Fine Soggy Faint Weak

Notes

[1] The lung is the "delicate viscus." Governing the skin and the body hair, it is the viscus most closely related to the exterior. Located in the upper body, it is the most yang of all the viscera, and thus corresponds to the exterior, which is also yang.

[2] A popular remedy for exterior cold patterns (common cold) is fresh ginger (one medium-sized root per cup) boiled in water for 15 minutes, with sugar to taste. Scallions may be added; or they may be prepared alone in a bouillon to produce a similar effect.

[3] ‡ after acupoints indicates that moxibustion may be used on the point if required.

[4] In this formula name, the word heart refers to the region of the heart.

Chapter 8
Qi—Blood Pattern Identification

The health and normal functioning of all the organs and tissues is dependent on the flow of qi and blood throughout the body. *Essential Questions* states, "When qi and blood fall into disharmony, a hundred diseases may arise." At the same time, the production and activity of qi and blood is dependent on the normal functioning of the bowels and viscera. For this reason, disease in a given organ may give rise to disorders of its own qi and blood, and may also affect the qi and blood of the whole body.

Qi-blood pattern identification, like eight parameter pattern identification, represents a basic element of diagnosis, and is applicable to exogenous heat diseases, endogenous damage, and miscellaneous diseases. In general, the qi aspect is affected during the initial stages of disease, while it is usually some time before the blood aspect is affected. Thus *The Canon of Perplexities* states, "When qi is affected first, it lodges and does not move; when the blood is subsequently affected, it congests and fails to supply nourishment." However, the order in which qi and the blood are affected conforms to no absolute laws. Some enduring diseases never affect the blood aspect, while others are characterized by blood-aspect disorders at onset.

In qi-blood pattern identification, it is important to identify not only general patterns, but also the organ or organs affected.

In exogenous heat diseases, qi-blood pattern identification is the basis of the four-aspect pattern identification applicable to thermic diseases. This is discussed in Chapter 11, "Exogenous Heat Disease Pattern Identification." The present chapter deals only with qi and blood disorders in endogenous damage and miscellaneous diseases.

The fluids also form part of the material basis of the body, and flow with the blood around the body. However, fluid pathologies such as insuffficiency of the fluids (damage to liquids, damage to yin) and untransformed accumulations of fluids (water swelling, phlegm-rheum, etc.), are dealt with in other chapters.

Disease Patterns of Qi

Since qi pathologies account for a wide variety of diseases, qi pattern identification is of general significance. Disorders fall into two major categories: qi vacuity and qi stagnation.

Qi vacuity

Pattern identification
The most important signs of qi vacuity are fatigue and weakness, and a weak, fine, soft pulse. Other signs include low voice, shortness of breath, and spontaneous sweating.

Qi vacuity is due to insufficiency of original qi giving rise to organic hypofunction and reduced resistance to pathogens. The information derived through organ pattern identification must be carefully correlated to determine the which organ's qi is affected. (See Table 8-1.)

Qi vacuity of a given organ is related to disturbance of its normal function. For example, lung qi vacuity is associated with debilitation of pulmonary governance of qi. Cardiac qi vacuity is associated with impairment of the heart's functions of governing the blood vessels and storing the spirit. Splenogastric qi vacuity is associated with diminished movement and transformation of the digestate, and with center-qi fall. Kidney qi vacuity is associated with debilitation of essence storage, marrow production, and the transformative action of kidney qi. Organ qi vacuities are described in detail in Chapter 9, "Organ Pattern Identification."

Since qi is yang in nature, qi and yang vacuities are similar in nature and manifestation. The major difference is that yang vacuity, producing cold, is associated with far more pronounced cold signs. Thus, the presence of such signs as frigid limbs, aversion to cold, cold sweating, and slow pulse (in addition to the regular signs of qi vacuity) point to yang vacuity.

Treatment

Drug therapy

"Vacuity is treated by supplementation." Hence, qi vacuity is treated by supplementing, or boosting, qi. Commonly used drugs include:

Qi Supplementers	
Radix Codonopsis Pilosulae	*dǎng shēn*
Radix Astragali	*huáng qí*
Radix Glycyrrhizae	*gān cǎo*

Since the spleen and stomach are the root of the acquired constitution, qi supplementers are often complemented by spleen strengtheners such as:

Spleen Strengtheners	
Rhizoma Atractylodis Macrocephalae	*bái zhú*
Sclerotium Poriae	*fú líng*

Four Nobles Decoction *(sì jūn zǐ tāng)* is a formula that treats any form of qi vacuity.

Acumoxatherapy

Qi vacuity is generally treated with such points as SP-6‡, ST-36‡, LI-4‡, CV-4, and BL-20‡. The degree of yang vacuity will determine the amount and method of moxibustion.

Qi stagnation

A disorder arising in any organ, channel, or part of the body frequently affects the flow of qi first, giving rise to what is termed qi stagnation. The phrase, "qi is affected at the onset of disease" mainly refers to qi stagnation. Essence-spirit and emotional disturbances, dietary irregularities, contraction of exogenous pathogens, and trauma are all frequent causes of disruption of qi dynamic manifesting as stagnant qi. Feeble flow of qi may also give rise to stagnation. Qi stagnation due to essence-spirit and emotional factors manifests as binding depression of liver qi.

Pattern identification

The chief observable signs of qi stagnation are pain and distention accompanied by sensations of oppression. Thus stagnation in the chest and lateral costal region is characterized by local distention and pain while gastrointestinal qi stagnation is characterized by painful distention in the abdomen. "Where there is stoppage, there is pain," and the pain associated with qi stagnation characteristically varies in intensity and is related to emotional factors. It is acute or scurrying, and of unfixed location. The sensation of oppression in the chest and abdominal distention is often temporarily relieved by eructation or passing of wind. Qi stagnation sometimes produces abdominal lump glomi that are soft to the touch and disperse and reform periodically. Liver-channel qi stagnation may be characterized by distended breasts, and large intestine qi stagnation may give rise to tenesmus. Qi stagnation is commonly seen in diseases classified by Western medicine as gastrointestinal neurosis, chronic gastritis, chronic enteritis, ulcers, diseases of the biliary tract, and chronic hepatitis.

Treatment

Drug therapy

Qi stagnation is treated by the methods of rectifying and moving qi. Agents such as those listed below may be used for all forms of qi stagnation, and are especially suitable for gastrointestinal qi stagnation:

Qi-Rectifying and Moving Agents	
Rhizoma Cyperi	*xiāng fù*
Radix Saussureae	*mù xiāng*
Fructus Citri	*zhǐ ké*
Pericarpium Citri Reticulatae	*chén pí*

The following substances are mostly used for binding depression of liver qi and for liver-channel qi stagnation:

Agents for Treating Binding Depression of Liver Qi and Liver-Channel Qi Stagnation	
Pericarpium Citri Reticulatae Viride	qīng pí
Tuber Curcumae	yù jīn
Fructus Meliae Toosendan	chuān liàn zǐ

Since most incidences of qi stagnation are related to failure of hepatic free-coursing, formulae often contain qi rectifiers and liver coursers, such as Radix Bupleuri *(chái hú)*. Commonly used liver-coursing, qi-rectifying formulae include:

Liver-Coursing Qi-Rectifying Formulae	
Counterflow Cold Powder	sì nì sǎn
Bupleurum Liver-Coursing Decoction	chái-hú shū gān tāng

Formulae used for treating qi stagnation caused by binding depression of liver qi, characterized by glomus blockage in the chest and diaphragm, and in severe cases, by block inversion, should contain qi breakers and qi downbearers such as: Semen Arecae *(bīn láng)* and Lignum Aquilariae *(chén xiāng)*. An example of such a formula is Five Torrents Cool Decoction *(wǔ mó yǐn zǐ)*, which precipitates qi, downbears counterflow, dissipates binding, and opens blocks.

Acumoxatherapy

Qi stagnation related to the liver is treated with points such as LV-3, LV-2, TB-6, GB-34, and LV-14. LI-11, LI-4, and ST-36 also help move qi. In general, a strong stimulus is desired, but the age and condition of the patient must be considered.

Disease Patterns of the Blood

Vacuity, stasis, and heat are the three major pathologies of the blood. All three are related to bleeding, since bleeding may give rise to blood vacuity or stasis, while blood heat and stasis may both give rise to bleeding.

Blood vacuity

Blood vacuity is the pathologic manifestation of blood insufficiency. It may develop as a result of excessive loss of blood before replenishment is complete. It may also be caused by splenic movement and transformation failure causing insufficiency of blood formation. A further cause is failure to eliminate static blood and engender new blood.

Pattern identification

Blood vacuity is characterized by pale white or withered yellow complexion, mental dizziness, flowery vision, relatively pale tongue, and a fine pulse. Other commonly observed signs include palpitations, racing of the heart, insomnia, and numbing of the extremities.

Blood vacuity signs reflect the insufficient supply of nutrifying blood to the organs and channels, caused by depletion of the blood. However, these general signs must be correlated with organ-specific data to determine the exact location of the vacuity. (See Table 8-2.)

Since the blood is governed by the heart, stored by the liver, and produced and managed by the spleen, blood vacuity is intimately related to these viscera. Vacuity of heart blood is characterized by signs of insufficiency of heart blood and disquieting of the heart spirit. Cardiosplenic blood vacuity is characterized by signs of insufficiency of heart blood and failure of splenic management of the blood. Vacuity of liver blood is characterized by such signs as insufficient supply of nourishment to the eyes and sinews, and disorders of the penetrating and conception vessels. These three specific forms of blood vacuity are discussed in the context of organ pattern identification in Chapter 9.

Since blood is yin in nature, blood vacuity and yin vacuity have much in common, both presenting such symptoms as mental dizziness, flowery vision, palpitations, and a fine pulse. Some differences nevertheless exist. Generally, blood vacuity is not associated with heat signs, and may even be accompanied by cold signs when occurring in conjunction with qi vacuity. Yin vacuity, which essentially refers to vacuity of the fluids, is characterized by signs of heat and dryness, such as upbearing fire flush, a rapid, fine, wiry pulse, and a distinctly red tongue, all of which indicate endogenous heat or hyperactivity of yang.

Treatment

Drug therapy

The following drugs are used in the treatment of all forms of blood vacuity:

Blood Supplementers	
Radix Angelicae Sinensis	dāng guī
Radix Rehmanniae Conquita	shóu dì
Radix Paeoniae Albae	bái sháo
Radix Polygoni Multiflori	shǒu wū
Gelatinum Corii Asini	lǘ pí jiāo
Herba Ecliptae	hàn lián cǎo

Spirit-quieting blood nourishers used to treat heart blood vacuity include:

Blood-Nourishing and Spirit-Quieting Agents	
Radix Salviae Miltiorrhizae	*dān shēn*
Semen Zizyphi Jujubae	*zǎo rén*
Arillus Euphoriae Longanae	*lóng yǎn*

The same agents may be used in combination with spleen fortifiers to treat cardiosplenic blood vacuity. Formulae containing blood-supplementing liver nourishers used to treat liver blood vacuity include:

Blood-Supplementing and Liver-Nourishing Agents	
Fructus Lycii	*qǐ zǐ*
Fructus Mori	*sāng shēn zǐ*
Radix et Caulis Chi Hsüeh T'eng	*jī xuè téng*

General blood-supplementing formulae include:

Blood-Supplementing Formulae	
Four Agents Decoction	*sì wù tāng*
Celestial Emperor Heart-Supplementing Elixir	*tiān wáng bǔ xīn dān*
Angelica Splenic Decoction	*guī pí tāng*

Four Agents Decoction also possesses a blood-quickening liver-nourishing action, and with its variants provides a standard remedy for liver blood insufficiency and menstrual disorders. Celestial Emperor Heart-Supplementing Elixir *(tiān wáng bǔ xīn dān)* nourishes yin-blood and quiets the heart spirit, and is thus used to supplement heart blood. Angelica Splenic Decoction *(guī pí tāng)* is a composite formula that treats cardiosplenic blood vacuity with spirit-quieting blood nourishers and spleen-fortifying qi boosters.

Acumoxatherapy

Points such as SP-6‡, SP-10‡, BL-20, and LV-8 have the general property of supplementing the blood. For heart blood vacuity, HT-7, PC-6, GB-20, and GV-25 may be added. Liver blood vacuity calls for the addition of points such as BL-18, GB-34, and LV-3. For menstrual disorders, the addition of points such as SP-8, CV-6‡, SP-6‡, CV-4‡, SP-4, and ST-29 can be beneficial.

Blood stasis

Under normal conditions the blood flows freely and unhindered around the entire body. However, impact trauma, hemorrhage, qi stagnation, qi vacuity, blood cold, and blood heat may impair free flow, causing blood to stagnate locally to give rise to what is termed blood stasis. Diseases classified in Western medicine as cardiovascular disorders, hepatosplenomegaly, menstrual disease, heterotopic pregnancy, and postpartum disorders often present as blood stasis.

Pattern identification

The observable signs of blood stasis may be discussed under four headings:

Pain

Static blood obstructs the channels impeding the flow of blood. Since "when there is stoppage, there is pain," pain is the outstanding feature of this pathology. The pain associated with blood stasis differs from the acute and scurrying pain characterizing qi stagnation as it is of fixed location and confined to the locality of the obstruction. Stabbing pain is rare.

Masses and swellings

When static blood accumulates, it forms into masses and swellings. Occurring as a result of impact trauma, it gives rise to local cyan-purple swellings (bruises). Occurring internally, it may give rise to relatively hard swellings that can develop into concretions and accumulations.

Bleeding

Since static blood obstructs the vessels, the blood may be unable to pursue its normal course and extravasate. Paroxysmal hemorrhage is thus a commonly observed sign of blood stasis, particularly in menstrual irregularities and postpartum disorders, and is generally characterized by dark, purple, clotted blood.

General signs

The complexion tends to be soot-black. The tongue is dark and purple, with stasis speckles. The pulse is fine and rough. The skin may be dry, rough, and lusterless (cutaneous cornification), with red speckles and purple macules (both due to subcutaneous hemorrhage), filiform red marks (spider nevi), and caput medusae. Such signs are particularly common in enduring sickness.

When blood stasis overwhelms the heart, raving, delirious speech and mania are observed. Static blood obstructing the vessels may also affect the free flow of fluids, giving rise to internal water accumulations, e.g., blood tympany. The etiology of such conditions is described in *Essential Prescriptions of the Golden Coffer* by the phrase, "inhibited blood flow may give rise to water."

Treatment

Drug therapy

Blood stasis is treated by quickening the blood and transforming stasis. Commonly used agents include:

Blood-Quickening Stasis-Transforming Agents	
Semen Persicae	*táo rén*
Flos Carthami	*hóng huā*
Radix Angelicae Sinensis	*dāng guī*
Radix Salviae Miltiorrhizae	*dān shēn*
Radix Paeoniae Rubrae	*chì sháo*
Herba Leonuri	*yì mǔ cǎo*
Herba Lycopi	*zé lán*

In severe, enduring conditions, blood-breaking hardness dispersers may be employed, such as:

Blood-Breaking and Hardness-Dispersing Agents	
Rhizoma Sparganii	*sān léng*
Rhizoma Curcumae Zedoariae	*é zhú*
Squama Manitis	*shān jiǎ*
Eupolyphaga	*dì biē chóng*

If necessary, Rhizoma Rhei *(dà huáng)* and Mirabilitum *(máng xiāo)* may be used to restore free flow and expel static blood. Where blood stasis gives rise to persistent hemorrhage, blood-quickening stasis transformers should still be used. Many agents, such as the following, serve the dual purpose of quickening the blood and arresting hemorrhage:

Hemorrhage-Arresting Blood Quickeners	
Radix Pseudoginseng	*sān qī*
Pollen Typhae	*pú huáng*
Herba Cephalanoploris	*xiǎo jì cǎo*
Radix Rubiae	*qiàn cǎo*

Formulae used to treat static blood include:

Static Blood Formulae	
Four Agents Decoction with Persica and Carthamus	*táo hóng sì wù tāng*
Sanguine Mansion Stasis-Expelling Decoction	*xuè fǔ zhú yū tāng*
Peach Pit Purgative Decoction	*táo-rén chéng qì tāng*
Rhizoma Rhei and Eupolyphaga Pills	*dà-huáng zhè-chóng wán*

There are also variants of these formulae. The first two are general blood-quickening stasis-transforming formulae, varied to suit different pathology locations. The third, which restores free flow and expels stasis, treats conditions characterized by essence-spirit and emotional disturbance. The last, a pre-prepared medicament that breaks blood and disperses hardness, treats enduring blood stasis.

Acumoxatherapy

General stasis-transforming points include LV-2, BL-60, LV-3, SP-8, LI-11, SP-6, and PC-5. LV-1‡ and SP-1‡ are often used along with SP-10 to arrest hemorrhage. In diseases characterized by essence-spirit and emotional disturbance, points such as HT-7, PC-7, and GV-26 are also suitable.

Blood heat

Blood heat mostly occurs in exogenous heat diseases, though it is common in miscellaneous diseases. It may manifest in disease conditions classified by Western medicine as anaphylactoid and thrombocytopenic purpura, aplastic anemia, and leukemia.

Pattern identification

Blood heat can scorch the vessels causing extravasation of the blood. This pathology is known as frenetic blood heat, manifesting itself as retching of blood, expectoration of blood, hemafecia, hematuria, nosebleed, and menorrhagia. Bleeding is often profuse and the blood is either bright red or purple-black in color. Red paples and macules may also occur. Other general symptoms, such as restlessness, thirst, red or deep red tongue, and rapid pulse, all indicate heat. Coma may occur in severe cases.

Treatment

Drug therapy

Since blood heat is usually caused by a heat toxin, it is treated by such methods as blood cooling, heat clearage, and detoxification. Commonly used agents include:

Blood Heat Agents	
Radix Rehmanniae Viva	*xiān shēng dì*
Rhizoma Imperatae Vivum	*xiān máo gēn*
Radix Lithospermi	*zǐ cǎo*
Cortex Radicis Mu Tan	*mǔ dān pí*
Radix Paeoniae Rubrae	*chì sháo*
Pollen Typhae	*pú huáng*
Radix Sanguisorbae	*dì yú*
Herba Cephalanoploris	*xiǎo jì cǎo*

Rhinoceros Horn and Rehmannia Decoction *(xī-jiǎo dì-huáng tāng)* and Cephalanoploris Cool Decoction *(xiǎo jì yǐn zi)*, are commonly used blood-cooling, heat-clearing formulae. Rhinoceros Horn and Rehmannia Decoction is primarily a blood-cooling, detoxifying formula, and may be used where generalized symptoms of toxic heat such as clouding of the spirit, delirious mania, red or crimson tongue, and maculopapular eruptions are pronounced. It may be combined with Coptis Detoxifying Decoction *(huáng-lián jiě dú tāng)* for stronger heat-clearing detoxifying action. Cephalanoploris Cool Decoction is a general antihemorrhagic blood-cooling formula.

Acumoxatherapy

It is common to bleed the capillaries around BL-54 and use such points as SP-6‡, CV-6, LI-11, and LV-3. If there is hemorrhage, moxibustion at SP-1 and LV-1 is the initial treatment. BL-20 and BL-18 can also be selected due to their relation to the spleen and liver.

Dual Disease Patterns of Qi and Blood

Since a close physiological relationship exists between qi and the blood, diseases of one may easily affect the other. The three most common forms of dual disorders are discussed below.

Qi stagnation and blood stasis

Qi stagnation and blood stasis commonly occur together in conditions characterized by amenorrhea, static clots in the menstrual discharge, abdominal pain at the onset of menstruation, or painful distention of the breasts. They may also arise together as a result of trauma. When qi fails to move the blood, qi stagnation may give rise to, and be further exacerbated by, blood stasis. This frequently occurs in syndromes Western medicine terms chronic nephritis and ulcerative diseases. Dual patterns of qi stagnation and blood stasis are treated with blood quickeners and qi rectifiers. A commonly used formula that relieves pain is Melia Toosendan Powder *(jīn-líng-zǐ sǎn)*.

Dual vacuity of qi and blood

Qi vacuity and blood vacuity also commonly concur. Because "blood is the mother of qi," blood vacuity gives rise to qi vacuity. Thus, blood vacuity patients often display qi vacuity signs such as shortness of breath and lack of strength. Dual vacuity is treated by dual supplementation of qi and blood, and since "qi engenders blood," the accent is placed on supplementing qi. Thus, the condition Western medicine identifies as anemia is characterized by classic blood vacuity signs such as lusterless complexion, pale-colored nails, mental dizziness, and palpitations, as well as qi vacuity signs such as shortness of breath and exhaustion. Its treatment involves supplementing both qi and blood, using such formulae as:

Qi and Blood-Supplementing Formulae	
Eight Jewel Decoction	bā zhēn tāng
Angelica Blood-Supplementing Decoction	dāng-guī bǔ xuè tāng

In the latter formula, Radix Astragali *(huáng qí)* should exceed in quantity Radix Angelicae Sinensis *(dāng guī)* to place the emphasis on fortifying qi.

Dual vacuity of qi and blood may also develop from failure of vacuous qi to contain the blood. In such cases, the resulting persistent hemorrhage gives rise to such signs as exhaustion, pale tongue, and a soft, soggy pulse. Blood containment failure is second only to blood heat as a cause of hemorrhagic disorders. It is treated with heavy doses of qi boosters:

Qi Boosters	
Radix Codonopsis Pilosulae	dǎng shēn
Radix Astragali	huáng qí
Radix Glycyrrhizae	gān cǎo

These are combined with smaller quantities of blood supplementers:

Blood Supplementers	
Radix Angelicae Sinensis	dāng guī
Radix Rehmanniae Conquita	shóu dì
Gelatinum Corii Asini	lǘ pí jiāo

The following formulae, and their variants, are used:

Qi and Blood-Supplementing Formulae	
Angelica Splenic Decoction	guī pí tāng
Center-Supplementing Qi-Boosting Decoction	bǔ zhōng yì qì tāng

Acumoxatherapy

Treatment by acupuncture and moxibustion uses qi-supplementing points such as SP-6‡, ST-36‡, CV-4 (moxa), and CV-6‡, with the addition of blood-supplementing points such as SP-10‡, BL-20‡, and BL-17‡.

Sequential desertion of blood and qi

Sequential desertion of blood and qi arises as a result of heavy blood loss. Original qi, deprived of the support of the blood, becomes vacuous and deserts. This condition may be characterized by a drained white complexion, a rapid pulse that is feeble at the deeper levels, or a scallion-stalk pulse, reduced blood pressure, cold sweating, and even clouding inversion. Since it is said that "when essence-blood cannot be produced at a sufficiently rapid rate, original qi must be swiftly secured," treatment involves boosting qi with formulae such as Ginseng Solo Decoction *(dú shēn tāng),* which both checks vacuity desertion and, by promoting blood containment, helps arrest bleeding. In acumoxatherapy, emergency acupuncture points such as ST-36‡, GV-26, GV-20‡, KI-1 and LI-4 revive the patient, and moxibustion at LV-1, SP-1, and SP-10 can help arrest bleeding.

Table 8-1

Please see following page.

Common Qi Vacuity Patterns	
Pattern	Symptoms
General Qi Vacuity	*These symptoms accompany all specific qi vacuities.* General fatigue and lack of strength Devitalized essence-spirit Short, shallow breathing No energy to speak Disinclination for physical movement Faint, low voice Spontaneous sweating Pale or enlarged tongue Soggy, forceless pulse

Lung Qi Vacuity	Cough and expectoration of phlegm
	  in addition to relatively pronounced
	  general symptoms such as:
	  Short, rapid, distressed breathing
	  No energy to speak
	  Low voice

Heart Qi Vacuity	Slow, rapid or slow, irregularly interrupted pulse
	Palpitations or racing of the heart
	Disquieting of essence-spirit
	  in addition to relatively pronounced
	  shortness of breath
	Lethargy of essence-spirit

Gastrosplenic Qi Vacuity	Abdominal distention and oppression
	Indigestion
	Thin stool
	Center qi fall
	Prolapse of the rectum and urinary
	  frequency and urgency in addition
	  to relatively pronounced withered yellow
	  complexion, exhaustion of
	  essence-spirit, and fatigued limbs

Kidney Qi Vacuity	Limp, aching knees and lumbar region
	Long micturition with clear urine
	Dribbling incontinence, enuresis,
	  urinary block, and vacuity of reproductive
	  functions, together with a drained white
	  or dull gray complexion, visual dizziness,
	  mental clouding, tinnitus, deafness

Table 8-2

Common Blood Vacuity Patterns	
Pattern	Symptoms
General Blood Vacuity	*These symptoms accompany all specific qi vacuities.* Lusterless or withered yellow complexion Mental dizziness Flowery vision Pale tongue Pale nails Fine pulse
Heart Blood Vacuity	Excessive dreaming and insomnia, in addition to the general blood vacuity symptoms Palpitations or racing of the heart Poor memory
Cardiosplenic Blood Vacuity	General blood vacuity symptoms and heart blood vacuity symptoms, with: Loss of appetite Spiritual fatigue Menstrual irregularity Metrorrhagia Loss of blood
Liver Blood Vacuity	Dizziness Flowery or blurred vision Tingling in the limbs Hypertonicity of the limbs Dry nails Restless sleep Menstrual irregularity Amenorrhea or marked oligomenorrhea

Chapter 9
Organ Pattern Identification

Organ pattern identification involves the correlation of information derived from the four examinations with visceral manifestation theory. Its aim is to determine what organs are affected by disease, and identify morbid changes in their qi-blood and yin-yang aspects. This then provides the basis for selection of appropriate treatment.

The first step of organ pattern identification involves identifying the affected organ on the basis of its physiopathologic characteristics. The heart governs the blood vessels and stores the spirit. Therefore, palpitations, interrupted pulses, and derangement of the heart spirit all point to disease of the heart. The lung is connected with the surface skin and governs qi, and lung qi diffuses, depurates, and bears downwards; hence symptoms such as cough, dyspnea, and insecurity of the defensive exterior are seen to be lung disorders. The spleen governs movement and transformation of the digestate, the stomach governs ingestion, and the intestines govern the conveyance and transformation of waste; hence vomiting, abdominal distention and fullness, and diarrhea are associated with diseases of the spleen, stomach and intestines. The liver governs free-coursing and stores blood, and liver yang is prone to upstirring; hence pain in the lateral costal region, jaundice, blood loss, dizziness, and spasms are symptomatic of liver disease. Finally, the kidney governs water, stores essence, governs the bones and engenders marrow; hence water swelling, urinary block, enuresis, seminal emission, pain in the knees and lower back, and sluggish movement are associated with kidney disorders.

Once the affected organ has been identified, the relative states of yin, yang, qi, and blood can be determined with the information derived from eight parameter and qi-blood pattern identification. Each organ is associated with characteristic pathologies of yin, yang, qi, and blood. The heart and the liver are associated with disease of all four aspects, whereas the lung is mainly susceptible to pathologies of yin and qi; the spleen is primarily affected by disorders of qi and yang, while kidney diseases include yin-yang and essential qi pathologies. Determining the affected aspect of an organ is of vital importance in treatment. Thus, identifying palpitations as a sign of heart disease provides an inadequate basis for prescribing treatment, since they may be attributable to vacuity of heart yin, heart blood, heart yang, or heart qi. The bowels and viscera are each closely related not only to one another but also to the minor organs and tissues of the body. Therefore, understanding the development of diseases, making a correct diagnosis, and determining appropriate treatment are all dependent on a holistic approach. For example, once insomnia has been identified as the result of heart blood or heart yin vacuity, it is important to determine whether the spleen or kidney is also affected, since the dual disorders, cardiosplenic blood vacuity and breakdown of cardiorenal interaction, are treated in different ways.

Disease Patterns of the Heart

The heart governs the blood vessels and stores the spirit. Disorders of heart yin, yang, qi, and blood are thus commonly characterized by blood flow disturbance and essence-spirit and emotional disturbances.

Heart qi and heart yang vacuity

Heart qi and heart yang vacuities are characterized not only by signs of general qi and yang vacuity, but also inhibited movement of blood and hebetude (dullness, lethargy) of essence-spirit. In most cases, they represent gradually developing, enduring disorders. Pathomechanisms include: insufficiency of ancestral qi preventing it from adequately penetrating the heart and vessels and driving respiration; intimidation of the heart by water qi resulting from kidney yang vacuity; wind-cold-damp obturation settling in the the heart; and damp turbidity or static blood obstructing the heart and vessels. Acute forms are the result of fulminant desertion of yang qi. Heart qi and heart yang vacuities may occur in conjunction with lung qi or kidney yang vacuities, the resulting conditions being referred to as cardiopulmonary qi vacuity and cardiorenal yang vacuity. They may also present with cold-damp, damp turbidity, and static blood complications.

These forms of heart vacuity correspond roughly to diseases designated by Western medicine as cardiac failure, angina pectoris, arrhythmia, general asthenia, and neurosis.

Pattern identification

Heart qi vacuity is characterized by white complexion, spiritual lassitude, dizziness, palpitations and racing of the heart, shortness of breath, and spontaneous sweating. The pulse is weak, fine, and slow or interrupted. These signs all reflect insufficiency of heart qi, and its consequent inability to warm and propel the blood adequately, as well as essence-spirit debilitation. Inhibition of blood flow due to insufficiency of heart qi is identified by oppression in the region of the heart, interrupted pulses, and cardiac pain.

Heart yang vacuity may be characterized by signs of heart qi vacuity, and by relatively pronounced cold signs such as inversion frigidity of the limbs, dark, gray, or cyan-purple complexion, and signs of static blood obstruction. In the advanced stages, profuse, streaming perspiration, swelling of the limbs and facial edema, cyan lips and frigid limbs, clouding of spirit-disposition, and a faint, fine pulse verging on expiry indicate yang qi vacuity desertion.

Cardiopulmonary qi vacuity is characterized by cough, dyspnea, and counterflow qi, in addition to signs of heart qi vacuity. In cardiorenal yang vacuity, the cold form and frigid limbs are more pronounced, and are accompanied by hematuria or water swelling.

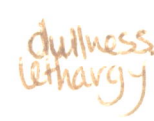

Treatment

Drug therapy

Boosting heart qi and warming heart yang are the basic methods of treatment. Commonly used agents include:

Heart Qi Boosters	
Radix Glycyrrhizae mix-fried	zhì gān cǎo
Radix Astragali	huáng qí
Radix Codonopsis Pilosulae	dǎng shēn
Radix Ginseng	rén shēn

Heart Yang Warmers	
Ramulus Cinnamomi	guì zhī
Radix Aconiti Fu Tzu	fù zǐ

Since the qi and blood of the heart are mutually dependent, agents that nourish the blood and quiet the spirit are also commonly used:

Blood Nourishers and Spirit Quietants	
Radix Salviae Miltiorrhizae	dān shēn
Semen Zizyphi Jujubae	zǎo rén
Poria cum Radice Pini	fú shén
Cinnabaris	zhū shā

General formulae used to treat both heart qi and heart yang vacuity include:

Heart Qi and Heart Yang Vacuity Formulae	
Honeyed Liquorice Decoction	zhì gān cǎo tāng
Heart-Nourishing Decoction	yǎng xīn tāng

Yang qi vacuity desertion patterns are treated by the method of salvaging yang ang securing against desertion, using formulae such as:

Yang Salvage Formulae	
Ginseng and Aconite Decoction	shēn fù tāng
Ginseng Solo Decoction	dú shēn tāng

Drugs such as Magnetitum (*cí shí*), Os Draconis (*lóng gǔ*), and Concha Ostreae (*mǔ lì*) may be added to formulae to settle the heart and quiet the spirit.

Finally, cardiopulmonary qi vacuity may be treated with formulae such as Ginseng and Gecko Powder *(shēn jiè sǎn)* while cardiorenal yang vacuity is treated with True Warrior Decoction *(zhēn wǔ tāng)* or Life-Saver Kidney Qi Pills *(jì shēng shèn qì wán)*.

Acumoxatherapy

Treatment of heart yang and qi vacuity is directed towards supplementing the kidney by use of points such as BL-23‡ and GV-4‡, supplementing the heart with points such as BL-15‡ and HT-7, and quieting the heart and spirit with points such as HT-7 and PC-6.

Supplementary treatment is aimed at boosting the qi of the entire body, using ST-36‡, CV-4‡, and CV-6‡. BL-38‡ supplements heart and lung qi, and is thus particularly effective for cardiopulmonary qi vacuity. LU-9 may also be added to regulate the qi of the upper burner.

Heart blood and yin vacuities

The outstanding common features of heart blood and heart yin vacuities are disquieting of the heart spirit and yin-blood insufficiency. Both disorders may occur when fire forming as a result of dispositional excess (excess of one or more of the five dispositions) damages yin, or when enduring illness causes damaging wear on yin-blood. Heart blood vacuity is mostly accompanied by signs of splenic vacuity while heart yin vacuity regularly occurs with kidney yin vacuity symptoms, the former being known as cardiosplenic blood vacuity and the latter as cardiorenal yin vacuity.

Heart blood vacuity and heart yin vacuity may occur in conditions that Western medicine terms nutritional disturbance, neurosis, tachycardia, arrhythmia, anemia, and hyperthyroidism.

Pattern identification

Signs associated with heart blood vacuity include a pale white complexion with little luster, distinctly pale tongue, fine pulse, palpitation and racing of the heart, dizziness, and mental disorders such as poor memory, insomnia, excessive dreaming, and emotional disturbance. Heart yin vacuity may also be characterized by palpitations and racing of the heart, dizziness, and insomnia, but is differentiated by the presence of signs of yin vacuity fire effulgence such as fever in the five hearts, upbearing fire, night sweating, distinctly red tongue, and a fine, rapid pulse.

Treatment

Drug therapy

Heart blood vacuity and heart yin vacuity are treated by supplementing blood and enriching yin, and by quieting the heart and spirit. Drugs used include heart blood supplementers such as:

Heart Blood Supplementers	
Radix Salviae Miltiorrhizae	dān shēn
Radix Rehmanniae Conquita	shóu dì
Radix Angelicae Sinensis	dāng guī
Arillus Euphoriae Longanae	lóng yǎn

These agents may be used with heart yin enrichers:

Heart Yin Enrichers	
Radix Rehmanniae Cruda	shēng dì
Tuber Ophiopogonis	mài dōng
Semen Tritici	huái xiǎo mài
Semen Biotae	bó zǐ rén
Bulbus Lilii	bǎi hé

Heart and spirit quietants may also be used in these formulae:

Heart and Spirit Quietants	
Semen Zizyphi Jujubae	zǎo rén
Radix Polygalae	yuǎn zhì
Poria cum Radice Pini	fú shén
Cinnabaris	zhū shā
Magnetitum	cí shí
Caulis Polygoni Multiflori	yè jiāo téng

Since heart blood vacuity is most commonly encountered in conjunction with splenic vacuity, treatment usually involves the use of formulae that act on both viscera, such as Angelica Splenic Decoction *(guī pí tāng)*. Heart yin vacuity may usually be treated with Wheat and Jujube Decoction *(gān-mài dà-zǎo tāng)*, which eliminates dryness. When heart yin vacuity occurs in combination with kidney yin vacuity, as is often the case, the basic method of treatment is nourishing heart and kidney yin, assisted by clearing the heart and downbearing fire. Celestial Emperor Heart-Supplementing Elixir *(tiān wáng bǔ xīn dān)* is commonly used to treat cardiorenal yin vacuity.

Acumoxatherapy

Points such as SP-6, BL-20, and BL-17 supplement the blood, while HT-7, PC-6, and BL-15 are used to quiet the spirit. GV-25 clears fire and KI-3 enriches yin. Special points for insomnia are M-LE-5 *(shi-mian)* and N-HN-54 *(an-mian),* among others.

Upflaming of heart fire

Upflaming of heart fire usually constitutes a repletion pattern. Where effulgent liver fire is also present, the condition is termed cardiohepatic fire effulgence. Sometimes, heart fire may spread to the small intestine. Upflaming of heart fire may occur in conjunction with kidney yin vacuity. This pattern, which is known as breakdown of cardiorenal interaction, is one of yin vacuity fire effulgence.

Pattern identification

Signs mainly associated with upflaming of heart fire include reddening of the tip of the tongue, restlessness, cracking of the tongue, and erosion of the oral and glossal mucosa. The pulse is rapid. Breakdown of cardiorenal interaction is characterized by restlessness, insomnia, and occasionally by dryness of the pharynx and mouth, upbearing fire flush, a red, mirror tongue, and a fine, rapid pulse. Signs associated with cardiohepatic fire effulgence include headache, ocular rubor, agitation, and irascibility, in addition to the general signs of upflaming heart fire. Heart fire spreading to the small intestine is characterized by painful, dribbling micturition with dark-colored urine.

Treatment

Drug therapy

Upflaming of heart fire is treated by clearing the heart and draining fire. Commonly used agents are:

Heart-Clearing and Fire-Draining Agents	
Rhizoma Coptidis	*huáng lián*
Embryon Nelumbinis	*lián zǐ xīn*
Fructus Forsythiae	*lián qiào*
Radix Glycyrrhizae Recens	*shēng gān cǎo*
Folium Bambusae	*zhú yè*
Caulis Mu T'ung	*mù tōng*
Medulla Junci	*dēng xīn*

Effective formulae include:

Upflaming Heart Fire Formulae	
Heart-Draining Decoction	*xiè xīn tāng*
Heat-Abducting Powder	*dǎo chì sǎn*

Heat-Abducting Powder may be combined with Heart-Draining Decoction or its variants to abduct the cardiac heat downwards. Breakdown of cardiorenal interaction may be treated with Coptis and Ass-Hide Glue Decoction *(huáng-lián ē-jiāo tāng)*, supplemented with heart and spirit quietants. Where signs of cardiohepatic fire effulgence are pronounced, heart-clearing fire drainers may be used with judicious admixture of liver clearers such as Cortex Radicis Mu Tan *(mǔ dān pí)*, Fructus Gardeniae *(zhī zǐ)*, Radix Gentianae *(lóng dǎn cǎo)*, and Folium Mori *(sāng yè)*. Heat spreading from the heart to the small intestine may be treated with Heat-Abducting Powder *(dǎo chì sǎn)*, which abducts the heat downwards and out through the bowels.

Acumoxatherapy

The source point of the heart, HT-7, may be combined with BL-15 and HT-5 to drain heart fire and quiet the spirit. KI-3 nourishes yin, while PC-6 and PC-7 clear the heart. The latter two points are also effective when cardiac heat spreads to the small intestine, presenting signs such as dark urine and tongue ulcers. In this situation they would be combined with BL-27, HT-5, ST-39, HT-6, and local points in the lower burner.

Other points, such as PC-8, HT-8, and CV-14, also have certain properties that make them effective in treating upflaming of heart fire.

Cardiac obturation

Essential Questions states, "Cardiac obturation is caused by stoppage in the vessels," that is, stasis obstruction in the heart or vessels. The cause may be either inadequate warming and propulsion of the blood as a result of insufficiency of yang qi or obstruction of the heart vessels by static blood forming when inner-body phlegm turbidity impedes blood flow. It may occur in conditions described in Western medicine as angina pectoris and myocardiac infarction.

Pattern identification

Signs mainly associated with cardiac obturation include dull pain and oppression in the area anterior to the heart, attributed to impaired yang qi perfusion or obstruction of the connecting channels by phlegm stasis (stasis arising as a result of the presence of phlegm). Paroxysms are characterized by angina pectoris, cyan-purple complexion, frigid limbs, and a fine, faint pulse verging on expiry, indicating severe obstruction of heart qi and heart yang. Palpitations, racing of the heart, spiritual fatigue, and shortness of breath are general signs of heart qi vacuity characterizing the non-paroxysmal condition.

Treatment

Drug therapy

Insufficiency of heart yang is treated by perfusing heart yang, while phlegm stasis is treated by quickening the blood and transforming stasis, and by transforming turbidity with pungent and aromatic agents. Commonly used agents that promote heart yang perfusion include:

Heart Yang Perfusers	
Ramulus Cinnamomi	guì zhī
Bulbus Allii Macrostemi	xiè bái
Fructus Trichosanthis	guā lóu

Agents that quicken the blood and transform stasis are:

Blood-Quickening and Stasis-Transforming Agents	
Radix Salviae Miltiorrhizae	dān shēn
Radix Angelicae Sinensis	dāng guī
Semen Persicae	táo rén
Flos Carthami	hóng huā
Fructus Crataegi	shān zhā

Pungent, aromatic turbidity transformers are:

Pungent, Aromatic Turbidity Transformers	
Styrax Liquidis	hé xiāng
Lignum Dalbergiae Odoriferae	jiàng xiāng
Rhizoma Acori Graminei	chāng pú
Tuber Curcumae	yù jīn

Phlegm-damp patterns, usually characterized by an enlarged tongue with white, slimy fur, are treated with Trichosanthes, Allium, and Pinellia Decoction *(guā-lóu xiè-bái bàn-xià tāng)* and its variants, which transform phlegm-damp with warm agents. Oppression in the region of the heart with frequent attacks of pain generally indicates obstruction of heart yang, and is mainly treated with Liquid Styrax Pills *(sū hé xiāng wán)*, which repel turbidity and open the portals. Dark, purple tongue, or cyan-purple lips and tongue generally indicate blood stasis and are treated with Portal-Opening Blood-Quickening Decoction *(tōng qiào huó xuè tāng)* and its variants, which quicken the blood and transform stasis. Cases presenting with such signs as a distinctly pale tongue, drained white complexion, and slow pulse, indicating yang qi insufficiency, may be treated with formulae containing drugs that boost qi and warm yang:

Qi Boosters and Yang Warmers	
Radix Codonopsis Pilosulae	*dǎng shēn*
Radix Glycyrrhizae	*gān cǎo*
Radix Aconiti Fu Tzu	*fù zǐ*
Cortex Cinnamomi	*ròu guì*
Rhizoma Zingiberis Recens	*shēng jiāng*

Acumoxatherapy

PC-6 and SP-4 are often combined to treat cardiac obturation. They are used with HT-8 and CV-17 to loosen the chest and open the portals. The M-UE-1 *(shi-xuan)* points are bled in acute conditions in order to open the portals and clear heat. If phlegm is present, ST-40 may be added. Other points used in cardiac obturation patterns include CV-13, CV-14, CV-15, and HT-1 (cf. Table 9-1).

Disease Patterns of the Lung

Diffusion and depurative downbearing of lung qi represent the chief functional characteristics of the lung. Non-diffusion of lung qi and impairment of depurative downbearing, together with lung qi and lung yin vacuities, are the most common of pulmonary pathologies. *Essential Questions* states, "Patterns characterized by respiratory distress and thoracic depression are associated with the lung."

Disorders of other organs may disrupt the diffusion and depuration of lung qi, causing cough and dyspnea. Hence, *Essential Questions* states, "Cough may be the result of disease not only of the lung but of any of the five viscera and six bowels."

Non-diffusion of lung qi

Non-diffusion of lung qi is generally attributable to invasion of the lung or fettering of the exterior by exogenous pathogens. Pathogenic heat or cold rheum congesting the lung may not only interfere with lung qi diffusion, but may as well cause counterflow ascent of lung qi, manifesting as cough (ascendant counterflow qi cough). Cough and rapid breathing from exogenous diseases and acute inflammation of the lung generally fall within this category.

Pattern identification

Non-diffusion of lung qi usually occurs in initial-stage invasion of the lung by wind-cold or wind-heat pathogens. The main signs are cough with varying amounts of phlegm, itchy throat, and loss of voice, frequently occurring with exterior signs. Pathogenic heat congesting the lung may be characterized by the additional presence of high fever, flaring nostrils, dyspnea with rough, rapid respiration, and thick, yellow, sticky phlegm, sometimes finely streaked with blood. The tongue is deep red with rough, yellow fur, while the pulse is rapid and slippery. If pre-existing cold-rheum ascends and invades the lung following contraction of an exogenous pathogen, such signs as cold form and frigid limbs, cough and dyspnea, white foaming phlegm and a "frog rattle" may also be observed. Such a pattern also includes somber white complexion, glossy white tongue fur, and wiry pulse.

Treatment

Drug therapy

The basic method of treatment is promoting lung qi diffusion with pungent agents, which, if necessary, may be combined with that of clearing heat and transforming phlegm, or transforming cold-rheum with warm agents. Where the pattern occurs as a result of invasion of the lung or fettering of the exterior by an external pathogen, as is commonly the case, the method of coursing the exterior and outthrusting the pathogen assists the restoration of lung qi diffusion. Commonly used drugs include:

Lung Diffusers	
Herba Ephedrae	má huáng
Radix Platycodi	jié gěng
Fructus Arctii	niú bàng zǐ
Bulbus Fritillariae Thunbergii	xiàng bèi mǔ

Defiant Three Decoction *(sān ào tāng)* is a basic formula that may used in variant forms to suit individual cases. Exterior resolvents are added where fettering of the exterior by wind-cold presents as an adiaphoretic exterior repletion pattern. Lonicera and Forsythia Powder *(yín qiào sǎn)* is often used for wind-heat invading the lungs. Counterflow ascent of lung qi, which calls for the use of lung-clearing, counterflow-downbearing and dyspnea-calming agents, is often treated with Ephedra, Apricot, Gypsum, and Liquorice Decoction *(má xìng shí gān tāng)* or Lonicera and Phragmites Combination *(yín wěi hé jì)*. Non-diffusion of lung qi from a complicating contraction of the cold pathogen in patients regularly suffering from cold-rheum should be treated by warming the lung and transforming rheum, using Minor Cyan Dragon Decoction *(xiǎo qīng lóng tāng)* and its variants.

Acumoxatherapy

LU-7 and LU-1 are major points used to diffuse lung qi. CV-17 can downbear counterflow, transform phlegm, and loosen the chest. These points are combined with BL-13 when combatting an exogenous pathogen invading the lung. If heat is present, points such as GV-14 and LU-5 are included, while wind-cold calls for BL-12‡, BL-13‡, and GB-20‡.

Impaired depurative downbearing of lung qi

Lung qi depuration and downbearing can be impaired by heat arising through transformation of exogenous pathogens or by brewing phlegm-damp. It is often characterized by, and is the most common cause of, persistent cough and qi counterflow.

Pattern identification

Cough is the chief symptom of impaired depurative downbearing of lung qi. Other signs vary depending on whether the cause is dampness or dryness. Dryness-heat patterns are characterized by a dry cough with little or no phlegm, dry pharynx, and loss of voice. This pattern, which tends to develop into lung yin vacuity, is often seen in pulmonary tuberculosis. Brewing phlegm-damp is characterized by cough, thick, sticky phlegm, and oppression in the chest. The tongue fur is slimy and the pulse is slippery. Severe cases present with dyspnea. Brewing phlegm-damp is commonly seen in what Western medicine terms chronic bronchitis, and when persistent may develop into lung qi vacuity.

Treatment

Drug therapy

Treatment is based on the method of promoting depurative downbearing of lung qi, which may be used in combination with the methods of clearing the lung, moistening dryness, and transforming phlegm-damp according to need. Where an exterior pattern is present, formulae may include exterior resolvents. Some lung qi depurative downbearers have a lung-clearing effect, and may be used for dryness-heat cough:

Lung-Clearing Depurative Downbearers	
Cortex Radicis Mori	*sāng bái pí*
Folium Mori	*sāng yè*
Folium Eriobotryae	*pí pa yè*
Fructus Aristolochiae	*mǎ dōu líng*
Radix Stemonae	*bǎi bù*
Bulbus Fritillariae Cirrhosae	*chuān bèi mǔ*

Where heat signs are pronounced, Radix Scutellariae (*huáng qín*) may be added, while patterns in which dryness symptoms are the more prominent may be treated with admixture of agents such as:

Lung-Moistening Depurative Downbearers	
Exocarpium Pyri	lí pí
Radix Adenophorae	shā shēn
Tuber Ophiopogonis	mài dōng

Other lung qi depurative downbearers possess a lung-warming action and may be used to treat phlegm-damp cough:

Lung-Warming Depurative Downbearers	
Fructus Perillae Crispae	sū zǐ
Semen Pruni Armeniacae	xìng rén
Radix Asteris	zǐ wǎn
Flos Tussilagi Farfarae	kuǎn dōng huā

Phlegm-damp cough patterns may also be treated with formulae supplemented by phlegm-transforming agents such as:

Phlegm-Transforming Agents	
Rhizoma Pinelliae	bàn xià
Pericarpium Citri Reticulatae	chén pí
Semen Sinapis Albae	bái jiè zǐ

Lung qi depurative downbearing formulae include:

Lung Qi Depurative Downbearing Formulae	
Lung-Draining Powder	xiè bái sǎn
Mulberry and Apricot Kernel Decoction	sāng xìng tāng
Dryness-Clearing Lung-Restorative Decoction	qīng zào jiù fèi tāng
T.B. Tested Formula	fèi láo yàn fāng
Three Seed Filial Devotion Decoction	sān zǐ yǎng qīn tāng
Perilla Fruit Qi-Downbearing Decoction	sū-zǐ jiàng qì tāng

Perilla Fruit Qi-Downbearing Decoction and its variants may be used for phlegm-damp. T.B. Tested Formula may be used for dryness-heat cough.

Since lung qi diffusion and depurative downbearing really represent two aspects of the same function, they are susceptible to simultaneous disruption. The dual condition is known as impaired diffusion and depuration of lung qi and is treated by combinations of the methods described above. One formula used is Phlegm-Cough Powder (zhǐ sòu sǎn). Primarily a depurative downbearing formula, it can treat most types of cough by dint of its additional diffusion-promoting action. Nevertheless, in clinical practice, it is still necessary to determine the prominence of non-diffusion and impaired depurative downbearing to ensure an effective drug-mix. When treating cough due to exogenous disease, it is inadvisable to use some lung qi depurative downbearers at too early a stage, since they may prevent pathogen expulsion and thereby cause the cough to persist.

Contraindicated Agents	
Fructus Aristolochiae	mǎ dōu líng
Folium Eriobotryae	pí pa yè
Bulbus Fritillariae Cirrhosae	chuān bèi mǔ
Flos Tussilagi Farfarae	kuǎn dōng huā

Acumoxatherapy

LU-9 helps depurate the upper burner, while LU-5 promotes downbearing and clears heat from the upper burner. When the heat is extreme, LU-10 is commonly employed. Points such as KI-3, KI-6, and KI-7 are used when there is lung dryness, and CV-22 and BL-13 aid qi diffusion. Where phlegm is a major factor, ST-40 and CV-12 are often added.

Lung qi vacuity

Lung qi vacuity is most commonly attributable to repeated impairment of lung qi diffusion and depuration over a long period of time, although it may also be caused by general qi vacuity. Lung qi vacuity may affect movement of essence to the surface skin and body hair, giving rise to insecurity of the defensive exterior. Since lung qi has its root in the kidney, and ancestral qi penetrates the heart and vessels to drive respiration, when lung qi vacuity reaches a certain degree, it can cause cardiopulmonary qi vacuity, qi absorption failure, or cardiorenal yang vacuity.

Pattern identification

Signs characterizing lung qi vacuity include general physical weakness, feeble speech, low timorous voice, cough, and shortness of breath. The tongue is pale and the pulse is weak and vacuous. Where exterior defense is insecure, spontaneous sweating and susceptibility to nasal congestion and to colds may be observed. Where there is detriment to heart and kidney yang qi, signs may include rapid breathing at the slightest exertion, pronounced frigidity of the limbs, cold form, facial edema, and swelling of the lower extremities. In severe cases, oppression in the chest with distressed, rapid breathing, palpitations, spontaneous sweating, and cyan-purple lips indicate cardiopumonary qi vacuity, qi absorption failure, or cardiorenal yang vacuity. (See "Heart qi and heart yang vacuity," and "Kidney yang vacuity" in the relevant sections of this chapter.)

Treatment

Drug therapy

Lung qi vacuity is treated by boosting lung qi. Commonly used drugs include:

Lung Qi Boosters	
Radix Codonopsis Pilosulae	dǎng shēn
Radix Astragali	huáng qí
Radix Glycyrrhizae	gān cǎo
Fructus Schisandrae	wǔ wèi zǐ

Lung-Supplementing Decoction *(bǔ fèi tāng)* and its variants are representative general formulae. Conditions also characterized by insecurity of the defensive exterior may be treated with the admixture of Jade Wind-Barrier Powder *(yù píng fēng sǎn)* and similar formulae. For treatment of cardiopulmonary qi vacuity, qi absorption failure, and cardiorenal yang vacuity, see the relevant sections of this chapter.

Acumoxatherapy

LU-9 is combined with BL-12‡ and BL-13‡ to boost lung qi. It is often advisable to fortify kidney qi with BL-23‡, and provide general supplementation of original qi using ST-36‡ and CV-4.

Lung yin vacuity

Lung yin vacuity presents as lung vacuity with heat signs. It is mostly the result of damage caused by long-lingering pulmonary heat, which frequently develops in patients suffering from either general debilitation from an enduring illness or impairment of pulmonary depuration. It sometimes arises as a result of invasion of the lung by the dryness pathogen, and mostly corresponds to what Western medicine sees as pulmonary tuberculosis. Lung yin vacuity frequently affects kidney yin, resulting in pulmorenal yin vacuity.

Pattern identification

General signs characterizing lung yin vacuity include emaciation and marked ill health. The cough is typically dry with little phlegm. Other signs include dry mouth and pharynx, low, hoarse voice, blood in the phlegm, and rapid breathing. Fire effulgence resulting from pulmorenal yin vacuity is characterized by red cheeks, tidal fever, night sweating, low back pain and seminal emission. The tongue is distinctly red, while the pulse is usually fine and rapid.

Treatment

Drug therapy

Lung yin vacuity is treated by enriching yin and moistening the lung. Commonly used agents include:

Yin-Enriching and Lung-Moistening Agents	
Radix Adenophorae	shā shēn
Tuber Ophiopogonis	mài dōng
Bulbus Lilii	bǎi hé
Bulbus Fritillariae Cirrhosae	chuān bèi mǔ
Rhizoma Polygonati Odorati	yù zhú
Radix Rehmanniae Cruda	shēng dì

Lily Bulb Metal-Securing Decoction (bǎi-hé gù jīn tāng) and similar formulae are used. Red tongue and thick, slimy tongue fur, together with thick, sticky phlegm, indicate stagnation and congestion of phlegm-damp. Where such signs are present, Six Nobles Metal and Water Decoction (jīn shuǐ liù jūn jiān) should be prescribed. Where damage to kidney yin is particularly pronounced, kidney yin enrichers such as the following should also be used:

Kidney Yin Enrichers	
Plastrum Testudinis	guī bǎn
Tuber Asparagi	tiān dōng
Radix Scrophulariae	xuán shēn
Gelatinum Corii Asini	lǘ pí jiāo

Pronounced signs of fire effulgence may call for the admixture of fire-draining agents such as:

Fire Drainers	
Radix Scutellariae	huáng qín
Rhizoma Anemarrhenae	zhī mǔ
Cortex Phellodendri	huáng bó

These agents drain the pulmorenal fire. Patterns including signs of invasion of the lung by the dryness-heat pathogen may be treated by Dryness-Clearing Lung-Restorative Decoction (qīng zào jiù fèi tāng) and its variants.

Lung qi and lung yin vacuities may both be caused by general physical vacuity or by repeated impairment of lung qi diffusion and depuration over a long period of time; one condition may give rise to the simultaneous occurrence of the other. Such patterns include spiritual fatigue, cough and shortness of breath, copious perspiration, tidal flushing of the cheeks, red tongue, and a rapid, vacuous pulse, and may be treated by boosting qi and constraining yin, using Pulse-Engendering Powder *(shēng mài sǎn)* with additions. (See Table 9-2.)

Acumoxatherapy

KI-3 and KI-7 are major points for enriching yin and supplementing water. If severe heat is present, LU-10 is used to drain fire. LU-9 and BL-13 used together will supplement the lung and diffuse lung qi. Other points commonly used to treat vacuous lung yin conditions include KI-6, TB-2, and TB-3.

Disease Patterns of the Spleen, Stomach, and Intestines

The main functions of the spleen, stomach, and intestines are the decomposition of food, movement and transformation of the essence of digestate, and conveyance and transformation of waste. Pathologies of these organs therefore chiefly involve disturbances of digestion, assimilation, distribution, and excretion.

The spleen is strong when its qi bears upwards, while the stomach is in harmony when its qi bears downwards. Splenic transformation failure and breakdown of gastric harmony and downbearing are disruptions of normal bearing. Splenic transformation failure occurs in a variety of forms: impairment of digestion and assimilation; accumulation of water-damp; and diminution of uplift. Advanced debilitation of splenic yang qi may affect the kidney and lead to splenorenal yang vacuity. Breakdown of gastric harmony and downbearing occurs in the forms of vacuity cold, depressed heat, insufficiency of yin humor, and damp turbidity digestate accumulations. Such disorders often occur in combinations, which must be precisely identified to ensure correct treatment. In general, splenic disorders involve disruption of the upbearing and transformative function of its yang qi, and present as vacuity patterns or vacuity-repletion complexes, with distinct cold signs. Disorders of the stomach, as a general rule, involve breakdown of stomach qi harmony and downbearing, and can present as cold, heat, vacuity, or repletion patterns.

Disorders of the intestines are closely related to those of the spleen and stomach. Diarrhea from impaired separation of the clear and the turbid in the small intestine is associated with splenic transformation failure. Breakdown of conveyance and transformation of waste in the large intestine leading to diarrhea or constipation is associated with both splenic transformation failure and breakdown of gastric harmony and downbearing. Most disorders of the intestines can be traced to splenogastric disease.

Finally, since the stomach and spleen are the basis of qi and blood formation, insufficiencies of these two elements are associated with failure of splenic movement and transformation, and may be treated by restoring these functions. The spleen also manages the blood, so that some cases of qi vacuity and blood containment failure, such as hemafecia and metrorrhagia, are termed blood-management failure (failure of the spleen to manage the blood).

Splenic transformation failure

Failure of splenic transformation occurs when dietary irregularities, essence-spirit and emotional disturbances, debilitation following illness, or taxation fatigue cause damage to splenic yang qi. It presents in a variety of forms including digestive disorders and impotence of uplift, and occurs in what Western medicine describes as chronic gastritis, cholecystic diseases, and nutritional disturbances, as well as general asthenia and prolapse.

The chief forms of splenic transformation failure are spleen qi vacuity, devitalization of splenic yang, and center qi fall.

Splenic qi vacuity

Pattern identification

Spleen qi vacuity is the most common form of splenic transformation failure and is associated with deficient digestion and assimilation. It is characterized by discomfort or dull pain in the abdomen, as well as thin stool or diarrhea. Occurring in conjunction with disharmony of stomach qi, there may also be reduced food intake, discomfort after eating, clamoring stomach, and eructation. The insufficiency of blood and qi supply that attends these disorders is characterized by lusterless complexion, exhaustion, relatively pale tongue, and a soft soggy pulse.

Treatment

Drug therapy

Spleen qi vacuity is treated by fortifying the spleen and boosting qi. Commonly used agents include:

Spleen Fortifiers	
Rhizoma Atractylodis Macrocephalae	*bái zhú*
Radix Dioscoreae	*shān yào*
Semen Dolichoris	*biǎn dòu*

Qi Boosters	
Radix Codonopsis Pilosulae	*dǎng shēn*
Radix Glycyrrhizae	*gān cǎo*

Concurrent disharmony of stomach qi calls for admixture of stomach harmonizers such as:

Stomach Harmonizers	
Pericarpium Citri Reticulatae	*chén pí*
Fructus Amomi	*shā rén*

Four Nobles Decoction *(sì jūn zǐ tāng)* represents a general formula that may be varied according to need. Where diarrhea is prominent, Atractylodes Seven Powder *(qī wèi bái-zhú sǎn)* may be used. Where indigestion and thin stool are prominent, Ginseng, Poria, and Atractylodes Powder *(shēn líng bái-zhú sǎn)* may be prescribed. Where there is concurrent disharmony of stomach qi, Saussurea and Amomum Six Nobles Decoction *(xiāng shā liù jūn zǐ tāng)* may be used.

Acumoxatherapy

BL-20‡, SP-6‡, and ST-36‡ are used to supplement spleen qi. ST-25‡ courses and regulates the large intesting and harmonizes the stomach; it is therefore useful in cases of diarrhea or thin stool. CV-12‡ is a major point for harmonizing the stomach. LI-4 is also often added.

Devitalization of splenic yang

Pattern identification

Splenic yang devitalization represents a further development of spleen qi debilitation, in which kidney yang is often affected. It presents with pronounced cold signs in addition to splenic vacuity symptoms. It may thus be differentiated from the latter pattern by the presence of drained white complexion, spiritual fatigue, cold form, abdominal pain relieved by warmth and pressure, and diarrhea with undigested food in the stool. The pulse is deep and weak, while the tongue is pale with white fur.

Treatment

Drug therapy

Treatment of splenic yang devitalization involves warming yang and promoting splenic movement. This method uses spleen fortifiers together with yang warmers such as:

Yang Warmers	
Rhizoma Zingiberis blast-fried	*pāo jiāng*
Cortex Cinnamomi	*ròu guì*
Radix Aconiti Fu Tzu	*fù zǐ*

Formulae for treating devitalized splenic yang include Center-Rectifying Pills *(lǐ zhōng wán)* and Aconite Center-Rectifying Pills *(fù-zǐ lǐ zhōng wán)* and variants.

Acumoxatherapy

The points used to treat spleen qi vacuity, mentioned in the previous section, may also be used to treat splenic yang devitalization, with the addition of BL-23‡, CV-4‡, CV-6‡, and GV-4‡. Moxibustion is particularly appropriate in this condition.

Because of impaired transformation of water-damp, both splenic qi vacuity and devitalization of splenic yang may give rise to water swelling, which is treated with water disinhibitors. Water swelling caused by vacuous splenic qi may be treated with Poria Four Powder *(sì líng sǎn)* and Five Cortices Cool Decoction *(wǔ pí yǐn)*, which together fortify the spleen and disinhibit water, or with Fang Chi and Astragalus Decoction *(fáng-jǐ huáng-qí tāng)*, which boosts qi and moves water. Since spleen qi vacuity affects kidney yang in nearly every case, and thus leads to splenorenal yang vacuity, water swelling caused by spleen qi vacuity may be treated with Spleen-Reinforcing Cool Decoction *(shí pí yǐn)* or True Warrior Decoction *(zhēn wǔ tāng)*. These warm and strengthen the yang qi of the spleen and kidney, dissipate cold-damp, and disinhibit water.

Acumoxatherapy

Acumoxatherapy uses points such as SP-9‡, KI-7, ST-28, and CV-9 to treat water swelling, together with BL-23‡ and GV-4‡, which warm kidney yang.

Center qi fall

Pattern identification

Center qi fall refers to diminished uplift of splenic yang qi, and often occurs as one aspect of general qi vacuity. Symptoms may be differentiated accordingly: qi vacuity is characterized by emaciation, weakness, soggy pulse, and a pale, enlarged tongue, while qi fall is characterized by sagging and distention in the abdomen, and by distention after eating, or by enduring diarrhea, and prolapse of the rectum or uterus.

Treatment

Drug therapy

Center qi fall is treated by fortifying the spleen and supplementing the center, or by upbearing yang and boosting qi. Spleen-fortifying and qi-boosting agents are used with upraisers such as Radix Bupleuri *(chái hú)* and Rhizoma Cimicifugae *(shēng má)*. A frequently prescribed formula is Center-Supplementing Qi-Boosting Decoction *(bǔ zhōng yì qì tāng)*. Since center qi fall is a form of insufficiency of splenic yang qi, signs of water-rheum accumulations are commonly observed (such as digestate stagnation due to prolapse of the stomach). Such conditions call for the admixture of rheum-transforming water-disinhibiting formulae, such as Poria, Cinnamon, Atractylodes and Liquorice Decoction *(líng guì zhú gān tāng)*.

Acumoxatherapy

Primary treatment is aimed at supplementing splenorenal yang with such points as SP-6‡, BL-20‡, BL-23‡, ST-36‡, and GV-4‡. In addition, GV-20‡ can have a positive effect on prolapse, and in cases of water-rheum accumulation, points such as SP-9 and CV-9 are commonly needled.

Blood Management Failure

Impairment of the spleen's function of managing the blood, resulting in hemorrhage, is known as blood management failure. Since the spleen is the basis of blood and qi formation, the pathomechanism of this disorder may be explained as failure of qi to contain the blood. Although blood management failure and containment failure are technically considered to be interchangeable terms, hemafecia and metrorrhagia are conventionally attributed to blood management failure.

Pattern identification

Hemorrhage resulting from blood management failure includes hemafecia and metrorrhagia. Other signs include somber white or withered yellow complexion, weakness and spiritual fatigue, dizziness, palpitations, and shortness of breath. The tongue is generally pale and the pulse is fine and soggy. Such signs indicate splenogastric vacuity and insufficiency of blood and qi. Splenic yang vacuity signs may also be observed.

Treatment

Drug therapy

Blood management failure is treated by boosting qi to contain blood. This may be combined with spleen warming where signs of splenic yang vacuity are present. Commonly used drugs that boost qi and restore blood containment are:

Blood-Containing Qi Boosters	
Radix Codonopsis Pilosulae	*dǎng shēn*
Radix Astragali	*huáng qí*
Radix Glycyrrhizae	*gān cǎo*

Concurrent splenic yang vacuity calls for admixture of spleen warmers such as:

Spleen Warmers	
Terra Flava Usta	*zào xīn tǔ*
Rhizoma Zingiberis blast-fried	*páo jiāng*
Radix Aconiti Fu Tzu	*fù zǐ*

Yellow Earth Decoction *(huáng tǔ tāng)* warms the spleen and enhances blood management, and is used where splenic vacuity hemafecia is accompanied by cold signs. Angelica Splenic Decoction *(guī pí tāng)*, which not only nourishes the heart and spleen but also boosts qi and contains the blood, is more suitable for metrorrhagia.

Since blood management failure is pathomechanically the same as failure of qi to contain the blood, boosting qi represents the basis of treatment. However, given the danger that hemorrhage may lead to blood vacuity, admixture of blood nourishers such as Radix Rehmanniae Cruda *(shēng dì)* and Gelatinum Corii Asini *(lǘ pí jiāo)* is advisable. If hemorrhage presents symptoms of disquieting of the heart spirit such as palpitations and insomnia, blood nourishers and spirit quietants such as Radix Polygalae *(yuǎn zhì)* and Semen Zizyphi Jujubae *(zǎo rén)* may be added. Admixture of blood quickeners may be indicated where blood stasis occurs in the course of an enduring hemorrhagic disorder.

Acumoxatherapy

The yang qi of the spleen and kidney can be supplemented by moxibustion on SP-6, CV-4‡, BL-20, and BL-23. GV-20‡ is used to upbear yang and boost qi. SP-1‡ is a special point for metrorrhagia and is often combined with LV-1‡ in treatment. Hemafecia accompanied by cold signs is treated by moxibustion on GV-4. Moxibustion on CV-2 dissipates cold in the uterus. HT-7 is added when hemorrhage leads to disquieting of the heart spirit.

Gastric qi vacuity cold

Gastric qi vacuity cold can be the result of damage to stomach qi by excessive consumption of raw and cold foods or other dietary irregularities. It may also occur when emotional constraint causes liver qi to invade the stomach and, in time, damages its qi. Contraction of an exogenous pathogen often represents a precipitating factor. Gastric qi vacuity cold is often seen in diseases described by Western medicine as ulcers and gastric neurosis.

Pattern identification

The ventral pain associated with gastric qi vacuity cold usually occurs on an empty stomach, and is relieved by eating or by pressure. Vomiting of clear, cold, sour fluid is sometimes observed. General symptoms include lusterless complexion, aversion to cold, lack of warmth in the extremities, and a pale, enlarged tongue. The pulse is soggy, but may become wiry or tight during pain attacks. Vacuity cold gives rise to symptoms of stomach qi disharmony such as eructation and acid upflow. Gastric qi vacuity cold characterized by pain in the venter may be precipitated by contraction of exogenous cold, but differs from that of a sudden invasion of the cold pathogen (from catching cold or from excessive consumption of raw or cold foods), as it is less sudden and violent in onset, of longer duration, and characterized by a prominence of vacuity signs. Sudden invasion of the cold pathogen is associated with pronounced cold signs, less pronounced vacuity signs, and a more sudden onset.

Treatment

Drug therapy

Gastric qi vacuity cold is treated by fortifying the center and warming the stomach. Center fortifiers include:

Center Fortifiers	
Saccharum Granorum	*yí táng*
Radix Paeoniae Albae	*bái sháo*
Radix Glycyrrhizae	*gān cǎo*
Fructus Zizyphi Jujubae	*dà zǎo*

Stomach warmers include:

Stomach Warmers	
Ramulus Cinnamomi	*guì zhī*
Rhizoma Zingiberis Recens	*shēng jiāng*
Rhizoma Alpiniae Officinari	*liáng jiāng*
Fructus Evodiae	*wú zhū yú*

A basic formula is Minor Center-Fortifying Decoction *(xiǎo jiàn zhōng tāng)*, which fortifies the center and warms the stomach, and as well harmonizes construction and relieves pain. Patterns with prominent qi vacuity may be treated with admixture of Radix Astragali *(huáng qí)*. For example, with Astragalus Center-Fortifying Decoction *(huáng-qí jiàn zhōng tāng),* where qi stagnation and pain is prominent, admixture of qi rectifiers such as the following is indicated:

Qi Rectifiers	
Rhizoma Cyperi	*xiāng fu*
Fructus Meliae Toosendan	*chuān liàn zǐ*
Rhizoma Corydalis	*yán hú suǒ*
Radix Saussureae	*mù xiāng*
Pericarpium Citri Reticulatae	*chén pí*

Admixture of antacids such as Os Sepiae *(wū zéi gǔ)* and Concha Arcae *(wǎ léng zǐ)* are required where acid upflow is prominent.

Acumoxatherapy

PC-6, a commonly used point acting on the stomach, chest, and heart, is a major point in treating gastric diseases. Gastric qi may be fortified by moxibustion at BL-20 and BL-21, and moxibustion at CV-4 will enhance the effect. CV-12 may be added to harmonize the stomach and regulate the middle burner. LV-3, the source point of the liver channel, can be used to calm liver qi, and if qi stagnation is prominent, point combinations such as ST-36‡, CV-12‡, BL-20‡, and BL-21‡ should be used. ST-36‡ is an appropriate point to use in most cases of vacuous gastric qi, and local points such as ST-21 are also added when there is qi stagnation and abdominal pain.

Stomach heat

Stomach heat represents a commonly observed interior heat pattern. It may be caused by interiorization of pathogenic heat (see Chapter 11, "Exogenous Heat Disease Pattern Identification"), damage to the stomach by overconsumption of rich or hot, spicy foods, or invasion of the stomach by liver fire. Such factors generally lead to repletion heat patterns. Vacuity heat patterns arising as a result of stomach yin vacuity are dealt with below.

Stomach heat occurs in diseases classified by Western medicine as gastritis, ulcers, diabetes mellitus, and gingivitis.

Pattern identification

Stomach heat occurs in a variety of forms. Affecting ingestion, it may cause hyperpepsia with rapid hungering. Affecting gastric downbearing, it is characterized by pain or burning sensations in the venter, vomiting, clamoring stomach, and hard stool. Upsteaming of stomach heat is characterized by painful swelling, cracking, and putrefaction of the gums, or periodontal *xuan* with bleeding gums. All forms of stomach heat may be characterized by bitter taste in the mouth, halitosis, dry mouth, a distinctly red tongue with dry, yellow fur, and a slippery pulse.

Treatment

Drug therapy

Stomach heat is treated by clearing the stomach and draining fire. Commonly used agents include:

Stomach-Clearing and Fire-Draining Agents	
Rhizoma Coptidis	*huáng lián*
Gypsum	*shí gāo*
Rhizoma Phragmitis	*lú gēn*
Fructus Gardeniae	*zhī zǐ*
Radix Scutellariae	*huáng qín*
Rhizoma Rhei	*dà huáng*

Formulae such as the following, or variants of same, may be used:

Stomach-Clearing Formulae	
Stomach-Clearing Powder	*qīng wèi sǎn*
Jade Lady Decoction	*yù nǔ jiān*

Intense stomach fire invariably causes damage to the yin fluids of the stomach, so that the judicious admixture of agents that nourish yin and engender liquid is indicated:

Yin-Nourishing and Liquid-Engendering Agents	
Radix Rehmanniae Cruda	*shēng dì*
Tuber Ophiopogonis	*mài dōng*
Rhizoma Anemarrhenae	*zhī mǔ*
Radix Scrophulariae	*xuán shēn*

Ascendant exuberance of stomach fire is invariably associated with constipation or accumulation and stagnation in the intestinal tract, and is treated by the method of clearing the upper body and draining the lower body, to free the bowels and drain heat. Diaphragm-Cooling Powder *(liáng gé sǎn)* and Stomach-Regulating Purgative Decoction *(tiáo wèi chéng qì tāng)* may be prescribed in such cases.

Acumoxatherapy

ST-43, ST-44, and ST-45 are the main points used to drain stomach fire. PC-6 calms and harmonizes the stomach, relieves pain, and rectifies qi. If there are also signs of intestinal heat, LI-4, ST-25, and ST-37 are among the points often chosen to drain the lower body. Other points commonly used in treating stomach heat conditions include ST-40, ST-41, BL-21, and CV-13.

Insufficiency of stomach yin

Insufficiency of stomach yin mainly occurs during the recovery stage of exogenous heat diseases when stomach yin may be damaged by residual heat. Another common cause is yin humor depletion in the course of enduring illness, where deprivation of the nourishing and moistening effect of yin humor may affect the downbearing of stomach qi. Insufficiency of stomach yin is commonly associated with breakdown of gastric harmony and downbearing.

Pattern identification

Insufficiency of stomach yin is characterized by signs of yin vacuity and heat, such as no thought of food, dry mouth, and a red, mirror tongue, together with symptoms of breakdown of gastric harmony and downbearing such as vacuity glomus in the venter, retching, and constipation.

Treatment

Drug therapy

Insufficiency of stomach yin is treated by the method of nourishing stomach yin, combined where necessary with clearing heat and harmonizing the stomach. Commonly used agents include:

Stomach Yin Nourishers	
Tuber Ophiopogonis	mài dōng
Rhizoma Polygonati Odorati	yù zhú
Radix Adenophorae	shā shēn
Herba Dendrobii	shí hú
Radix Rehmanniae Cruda	shēng dì
Radix Trichosanthis	tiān huā fěn

Formulae include:

Stomach-Yin-Nourishing Formulae	
Ophiopogon Decoction	mài-mén-dōng tāng
Stomach-Nourishing Decoction	yǎng wèi tāng

Ophiopogon Decoction clears counterflow ascent of qi and fire, while Stomach-Nourishing Decoction restores stomach yin with sweet, cool, and moistening agents.

Acumoxatherapy

This pattern is rarely mentioned in acupuncture texts, perhaps because supplementing of yin humor is achieved by draining fire while supplementing water, rather than direct nourishment of yin. A few points are given for nourishing kidney yin (KI-3, BL-46), but seldom for the yin of the other organs. In treating this condition, points such as ST-36 and CV-12 are used to supplement and harmonize the stomach, ST-25 and TB-6 are used to drain stomach heat, and HT-6 helps check yang hyperactivity. ST-21 may be added to harmonize the stomach and large intestine.

Counterflow ascent of stomach qi

Counterflow ascent of stomach qi is the chief form of breakdown of gastric harmony and downbearing, and may be caused by a wide variety of factors including cold, heat, phlegm, foul turbidity, digestate stagnation, and gastrointestinal qi stagnation. Counterflow ascent of stomach qi is a pattern that can occur in any stomach disease.

Pattern identification

The principal signs are nausea, vomiting, eructation, and hiccough. Counterflow occurring in a cold pattern is usually characterized by a pale tongue, white complexion, vomiting of clear fluid, or vomiting in the evening of food ingested in the morning. Where heat is present, signs include red tongue with yellow fur, vomiting of sour or bitter fluid, and immediate vomiting of ingested food. If phlegm is the cause, a slimy tongue fur, repeated ejection of phlegm-drool, and occasionally dizziness are observed. Counterflow ascent of stomach qi due to foul turbidity usually occurs in hot weather, is sudden in onset, and characterized by abdominal pain, ungratified desire to vomit, and agonizing distention and oppression in the venter. Where a result of digestate stagnation, there is usually history of ingesta damage, and signs include sour, putrid vomitus, with improvement brought by vomiting. Finally, counterflow ascent of stomach qi from gastrointestinal qi stagnation is characterized by thoracic glomus, abdominal pain, and eructation.

Treatment

Drug therapy

Harmonizing the stomach and downbearing counterflow is the basic method of treatment. Frequently used agents include:

Stomach Harmonizers and Counterflow Downbearers	
Rhizoma Pinelliae	*bàn xià*
Pericarpium Citri Reticulatae	*chén pí*
Fructus Evodiae	*wú zhū yú*
Rhizoma Zingiberis Recens	*shēng jiāng*
Rhizoma Coptidis	*huáng lián*
Caulis Bambusae in Taenis	*zhú rú*
Flos Inulae	*xuán fù huā*
Haematitum	*dài zhě shí*

Treatment should also be directed toward eliminating the relevant disease factor, using methods such as warming the stomach, clearing heat, transforming phlegm, repelling turbidity, abductive dispersion, and rectifying qi. Counterflow ascent of stomach qi due to stomach cold may be treated with Evodia Decoction *(wú-zhū-yú tāng)* or Clove and Persimmon Decoction *(dīng-xiāng shì-dì tāng)*. These are suitable for patterns with pronounced hiccough. Where the cause is stomach heat, Coptis and Evodia Pills *(zuǒ jīn wán)* may be used. Minor Pinellia Decoction with Poria *(xiǎo bàn-xià jiā fú-líng tāng)* or Gallbladder-Warming Decoction *(wēn dǎn tāng)* may be used to treat patterns caused by phlegm, and Gallbladder-Warming Decoction supplemented with Rhizoma Coptidis *(huáng lián)* may be used if an added heat complication is identified. Foul turbidity patterns are treated with Jade Axis Elixir *(yù shū dān)*. Harmony-Preserving Pills *(bǎo hé wán)* are most appropriate for digestate stagnation. Inula and Hematite Decoction *(xuán fù dài-zhě tāng)* and its variants may be used where qi stagnation is the cause.

Acumoxatherapy

Treatment varies according to the symptoms. Wind-cold contraction may be treated by combining BL-21 and BL-22 with TB-5 to supplement the stomach and resolve the exterior. Stomach-heat vomiting may be treated by needling CV-12, BL-21, ST-41, and PC-6, in order to stop vomiting as well as drain fire. Phlegm heat calls for the addition of ST-40 to transform phlegm turbidity and CV-17 with CV-6 to move water. Digestate accumulation vomiting can be treated with ST-36 and CV-21, which downbear qi and disperse accumulation. The addition of BL-20 and SP-4 can aid digestion. Vomiting caused by "wood rebelling against earth" is treated by draining at LV-2, which will course the liver (wood), and supplementing SP-4 to support the spleen (earth). ST-36 may be added to help supplement earth and harmonize the stomach. In cases of gastric qi vacuity, moxibustion at CV-12 and LV-13 will fortify the center. It should be accompanied by moxibustion at BL-20, to supplement spleen qi, and at CV-4, to boost fire and thus engender earth. PC-6 may be added to harmonize the stomach and stop vomiting.

Intestinal vacuity efflux desertion

When enduring diarrhea culminates in reduced uplift of yang qi, the resulting pattern is known as intestinal vacuity efflux desertion.

Pattern identification

The main characteristic of this disorder is persistent diarrhea with periodic incontinence or prolapse resulting from bowel movements. Generally there is dull abdominal pain, overall physical debilitation, and vacuity cold signs.

Treatment

Drug therapy

The method of treatment used is astringing the intestines and securing against desertion. Commonly used agents include:

Intestinal Astringents	
Halloysitum Rubrum	chì shí zhī
Limonitum	yǔ yú liáng
Pericarpium Punicae Granati	shí liú pí
Fructus Terminaliae Chebulae	hē zǐ
Semen Myristicae	ròu dòu kòu
Pericarpium Papaveris	yīng sù ké

Formulae include:

Intestinal Vacuity Formulae	
Peach Blossom Decoction	táo huā tāng
True Man Viscera-Nourishing Decoction	zhēn rén yǎng zàng tāng

Although intestinal insecurity is primarily treated with antidiarrheic intestinal astringents, qi rectifiers are used to prevent stagnation:

Qi Rectifiers	
Radix Saussureae	mù xiāng
Fructus Citri	zhǐ ké
Pericarpium Citri Reticulatae	chén pí

Upraisers, qi supplementers, and yang warmers are also employed.

Acumoxatherapy

Large intestine yang qi may be warmed and supplemented by combining the front-alarm and back-associated points of the large intestine, ST-25‡ and BL-25‡ respectively. CV-12‡ warms and moves spleen and stomach yang, and ST-36 combined with CV-6‡ boosts qi. GV-20‡ is often used in cases of prolapse because it promotes uplift of yang qi.

To supplement the yang of the spleen and kidney, BL-20, BL-23, GV-4‡ and SP-6‡ should be supplemented.

CV-8 (moxa only) and GV-1‡ are included when there is vacuity prolapse of the rectum.

Intestinal humor depletion

Intestinal humor depletion is caused by general lack of liquid and blood in the body. It is observed in postpartum blood vacuity, liquid depletion in the aged, and in enduring and severe diseases. It may also occur in exogenous heat disease prior to replenishment of the fluids.

Pattern identification

Signs comprise dry, hard stool and evacuative difficulty. Generally, no pronounced abdominal distention or pain is observed. The patient is in a weak state of health.

Treatment

Drug therapy

Intestinal humor depletion is treated by the method of increasing humor and lubricating the intestine. Commonly used agents include:

Intestinal Lubricants	
Radix Polygoni Multiflori Viva	*xiān shǒu wū*
Radix Rehmanniae Viva	*xiān shēng dì*
Radix Scrophulariae	*xuán shēn*
Tuber Ophiopogonis	*mài dōng*
Herba Cistanches	*cōng róng*
Semen Trichosanthis	*guā lóu rén*
Semen Biotae	*bó zǐ rén*
Semen Cannabis	*má rén*
Semen Persicae	*táo rén*

Although these agents lubricate the intestines, some are warm and others are cool in nature, so that selection is determined by the presence of heat or cold. Small quantities of precipitants and qi movers may be admixed to ease defecation. Examples of formulae include Five Kernel Pills *(wǔ rén wán)* and Cannabis Pills *(má-zǐ-rén wán)*.

Acumoxatherapy

General points used to treat constipation include ST-25, SP-15, and BL-25. If there is heat, ST-44, KI-6, and LI-11 are commonly used. Blood vacuity is treated with points such as BL-17, BL-20, BL-18, and SP-6. TB-6 and LI-4 may also be used to treat constipation due to humor depletion. (See Table 9-3.)

Disease Patterns of the Liver & Gallbladder

The liver governs free-coursing and stores blood. Disturbances of these two functions account for virtually all the many disease patterns associated with both the liver and the gallbladder.

Liver disorders may be analyzed in terms of superabundance and insufficiency. Impaired free-coursing may provoke binding depression of liver qi, a condition of superabundance. Excessive upstirring of liver yang, known as ascendant hyperactivity of liver yang, is also a condition of superabundance. By contrast, blood storage failure is an insufficiency disorder. It is characteristic of the liver that its yang and qi tend toward superabundance while its yin and blood tend toward insufficiency. However, liver yang commonly becomes hyperactive when liver yin is insufficient and fails to keep it in check. Also, when liver qi is depressed, it may transform into fire, which damages both yin and blood. In extreme cases, when check is lost over yang, liver wind may stir in the inner body.

Treatment of liver and gallbladder disorders invariably involves restoration of hepatic storage of blood and governance of free-coursing. Only in the case of hepatocystic damp-heat should pathogen elimination be chosen. Coursing the liver and rectifying qi, and calming the liver and draining fire are two treatment methods designed to restore free-coursing. Nourishing the blood and emolliating the liver, and enriching the liver and supplementing the kidney, are two examples of methods used to restore blood storage. Other methods include nurturing yin and subduing yang, harmonizing the blood and coursing the liver, and nourishing the blood and extinguishing wind, all of which correct superabundance of liver yang and qi and insufficiency of liver yin and blood. The gallbladder is closely related to the liver, bile being formed from excess liver qi. Most diseases of the gallbladder are thus treated as impaired free-coursing.

Identification of the major disease patterns of the liver and gallbladder are dealt with below. Hepatocystic damp-heat is dealt with in Chapter 10.

Binding depression of liver qi

Binding depression of liver qi is the most common form of impaired free-coursing. It is a qi dynamic disorder of the depression or stagnation type. It may be caused by essence-spirit and emotional disorders, invasion of exogenous damp-heat, or insufficiency of yin blood depriving the liver of nourishment. It manifests as mental depression, bile secretion disorders, qi dynamic disorders, or combinations of these, and may be observed in diseases of the liver and gallbladder proper, of the liver channel (plum-stone globus, struma, or breast swellings), in ulcerative diseases, gastrointestinal disturbances, neurosis, and irregular menses.

Severe depression may lead to fire formation and the emergence of an upflaming liver fire pattern, or to damage to liver yin-blood, which manifests as a a vacuity pattern. Extreme depression may cause a counterflow upsurge of liver qi, one form of qi inversion.

Pattern identification

The essence-spirit and emotional symptoms of binding depression of liver qi are depression or rashness, impatience, and exaggerated emotional response.

The main signs of qi dynamic disruption include scurrying pains or painful distention in the chest and lateral costal region, oppression in the chest, and a wiry pulse.

Symptoms of bile secretion disruption, which are dealt with in greater detail under the heading "Hepatocystic Damp-Heat" in Chapter 10, include jaundice and vomiting of bitter fluid or yellow bile.

Other forms of binding depression of liver qi involve organs related to the liver and gallbladder, or parts of the body to which they are linked by their channels. Liver qi may invade the spleen and stomach, resulting in two possible conditions: invasion of the stomach by liver qi, characterized by nausea, vomiting, acid regurgitation, and acute abdominal pain and distention, or hepatosplenic disharmony, indicated by painful distention and diarrhea. Liver qi may also ascend counterflow, carrying phlegm upwards. This may cause plum-stone globus, characterized by the sensation of a lump in the throat, with inability to swallow or vomit. If qi and phlegm obstruct each other and accumulate in the neck, it gives rise to struma (thyroid enlargement), characterized by soft swellings on both sides of the laryngeal prominence that move up and down when the patient swallows. Binding liver qi depression may also affect the penetrating and conception vessels, leading to menalgia, menstrual block, cyclical swelling of the breasts, breast lumps, and irregular menses.

Treatment

Drug therapy

Coursing the liver and rectifying qi is the basic method of treating binding depression of liver qi, though this may be varied depending on the symptomatic manifestation. If occurring as emotional disturbances, it may be treated by coursing the liver and resolving depression, and by appropriate psychiatric treatment. If it manifests as disruption of qi dynamic, the accent is placed on rectifying qi. When it presents as a bile secretion disorder, the emphasis is placed on disinhibiting bile.

Commonly used liver-coursing and qi rectifying agents include:

Liver Coursers	
Radix Bupleuri	chái hú
Tuber Curcumae	yù jīn
Pericarpium Citri Reticulatae Viride	qīng pí
Fructus Citri	zhǐ ké
Rhizoma Cyperi	xiāng fù
Fructus Meliae Toosendan	chuān liàn zǐ
Rhizoma Corydalis	yán hú suǒ
Caulis Perillae	sū gěng
Fructus Akebiae	bā yuè zhā
Fructus Liquidambaris	lù lù tōng
Radix Linderae	wū yào
Semen Citri	jú hé

A basic formula is Bupleurum Liver-Coursing Decoction (chái-hú shū gān tāng), which may be varied according to need. Invasion of stomach by liver qi further requires the additional use of the stomach-harmonizing method, for which formulae such as Coptis and Evodia Pills (zuǒ jīn wán) may be prescribed. Disharmony between the liver and spleen disharmony is treated by hepatosplenic harmonization, using Free Wanderer Powder (xiāo yáo sǎn) or Pain and Diarrhea Formula (tòng xiè yào fāng).

Plum-stone globus is treated by downbearing qi and transforming phlegm, using Four-Seven Decoction (sì qī tāng) and similar formulae. Struma is generally treated by qi-rectifying dispersion, using such formulae as Sargassium Jade Teapot Decoction (hǎi-zǎo yù hú tāng). Finally, disorders of the penetrating and conception vessels resulting from binding depression of liver qi are mainly treated with such formulae as Free Wanderer Powder.

Most liver-coursing qi rectifiers are aromatic and dry, and may readily damage yin and blood. To prevent the complications this may cause in weaker patients, they are combined with agents that nourish the blood and emolliate the liver, such as:

Liver Emollients	
Radix Paeoniae Albae	*bái sháo*
Radix Angelicae Sinensis	*dāng guī*
Radix Rehmanniae Cruda	*shēng dì*
Fructus Lycii	*qǐ zǐ*

Acumoxatherapy

Acupuncture uses points to move the blood and qi as the primary treatment of binding depression of liver qi. LV-2, LV-3, LV-8, LV-13, GB-40, and GB-34 are some of the points often chosen to course the liver and move liver qi and blood.

SP-8 is a major point for moving uterine blood, and is combined with points such as SP-6, LV-8, LV-2, ST-30, ST-29, BL-32, CV-3, and SP-10 to treat menstrual disturbances related to liver qi depression. GB-41 is often used for cyclical swelling of the breasts.

Liver qi disruption resulting in pain and distention in the lateral costal region is often treated with points such as LV-13, LV-14, LV-2, and GB-40, which move hepatocystic qi. They may be combined with PC-6, which soothes the chest and resolves depression. SI-5, TB-6, CV-17, and GB-34 are also effective, depending on the particular symptom pattern.

Invasion of the stomach by liver qi is treated with points that supplement stomach qi and harmonize the spleen and stomach, exemplified by CV-12, ST-36, PC-6, and SP-6. These may be combined with points that calm the liver and course liver qi, such as LV-2, LV-13, and LV-3. Points such as BL-20, BL-21, and SP-4 are often used to help fortify the spleen and stomach. Similar points are used in treatment of hepatosplenic disharmonies.

CV-23 is a major point in the treatment of plum-stone globus. Neck swellings due to binding depression of liver qi are treated with local points such as TB-13, LI-17, CV-22, and local paravertebral *jia-ji* points lateral to the third, fourth, and fifth cervical vertebrae, in combination with distal points such as LI-4, LI-11, ST-36, and LI-10, which all belong to channels that pass through the neck and have the ability to move channel qi. Moxibustion on the contralateral olecranon process is a special technique used to treat neck swellings.

Upflaming of liver fire

Upflaming of liver fire is a hepatocystic heat depression pattern. It may be caused by transformation of depressed liver qi into fire, by severe emotional disturbance, or by depressed damp-heat pathogens in the inner body.

Pattern identification

Upflaming of liver fire is characterized by qi and fire rising to the head, and pronounced heat signs. Blood storage is frequently affected, which leads to hemorrhage. The chief symptoms are severe headache, red complexion, ocular rubor, dry mouth, sudden tinnitus or deafness, and vomiting of sour or bitter fluid. The stool is dry or hard. The pulse is generally slippery and wiry, and the tongue is red with dry, yellow fur. Emotional signs include irascibility, rashness, and impatience. If blood storage is affected, there may be expectoration of blood, hematemesis, and nosebleed, as well as menorrhagia. The essential characteristic of upflaming liver fire is exuberant fire in the upper body. In general, no lower-body pattern indicating yin-blood insufficiency is observed. In this respect, it differs from liver yin vacuity and ascendant hyperactivity of liver yang, which are both characterized by upper-body exuberance and lower-body vacuity.

Treatment

Drug therapy

Clearing the liver and draining fire is the method classically employed to treat upflaming of liver fire. Commonly used agents include:

Liver Clearers and Fire Drainers	
Radix Gentianae	*lóng dǎn cǎo*
Fructus Gardeniae	*zhī zǐ*
Radix Scutellariae	*huáng qín*
Spica Prunellae	*xià kū cǎo*
Folium Mori	*sāng yè*
Flos Chrysanthemi	*jú huā*
Semen Celosiae	*qīng xiāng zǐ*

Gentian Liver-Draining Decoction *(lóng dǎn xiè gān tāng)* and its variants may be used. Where frenetic blood flow is present, blood coolers may be admixed:

Blood Coolers	
Radix Rehmanniae Cruda	*shēng dì*
Cortex Radicis Mu Tan	*mǔ dān pí*
Radix Paeoniae Rubrae	*chì sháo*

Where counterflow rising of qi and fire causes expectoration of blood or hematemesis, qi downbearers may be employed:

Qi Downbearers	
Lignum Aquilariae	*chén xiāng*
Haematitum	*dài zhě shí*

Precipitant formulae may be added for inner-body liver-fire bind that leads to hard, dry stool.

Precipitant Formulae	
Toilette Pills	*gēng yī wán*
Clear and Quiet Pills	*qīng níng wán*

Acumoxatherapy

LV-2 and LV-3 are main points for draining liver fire. If the eyes are bloodshot, GB-41 may be added. Points on the head, such as GV-20, M-HN-9 *(tai-yang)*, GB-1, and SI-19 are used to drain fire.

Blood heat may be cooled by the addition of points such as BL-17, SP-10, and BL-54. LI-4 and points on the governing vessel channel are often needled to eliminate superabundance of yang.

Ascendant hyperactivity of liver yang

Ascendant hyperactivity of liver yang represents an imbalance of the liver's yin and yang aspects. It occurs when hepatorenal yin vacuity causes excessive upstirring of liver yang.

Though possessing distinct characteristics, this disorder is closely related to the liver qi and yang patterns previously discussed. Ascendant hyperactivity of liver yang occurs when liver yin is insufficient and unable to counterbalance the upstirring of its complement. Upflaming of liver fire is essentially a further development of binding depression of liver qi, since it occurs when depressed liver qi transforms into fire and rises. Binding depression of liver qi itself stems from disruption of free-coursing, and since in severe cases it may entail damage to liver yin, it is a potential cause of both liver yang and liver fire disorders. The characteristics of these three disorders may be summed up as follows: liver qi is associated with depression; liver yang is associated with floating and ascendant hyperactivity; and liver fire is associated with transformation of depressed qi.

Pattern identification

Ascendant hyperactivity is identifiable by signs of upper-body exuberance, and by symptoms of the yin-blood insufficiency from which this condition springs. Thus, symptoms include: essence-spirit excitation, irascibility, dizziness, pressure and pain in the head, upbearing fire flush, blurred vision, reddening of the ears, ocular rubor, tinnitus, insomnia, palpitations, low back pain, and weakness in the legs. The pulse is wiry and may also be fine, and frequently the tongue is distinctly red. Prominence of yang hyperactivity and yin vacuity signs varies from case to case. In some cases, both are equally pronounced.

Treatment

Drug therapy

Treatment involves enriching yin, calming the liver, and subduing yang. Yin enrichers include:

Yin Enrichers	
Radix Rehmanniae Cruda	*shēng dì*
Fructus Lycii	*qǐ zǐ*
Fructus Ligustri Lucidi	*nǚ zhēn zǐ*
Plastrum Testudinis	*guī bǎn*
Carapax Amydae	*biē jiǎ*
Tuber Asparagi	*tiān dōng*
Tuber Ophiopogonis	*mài dōng*

Liver calmatives include:

Liver Calmatives	
Ramulus et Uncus Uncariae	*gōu téng*
Rhizoma Gastrodiae	*tiān má*
Fructus Tribuli	*jí lí*
Radix Paeoniae Albae	*bái sháo*
Concha Haliotidis	*shí jué míng*
Cornu Antelopis	*líng yáng jiǎo*

Yang subduers include:

Yang Subduers	
Concha Ostreae	*mǔ lì*
Concha Haliotidis	*shí jué míng*
Concha Margaritifera	*zhēn zhū mǔ*
Dens Draconis	*lóng chǐ*

Prominence of hyperactivity is treated with formulae such as Gastrodia and Uncaria Cool Decoction *(tiān-má gōu-téng yǐn)*, whose action of enriching yin and boosting the kidney is secondary to that of calming the liver. Prominence of yin vacuity is treated with formulae such as Lycium, Chrysanthemum and Rehmannia Pills *(qǐ jú dì-huáng wán)* whose principal action of enriching the kidney and nourishing the liver is assisted by liver clearage. Severe yin vacuity and yang hyperactivity can lead to the stirring of endogenous liver wind. This may be treated with Great Wind-Stabilizing Pills *(dà dìng fēng zhū)* and similar yin-fostering yang-subduing formulae, which may be supplemented with wind-extinguishing *chong* products.

Acumoxatherapy

Treatment is similar to that for upflaming of liver fire, except that emphasis is placed on enriching yin with points such as KI-3, SP-6, and TB-3, and calming the liver with LV-3, LV-8, LV-14, BL-18, etc.. Wind-extinguishing points such as GB-20 are used if wind signs are present. Points such as GV-20 and LI-4 can be used to reduce yang superabundance. Various local points may be added according to the symptoms.

Liver wind

Liver wind is a form of endogenous wind, an unchecked upstirring of liver yang resulting from depletion of hepatorenal yin humor. *Case Studies for Clinical Guidance* states, "Endogenous wind is movement of the body's yang qi," and is the result of "depleted stocks of yin in the viscera." Liver wind arises from extreme yin-yang and qi-blood imbalance. Ascending hyperactivity of liver yang, upflaming of liver fire, and insufficiency of liver yin and/or blood may all, in extreme cases, stir liver wind.

Pattern identification

The chief signs of liver wind are severe dizziness and headache, iron-band sensation, tension and stiffness in the neck, tingling or numbness in the limbs, or twitching of the sinews and flesh. In serious cases, there may be tautness of the face and eye muscles, trembling lips and fingers, inhibited speech, or unsteady gait. In more severe cases there may be convulsive spasm or tetanic inversion. *Essential Questions* states, "Wind patterns characterized by shaking and visual dizziness are associated with the liver." Usually, the pulse is wiry, the tongue is red, and the tongue fur is dry.

Treatment

Drug therapy

Liver wind can be treated symptomatically by calming the liver and extinguishing wind, and radically by fostering yin and subduing yang. These agents calm the liver and extinguish wind:

Liver-Calming and Wind-Extinguishing Agents	
Rhizoma Gastrodiae	tiān má
Ramulus et Uncus Uncariae	gōu téng
Cornu Antelopis	líng yáng jiǎo
Lumbricus	dì lóng
Buthus	quán xiē
Bombyx Batryticatus	jiāng cán

Agents that nurture yin and check yang are also potentially indicated:

Yin-Fostering and Yang-Subduing Agents	
Radix Rehmanniae	dì huáng
Radix Paeoniae Albae	bái sháo
Gelatinum Corii Asini	lǘ pí jiāo
Plastrum Testudinis	guī bǎn
Carapax Amydae	biē jiǎ
Concha Ostreae	mǔ lì

Lumbricus *(dì lóng)* and other *chong* products also transform static blood and free the connecting channels, so that windstroke aftereffects and cerebrovascular disorders are often treated by the method of freeing the connecting channels and extinguishing wind. Two commonly used formulae are Great Wind-Stabilizing Pills *(dà dìng fēng zhū)* and Antelope Horn Decoction *(líng-yáng-jiǎo tāng)*. Both of these treat both root and branches, although in the former, emphasis is placed on nurturing yin and subduing yang, while in the latter it is placed on calming the liver and extinguishing wind.

Acumoxatherapy

Liver wind is treated with such points as BL-18, LV-2, and GB-20, all needled with strong stimulation to expel wind and drain the liver and gallbladder. KI-3 and BL-23 are used to enrich water (kidney) and moisten wood (liver). KI-1 is warmed with indirect moxibustion to bring down floating yang. Local points, such as M-HN-9 *(tai-yang)* and GV-20 are used for dizziness and headache.

Points used to treat liver wind numbness in the limbs are PC-6, LI-11, which also loosen the chest and abdomen and relieve depression, and LV-2, which courses the liver. Local points are added according to the location of the numbness. Wind-extinguishing points (such as GB-20) and yin-fostering points are added to complete the treatment.

Tension and stiffness in the neck are treated by using many of the points previously mentioned to calm the liver and extinguish wind, in combination with points that have a special effect on the neck region, such as

SI-3 and GB-39. Local points, such as GB-21, TB-10, GV-14, and BL-10, or any particularly sensitive points in the affected area, may be added.

Liver blood vacuity

Two causes of liver blood vacuity are commonly observed: damage to yin-blood in the course of enduring illness which deprives the liver of blood for storage and of adequate nourishment; and continual expectoration of blood, nosebleed, or menorrhagia due to blood storage failure.

Pattern identification

In addition to general blood vacuity signs, liver blood vacuity is associated with a variety of patterns: blood failing to nourish the liver, blood failing to nourish the sinews or eyes, and penetrating and conception vessel disorders. Signs include dizziness, insomnia, excessive dreaming, flowery vision, blurred vision, inhibited sinew-vascular movement, lusterless nails, reduced menstrual flow, or alternating menstrual block and metrorrhagia. In severe cases, the kidney may be affected, resulting in hepatorenal essence-blood depletion, and thereby such symptoms as low back pain, seminal emission, sterility, menstrual block, emaciation, and tidal fever, in addition to the above-mentioned symptoms.

Treatment

Drug therapy

Since liver blood and kidney essence are mutually engendering, treatment usually involves dual treatment of liver and kidney. The basic method of treatment is supplementing the blood and nourishing the liver. Commonly used agents that supplement both liver and kidney include:

Liver and Kidney Supplementers	
Radix Rehmanniae	dì huáng
Radix Paeoniae Albae	bái sháo
Radix Angelicae Sinensis	dāng guī
Fructus Lycii	qǐ zǐ
Mesocarpium Corni	yú ròu
Fructus Ligustri Lucidi	nǚ zhēn zǐ
Herba Ecliptae	hàn lián cǎo
Fructus Mori	sāng shēn zǐ
Radix Polygoni Multiflori	shǒu wū
Gelatinum Corii Asini	lǘ pí jiāo
Plastrum Testudinis	guī bǎn
Carapax Amydae	biē jiǎ

For most simple cases of liver blood insufficiency the following formulae, or their variants, may be used:

Liver Blood Insufficiency Formulae	
Liver-Supplementing Decoction	bǔ gān tāng
Four Agents Decoction	sì wù tāng

For blood failing to nourish the sinews or connecting vessels, characterized by signs such as numbness in the extremities or impaired locomotion, blood-nourishing and connecting-channel-freeing agents such as the following are indicated:

Blood Nourishers and Connecting-Channel Freers	
Radix et Caulis Chi Hsüeh T'eng	jī xuè téng
Flos Carthami	hóng huā
Ramus Loranthi	sāng jì shēng
Radix Dipsaci	xù duàn
Radix Achyranthis Bidentatae	niú xī

Blood failing to nourish the head and eyes, characterized by such symptoms as loss of visual acuity and dizziness, may be treated with Lycium, Chrysanthemum and Rehmannia Pills *(qǐ jú dì-huáng wán)* or similar formulae. Disorders of the penetrating and conception vessels due to liver blood vacuity may be treated with Black Free Wanderer Powder *(hēi xiāo yáo sǎn)* (Free Wanderer Powder with Radix Rehmanniae Conquita), and its variants. Depletion of hepatorenal essence-blood is generally treated with such formulae as Kidney Pills *(zuǒ guī wán)* and their variants, which supplement kidney essence and nourish liver blood.

Acumoxatherapy

SP-10‡, SP-6‡, and BL-17‡ are used to supplement the blood. KI-3 and BL-23 nourish kidney yin. Points such as these are the basis for treating insufficiency of liver blood.

Dizziness calls for the addition of points such as M-HN-9 *(tai-yang)* and GV-20. Insomnia is treated by adding HT-7 and PC-7. LV-8, the water point of the liver (wood) channel, and GB-34, the meeting point for the sinews, are major points used for blood failing to nourish the sinews.

Menstrual disorders are treated with points such as SP-6 and PC-6, along with points such as BL-18‡ and BL-20‡, the back-associated points of the liver and spleen, and CV-3, a major conception vessel point where the three leg yin channels intersect. Other points that may be used to treat this type of disorder include LV-5 and M-CA-18 *(zi-gong)*.

Because of the relationship between qi and blood production, points such as ST-36‡, CV-6‡, and BL-20‡ are frequently included in the treatment of insufficiency of liver blood. (See Table 9-4.)

Disease Patterns of the Kidney and Bladder

The kidney stores essential qi, governs the bones, engenders marrow, and is the basis of reproduction. The transformative action of kidney qi regulates the fluid metabolism of the body. Therefore, diseases of the kidney usually occur in the form of insufficiency of essence-marrow, deficiency of the reproductive function, and disruption of fluid metabolism.

The essential qi that is stored by the kidney is constantly being replenished by the essential qi of the digestate. At the same time, kidney yin and kidney yang, the yin and yang aspects of kidney essential qi, are the root of yin and yang of all the organs. The yang of all organs is warmed by kidney yang, while their yin is nourished by kidney yin. Therefore, when kidney yin or yang is vacuous, the corresponding aspect of all the other organs may be affected. Conversely, when yin and yang vacuity of the other organs reaches a certain degree, kidney yin and yang may be affected. This explains why it is said, "Enduring illness affects the kidney." However, since the organs are each particularly susceptible to specific vacuities — the liver to yin vacuity and the spleen to yang vacuity — each has its own characteristic relationship to the kidney yin and yang. Thus, kidney yang is most closely related to splenic yang, since splenic movement and transformation supports the kidney in performing its function of supplying the body with essential qi and regulating water metabolism. Kidney yin is most closely related to liver yin; the kidney essence and liver blood nourish each other: "The liver and kidney are of the same source." Splenorenal yang vacuity and hepatorenal yin vacuity are commonly observed dual vacuity patterns.

Kidney yin and yang are regarded as being interdependent and complementary aspects of kidney essential qi. When vacuity of kidney yin or yang reaches a certain degree, it may affect its complement, since detriment to yang affects yin, and vice versa. The principle of interdependence of yin and yang is also of great importance when treating kidney yin-yang imbalances. *Jing Yue's Complete Compendium* states:

> Yang, when requiring supplementation, should be sought in yin, since with the help of yin, it can arise infinitely; yin, when requiring supplementation, must be sought in yang, since with the help of yang, its source is never ending.

Except for downpour of damp-heat, which is characterized by urinary frequency, painful urination, and dark-colored urine, most disorders of the bladder, such as urinary block, enuresis, and incontinence, are associated with disruptions of the transformative action of kidney yang, and are thus treated through the kidney.

Kidney yin vacuity

Kidney yin is the root of all yin of the body. It is most closely related to the heart, liver and lung. Thus kidney yin depletion frequently leads to vacuity of heart, liver, or lung yin. Conversely, persistent yin vacuity in the three related viscera may culminate in depletion of kidney yin. Hence in clinical practice, kidney yin vacuity most commonly occurs in dual vacuity patterns. Correspondence to Western medical disease categories varies accordingly. Hepatorenal yin vacuity is seen in some forms of hypertension, neurosis, and menstrual diseases. Cardiorenal yin vacuity may occur in tachycardia, hyperthyroidism, and neurosis. Finally, pulmorenal yin vacuity is seen in pulmonary tuberculosis.

Pattern identification

Kidney yin vacuity is characterized by vacuity and heat signs, and varies greatly in severity. Mild cases are characterized by dizziness, tinnitus, dry pharynx, dry mouth, steady fever, low back pain, seminal emission and spontaneous sweating. The pulse is fine and rapid, and the tongue is distinctly red in color. Severe cases are marked by the additional presence of emaciation, drastic loss of muscle mass, and a red, mirror tongue.

The dual patterns are identified by additional symptoms. Hepatorenal yin vacuity is characterized by headache, blurred or flowery vision, and loss of visual acuity, as well as irregular menses and sterility. Cardiorenal yin vacuity is characterized by such symptoms as insomnia, palpitations, poor memory, and excessive dreaming. Cough, expectoration of blood, and steaming bone tidal fever are observed in pulmorenal yin vacuity.

Treatment

Drug therapy

"Invigorating the governor of water to counteract the brilliance of yang" is the principle of treatment applicable to kidney yin vacuity. Commonly used drugs that enrich kidney yin include:

Kidney Yin Enrichers	
Radix Rehmanniae	*dì huáng*
Plastrum Testudinis	*guī bǎn*
Tuber Asparagi	*tiān dōng*
Carapax Amydae	*biē jiǎ*
Radix Scrophulariae	*xuán shēn*

Kidney Yin Enrichers (continued)	
Radix Polygoni Multiflori	shǒu wū
Mesocarpium Corni	yú ròu
Fructus Ligustri Lucidi	nǚ zhēn zǐ
Herba Ecliptae	hàn lián cǎo

Rehmannia Six Pills *(liù wèi dì-huáng wán)* represent the basic formula prescribed. For mild cases, Double Supreme Pills *(èr zhì wán)* may be used. Where effulgent fire symptoms are prominent, Anemarrhena, Phellodendron and Rehmannia Pills *(zhī bó dì-huáng wán)* may be prescribed. Hepatorenal yin vacuity may be treated with Lycium, Chrysanthemum and Rehmannia Pills *(qǐ jú dì-huáng wán)* and similar formulae. Heart-Supplementing Pills *(bǔ xīn wán)* treat cardiorenal yin vacuity. Lily Bulb Metal-Securing Decoction *(bǎi-hé gù jīn tāng)* treats pulmorenal yin vacuity. Where signs of essence-blood depletion are present, kidney essential qi must also be supplemented.

Acumoxatherapy

BL-47, KI-3, and BL-23 are major points used to treat kidney yin vacuity. KI-7 is the "metal point" of the kidney (water) channel, and thus according to five-phase theory engenders water. KI-3 is the most commonly used point, while BL-47 is used primarily in the treatment of nephritis and urogenital problems. KI-6 and LU-7 are often combined to treat sore throat caused by yin vacuity fire effulgence.

Treatment of dual vacuities involves combined use of fire-draining and yin-nourishing points. For example, hepatorenal yin vacuity with symptoms such as headache and blurred vision may be treated with yin-nourishing points such as BL-47, KI-3, and BL-23, combined with points such as LV-2, which downbears counterflow, and M-HN-9 *(tai yang)*, which diffuses and drains channel qi at the vertex.

Cardiorenal and pulmorenal yin vacuities are treated by needling points such as BL-47, TB-3, BL-23, KI-3, KI-10, and KI-7. These points are also indicated for heart and lung yin vacuities.

Kidney yang vacuity

Kidney yang is the root of the yang of the entire body, and is related most closely to the yang qi of the spleen, lung and heart. Kidney yang vacuities may cause, or be caused by, vacuities of the yang qi of the three related viscera. As with kidney yin vacuity, correspondence to Western medical categories varies according to the type of pattern. Simple kidney yang vacuity may be seen in diseases described in Western medicine as chronic nephritis, general asthenia, and neurasthenia sexualis. Splenorenal yang vacuity is associated with chronic nephritis and chronic diarrhea. Qi absorption failure is seen in pulmonary emphysema. Cardiorenal yang debilitation is observed in cardiac failure.

Pattern identification

Kidney yang vacuity is characterized by both vacuity and cold signs, such as drained white complexion, hebetude of essence-spirit, aversion to cold, lack of warmth in the extremities, dizziness, tinnitus, limpness of the knees and lumbar region, and an enlarged, pale tongue. Where the reproductive function is affected, spermatorrhea, impotence, sterility, and irregular menses may be observed. Where the transformative function of kidney qi is impaired, signs include long micturition with copious, clear urine, nocturia or oliguria, urinary block, and water swelling. In serious cases water-rheum may flood upward, intimidating the heart and shooting into the lung. Such cases are characterized by palpitations, dyspnea with rapid breathing, and inability to assume a recumbent posture.

Splenorenal yang vacuity is characterized by pronounced water swelling or enduring diarrhea, clear-food diarrhea, or daybreak diarrhea. Qi absorption failure, which generally stems from lung qi vacuity, is characterized by rapid breathing at the slightest exertion. Cardiorenal yang debilitation is identified by the presence of palpitations, dyspnea, water swelling, and in serious cases, by inversion frigidity of the limbs, oily perspiration, and other critical signs.

Treatment

Drug therapy

"Boosting the source of fire to eliminate the entrenched surfeit of yin" is the method used to treat kidney yang vacuity. Commonly used are agents that warm and supplement kidney yang, such as

Kidney Yang Warming Supplementers	
Radix Aconiti Fu Tzu	*fù zǐ*
Cortex Cinnamomi	*ròu guì*
Semen Trigonellae	*hú lú bā*
Fructus Psoraleae	*bǔ gǔ zhǐ*
Fructus Alpiniae Oxyphyllae	*yì zhì rén*
Rhizoma Curculiginis	*xiān máo*
Herba Epimedii	*xiān líng pí*

Formulae include Aconite and Cinnamon Eight Pills *(fù guì bā wèi wán)*. These warm the lower burner and are used for general kidney yang vacuities. Splenorenal yang vacuity presenting with enduring, clear-food, or daybreak diarrhea may be treated with Four Divinity Pills *(sì shén wán)*

and variants, which warm and supplement the spleen and kidney. Where water swelling is pronounced, True Warrior Decoction *(zhēn wǔ tāng)* or Life-Saver Kidney Qi Pills *(jì shēng shèn qì wán)* may be used to warm yang and disinhibit water. Qi absorption failure may be treated with combinations including such formulae as Ginseng and Gecko Powder *(shēn jiè sǎn)* or Black Tin Elixir *(hēi-xí dān)*, which warm the kidney and promote qi absorption. Impending desertion due to cardiorenal yang debilitation should be treated with such anti-desertive yang-salvaging formulae as Ginseng and Aconite Decoction *(shēn fù tāng)*. Kidney yang vacuity occurring in combination with insufficiency of essence-blood may be treated according to the principle that the "essence promotes qi formation" using formulae that replenish essence and supplement the kidney, such as Vital Gate Pills *(yòu guī wán)*.

Acumoxatherapy

Moxibustion at GV-4, BL-23, CV-4, KI-3, and ST-36 helps supplement kidney yang. At SP-9 and CV-9 it will disinhibit water, where severe water swelling is present.

Splenorenal yang vacuity with cold diarrhea calls for the addition of points such as BL-20, SP-6, BL-25, and ST-25 to supplement the spleen and large intestine. Cardiorenal yang vacuity may be treated with the back-associated point of the heart, BL-15, which will supplement the heart, and points such as HT-7 and PC-6 which quiet the spirit and heart respectively.

Insufficiency of kidney essence

Popularly referred to in China as kidney depletion or kidney vacuity, insufficiency of kidney essence arises from depletion of kidney essence because of enduring illness or as a result of improper development during the fetal stage. It differs from kidney yin and yang vacuity in that vacuity symptoms are accompanied by neither cold nor heat signs of any marked degree. The kidney governs the bones and engenders marrow, and the brain is the sea of marrow. Only when kidney essential qi is abundant can the bone, marrow and brain fulfill their functions. Insufficiency of kidney essence may thus lead to signs of essence-marrow depletion and sea-of-marrow vacuity, such as impaired intellect, osteodystrophy, and deficiency of the reproductive function.

Pattern identification

Insufficiency of kidney essence is generally characterized by dizziness, tinnitus, pain and limpness in the lumbar region and knees, deficient reproductive function and loss of head hair, and loosening of the teeth. Insufficiency of essence-marrow or sea-of-marrow vacuity manifests in different ways according to age. In children, it can result in retarded growth and development, short stature, sluggish intellection and movement, weak bones, or retarded closure of the fontanels. In adults, it may lead to premature senility, or weakness in the legs, difficulty in walking, dulling of essence-spirit, and sluggish movement.

Treatment

Drug therapy

"Insufficiency of essence is treated by supplementation with sapor." Commonly used drugs include:

Essence-Replenishing and Marrow-Boosting Agents	
Placenta Hominis	zǐ hé jū
Cornu Cervi	lù jiǎo
Plastrum Testudinis	guī bǎn
Cortex Eucommiae	dù zhòng
Fructus Lycii	qǐ zǐ
Herba Cistanches	cōng róng
Radix Morindae	bā jǐ ròu
Herba Cynomorii	suǒ yáng
Mesocarpium Corni	yú ròu
Semen Cuscutae	tù sī zǐ
Radix Rehmanniae Conquita	shóu dì

Formulae include:

Kidney Depletion Formulae	
Kidney Pills	zuǒ guī wán
Placenta Solo Powder	dān wèi hé-jū fěn

Where cold signs are present, Vital Gate Pills *(yòu guī wán)* may be used to replenish essence and warm the kidney. The presence of heat signs calls for Greatly Fortifying Placenta Pills *(hé-jū dà zào wán)*, which enrich the kidney and boost essence.

Acumoxatherapy

Major treatment points are those related to the kidney, such as BL-23‡, KI-3‡, and GV-4‡, and those related to original qi, such as CV-4‡ and CV-6‡. Moxibustion is used when cold signs are present. It is often appropriate to quiet the heart with HT-5 or HT-7, and supplement center qi with CV-12‡ and ST-36‡.

Insecurity of kidney qi

Kidney qi is said to be "insecure" when it fails to perform its function of regulating discharge of urine and semen. Insecurity results from senile debilitation or juvenile maldevelopment of kidney qi, or from damage through sexual intemperance or early commencement of sexual activity.

Pattern identification

Insecurity of kidney qi is characterized by signs of general kidney vacuity such as spiritual fatigue, low back pain, limpness of the knees, distinctly pale tongue, and a weak, fine pulse. Mild cold signs are also observed. Specific features include urinary disturbances such as frequent and long micturition with clear urine, or incontinence, enuresis, and dribbling, and disruptions of the reproductive function such as seminal emission, seminal efflux, and premature ejaculation.

Treatment

Drug therapy

The method of treatment is that of securing the kidney and astringing essence. General kidney supplementers are combined with agents that astringe essence and check enuresis.

Essence-Astringing and Urine-Controlling Agents	
Fructus Rosae Laevigatae	jīn yīng zǐ
Semen Euryalis	qiàn shí
Os Draconis	lóng gǔ
Concha Ostreae	mǔ lì
Semen Astragali Complanati	tóng jí lí
Stamen Nelumbinis	lián xū
Radix Dioscoreae	shān yào
Oötheca Mantidis	sāng piāo xiāo

Golden Lock Essence-Securing Pills *(jīn suǒ gù jīng wán)* are used to treat seminal emission. Stream-Reducing Pills *(suō quán wán)* treat polyuria and urinary frequency, and incontinence in the aged. Oötheca Mantidis Powder *(sāng-piāo-xiāo sǎn)* is used to treat enuresis in children.

Acumoxatherapy

GV-4‡, LI-4‡, BL-23‡, and GV-20‡ are used to assist yang in its function of containing essence. BL-30‡ is often added. KI-3 is also effective, and in cases of urinary dysfunction CV-2‡ and SP-9‡ are often used. ST-36‡ and SP-6‡ are used with any type of vacuity to aid the middle burner and increase the transformative action of qi. (See Table 9-5.)

Table 9-1 page 1

Identification and Treatment of Heart Disease Patterns

Pattern Type	Principal Signs	Treatment Method	Commonly Used Formulae	Acupoints
Heart Qi Vacuity	Racing of the heart; Palpitations; Dizziness; Lusterless complexion; Shortness of breath; Rapid breathing (at slight movement); Essence-spirit fatigue; Tendency to sweat; Interrupted or slow, fine, weak pulse; Pale, enlarged tongue	Supplementing heart qi; nourishing the heart and quieting the spirit.	Heart-Nourishing Decoction	PC-3 BL-15 PC-6
Heart Yang Vacuity	Shortness of breath; Interrupted pulses; Dull grey or cyan-purple complexion; Frigidity of limbs; Dull, pale tongue; Yang vacuity cold signs such as: water swelling, cold sweating; Heart qi vacuity signs	Warming and freeing heart yang; nourishing the heart and quieting the spirit; in serious cases, salvaging yang and securing against desertion.	Honeyed-Liquorice Decoction; Ginseng and Aconite Decoction; Ginseng, Aconite, Dragon Bone and Oystershell Decoction.	PC-6 GV-14‡ GV-4‡

Table 9-1 page 2

Identification and Treatment of Heart Disease Patterns

Pattern Type	Principal Signs	Treatment Method	Commonly Used Formulae	Acupoints
Heart Blood Vacuity	Dizziness Palpitations Racing of the heart Insomnia Poor memory Pale tongue Forceless, fine pulse Lusterless complexion	Supplementing the blood, boosting qi; nourishing the heart and quieting the spirit.	Angelica Splenic Decoction	PC-6 SP-6 HT-7
Heart Yin Vacuity	Dizziness Palpitations Racing of the heart Insomnia Upbearing fire-flush Restlessness Fever in the five hearts Night sweating *Usually:* Fine, rapid pulse Red tongue Palpitations Racing of the heart Shortness of breath Interrupted pulse	Enriching yin; quieting the heart and spirit	Celestial Emperor Heart-Supplementing Elixir	KI-3 HT-7 SP-6

251

Table 9-1 page 3

Identification and Treatment of Heart Disease Patterns

Pattern Type	Principal Signs	Treatment Method	Commonly Used Formulae	Acupoints
Upflaming of Heart Fire	Cracked tongue Restlessness Red tongue tip In breakdown of cardiorenal interaction there may be: insomnia, upbearing fire, furless red tongue, and a fast, fine pulse Heart heat spreading to the small intestine is characterized by: painful strangury with dark-colored urine	Draining heart fire Breakdown of cardiorenal interaction is treated by enriching yin and downbearing fire	Heart-Draining Decoction Coptis and Ass-hide Glue Decoction	PC-7 HT-5 SP-9 KI-3 ST-39 HT-6
Cardiac Obturation	Stifling oppression and dull pain in the precordial region Paroxysms characterized by angina pectoris, cyan-purple complexion, cold sweat Faint, fine pulse verging on expiry	Perfusing heart yang Quickening the blood and transforming stasis Transforming turbidity with pungent aromatics	Trichosanthes, Allium and Pinellia Decoction Portal-Opening, Blood-Quickening Decoction Liquid Styrax Pills	HT-8 SP-4 PC-6 CV-17

Table 9-2

Identification and Treatment of Lung Disease Patterns

Pattern Type	*Principal Signs*		*Treatment Method*	*Commonly Used Formulae*	*Acupoints*
Non-Diffusion of Lung Qi	Cough and rapid breathing	Usually occurs in acute paroxysms or is accompanied by exogenous contraction exterior patterns. Dyspnea occurs when pathogenic heat or cold phlegm congests the lung.	Diffusing the lung with pungent dissipators	Defiant Three Decoction	LU-1 BL-13 LU-7 CV-17
Impaired Depurative Downbearing of Lung Qi		Usually because of long-lingering pathogens. There is generally no exterior pattern.	Depurating and downbearing lung qi	Lung-Draining Powder Perilla Fruit Qi-Downbearing Decoction	LU-7 KI-6 CV-22 LU-9
Lung Qi Vacuity		Shortness of breath Thin, clear phlegm-drool Low voice and weak enunciation Pale tongue Vacuous, weak pulse	Supplementing yang qi	Lung-Supplementing Decoction	BL-13 BL-12 LU-9
Lung Yin Vacuity		Dry cough Hoarse voice Dry mouth and pharynx Night sweating Emaciation Flushed cheeks Tidal fevers	Enriching yin and moistening the lung	Lily-Bulb Metal-Securing Decoction	LU-10 TB-2 KI-7

Table 9-3 page 1

Identification of Splenic Disease Patterns

Pattern Type	Principal Signs	Treatment Method	Commonly Used Formulae	Acupoints
Spleen Qi Vacuity	Lusterless complexion Diarrhea or thin stool Abdominal discomfort Soggy pulse Fatigue Lack of strength Pale tongue	Fortifying the spleen and boosting qi	Four Nobles Decoction	SP-6‡ BL-20‡ ST-36‡
Devitalization of Splenic Yang	Drained white complexion Abdominal pain relieved by warmth or pressure Clear-food diarrhea Deep pulse	Warming yang and reinforcing movement	Aconite Center-Rectifying Decoction	SP-6‡ BL-20‡ GV-4‡
Center Qi Fall	Emaciation Sagging and distention of the abdomen Bloating after eating Soggy pulse	Fortifying the spleen Upbearing yang and boosting qi	Center-Rectifying Pills Center-Supplementing Qi-Boosting Decoction	GV-20 CV-6‡ CV-4‡

All three patterns are forms of splenic transformation failure.

Table 9-3 page 2

Identification of Stomach and Spleen Disease Patterns

Pattern Type	Principal Signs	Treatment Method	Commonly Used Formulae	Acupoints
Blood Management Failure	Hemorrhage (mainly hemafecia and metrorrhagha) occurring with: somber white or withered yellow complexion lack of strength shortness of breath pale tongue fine, soggy pulse	Boosting the qi and containing the blood Warming the spleen	Angelica Splenic Decoction Yellow Earth Decoction	SP-1 LV-1 SP-6‡ BL-17‡ BL-20‡
Gastric Qi Vacuity Cold	Ventral pain relieved by pressure and eating	Fortifying the center and warming the stomach	Minor Center-Fortifying Decoction	ST-36‡ CV-12‡ CV-4‡
Stomach Heat	Painful swelling of gums Dental *xuan* and bleeding gums Hyperpepsia with rapid hungering or burning sensation in venter Red tongue Halitosis Constipation	Clearing the stomach and draining fire	Stomach-Clearing Powder Jade Lady Decoction	ST-44 CV-13 BL-21 ST-41 ST-45
Insufficiency of Stomach Yin	Red mirror tongue Dry mouth No thought of food or drink Vacuity glomus of the venter, retching	Nourishing stomach yin	Ophiopogon Decoction Stomach-Nourishing Decoction	ST-36 HT-6 ST-25 TB-6 CV-12

Table 9-3 page 3

Identification of Stomach Disease Patterns

Pattern Type	Principal Signs	Treatment Method	Commonly Used Formulae	Acupoints
Stomach Cold	Pale tongue	Warming the stomach and downbearing counterflow	Evodia Decoction Clove and Persimmon Decoction	CV-6 ST-36‡ CV-12‡
Stomach Heat	Red tongue Dry mouth Constipation	Draining fire and downbearing counterflow	Coptis and Evodia Pills	CV-13 PC-6 ST-44
Phlegm Turbidity	Nausea, Vomiting, Eructation, or Hiccough — Repeated vomiting Turbid, slimy tongue fur	Transforming phlegm and repelling turbidity	Minor Pinellia Decoction with Poria Jade Axis Elixir	CV-12 SP-4‡ ST-40‡
Qi Stagnation	Thoracic glomus Abdominal pain, often associated with essence-spirit factors	Precipitating qi and downbearing counterflow	Inula and Hematite Decoction	PC-6 CV-12 ST-44

All four patterns are associated with counterflow ascent of stomach qi.

Table 9-4 page 1

Identification and Treatment of Liver Disease Patterns

Pattern Type	Principal Signs	Treatment Method	Commonly Used Formulae	Acupoints
General Binding Depression of Liver Qi	Essence-spirit depression Painful distention of lateral costal region Wiry pulse	Coursing the liver and rectifying qi	Bupleurum Liver-Coursing Decoction	LV-3 LV-2 GB-34 GB-40
Invasion of the Stomach by Liver Qi	Ventral pain Eructation Acid upflow Nausea Vomiting	Coursing the liver and harmonizing the stomach	Coptis and Evodia Pills	ST-36 LV-3 CV-12 PC-6
Hepatosplenic Disharmony	Abdominal pain Diarrhea, exacerbated by emotional factors	Hepatosplenic harmonization	Pain and Diarrhea Formula	LI-4 SP-4 BL-20 SP-6

All three patterns are forms of binding depression of liver qi.

Table 9-4 page 2

Identification and Treatment of Liver Disease Patterns

Pattern Type	Principal Signs	Treatment Method	Commonly Used Formulae	Acupoints
Plumstone Globus	Sensation of lump in the throat that can be neither swallowed nor brought-up	Downbearing qi and transforming phlegm	Four-Seven Decoction	CV-22 LI-4
Struma	Softer lumps either side of the throat that move up and down when swallowing	Rectifying qi and transforming phlegm Dispersing struma	Sargassium Jade Teapot Decoction	LI-11 CV-22 ST-6 TB-3
Disorders of the Governing and Penetrating Vessels	Irregular menses Painful distention of the breasts Breast lumps	Regulating the governing and penetrating vessels	Free Wanderer Powder	SP-4 SP-16 CV-6 CV-4

All three patterns are forms of binding depression of liver qi.

Table 9-4 page 3

Identification and Treatment of Liver Disease Patterns

Pattern Type	Principal Signs	Treatment Method	Commonly Used Formulae	Acupoints
Upflaming of Liver Fire	Rashness Impatience Anger Headache Red complexion Ocular rubor Dry mouth Sudden tinnitus or deafness Fecal block Rapid wiry pulse Rough yellow tongue fur	Clearing the liver and draining fire	Gentian Liver-Draining Decoction	LV-3 LV-2 ST-36 SP-6
Ascendant Hyperactivity of Liver Yang	Dizziness Insomnia Palpitations Pain in the lumbar region Limp legs Wiry pulse Red tongue Rapid, fine pulse	Enriching yin and calming the liver	Gastrodia and Uncaria Cool Decoction Lycium, Chrysanthemum and Rehmannia Pills	LV-3 TB-3 ST-36 SP-6 KI-3

Table 9-4 page 4

Identification and Treatment of Liver Disease Patterns

Pattern Type	Principal Signs	Treatment Method	Commonly Used Formulae	Acupoints
Liver Wind	Rigidity of the neck Tremor of the eyes, face lips, tongue, and hands Inhibited speech Tingling numbness of the limbs Jerking sinews In serious cases: convulsive spasms and tetanic inversion	Calming the liver and extinguishing wind Nurturing yin and subduing yang	Antelope Horn Decoction Great Wind-Stabilizing Pills	LV-3 SI-19 GV-20 GV-14 GB-20 BL-18
Liver Blood Vacuity	Dizziness Flowery vision Scant menstrual flow Amenorrhea Insomnia Excessive dreaming Tingling numbness of the limbs Inhibited sinew-vascular movement	Nourishing liver blood Enriching kidney yin	Liver-Supplementing Decoction Four Agents Decoction Lycium, Chrysanthemum and Rehmannia Pills Black Free-Wanderer Powder	SP-10 SP-6 LV-3 KI-3

Table 9-5 page 1

Identification and Treatment of Kidney Disease Patterns

Pattern Type	Principal Signs	Treatment Method	Commonly Used Formulae	Acupoints
Kidney Yin Vacuity	(see left)	Enriching the kidney and nourishing yin	Rehmannia Six Pills	KI-3, BL-47, TB-3
Cardiorenal Yin Vacuity	Palpitations, Insomnia, Excessive dreaming, Poor memory (all relatively pronounced)	Enriching the kidney and nourishing the heart	Celestial Emperor Heart-Supplementing Elixir	HT-7, KI-3, PC-7
Hepatorenal Yin Vacuity	Pronounced dizziness, Headache, Flowery vision, Tinnitus	Enriching the kidney and calming the liver	Lycium, Chrysanthemum and Rehmannia Pills	BL-23, KI-3, LV-3, BL-47
Pulmorenal Yin Vacuity	Dry cough, Tidal fever, Night sweating (all relatively pronounced)	Enriching the kidney and nourishing the lung	Lily-Bulb Metal-Securing Decoction	KI-3, KI-6, KI-7, LU-9

Principal signs for Kidney Yin Vacuity (see left column): Dizziness, Tinnitus, Dry throat and lips, Steady fever, Pain in the lumbar region, Seminal emmission, Fine, rapid pulse, Red tongue

Table 9-5 page 2

Identification and Treatment of Kidney Disease Patterns

Pattern Type	Principal Signs	Treatment Method	Commonly Used Formulae	Acupoints
Kidney Yang Vacuity	Dizziness Tinnitus Frigidity of the limbs Cold form Spiritual fatigue Drained white complexion Painful, limp knees, lumbar region Weak, soggy pulse Pale, fat tongue Impotence Seminal efflux Sterility Polyuria and urinary frequency or nocturia	Warming the kidney and restoring yang	Aconite and Cinnamon Eight Pills	GV-4‡ CV-4‡ BL-23‡ ST-36‡
Splenorenal Yang Vacuity	Persistent diarrhea or fifth-watch diarrhea	Warming and supplementing the spleen and kidney	Four Divinity Pills	ST-36‡ BL-20‡ BL-23‡ SP-6‡ GV-4‡
Qi-Absorption Failure	Dyspnea with distressed, rapid breathing Rapid breathing (at the slightest movement)	Warming the kidney and promoting qi absorption	Black Tin Elixir Ginseng and Gecko Powder	CV-22 CV-4 CV-17
Cardiorenal Yang Debilitation	Water swelling Palpitations Dyspnea with rapid breathing Frigid limbs	Salvaging yang and securing against desertion	Ginseng and Aconite Decoction	BL-15 HT-7 PC-6

Table 9-5 *page 3*

Identification and Treatment of Kidney Disease Patterns

Pattern Type	Principal Signs	Treatment Method	Commonly Used Formulae	Acupoints
Yang Vacuity Water Flood	Oliguria Water swelling Pale, fat tongue Water-rheum intimidating the heart and shooting into the lung, characterized by palpitations and rapid breathing	Warming Yang and disinhibiting water	True Warrior Decoction	GV-4 BL-23 CV-4 SP-9 CV-9
Insufficiency of Kidney Essence	Diminished intellection Deficient reproductive function Hair loss; losening of the teeth poor development in children soft bones, delayed closure of the fontanels	Supplementing the kidney and boosting essence	Life-Saver Kidney Qi Pills Kidney Pills	GV-4 KI-3 BL-23 CV-4 CV-6
Insecurity of Kidney Qi	Enuresis Polyuria Urinary frequency or incontinence Seminal emission or seminal efflux Low back pain Limp knees	Securing the kidney and astringing essence	Golden Lock Essence-Securing Pills Stream-Reducing Pills Ootheca Mantidis Powder	GV-4 KI-3 BL-23 CV-4 CV-6

Chapter 10
Pathogen Pattern Identification

Pathogen pattern identification involves determining what pathogen is the cause of a particular disease, using the information gathered through the four examinations. This process falls within the scope of identifying the pattern and determining the cause. Once the pathogen has been determined, appropriate treatment may be prescribed to achieve its elimination. Thus, when the wind pathogen is identified, wind-dispelling treatment is prescribed, and when the heat pathogen is identified, heat-clearing treatment may be prescribed, etc. This process is known as ascertaining the disease factor and prescribing appropriate treatment.

The pathogen represents only one aspect of a disease, and does not explain its whole etiology. For example, the wind pathogen may cause coughing, but may also cause a severe headache. Although the two conditions are both attributable to the presence of the wind pathogen, they have different pathomechanisms, and are therefore treated in different ways. Wind cough is explained by non-diffusion of lung qi due to invasion of the lung by the wind pathogen, and is treated by dissipating wind and diffusing the lung. Headache, by contrast, is explained by the pathogen rising to the vertex of the head where it inhibits flow through the connecting channels, and its treatment is based on dispelling wind. Pathogen pattern identification provides inadequate data for a complete diagnosis, and it is only by correlating the information derived from the other methods of pattern identification that a sufficiently clear picture of the disease can be established and treatment be prescribed.

Although disease factors include the six environmental excesses, affect damage (damage due to excesses of one or more of the seven affects), dietary irregularities, sexual intemperance, taxation fatigue, trauma, parasites, phlegm, and static blood, pathogen pattern identification involves identification of substantial pathogens only — the six environmental excesses, dietary irregularities, phlegm, and blood stasis. These pathogens are dealt with in this chapter, with the exception of static blood, discussed in Chapter 8.

Wind Disease Patterns

Wind is swift and changeable, capable of rapid movement and frequent change, and often invades the body in conjunction with other pathogens. It is said, "Wind is the chief of the hundred diseases." It bears the following characteristics:

Wind is light and buoyant by nature, and most easily invades the upper body and the muscular exterior. It easily affects the head and face, causing headache, mental dizziness, and swelling and redness of the face and eyes. Often, wind will initially invade the lung, presenting such symptoms as nasal congestion, sore pharynx, and cough. Usually, wind enters the body through the exterior, causing symptoms such as aversion to wind, fever, and floating pulse.

Wind is swift and changeable by nature. Thus wind diseases are characterized by changeability and symptoms of unfixed location. Migratory pain in the muscles and joints, itching of unfixed location, and sudden, remittent papular outthrusts are commonly indicative of the presence of wind.

Wind is blusterous, violent, and impetuous, and can cause severe damage within a short space of time. The sudden appearance of symptoms such as wry mouth and eyes, trismus, rigidity of the limbs, opisthotonos, and convulsive spasm of the limbs generally indicates wind.

Distinction is made between exogenous and endogenous wind. Exogenous wind denotes the wind pathogen that enters the body from outside; endogenous wind refers to wind that arises from within the body. Excessive upstirring of liver yang transforming into wind, characterized by mental and visual dizziness, tremor, and convulsive spasms, and extreme heat engendering wind, characterized by tetanic inversion and convulsive spasm in the limbs, are both forms of endogenous wind. Endogenous wind is closely associated with the liver. The phrase, "wind patterns characterized by shaking and visual dizziness are associated with the liver" mainly refers to this. Finally, blood vacuity engendering wind, characterized by itchy skin, also falls with the scope of endogenous wind. Identification and treatment of wind patterns are also discussed in Chapters 2, 9, and 11.

Exogenous Wind Contractions

Exogenous wind enters the body through the muscular exterior. Contraction of exogenous wind is invariably characterized by exterior signs such as fever, aversion to wind, and headache. There may also be signs of non-diffusion of lung qi, such as cough, itchy throat, expectoration of phlegm, and, in serious cases, rapid breathing. The pulse is usually floating, and may also be rapid. Conditions characterized by pronounced exterior signs are termed wind pathogen assault on the exterior. Patterns in which respiratory tract signs are prominent are known as fettering of the lung by the wind pathogen. The terms wind-heat and wind-cold denote commonly occurring pathogen combinations and the diseases they effect.

Wind-cold

Pattern identification

Headache, generalized pain, and aversion to wind are pronounced. There may also be absence of sweating; cough; clear, thin phlegm; absence of thirst; white, glossy tongue fur; and a tight, floating pulse.

Wind-cold is characterized by the presence of wind signs and pronounced cold signs, and therefore presents as an exterior cold pattern. (See Chapter 7, "Eight-Parameter Pattern Identification".)

Treatment

Drug therapy

The methods of treatment applicable to wind-cold are resolving the exterior with warm, pungent agents, dissipating wind-cold, and diffusing lung qi. The first two methods make use of warm, pungent agents such as:

Warm, Pungent Exterior Resolvents	
Herba Schizonepetae	jīng jiè
Rhizoma et Radix Notopterygii	qiāng huó
Radix Ledebouriellae	fáng fēng
Folium Perillae	sū yè
Herba Ephedrae	má huáng
Ramulus Cinnamomi	guì zhī

Lung diffusers include:

Lung Diffusers	
Herba Ephedrae	má huáng
Semen Pruni Armeniacae	xìng rén
Radix Peucedani	qián hú
Radix Platycodi	jié gěng
Bulbus Fritillariae Thunbergii	xiàng bèi mǔ

Schizonepeta and Ledebouriella Detoxifying Powder *(jīng fáng bài dú sǎn)* and its variants treat patterns exhibiting prominent signs such as headache, generalized pain, fever, and aversion to wind. Ephedra Decoction *(má-huáng tāng)* and its variants treat patterns with pronounced symptoms of cough, rapid breathing, and absence of sweating. Where the headache is particularly severe, Tea-Blended Ligusticum Powder *(chūan-xiōng chá tiáo sǎn)* may be prescribed.

Acumoxatherapy

Wind-cold diseases are commonly treated with GB-20‡, GV-16, BL-12‡, and TB-5, all of which help resolve the exterior and dissipate wind and cold. LU-7 and LU-9 may be added to diffuse lung qi. Wind-cold headache is treated with LI-4, M-HN-9 *(tai-yang)*, and M-HN-3 *(yin-tang)*, combined with some of the previously mentioned points, particularly GB-20. LI-4 is often combined with KI-7 to promote diaphoresis, if necessary. Points used to treat wind-cold nasal congestion include BL-7 and LI-20. Other points that may be used to treat wind-cold exterior diseases include BL-13‡, SI-3, BL-10‡, and SP-6‡, applied according to the presenting symptoms.

Wind-heat

Pattern identification

Heat signs such as cough, sticky or yellow phlegm, sore pharynx or red, swollen tonsils, dry mouth, red tongue, and a rapid, floating pulse are pronounced. At the same time, exterior signs such as fever, aversion to wind, headache, absence of sweating, or impeded sweating may be observed. Most wind-heat diseases present as exterior heat patterns. (See Chapter 7, "Eight-Parameter Pattern Identification".)

Treatment

Drug therapy

Methods of treatment include resolving the exterior with cool, pungent agents, dissipating wind-heat, and diffusing lung qi. The first two methods use cooling, pungent agents such as:

Cool, Pungent Exterior Resolvents	
Herba Menthae	bò hé
Folium Mori	sāng yè
Fructus Arctii	niú bàng zǐ
Semen Sojae Praeparatum	dòu shǐ

To promote lung qi diffusion, the agents discussed under "wind-cold" may be used, in addition to heat-clearing detoxicants such as:

Heat Clearers	
Flos Lonicerae	yín huā
Fructus Forsythiae	lián qiào
Herba et Radix Taraxaci	pú gōng yīng
Radix Isatidis	bǎn lán gēn
Folium Ta Ch'ing Yeh	dà qīng yè

Lonicera and Forsythia Powder *(yín qiào sǎn)* and variants are used for severe wind-heat contractions, while Mulberry and Chrysanthemum Cool Decoction *(sāng jú yǐn)* and variants are used for milder contractions.

Acumoxatherapy

GV-20 and LV-4 are among the major points used to expel wind and resolve the exterior. LU-5 clears heat from the upper burner, and GV-14, the point of intersection of all the yang channels of the body, may also be needled or bled to drain heat. LU-7 is a major point for diffusing lung qi. Other points useful in treatment of exterior wind-heat diseases include SI-3, LI-10, LI-11, and TB-5.

Wind-cold and wind-heat patterns largely correspond to diseases referred to in Western medicine as colds, influenza, and upper respiratory tract infections, though wind-heat sometimes corresponds to tonsilitis and pneumonia as well. Other forms of wind-heat have specific names in Chinese medicine, such as wind-fire ocular rubor (acute conjunctivitis) and wind-fire toothache (acute gingivitis). These may be treated by the above methods. Most conditions characterized by redness and swelling of head and face are wind-heat conditions, and may be treated with formulae that dissipate wind, clear heat, and detoxify, such as the well-known Universal Salvation Detoxifying Cool Decoction *(pǔ jì xiāo dú yǐn)* which treats balloon-head scourge (corresponding to diseases including facial erysipelas in Western medicine) and toad-head scourge (corresponding to diseases including parotitis).

Acumoxatherapy

Wind-fire ocular rubor is treated with points known to have a special effect on the eyes, such as GB-42, LI-2, and GB-15, combined with local points such as BL-1, BL-2, and GB-1. Wind-heat dispersing points, such as LI-4 and GB-20, are often added.

A sample formula for treating wind-fire toothache might include LI-4 and TB-5, both of which clear wind-heat. LI-4 is particularly appropriate because it belongs to the hand yang ming large intestine channel, which encircles the teeth and gums. Local points, such as ST-6 and CV-24, could also be added.

Redness and swelling in the head area can be treated through points that disperse heat in the upper burner, such as LI-11 and GV-14 (bleed), combined with points that disperse fire, such as LI-2 and ST-41. Other points are added according to the symptoms: BL-54 (bleed) to cool the blood, SP-9 to drain heat by disinhibiting urine, and local points such as GV-20 (bleed), GB-20, and M-HN-9 *(tai-yang)* (bleed) to dissipate repletion in the head.

Wind pathogen invasion of the channels

Pattern identification

When the wind pathogen invades the channels and sinews, causing obstruction of the channels and impeded movement of the sinews, three outcomes are possible. One would be localized paralysis or palsy, wryness of the mouth and eyes, or facial paralysis. A second outcome would be rigidity of the neck and back, trismus, and convulsive spasm of the limbs. These symptoms are what is referred to by the word "rigidity" in the phrase, "Fulminant rigidity is associated with wind." The classical example of such pathologies is tetanus. The third outcome would be general or localized muscular or articular pain, numbness, and impeded movement. Such conditions, classified under the general heading of obturation disease, are caused by a combination of the wind, cold, and damp pathogens. "When wind, cold, and damp pathogens concur and combine, they give rise to obturation disease." Patterns in which wind is most prominent are characterized by migratory symptoms.

Treatment

Drug therapy

Wind pathogen invasion of the channels is treated by the method of dispelling wind and freeing the connecting channels. However, drug therapy is used only as a complement to acupuncture, moxibustion, and massotherapy. Commonly used drugs include:

Wind-Dispelling and Connecting-Channel-Freeing Agents	
Rhizoma et Radix Notopterygii	*qiāng huó*
Radix Ledebouriellae	*fáng fēng*
Rhizoma Aconiti Coreani	*bái fù zǐ*
Scolopendra	*wú gōng*
Buthus	*quán xiē*
Lumbricus	*dì lóng*
Zaocys	*wū shāo shé*
Periostracum Cicadae	*chán yī*

Treatment of obturation patterns may also include wind-damp dispellants such as:

Wind-Damp Dispellants	
Ramulus Mori	*sāng zhī*
Radix Clematidis	*wēi líng xiān*
Herba Siegesbeckiae	*xī xiān cǎo*
Folium Clerodendri Trichotoni	*chòu wú tóng*
Herba Gentianae Macrophyllae	*qín jiāo*
Radix Tu Huo	*dú huó*
Radix Caraganae Sinicae	*jīn què gēn*
Caulis Piperis Kadsurae	*hǎi fēng téng*

Anti-Contracture Powder *(qiān zhèng sǎn)* is often used to treat facial paralysis; Five-Tigers-Chasing-The-Wind Decoction *(wǔ hǔ zhuī fēng sǎn)* is often used for tetanus.[1] Anti-Obturation Decoction *(juān bì tāng)* is commonly used to treat obturation patterns.

Acumoxatherapy

Acupuncture, moxibustion, and massotherapy form the basis of treatment of many forms of invasion of the channels by the wind pathogen. Local points are primarily employed to dispel wind; these are combined with distal points that either move the qi of the affected channels, or have a special relationship to the affected area.

Generalized, migratory muscular pain is treated with points such as GB-20, GV-16, and GV-26. Distal points affecting specific body areas include:

Neck: SI-3, TB-3, and GB-39.

Shoulders: ST-38, LI-4, and TB-4.

Knees: BL-23, BL-60, and GB-39.

Local points are often warmed with moxa to dissipate cold and move qi. Massotherapy, employing local and distant acupuncture points and special techniques, is frequently effective in dissipating wind in the channels.

In order to prescribe proper treatment when using acupuncture, moxibustion, or massotherapy to dispel wind from the channels, particular attention must be paid to determining the channel or channels affected.

Many skin diseases may be caused by the wind pathogen. These are characterized by severe itching, and periodic papular outthrusts of unfixed location. Thus, the *Essential Prescriptions of the Golden Coffer* states, "Wind qi {the wind pathogen} striking the channels causes generalized itching and dormant papules." Such diseases occur as either wind-cold or wind-heat patterns. Wind-cold skin eruptions are whitish in color and are brought on by exposure to cold. Wind-heat skin eruptions are characterized by a slight reddening, and are precipitated by heat. Treatment centers on dispelling wind. Wind-cold is treated with warm-natured wind dissipators such as:

Warm-Natured Wind Dissipators	
Herba Schizonepetae	*jīng jiè*
Radix Ledebouriellae	*fáng fēng*
Rhizoma et Radix Notopterygii	*qiāng huó*

Wind-heat contractions are treated with cool-natured wind dissipators such as:

Cool-Natured Wind Dissipators	
Folium Mori	*sāng yè*
Flos Chrysanthemi	*jú huā*
Herba Menthae	*bò hé*
Periostracum Cicadae	*chán yī*
Herba Lemnae	*fú píng*

Wind pathogen skin diseases are mostly dry in nature, and are thus classically represented by urticaria. Complication by damp-heat gives rise to the additional presence of vesicles, pustules, erosion, and serous discharge. In such cases admixture of damp disinhibitors and heat-clearing detoxicants is called for. Senile blood vacuity may also lead to dry, rough skin and itching. This is known as blood vacuity engendering wind or dry blood engendering wind. These conditions are generally treated by dispelling wind and nourishing the blood.

Wind-numbness (leprosy) is also caused by the wind pathogen. When intractable and highly contagious, it is called "great wind disease" or "pestilential wind." It is treated by dispelling wind and resolving toxins, using agents such as the following:

Wind-Dispelling and Toxin-Resolving Agents	
Semen Hydnocarpi	*dà fēng zǐ*
Fructus Xanthii	*cāng ěr zǐ*
Agkistrodon	*fù shé*

Acumoxatherapy

Wind-cold skin diseases are treated by dispersing wind and cold from the exterior. Useful points include LI-4, LI-11‡, LI-10‡, BL-12‡, and GB-31‡.

Treatment of wind-heat skin diseases emphasizes points such as LI-11, LI-4, and LI-10, which dispel wind-heat from the hand yang ming large intestine channel. The capillaries surrounding BL-54 may be bled, and SP-10, PC-3, PC-7, and PC-8 may be needled to cool blood heat. For damp-heat skin diseases, add TB-10 and SP-9 to dissipate dampness.

Lung channel points, and the back-associated point of the lung, BL-13, are often chosen because of the lung's relationship to the surface skin. LU-10 and LU-7 are among the points commonly used. The seven-star or plum blossom needle is sometimes used at the site of morbidity to cause a small amount of bleeding to release local heat, or at points such as SP-10, to release the heat from the blood.

Identification and treatment of wind diseases

Wind pathogen characteristics

It is important to understand the characteristics of the wind pathogen. The respiratory tract symptoms associated with exogenous wind diseases are explained by the lightness and buoyancy of wind and the ease with which it assails the upper body and the muscular exterior. The migratory pain associated with obturation patterns in which wind signs are prominent is understood in the sense of wind being "swift and a changeable." This characteristic of wind also explains why wind-induced skin diseases are associated with severe itching.

Wind is "the chief of the hundred diseases," and commonly occurs in conjunction with other pathogens. Exogenous wind contractions and wind-induced skin diseases both occur in the forms of wind-heat and wind-cold. Obturation patterns are caused by a combination of the wind, cold, and damp pathogens.

Distinguishing exogenous and endogenous wind

Exogenous and endogenous wind patterns may be characterized by such symptoms as convulsive spasm or paralysis of the limbs, and wry mouth and eyes. Careful analysis of other symptoms is required to identify the exact nature of the pathogen. Exogenous wind is generally the result of contraction of wind-cold or trauma. Facial paralysis, obturation patterns, and tetanus are all attributable to contraction of exogenous wind, and are explained by the presence of the pathogen in the channels. Endogenous wind either occurs in chronic diseases (endogenous damage and miscellaneous diseases) or as a consequence of high fever in febrile diseases.

Some differences of symptoms are associated with the two forms of wind. Transformation of liver yang into wind, which is a classical example of endogenous wind, is associated with dizziness, shaking of the head, and tremor. It is generally attributed to yin humor depletion leaving the upbearing of yang unchecked. Extreme heat engendering wind is associated with extreme heat signs. Blood vacuity or dry blood engendering wind is associated with a general desiccation of blood and liquid.

Drug therapy

Exogenous and endogenous wind are treated in different ways. Exogenous wind is treated by dissipation (including coursing and dispelling). Endogenous wind is "extinguished" by calming the liver, clearing fire, nourishing the blood, and enriching yin. Tetany settlers may be used to treat both exogenous and endogenous wind:

Tetany Settlers	
Buthus	*quán xiē*
Scolopendra	*wú gōng*
Bombyx Batryticatus	*jiāng cán*
Lumbricus	*dì lóng*
Ramulus et Uncus Uncariae	*gōu téng*

For further review, see Table 10-1.

Cold Disease Patterns

Distinction is made between exogenous and endogenous cold. Exogenous cold is the result of catching cold or drinking cold beverages. Endogenous cold arises from debilitation of yang qi that warms the body. This is known as "cold arising from within." However, exogenous and endogenous cold are also mutually conducive. Individuals with yang vacuities have lowered resistance to exogenous cold, and easily contract this pathogen. Exogenous cold is yin in nature, and on entering the body may easily damage yang qi, giving rise to endogenous cold. Exogenous and endogenous cold share the following characteristics:

Cold signs

Generalized cold signs include cold form, aversion to cold, lack of warmth in the limbs, a dull, stagnant-looking, somber white complexion, desire for warmth, slow and/or tight pulse, and a pale tongue with glossy white fur. Localized symptoms include subjective sensations of cold in the abdomen, and cold and pain in the joints.

"When cold prevails there is pain."

Severe pain relieved by warmth may be experienced in the affected parts of the body. The cold pathogen is "congealing" by nature, and when settling in the body may easily effect qi stagnation and blood stasis. Since "stoppage gives rise to pain," pain is associated with cold patterns.

"Any disease characterized by thin, clear, frigid fluids is associated with cold."

Long micturition with clear urine, watery diarrhea containing undigested food, and clear, thin phlegm all indicate the presence of a cold pathogen.

Cold often invades the body in conjunction with the wind or damp pathogens. These combinations are wind-cold and cold-damp patterns. Commonly observed cold pathogen patterns are described below.

Exogenous cold contraction

Contraction of exogenous cold is often referred to as cold damage. The cold pathogen is most commonly observed in wind-cold combinations and is thus discussed in detail in the section, "Exogenous Wind Contractions."

Cold obturation

Cold obturation is a commonly observed obturation pattern. "When the wind, cold, and damp pathogens concur and combine, they give rise to obturation." Patterns in which the cold pathogen is prominent are known as cold obturation patterns.

Pattern identification

"When cold prevails there is pain." Severe articular and muscular pain is a principal characteristic of cold pathogen diseases; hence cold obturation patterns are sometimes referred to as dolorous obturation. Pain is often attended by hypertonicity and stiffness inhibiting normal movement. This is in keeping with the observation of the *Inner Canon*, "Cold is associated with contracture and tautness."

Treatment

Drug therapy

Cold obturation is treated by warming the channels and dissipating cold. Drug therapy makes use of potent hot, pungent agents that free the channels, enabling the cold to dissipate. These include:

Potent Hot, Pungent Agents	
Radix Aconiti Wu T'ou	*wū tóu*
Radix Aconiti Fu Tzu	*fù zǐ*
Herba Ephedrae	*má huáng*
Ramulus Cinnamomi	*guì zhī*
Herba Asari	*xì xīn*

Their action can be enhanced by the admixture of blood and qi supplementers. A formula possessing this dual action is Wu T'ou Aconite Decoction *(wū-tóu tāng)*.

Acumoxatherapy

Cold obturation is treated by acupuncture and moxibustion at local and distal points to warm the channels and dissipate cold. Commonly used local points are listed below:

Wrist: LI-5‡, TB-4‡, SI-4‡, PC-7‡, and SI-5‡.

Ankle: GB-40‡, SP-5‡, ST-41‡, and BL-60‡.

Hip: GB-31‡, GB-30‡, GB-29‡, and BL-49‡.

Knee: ST-36‡, SP-9‡, GB-34‡, ST-35‡, and GB-33‡.

Elbow: LI-11‡, LU-5‡, LI-10‡, TB-10‡, and HT-3‡.

Shoulder: LI-15‡, TB-14‡, and SI-9‡.

Fingers: M-UE-22 *(ba-xie)*, LU-5‡, SI-3‡, and LI-3‡.

Toes: M-LE-8 *(ba-feng)*, SP-4‡, KI-2‡, and BL-65‡.

Generalized aching: LI-4, GB-20, SI-3‡, and BL-62‡.

Enduring conditions may be aided with moxibustion at BL-23.

Cold pain

Pattern identification

By convention, the term "cold pain" generally refers to acute pain in the abdomen caused by catching cold or ingesting cold food or beverages. The pain is exacerbated by exposure to cold and relieved by warmth. There may be vomiting of clear fluid. The stool may be clear and thin, or there may be constipation. The pulse is usually wiry, tight, deep, and slow, and in severe cases, hidden. The tongue is pale or dark, while the fur is white and glossy.

Treatment

Drug therapy

Since cold pain is a result of the cold pathogen striking the spleen and stomach, the accent is placed on dispelling the pathogen. The basic method is therefore dissipating cold and relieving pain. Commonly used agents include:

Cold Pain Dissipators	
Cortex Cinnamomi	ròu guì
Fructus Evodiae	wú zhū yú
Rhizoma Zingiberis blast-fried	pāo jiāng
Rhizoma Alpiniae Officinari	liáng jiāng
Flos Caryophylli	dīng xiāng
Fructus Zanthoxyli Szechuanensis	chuān jiāo
Fructus Cubebae	bì chéng

A frequently used formula is Alpinia and Cyperus Pills *(liáng fù wán)*.

Acumoxatherapy

Cold pain may be treated by warming the center and the large intestine by moxibustion at the front-alarm and back-associated points of the large intestine, ST-25 and BL-25 respectively, and by moxibustion on salt or warming with a moxa stick at CV-8. ST-37‡ is the lower uniting point of the large intestine, and so affects both the stomach and large intestine. Other points commonly used in treatment of cold-induced abdominal pain include CV-10‡, CV-12‡, ST-36‡, and BL-20‡.

Cold diarrhea

Pattern identification

Essential Questions states, "Thin, clear, frigid fluids are associated with cold." Accordingly, cold diarrhea is characterized by clear, watery diarrhea, sometimes with undigested food in the stool. There is abdominal pain that is relieved both by pressure and heat. There is lack of warmth in the extremities, and the body temperature is low. The tongue fur is white, and the pulse either wiry and tight or deep and slow.

Treatment

Drug therapy

Cold diarrhea is treated by warming the center and fortifying the spleen to dissipate the cold pathogen. Commonly used agents include:

Center-Warming and Spleen-Fortifying Agents	
Radix Aconiti Fu Tzu	*fù zǐ*
Rhizoma Zingiberis blast-fried	*pāo jiāng*
Cortex Cinnamomi	*ròu guì*
Rhizoma Atractylodis Macrocephalae	*bái zhú*
Herba Polygoni Hydropiperis	*là liǎo*

This pattern is commonly treated with Center-Rectifying Pills *(lǐ zhōng wán)* and variants.

Acumoxatherapy

Diarrhea is treated by moxibustion on points such as BL-20, SP-4, and SP-6, all of which strengthen the spleen. CV-12‡, CV-6‡, and ST-36‡ warm the center, and ST-25‡ and BL-25‡ are also commonly used, because of their relation to the large intestine. Other points commonly added include LI-4, CV-4‡, and ST-22‡. If kidney yang is vacuous, points such as BL-23‡, GV-4, and GV-20‡ should be added.

Cold shan

Pattern identification

Classically, the term cold *shan* referred to all forms of cold abdominal pain, and particularly lower abdominal pain. In modern usage, it is equivalent to cold *shan* qi pain which refers to painful sagging of the testicles. The pain, which reaches up into the lower abdomen, is exacerbated by cold and relieved by warmth. The pulse associated with this condition is deep, wiry, and tight. The tongue fur is white and glossy. Cold *shan* qi pain is caused by cold qi stagnation in the liver channel. Other forms of *shan* qi pain are caused by damp-heat pouring into the liver channel or qi vacuity fall.

Treatment

Drug therapy

Cold *shan* is treated by the methods of warming the liver and dissipating cold, and rectifying qi and relieving pain. Commonly used drugs include:

Liver Warmers and Qi Rectifiers	
Fructus Evodiae	wú zhū yú
Fructus Foeniculi	xiǎo huí xiāng
Cortex Cinnamomi	ròu guì
Semen Citri	jú hé
Semen Trigonellae	hú lú bā
Radix Linderae	wū yào

Formulae include:

Cold Shan Formulae	
Liver-Warming Decoction	nuǎn gān jiān
T'ien T'ai Lindera Powder	tiān-tái-wū-yào sǎn

Acumoxatherapy

Points such as CV-4‡, CV-3‡, LV-2‡, LV-1‡, SP-6‡, are used to course and move the qi of the liver and conception channels, thus relieving pain. Moxibustion at CV-4 can warm yang and dissipate cold. KI-6 courses the lower burner and expels yin cold. ST-33‡ is a special point for cold *shan* pain. Local points such as ST-29 and ST-28‡ are also commonly used.

Identification and treatment of cold disease patterns

Cold pathogen characteristics

Although the cold pathogen may invade the body through the exterior, the interior, the channels, and the organs, all forms of cold patterns are characterized by generalized cold signs. Exogenous cold pathogen diseases, cold obturation, cold pain, cold diarrhea, and cold *shan* are all characterized by a tight, wiry, or slow pulse, pale tongue with moist, white fur, and varying degrees of cold form, aversion to cold, and pronounced lack of warmth in the extremities.

Combinations of cold with other pathogens

Exogenous cold commonly enters the body in combination with the wind pathogen. However, a combination of cold and damp pathogens may also invade the muscular exterior and damage the organs. Both cold obturation and cold diarrhea are examples of cold-damp patterns. Where cold appears in combination with damp, it is usually the prominent pathogen.

Transformation of the cold pathogen into heat

If the cold pathogen remains depressed in the body for extended periods, it may transform into heat. This may be observed in a wind-cold contraction of the common cold or influenza type; when fever and aversion to cold subside, the white, moist tongue fur becomes yellow and dry, and thirst develops where previously there was none. Wind-cold-damp obturation may similarly transform into heat obturation. Thus, in cold pathogen diseases, attention must always be paid to possible conversion into a heat pattern.

Exogenous and endogenous cold

Exogenous cold diseases may be caused by contraction of wind-cold (common cold or influenza) or of cold-damp, or by ingestion of excessively cold or raw food. Such diseases are characterized by exuberance of pathogenic qi, and are treated by dispelling the pathogen.

Drug therapy

Treatment involves the use of warm-natured, cold-dissipating agents such as:

Cold Dissipators	
Herba Ephedrae	*má huáng*
Ramulus Cinnamomi	*guì zhī*
Herba Asari	*xì xīn*
Fructus Evodiae	*wú zhū yú*
Rhizoma Zingiberis Recens	*shēng jiāng*

Endogenous cold is caused by debilitation of the body's yang qi, and is always characterized by vacuity signs. Treatment aims to restore the correct, and hence uses agents that warm and supplement yang qi. Formulae are selected that contain such agents as:

Yang Warmers	
Radix Aconiti Fu Tzu	*fù zǐ*
Cortex Cinnamomi	*ròu guì*
Rhizoma Zingiberis Exsiccatum	*gān jiāng*

Qi Boosters	
Radix Codonopsis Pilosulae	*dǎng shēn*
Radix Astragali	*huáng qí*
Radix Glycyrrhizae	*gān cǎo*
Rhizoma Atractylodis Macrocephalae	*bái zhú*

Acumoxatherapy

Exogenous cold diseases are treated with points such as GB-20‡, BL-12‡, LU-7, and LI-4, which dispel the pathogen and promote lung qi diffusion. Endogenous cold is treated by warming yang and dispersing cold, burning moxa on BL-23, GV-4, BL-20, CV-4, CV-12, etc.

Heat, Fire, and Summerheat Disease Patterns

Although heat does not figure among the six environmental excesses, it embraces both fire and summerheat inasmuch as they give rise to heat signs. Heat, fire, and summerheat differ in name but are of one essence. In clinical practice, the terms heat and fire are to some degree used interchangeably. A more important distinction to be made is that of exogenous and endogenous fire. Summerheat may be regarded as an exogenous heat pathogen that is seasonal in nature. For further elaboration on the meanings of heat, fire, and summerheat, see the Appendix, "Glossary of Terms."

Heat and fire bear the following characteristics:

Heat signs

Generalized heat signs include high fever, aversion to heat, restlessness, short micturition with dark-colored urine, red complexion, red tongue with yellow fur, and a rapid pulse. Localized signs include ocular rubor, a painful, red tongue with erosion and cracking, and red, swollen lesions.

Damage to fluids

Fire and heat may easily damage the fluids, causing dry tongue without liquid, thirst with desire for fluids, and dry, hard stool.

Frenetic blood heat

Fire and heat easily scorch the vessels, and give rise to frenetic blood movement. This is characterized by hemorrhage or maculopapular eruptions.

Exogenous fire is mostly caused by contraction of thermic heat pathogens, and by the wind, cold, damp, and dry pathogens transforming into fire. Exogenous fire, manifesting as repletion heat patterns, accounts for a large proportion of exogenous heat diseases and is dealt with in Chapter 11. In the field of miscellaneous disease, dispositional excesses (severe emotional disturbances), qi depression, hyperactivity of yang, as well as accumulation of phlegm, digestate, and static blood may all lead to endogenous fire, presenting as either vacuity or repletion heat. Although heat and fire may be caused by a wide variety of factors, the most important clinical distinction is between vacuity and repletion. For summerheat, distinction is made between summerheat-heat and summerheat-damp.

Repletion heat

Pattern identification

Repletion heat is characterized by pronounced heat signs such as red complexion, essence-spirit excitation, and agitation. In serious cases there may also be delirious speech and mania. Hence *Essential Questions* states, "Excessive mania and agitation are associated with fire." Signs such as red tongue, yellow tongue fur, strong, rapid, surging pulse, high fever, aversion to heat, palpable heat in the chest and abdomen, thirst with desire for cold fluids, and reddish or dark-colored urine commonly occur together. Other patterns include expectoration of thick, yellow phlegm; hemorrhage, and maculopapular eruptions. Some repletion heat patterns include hard stool or diarrhea characterized by sticky, slimy, foul-smelling stool. This form of diarrhea is referred to in the *Essential Questions:* "Fulminant downpour and lower-body distress are associated with heat."

Treatment

Drug therapy

Repletion heat is explained as heat resulting from yang exuberance, i.e., exuberance of pathogenic qi. It is treated by the methods of clearing heat (or fire) and draining heat (or fire). Commonly used heat (fire) clearers include:

Heat Clearers	
Radix Scutellariae	huáng qín
Rhizoma Coptidis	huáng lián
Rhizoma Anemarrhenae	zhī mǔ
Flos Lonicerae	yín huā
Fructus Forsythiae	lián qiào
Fructus Gardeniae	zhī zǐ
Radix Isatidis	bǎn lán gēn
Folium Ta Ch'ing Yeh	dà qīng yè
Herba Andrographis	chuān xīn lián

These are sometimes used in combination with heat (or fire) drainers such as:

Fire Drainers	
Rhizoma Rhei	(dà huáng)
Mirabilitum	(máng xiāo)

Coptis Detoxifying Decoction *(huáng-lián jiě dú tāng)* and its variants may be used to clear heat (or fire), and Heart-Draining Decoction *(xiè xīn tāng)* and its variants may be used to drain heat (or fire).

Acumoxatherapy

Selection of heat-draining points is dependent on the location of the heat pathogen. General points used to drain heat include GB-34, LI-11, LU-5, LU-10, HT-6, PC-8, GV-14, and ST-44. Repletion heat usually calls for strong needle stimulation, or letting of a few drops of blood at the point. Special points at the fingertips, M-UE-1 *(shi-xuan)*, are also bled in extreme cases.

Vacuity heat

Pattern identification

Vacuity heat is usually due to yin vacuity, i.e., insufficiency of yin humor. Signs include emaciation and dry throat and mouth. The tongue is red and fissured, with scant or peeling fur. The pulse is feeble, fine, and rapid. Signs of heat, which arises in the inner body as a result of the yin vacuity, include upbearing fire flush, steaming bone tidal fever, subjective feelings of heat in the inner body, restlessness, insomnia, and fever in the palms of the hands and soles of the feet.

Treatment

Drug therapy

Though heat signs are present in a vacuity heat condition, the pattern is at root one of vacuity and thus is treated primarily with yin enrichers and only secondarily with heat clearers. Commonly used agents include:

Vacuity Heat Clearers	
Radix Rehmanniae Cruda	*shēng dì*
Radix Scrophulariae	*xuán shēn*
Tuber Ophiopogonis	*mài dōng*
Herba Dendrobii	*shí hú*
Rhizoma Anemarrhenae	*zhī mǔ*
Cortex Phellodendri	*huáng bó*
Cortex Radicis Mu Tan	*mǔ dān pí*
Cortex Radicis Lycii	*dì gǔ pí*
Herba Artemisiae Apiaceae	*qīng hāo*

Great Yin Supplementation Pills *(dà bǔ yīn wán)* and their variants may be used to enrich yin and clear endogenous heat, while Two-A Decoction *(qīng-hāo biē-jiǎ tāng)* and its variants enrich yin and abate tidal fever.

Acumoxatherapy

KI-3 is the chief point used to supplement yin, and points such as LV-2, LV-3, ST-44, PC-8, HT-7, and LU-10 are commonly used to drain vacuity fire, depending on its location. TB-2 may be added for its moistening effect.

Summerheat-heat

Pattern identification

Summerheat-heat is caused by contraction of the exogenous summerheat pathogen and is thus seasonal in nature. It is characterized by pronounced heat signs such as high fever, thirst, oliguria, and restlessness. In serious cases there may be clouding of spirit and tetanic inversion. Other symptoms include either absence of sweating or profuse sweating, and a rapid, large, surging pulse. High fever poses the danger of damage to fluids and original qi, which is characterized by such symptoms as diminished qi, exhaustion, dry tongue fur, and a thin and rapid or large and vacuous pulse.

Treatment

Drug therapy

The method of treatment applied is that of clearing summerheat-heat. Commonly used agents include:

Summerheat Clearing Agents	
Gypsum	shí gāo
Rhizoma Anemarrhenae	zhī mǔ
Radix Glycyrrhizae	gān cǎo
Exocarpium Citrulli Vulgaris	xī guā cuì yī
Folium Bambusae Vivum	xiān zhú yè
Six-to-One Powder	liù yī sǎn
Rhizoma Coptidis	huáng lián

Where qi and yin are damaged, agents that may be added to boost qi and engender liquid include:

Qi Boosters and Liquid Engenderers	
Radix Adenophorae	shā shēn
Tuber Ophiopogonis	mài dōng
Herba Dendrobii	shí hú

Where clouding of the spirit occurs as a result of portal block, portal openers may be used. Formulae such as White Tiger Decoction *(bái hǔ tāng)* mainly treat patterns involving high fever, copious perspiration, thirst, and a large, rapid, surging pulse. Wang's Summerheat-Clearing Qi-Boosting Decoction *(wáng shì qīng shǔ yì qì tāng)* is mainly used for summerheat-heat with damage to qi and yin, characterized by copious perspiration, a dry, red tongue, thirst, restlessness and fever, and a large vacuous pulse. Purple Snow Elixir *(zǐ xuě dān)* is mainly used for patterns including high fever, coma, and tetanic inversion.

Acumoxatherapy

Mild summerheat is treated by applying strong needle stimulation at GV-14 to drain yang-heat. PC-7 and HT-7 are used to drain heart fire, and BL-54 and SP-10 are used to course and drain summerheat and cool the blood. In more severe cases, M-UE-1 *(shi-xuan)* and the capillaries around BL-54 are bled, while GV-20 and GV-26 may be needled to drain toxic summerheat and open the portals. Depending on the symptoms, PC-6, LI-4, LI-11, and SI-3 may also be used.

Summerheat-damp

Pattern identification

During hot, damp weather, the summerheat pathogen combines with the damp pathogen. Known as summerheat-damp, such diseases are characterized by enduring low fever, fatigued and cumbersome limbs, poor appetite, oppression in the chest, and nausea and vomiting. There is frequently thin-stool diarrhea, with evacuation bringing no relief from discomfort. Micturition is short with dark-colored urine. The pulse is soggy and the tongue fur thick and slimy.

Treatment

Drug therapy

Summerheat-damp is treated by clearing summerheat and transforming damp.

Damp Transformers	
Herba Agastaches	huò xiāng
Herba Eupatorii	pèi lán
Herba Artemisiae Apiaceae	qīng hāo
Six-to-One Powder	liù yī sǎn
Cortex Magnoliae	hòu pò
Rhizoma Atractylodis	cāng zhú
Sclerotium Poriae	fú líng
Rhizoma Pinelliae	bàn xià

These drugs are commonly used with Rhizoma Coptidis *(huáng lián)* and Radix Scutellariae *(huáng qín)*. Pronounced exterior patterns may be treated with formulae containing Herba Elsholtziae *(xiāng rú)* which clears summerheat and resolves the exterior. General summerheat-damp patterns may be treated with Artemisia Apiacea and Scutellaria GB-Clearing Decoction *(hāo qín qīng dǎn tāng)* and its variants. Summerheat-heat with pronounced exterior signs may be treated with Elsholtzia Cool Decoction *(xiāng-rú yǐn)* and its variants.

Acumoxatherapy

SP-9, ST-40, and SP-6 are all used to transform damp. GB-34 courses gallbladder damp-heat, and when combined with points such as BL-54 (bleed capillaries) and LI-11, can help clear summerheat. In extreme cases, GV-20, GV-26, and the twelve well-points at the extremities of the hand channels are added to free the portals and open blocks. Oppression in the chest and nausea are frequently treated with PC-6.

Identification and treatment of heat, fire, and summerheat disease patterns

Repletion fire, depressed fire, vacuity fire, and floating fire

Heat signs always accompany, but do not necessarily indicate, disease caused by the heat or fire pathogens.

Diseases caused by the heat or fire pathogens manifest as repletion heat (or fire) patterns, and are therefore treated with cold and cool agents that clear fire or drain fire. However, repletion fire also includes depressed fire that may arise under the following conditions:

> When fire is "enveloped" by an exogenous pathogen, (e.g., a cold enveloping fire), meaning when there is an unresolved exterior pattern together with exuberant inner-body heat manifesting symptoms such as a red, sore throat.
>
> When there is deep-lying inner-body heat prior to maculopapular eruption;
>
> Where phlegm or damp complications cause binding of phlegm and fire or constrained damp with deep-lying heat, characterized by thoracic glomus and restlessness.

Cold and cool agents alone are ineffective in eliminating depressed fire, and must be complemented either with the method of outthrust, or of upbearing and dissipation. Outthrusters include:

Outthrusters	
Herba Allii Fistulosi	*cōng bái*
Semen Sojae Praeparatum	*dòu shǐ*
Herba Menthae	*bò hé*
Fructus Gardeniae	*zhī zǐ*
Fructus Forsythiae	*lián qiào*
Fructus Arctii	*niú bàng zǐ*
Periostracum Cicadae	*chán yī*
Ramulus et Folium Tamaricis	*xī hé liǔ*

Upbearing dissipators include:

Upbearing Dissipators	
Rhizoma Cimicifugae	*shēng má*
Radix Puerariae	*gé gēn*
Radix Bupleuri	*chái hú*
Rhizoma et Radix Notopterygii	*qiāng huó*
Pericarpium Alpiniae	*kòu ké*
Semen Citri	*jú hé*
Radix Platycodi	*jié gěng*

The latter two drugs may also be used to open phlegm-damp. Hence the phrase, "Depressed fire is treated by effusion," which means that by effusion, fire is dissipated and heat discharged. Diaphoresis, papule outthrust, and transforming phlegm-damp are all important methods of dissipating fire.

Vacuity fire is caused not by the heat or fire pathogens, but by yin vacuity, and is treated by the method of enriching yin and clearing heat. Floating fire usually occurs in yang collapse vacuity desertion and is characterized by flushing of the cheeks, agitation, and thirst with desire for fluid. Although these are signs of heat, all other symptoms indicate cold due to yang vacuity. Careful observation reveals that since the thirst is allayed by intake of fluid and the complexion is the "floating red" characteristic of *dai yang* patterns, the heat signs are false and the vacuity signs are those of extreme yang vacuity (yang collapse). Floating fire is the manifestation of the overfloating of vacuity yang that results from exuberant inner-body yin cold. It is treated with warm agents such as:

Yang Salvagers	
Radix Aconiti Fu Tzu	*fù zǐ*
Cortex Cinnamomi	*ròu guì*
Radix Ginseng	*rén shēn*
Radix Glycyrrhizae	*gān cǎo*

These salvage yang and confine fire to its source, and may be combined with the following drugs that subdue yang and constrain qi:

Yang Subduing and Qi-Constraining Agents	
Os Draconis	*lóng gǔ*
Concha Ostreae	*mǔ lì*
Fructus Schisandrae	*wǔ wèi zǐ*
Magnetitum	*cí shí*

Timely use of qi boosting and yin enriching

Heat clearers and fire drainers are sufficient in themselves to treat repletion heat patterns, since they provide an adequate safeguard against damage to qi and liquid by eliminating the potential cause. Qi boosters and yin enrichers are only used where damage to qi and liquid has already occurred. If administered too early, they may exacerbate the heat and cause the pathogen to lodge in the body. Damage to qi and liquid is a common occurrence in diseases caused by heat and fire. Damage to original qi is of especially high incidence in diseases caused by the summerheat pathogen and is characterized by diminished qi and exhaustion. A clear example of such vacuity signs is seen in summerheat-strike (sunstroke) when the patient regains consciousness after the abatement of a high fever. However, supplementers should not be administered too soon if increase in fever and reoccurrence of coma is to be prevented. The summerheat pathogen is a form of heat. Heat is the radical characteristic, while the vacuity is only a secondary manifestation. In the initial stages of fever abatement, "although smoke ceases to rise from the hearth, there is still fire in the ashes." Treatment at this stage should be directed neither solely to eliminating vacuity nor solely to eliminating heat. Supplementers should only be given after careful assessment of the patient's condition, and should never be used in large doses. Wang's Summerheat-Clearing Qi-Boosting Decoction *(wáng shì qīng shǔ yì qì tāng)* is one summerheat-clearing formula that contains qi and yin nourishers.

Different considerations apply when summerheat strike leads to exhaustion of qi and yin. Here, a vacuous pulse and profuse sweating, together with severe dyspnea and thirst, indicate impending desertion. This is treated with Pulse-Engendering Powder *(shēng mài sǎn)* which boosts qi and constrains yin. Signs of severe damage left when fever has abated counsel against the use of either cool and cold agents, which can damage qi, or of cold, bitter agents, which can engender dryness and thereby cause further damage to liquid.

Organ involvement

In miscellaneous diseases, it is important to determine the organs involved in heat and fire patterns. Fire of each of the organs bears its own special marks. Heart fire is characterized by restlessness, insomnia, and cracking and lesions of the mouth and tongue. Liver fire is associated with headache, irascibility, restlessness, and ocular rubor. Stomach fire is characterized by halitosis, toothache, clamoring stomach, and hard stool. Lung fire is indicated by phlegm containing blood, coughing of blood, nosebleed, and dry nostrils with lesions. Kidney fire is characterized by steaming bone tidal fever, dream emissions, hyperactivity of the sexual functions, and unctuous strangury or hematuria. While each has its own characteristics, all organ fire falls within the scope of either vacuity or repletion heat. For further elaboration, see Chapter 9 and Table 10-3.

Damp Disease Patterns

Diseases caused by the damp pathogen are associated with damp as an environmental or climatic phenomenon. To this extent, they are either seasonal in nature or caused by living or working in damp localities. Damp bears the following characteristics:

Damp is a yin pathogen, i.e., it is clammy and viscous in nature, and difficult to eliminate. Damp diseases are usually of long duration.

Damp diseases have a tendency to stagnate. They are often characterized by a generalized sensation of heaviness, fatigued and cumbersome limbs, and "bag-over-the-head" sensation. Invasion of the channels and joints by damp, presenting such symptoms as pain of fixed location, labored movement, and leaden limbs, is known as damp obturation, or leaden obturation.

Damp easily invades the spleen, causing loss of appetite, indigestion, oppression in the chest, abdominal distention, thin stool, and short micturition with scant urine. The tongue fur is thick and slimy, and the pulse is either soggy or moderate.

Generalized or localized water-damp accumulations may take the form of water swelling, foot-qi disease, white vaginal discharge, damp papules (eczema), and lesions with copious serous discharge.

Distinction may be made between exogenous and endogenous damp. Exogenous damp is caused by contraction of the damp pathogen, but endogenous damp is the result of splenic failure to move and transform fluids. However, the two are mutually conducive. Splenic transformation failure represents an intrinsic factor facilitating the invasion of exogenous damp, while failure to eliminate exogenous damp may damage the spleen and thereby give rise to endogenous damp. The significance of the distinction between exogenous and endogenous damp lies in determining the relative importance of splenic vacuity and the pathogen. In treatment, it must be decided whether emphasis should be placed on transforming, drying, and disinhibiting damp, or on fortifying the spleen to move damp.

Damp frequently invades the channels in combination with wind and cold to become obturation disease. Combinations of damp with heat or with cold may effect other diseases. Of these, damp-heat is the most common.

Damp obstruction

Pattern identification

Damp obstruction denotes a frequently observed disease in which the spleen and stomach are obstructed by the damp pathogen. It mainly occurs in summer and is characterized by disturbance of splenogastric movement and transformation. Signs include oppression in the chest, no thought of food and drink, and a sickly, bland, or sweet taste in the mouth. The tongue fur is thick and slimy, while the pulse is soggy. Micturition is short with scant urine; the limbs are cumbersome and fatigued; sometimes a low fever is observed. Regular summer recurrence of loss of appetite, fatigue and weakness, and low fever, with gradual recovery in the autumn, indicates damp obstruction. The above symptoms together with thin stool or diarrhea are also signs of damp encumbering the spleen and stomach. A higher body temperature with more pronounced heat signs indicates summerheat-damp, which is a form of damp-heat (see previous section).

Treatment

Drug therapy

Damp obstruction is treated by the methods of transforming damp with aromatics and drying damp with warm, bitter agents. These may be combined with splenic fortification. Commonly used aromatic damp transformers and warm, bitter damp driers include:

Aromatic and Warm, Bitter Damp Driers	
Herba Agastaches	*huò xiāng*
Herba Eupatorii	*pèi lán*
Rhizoma Atractylodis	*cāng zhú*
Cortex Magnoliae	*hòu pò*
Rhizoma Pinelliae	*bàn xià*

Spleen fortifiers include:

Spleen Fortifiers	
Rhizoma Atractylodis Macrocephalae	*bái zhú*
Sclerotium Poriae	*fú líng*
Semen Dolichoris	*biǎn dòu*

Damp disinhibitors may also be used:

Damp Disinhibitors	
Sclerotium Poriae	*fú líng*
Semen Coicis	*yì yǐ rén*
Talcum	*huá shí*
Medulla Tetrapanacis	*tōng cǎo*
Semen Plantaginis	*chē qián zǐ*

One frequently used formula is Agastache, Magnolia, Pinellia and Poria Decoction *(huò pò xià líng tāng)*.

Acumoxatherapy

SP-9 is a major point used in transforming damp. Splenic movement and transformation can be fortified with SP-6, ST-36, and BL-20. LI-11 is used to drain heat and transform damp. ST-36 and CV-12 are commonly used to harmonize the spleen and stomach, and PC-6 can ease the chest. The above points may be used in conjunction with points such as GB-20, CV-2, or LI-4, depending on the presenting symptoms.

Damp-heat

Damp-heat can cause a variety of different diseases. It is associated with both damp and heat signs: fever, pain and distention in the chest and lateral costal region, pain and fullness in the abdomen, nausea and vomiting, poor appetite, thirst without appreciable fluid intake, hard stool or diarrhea, and short micturition with scant, yellow or dark-colored urine. The pulse is rapid and either soggy or slippery. The tongue fur is thick, yellow, and slimy. Damp-heat is treated by the combined method of clearing heat and transforming damp, emphasis being variously placed on each of its two components depending on whether damp or heat is prominent. (See Table 10-4.)

This broad range of diseases caused by damp-heat pathogens may be classified according to the organ or aspect of the organism affected, as discussed in the following sections.

Damp-heat lodged in the qi aspect

Pattern identification

Damp-heat lodged in the qi aspect, also known as damp-heat lodged in the triple burner, is attended by persistent fever that is relatively low or remittent; the limbs feel fatigued and there is oppression in the chest. Thirst without appreciable intake of fluid is accompanied by a bland, bitter, or sickly taste in the mouth. Micturition is short with dark-colored urine. The tongue fur is yellow and slimy. Summerheat-damp and damp obstruction may also be characterized by such symptoms.

Treatment

Drug therapy

Damp-heat lodged in the qi aspect is treated by perfusing the qi aspect and by transforming damp and clearing heat. Commonly used agents include:

Qi-Aspect Damp-Heat Agents	
Herba Agastaches	*huò xiāng*
Herba Eupatorii	*pèi lán*
Herba Artemisiae Apiaceae	*qīng hāo*
Semen Pruni Armeniacae	*xìng rén*
Fructus Amomi Cardamomi	*kòu rén*
Semen Coicis	*yì yǐ rén*
Rhizoma Pinelliae	*bàn xià*
Six-to-One Powder	*liù yī sǎn*
Radix Scutellariae	*huáng qín*
Fructus Gardeniae	*zhī zǐ*

Formulae such as Three Kernel Decoction *(sān rén tāng)* and its variants are mostly used where damp is prominent. Sweet Dew Toxin-Dispersing Elixir *(gān lù xiāo dú dān)* and variants are mostly used for heat-prominent patterns.

Acumoxatherapy

TB-6 is commonly used to clear the triple burner. BL-53 is the lower uniting point of the triple burner, and may be used to the same purpose. Other points used to transform damp and clear heat include CV-12, LI-11, LI-4, PC-6, SP-9, and SP-6.

Splenogastric damp-heat obstruction

Pattern identification

Obstruction of the spleen and stomach by damp-heat is characterized by pronounced digestive tract symptoms: painful distention and oppression in the chest and abdomen, or pain brought on by pressure; a sickly or bitter taste in the mouth; hard stool, or diarrhea with foul-smelling stool. The tongue is red at the tip and edges and the tongue fur is either white and slimy or thick, yellow, and slimy. Other signs include fever, thirst with no desire for fluids, and short micturition with dark-colored urine.

Treatment

Drug therapy

Drying damp and clearing heat is combined with the method of opening with pungent agents and discharging with bitter agents. Commonly used drugs include:

Pungent-Opening and Damp-Drying Agents	
Rhizoma Atractylodis	*cāng zhú*
Cortex Magnoliae	*hòu pò*
Herba Agastaches	*huò xiāng*
Rhizoma Pinelliae	*bàn xià*

These may be used together with cold, bitter heat dischargers such as:

Cold, Bitter Heat Dischargers	
Radix Scutellariae	*huáng qín*
Rhizoma Coptidis	*huáng lián*
Fructus Gardeniae	*zhī zǐ*

Frequently used formulae include Coptis and Magnolia Cool Decoction (*lián pò yǐn*) and its variants.

Acumoxatherapy

Treatment centers on clearing heat through points such as LI-11, LI-4, and ST-43. The spleen is supported with SP-4, SP-6, and BL-20. SP-9 is a typical point used to transform damp. Points such as CV-12 and PC-6 are used to transform damp, harmonize the center, and loosen the chest.

Brewing hepatocystic damp-heat

Pattern identification

Brewing hepatocystic damp-heat, or simply hepatocystic damp-heat, is a disturbance of hepatocystic free coursing due to either exogenous or endogenous damp-heat. Endogenous damp-heat is generally attributable to overconsumption of fatty or sweet foods. The principal signs are jaundice, painful distention of the lateral costal region, fullness and distention in the abdomen, retching and nausea, diminished food intake, fatigued limbs, hard stool or thin-stool diarrhea with discomfort unrelieved by evacuation. There may also be fever. Concurrence of hepatocystic and splenogastric damp-heat is known as splenogastric damp-heat sweltering the liver and gallbladder.

Treatment

Drug therapy

The method of treatment is coursing the liver and disinhibiting bile combined with treatment clearing and draining damp-heat. Commonly used agents include:

Hepatocystic Damp-Heat Agents	
Herba Artemisiae Capillaris	yīn chén
Radix Bupleuri	chái hú
Tuber Curcumae	yù jīn
Fructus Citri Immaturus	zhǐ shí
Radix Scutellariae	huáng qín
Cortex Phellodendri	huáng bó
Fructus Gardeniae	zhī zǐ
Rhizoma Rhei	dà huáng
Radix Gentianae	lóng dǎn cǎo
Radix Isatidis	bǎn lán gēn
Rhizoma Polygoni Cuspidati	hǔ zhàng
Herba Sedi Sarmentosi	chuí pén cǎo

Artemisia Capillaris Decoction *(yīn-chén-hāo tāng)* is used for damp-heat jaundice. Major Bupleurum Decoction *(dà chái-hú tāng)* is mainly used for hepatocystic damp-heat characterized by high fever or alternating fever and chills, painful distention in the lateral costal region, severe pain in the upper abdomen, bitter taste in the mouth, nausea and vomiting of bitter fluid, constipation, or jaundice.

Acumoxatherapy

SP-6 and SP-9 are the basic points used for many damp-related diseases. Hepatocystic damp-heat may be treated with LV-3, GB-34, LV-8, and GB-40, all of which clear damp-heat from the liver and gallbladder. BL-43 and BL-18 can be used to calm the liver and clear liver fire. CV-11 and PC-6 harmonize the stomach and free the flow of the center. Points such as BL-53 drain damp-heat by disinhibiting urine. If there is pain in the lateral costal region and upper abdomen, LV-13 and CV-13 may be added.

Downpour of damp-heat into the large intestine

Pattern identification

Downpour of damp-heat into the large intestine is generally characterized by abdominal pain, diarrhea with discomfort unrelieved by evacuation, and foul-smelling stool. An alternative pattern is dysentery characterized by frequent evacuation and blood and pus in the stool, abdominal pain, tenesmus, and a burning sensation in the rectum. In both cases, general symptoms include fever, bitter taste in the mouth, and slimy, yellow tongue fur.

Treatment

Drug therapy

This condition is treated by clearing heat and disinhibiting damp, and by resolving toxin, using agents such as:

Large Intestine Damp-Heat Agents	
Radix Pulsatillae	bái tóu wēng
Cortex Fraxini	qín pí
Rhizoma Coptidis	huáng lián
Radix Scutellariae	huáng qín
Cortex Phellodendri	huáng bó
Radix Sanguisorbae	dì yú
Herba Portulacae	mǎ chǐ xiàn

A basic formula is Pulsatilla Decoction *(bái-tóu-wēng tāng)*.

Acumoxatherapy

ST-25 and BL-25, the front-alarm and back-associated points of the large intestine, are combined with points such as BL-54 to drain heat and clear the large intestine. Other effective points are SP-4, SP-6, CV-12, LI-4, and LI-11.

Downpour of damp-heat into the bladder

Pattern identification

Signs include urinary frequency, urinary urgency, painful urination, and yellow to dark-colored urine. If the damp-heat gathers and binds, it can lead to sabulous or calculous strangury and hematuria, with low back pain, yellow tongue fur, and rapid pulse.

Treatment

Drug therapy

The method of clearing heat and disinhibiting damp and that of disinhibiting water and freeing strangury are both used to treat downpour of damp-heat into the bladder. Commonly used agents include:

Bladder Damp-Heat Agents	
Caulis Mu T'ung	mù tōng
Semen/Herba Plantaginis	chē qián zǐ/cǎo
Herba Polygoni Avicularis	biǎn xù
Talcum	huá shí
Herba Dianthi	qū mài
Fructus Gardeniae	zhī zǐ
Herba Chin Ch'ien Ts'ao	jīn qián cǎo
Folium Pyrrosiae	shí wěi
Herba Cephalanoploris	xiǎo jì cǎo
Pollen Typhae	pú huáng
Sclerotium Polypori Umbellati	zhū líng
Rhizoma Alismatis	zé xiè
Rhizoma Dioscoreae Pi Hsieh	bì xiè

A general formula is Eight Corrections Powder *(bā zhèng sǎn)*. Pyrrosia Powder *(shí-wěi sǎn)* and its variants treat calculus patterns.

Damp-heat downpour also includes disorders characterized by copious, thick, sticky, fishy-smelling vaginal discharge that is yellow in color or seen to contain blood, accompanied by dull pain or painful distention in the lower abdomen. Such patterns may be treated with Gentian Liver-Draining Decoction *(lóng dǎn xiè gān tāng)* and variants which clear and disinhibit liver channel damp-heat. It also includes lower-limb fireflow (erysipelas), characterized by redness, swelling, and pain. This may be treated with Mysterious Trinity Pills *(sān miào wán)* which, with the added agents, clear and disinhibit triple burner damp-heat.

Acumoxatherapy

BL-54 and CV-3 are used to clear bladder heat. KI-7 moistens kidney yin and clears the bladder, dispels damp and disperses stagnation. BL-28 frees the lower burner and promotes flow through the waterways. Other useful points include SP-9, SP-6, CV-4, ST-28, BL-32, and ST-44.

Damp-heat vaginal discharges are treated by combining local points such as GB-26 which, being located on the girdling vessel irregular channel, has a direct effect on the genitourinary system, and CV-3, the front-alarm point of the bladder, with such points as SP-6 and SP-9, which drain damp, and SP-10, which clears heat. GB-26 is used to stop leukorrhea and CV-3 to clear the lower burner of brewing heat. Other points commonly used to treat downpour of damp-heat into the bladder include CV-4, CV-6, BL-30, LV-2, and PC-5.

Lower-limb fire flow is treated by disinhibiting damp and clearing heat from the blood and the lower burner, using points such as SP-9, LV-2, ST-36, SP-10, ST-41, GB-38, SP-6, and BL-54 (bleed capillaries). LV-2 and GB-38 combined with SP-9 drain hepatocystic fire and extinguish wind. Seven-star or plum-blossom needle therapy on the above points and affected areas is also a commonly employed technique.

Identification and treatment of damp disease patterns

Location within the triple burner

Damp heat patterns may also be identified in terms of the location of the pathogen within the triple burner.

Damp clouding the upper burner is characterized by sensations of heaviness and pressure in the head, glomus and oppression in the chest and venter, no thought for food or drink, and a bland taste in the mouth.

Drug Therapy

Treatment, based on promoting qi perfusion and transforming phlegm, employs aromatic agents whose dry nature is not too pronounced. These include:

Mild Bitter, Pungent Agents	
Herba Agastaches	huò xiāng
Herba Eupatorii	pèi lán
Semen Pruni Armeniacae	xìng rén
Fructus Amomi Cardamomi	kòu rén
Epicarpium Citri Tangerinae	jú hóng
Radix Platycodi	jié gěng

By their slight bitterness and pungency, these drugs enhance qi dynamic and so promote transformation of damp.

Middle-burner damp obstruction is generally characterized by fullness and distention in the chest and abdomen, improper movement of digestate, thirst with no desire for fluids, thin stool, and fatigued and cumbersome limbs. The tongue fur is thick and slimy. This pattern is treated essentially by drying damp and fortifying the spleen using formulae in which Rhizoma Atractylodis *(cāng zhú)* and Cortex Magnoliae *(hòu pó)* are sovereign.

Downpour of damp into the lower burner is generally characterized by short micturition with yellow or dark-colored urine. Treatment centers on disinhibiting damp, using agents that disinhibit urine and abduct damp:

Damp-Abducting Diuretics	
Sclerotium Poriae	fú líng
Rhizoma Alismatis	zé xiè
Semen Plantaginis	chē qián zǐ
Medulla Tetrapanacis	tōng cǎo
Talcum	huá shí

Transformation, drying, and disinhibition represent the three major methods of treating damp. All three may be used together, but care must be taken to ensure that drugs selected act on the desired burner.

Identifying cold-damp and damp-heat

Damp usually occurs in combination with other pathogens. Apart from wind, cold, and damp, which unite to give rise to obturation diseases, the main combinations are cold-damp and damp-heat.

Cold-damp is usually of endogenous origin and arises when fluid transformation is impaired owing to devitalization of splenic yang, and the original condition of pronounced vacuity cold becomes one of both cold and damp. This process is known as damp forming with cold. Cold-damp is characterized either by abdominal fullness and diarrhea, or by phlegm-rheum and water swelling. *Essential Questions* describes this pathomechanism in the following way: "Damp, swelling, and fullness are associated with the spleen." Cold and damp are both yin pathogens and are treated by warming and transforming.

Damp-heat can be caused by direct contraction of exogenous damp-heat, but may also arise from within the body when intense stomach heat resulting from excessive consumption of sweet or fatty foods impairs fluid transformation. This process is known as "damp forming with heat." Damp is a yin pathogen, while heat is a yang pathogen. The two are thus opposite in nature. In clinical practice, one is invariably found to be more prominent than the other so that emphasis on damp transformation and heat clearing varies according to case.

Although cold-damp may stem from invasion by combined pathogens, it much more commonly arises when intrinsic factors or incorrect treatment cause damp to develop out of pre-existing heat or cold within the body. Damp easily forms with cold in a patient suffering from splenogastric vacuity cold or in one who is wrongly treated with cold and cool agents. Conversely, it may develop with heat in a patient who is suffering from pre-existing splenogastric heat accumulation or who is inappropriately treated with hot, pungent agents.

When damp forms with cold, yang is easily damaged; when it forms with heat, yin is readily damaged. Therefore, although damp is a yin pathogen for which yang agents are indicated, aromatic damp transformers, spleen fortifiers, and damp disinhibitors are often used instead of potent hot, pungent agents, in order to prevent dryness formation and damage to yin. Damp combined with heat should not be treated with soft, yin agents, since these may cause it to congeal and resist transformation. Where the damp pathogen has promoted cold formation and damaged yang, the resulting pattern, characterized by prevalence of damp and weakness of yang, should be treated with warm and hot agents to support yang and dry damp. When it forms heat and damages yin, moist but not sticky yin nourishers should be blended with cold, bitter agents to drain heat and dry damp while safeguarding yin.

As a yin pathogen, damp has yin characteristics and readily damages yang; it is eradicated by warm, bitter agents. Thus, even if it occurs in combination with heat, which is a potential threat to yin, the use of cold and cool agents alone, without dry, bitter agents, may fail to dispel damp, and may further cause damage to yang. "Damp arising from the center" as a result of splenogastric weakness should always be treated with spleen-fortifying and yang-freeing agents such as:

Spleen Fortifiers	
Ramulus Cinnamomi	*guì zhī*
Sclerotium Poriae	*fú líng*
Rhizoma Atractylodis Macrocephalae	*bái zhú*

By enhancing splenogastric transformation and the spread of yang qi, these help the body to eliminate water-damp naturally.

Damp-heat lodging in the qi aspect, summerheat-damp, and damp obstruction

Damp-heat lodging in the qi aspect is characterized by persistent remittent fever, and is seen in a wide range of exogenous heat diseases. Summerheat-damp may take the form of damp-heat lodging in the qi aspect, but only occurs in the height of summer. Damp obstruction is characterized by fatigued and cumbersome limbs, oppression in the chest, and loss of appetite, and its pathomechanism is explained as damp encumbering the spleen and stomach. If damp is combined with heat, the pattern is one of damp-heat, and if occurring in summer, summerheat-damp. Damp obstruction is treated by transforming damp with aromatics, drying damp, and disinhibiting damp. The two damp-heat patterns are treated by clearing summerheat and transforming damp. (See Table 10-5.)

Dryness Disease Patterns

Dryness is characterized by symptoms of dehydration that is mainly caused by damage to liquid and blood, but which may also be caused by contraction of the dryness pathogen. Thus there is both exogenous and endogenous dryness. Endogenous dryness is both more common and more serious than exogenous dryness.

Exogenous dryness contractions

Pattern identification

Contraction of exogenous dryness is mostly attributable to dry weather, and thus most commonly occurs in autumn, and in dry regions. The main symptoms are dry cough, with either little phlegm or thick, sticky phlegm that is difficult to expectorate, as well as dry throat, lips, tongue, and nostrils. Nosebleed may be symptomatic of dryness. Since all these signs are related to the respiratory tract, such patterns are sometimes described as invasion of the lung by the dryness pathogen. Further, since the lung is connected with the surface skin and body hair, and stands in interior-exterior relationship with the large intestine, other signs include dry, cracked skin and hard stool.

Treatment

Drug therapy

Exogenous dryness contractions are treated by the method of clearing the lung and moistening dryness. Commonly used agents include:

Lung Clearers and Dryness Moisteners	
Folium Mori	*sāng yè*
Exocarpium Pyri	*lí pí*
Bulbus Fritillariae Cirrhosae	*chuān bèi mǔ*
Fructus Arctii	*niú bàng zǐ*
Pericarpium Trichosanthis	*guā lóu pí*
Radix Trichosanthis	*tiān huā fěn*
Radix Adenophorae	*shā shēn*
Rhizoma Phragmitis	*lú gēn*
Rhizoma Imperatae	*máo gēn*

A frequently used formula is Mulberry and Apricot Kernel Decoction *(sāng xìng tāng)*, which may be varied according to need.

Acumoxatherapy

Treatment is based on clearing pulmonary and large intestinal heat through points such as LI-4, LI-11, LU-5, LU-10, and BL-13, and moistening dryness through points such as TB-2 and TB-6. Other points useful in treating exogenous dryness contractions include GV-14, ST-25, LU-6, and LU-9.

Damage to liquid and damage to yin

Pattern identification

Damage to liquid is generally associated with exogenous heat diseases, and may occur at any time during their course. It is the result of major depletion of fluids following high fever, excessive sweating, or profuse vomiting and diarrhea. Signs include thirst with urge to drink, and a red, dry tongue. Damage to yin, sometimes referred to as humor desertion, generally occurs in the later stages of exogenous heat diseases when the patient's general condition is poor, and is characterized by a desiccated or mirror tongue that is dull crimson in color. The throat and mouth are dry although the thirst is not pronounced. In severe cases, there may be clouding of the spirit and tetanic inversion indicating exhaustion of yin humor which is more serious than damage to liquid. Damage to liquid or to yin may also occur in endogenous damage and miscellaneous diseases when yin humor is depleted as a result of enduring illness, excessive loss of blood, excessive urination, or overuse of diuretic agents.

Treatment

Drug therapy

Damage to liquid is treated by the method of engendering liquid, whereby cold and sweet agents nourish the stomach liquid. Commonly used agents include:

Cold, Sweet Liquid Engenderers	
Radix Rehmanniae Viva	*xiān shēng dì*
Radix Adenophorae Viva	*xiān shā shēn*
Herba Dendrobii Viva	*xiān shí hú*
Rhizoma Phragmitis Vivum	*xiān lú gēn*
Radix Trichosanthis	*tiān huā fěn*

These cold, sweet, moistening agents not only enrich the fluids, but also clear heat. However, their application in exogenous heat diseases is limited, since damage to liquid is the result of exuberant heat that is treated by clearage. Exuberant heat stage diseases are treated by clearing heat and detoxifying, and draining fire with cold, bitter agents. These two methods are usually sufficient to safeguard liquid, and cold, sweet, liquid-engendering agents are added only where they do not jeopardize pathogen expulsion. Fluids Decoction *(jīn yè tāng)*, which moistens dryness and engenders liquid, treats dryness formation and damage to liquid occurring in both exogenous heat diseases and endogenous damage and miscellaneous diseases. Damage to liquid from exuberant heat may be treated with White Tiger Decoction *(bái hǔ tāng)*, which clears heat and safeguards liquid. The basic treatment for damage to yin is enriching yin with cold, sweet agents complemented with salty, moistening agents:

Cold, Sweet Yin Enrichers and Salty Moisteners	
Gelatinum Corii Asini	lǘ pí jiāo
Egg Yolk	jī zǐ huáng
Radix Scrophulariae	xuán shēn
Plastrum Testudinis	guī bǎn

Using these with liquid engenderers will enrich kidney yin. A commonly used formula possessing this effect is Pulse-Restorative Decoction *(fù mài tāng)*, which may be varied according to need. Diseases characterized by sirring of wind and tetanic inversion are treated by fostering yin and subduing yang, using Triple-Armored Pulse-Restorative Decoction *(sān jiǎ fù mài tāng)*.

Acumoxatherapy

Heat-clearing points such as LU-10, LI-11, and PC-7 can be combined with points that nourish yin and safeguard liquid, such as TB-2, KI-3, and KI-7. The location of the heat signs is the determining factor when selecting points to clear heat.

Blood dryness

Pattern identification

Blood dryness may occur when essence-blood is depleted in old age, or when nutritional disturbances or static blood binding in the inner body reduce the nutritive power of the blood. This disease is characterized by wasting of the muscles, dry, rough skin (cutaneous cornification), brittle nails, dry, lusterless hair, hard stool, and dry, unmoistened tongue. Itchy and scaling skin, either alone or with the above symptoms, is known as blood dryness (or blood vacuity) engendering wind.

Treatment

Drug therapy

Blood dryness is treated by the method of nourishing the blood and moistening dryness. Commonly used agents include:

Blood-Nourishing and Dryness-Moistening Agents	
Radix Rehmanniae Cruda	shēng dì
Radix Rehmanniae Conquita	shóu dì
Radix Polygoni Multiflori	shǒu wū
Radix Angelicae Sinensis	dāng guī
Radix Salviae Miltiorrhizae	dān shēn
Radix Paeoniae Albae	bái sháo
Fructus Lycii	qǐ zǐ
Semen Sesame Atrum	hēi zhī má

Formulae include Dryness-Moistening Construction-Nourishing Decoction (zī zào yǎng yíng tāng) and its variants.

Acumoxatherapy

Spleen and liver channel points, such as SP-6, SP-10, and LV-8, are chosen to support the spleen's blood-forming and the liver's blood-storing functions. The back-associated points of the liver and spleen, BL-18 and BL-20 respectively, are used for the same purpose. BL-54 and SP-10 may also be used to cool the blood.

Identification and treatment of dryness disease patterns

Cool and warm dryness

Classically, distinction was made between cool and warm dryness. Cool dryness is similar to wind-cold diseases of the cold and influenza type, except that it occurs only in the autumn. Most exogenous dryness pathogen diseases fall into the category of warm dryness. They are generally mild and are precipitated by lung yin vacuity. More severe cases may be characterized by hoarseness of voice, blood in the phlegm, and pain in the chest and costal region.

Treatment usually involves clearing dryness and restoring the lung, for which Dryness-Clearing Lung-Restorative Decoction (qīng zào jiù fèi tāng) is prescribed. Diphtheria is also attributable to contraction of the dryness pathogen, and is generally treated by the method of nourishing yin and clearing the lung. However, severe, contagious forms of diphtheria are considered to be caused by epidemic pestilence, which is different from general dryness, and is treated by the admixture of heat-clearing and toxin-resolving agents.

Upper, middle, and lower burner dryness patterns

Dryness patterns occurring in endogenous damage and miscellaneous diseases may be analyzed according to location in the triple burner. The classics state:

> When the upper body is dry, there is cough {dry cough};
> when the center is dry there is thirst;
> when the lower body is dry, binding occurs {dry, solid stool}.

The universal principle applied is dryness treated by moistening. Thus dryness in the upper, middle, and lower burners is treated by moistening the lung, nourishing the stomach, and moistening the intestines respectively. However, the lower burner is associated with the liver and the kidney, so that although dryness in the lower burner is characterized by desiccation of intestinal humor and dry, hard stool, in reality it stems from hepatorenal essence-blood vacuity. When intestinal lubricants are not adequately effective, agents such as the following are used to enrich hepatorenal yin-blood:

Hepatorenal Yin-Blood Enrichers	
Herba Cistanches	cōng róng
Radix Rehmanniae	dì huáng
Radix Polygoni Multiflori	shǒu wū
Radix Angelicae Sinensis	dāng guī
Radix Paeoniae Albae	bái sháo
Fructus Lycii	qǐ zǐ
Fructus Mori	sāng shēn zǐ

(See Table 10-6.)

Digestate Accumulation

Digestate accumulations may occur either when dietary irregularities place excessive strain on, and hence damage, the stomach and intestines, or when splenogastric transformation is so weak that even regular amounts of food, improperly transformed, accumulate in the stomach and intestines. Food is an essential requisite of the body, since it is the source of qi and blood. However, if it is not digested and accumulates in the stomach and intestines, it not only fails to benefit the body but even becomes a pathogen. Digestate accumulation patterns include ingesta damage, gastrointestinal accumulation, and spleen vacuity with ingesta damage complication.

Ingesta damage

Pattern identification

Ingesta damage is characterized by aversion to food, nausea and vomiting, eructation, putrid-smelling vomitus and gas, painful bloating of the abdomen, diarrhea or constipation, foul-smelling stool and flatus, and relief from pain and distention after defecation or passing of flatus. The tongue fur is slimy and either thick or yellow. This disorder is usually attributable to voracious eating. *Essential Questions* states, "Overeating causes damage to the stomach and intestines."

Treatment

Drug therapy

Ingesta damage is treated by dispersion and abduction. Commonly used agents are:

Abductive Dispersers	
Massa Fermentata	liù qū
Fructus Crataegi	shān zhā
Fructus Hordei Germinatus	mài yá
Semen Raphani	lái fú zǐ
Endothelium Gigeriae Galli	jī nèi jīn
Fructus Citri Immaturus	zhǐ shí
Semen Arecae	bīn láng

Formulae such as the ready-prepared Harmony-Preserving Pills *(bǎo hé wán)* are frequently used.

Acumoxatherapy

Points such as ST-25, BL-25, TB-6, LI-11, CV-12, ST-44, ST-36, PC-6, and ST-37 are used to move and expel stagnation from the stomach and large intestines. SP-4, SP-6, and BL-20 may be used to fortify splenic transformation, thereby dispersing accumulation. PC-6 is a primary point for easing nausea and vomiting. Many older texts cite the combination of CV-21 and ST-36 for treating ingesta damage and accumulation.

Gastrointestinal accumulation

Pattern identification

Gastrointestinal accumulation is usually more serious than most cases of ingesta damage. It is characterized by the same symptoms, with the addition of palpable accumulation lumps in the abdomen, painful distention exacerbated by pressure, diarrhea with discomfort unrelieved by defecation, or tenesmus. Causes include excessive consumption, especially of cold, raw, fried, rich, or fatty foods, and ingestion of unclean foodstuffs.

Treatment

Drug therapy

Gastrointestinal accumulation is treated according to the principle of "lodging is treated by attack," or offensive precipitation. Both abductive dispersers and offensive precipitants are used. Commonly used formulae include:

Offensive Precipitation Formulae	
Minor Purgative Decoction	xiǎo chéng qì tāng
Immature Citrus Stagnation-Abducting Pills	zhǐ-shí dǎo zhì wán
Saussurea and Areca Pills	mù-xiāng bīn-láng wán

Acumoxatherapy

Gastrointestinal accumulation is treated with the same points used for ingesta damage. A strong stimulation is preferable and electroacupuncture is also useful.

Splenogastric vacuity with ingesta damage complication

Pattern identification

Non-transformation of ingested food caused by splenogastric vacuity is characterized by bloating after eating, and thin stool containing undigested food. In general, there is no abdominal pain and the tongue fur may be completely normal. Signs such as no thought for food and drink and no enjoyment in eating indicate that the emphasis is on gastric vacuity. Non-transformation of ingested food indicates splenic vacuity. Yellow complexion, emaciation, and large appetite with poor digestation, indicate a strong stomach and weak spleen.

Treatment

Drug therapy

Treatment involves either increasing the appetite and fortifying the spleen, or simultaneous dispersion and supplementation. Frequently used agents that supplement the spleen and stomach are:

Gastrosplenic Supplementers	
Radix Codonopsis Pilosulae	dǎng shēn
Rhizoma Atractylodis Macrocephalae	bái zhú
Sclerotium Poriae	fú líng
Semen Dolichoris	biǎn dòu
Radix Dioscoreae	shān yào

The following drugs increase the appetite and disperse digestate accumulation:

Appetite-Increasing and Digestate-Dispersing Agents	
Pericarpium Citri Reticulatae	chén pí
Fructus Oryzae Sativae Germinatus	gǔ yá
Fructus Hordei Germinatus	mài yá
Fructus Citri Immaturus	zhǐ shí
Fructus Amomi	shā rén

Formulae such as Ginseng, Poria and Atractylodes Powder *(shēn líng báizhú sǎn)* are mainly used to supply splenogastric vacuity characterized by little thought for food and drink and non-transformation of ingested foods, with thin stool. Great Quieting Pills *(dà ān wán)* are mainly used for splenogastric vacuity with food accumulation.

Acumoxatherapy

Points that regulate the spleen and stomach, such as SP-2‡, CV-12‡, ST-36‡, and SP-6‡, are combined with points to fortify the spleen, such as BL-20‡.

Identification and treatment of digestate accumulation patterns

Simple digestate accumulation patterns are easily identified and treated. However, it should be remembered that stagnant digestate complication may attend a variety of diseases. Formulae used to treat such diseases should include accumulation-dispersing and stagnation-transforming drugs.

A strong stomach and weak spleen are often associated with parasite accumulations, and are frequently seen in *gan* accumulation patterns. Such cases are treated by first expelling the parasite and then regulating the spleen and stomach. (See Table 10-7.)

Phlegm Disease Patterns

The term "phlegm" has two meanings. In the narrow sense, it refers to expectorated matter, while in the broader sense it denotes phlegm lodging in the channels and organs, manifesting as phlegm patterns. For example, phlegm lodging in the lung gives rise to cough, dyspnea, and copious expectoration; phlegm lodging in the heart may give rise to palpitations and clouding of the spirit, or mania and withdrawal; phlegm lodging in the stomach causes nausea and vomiting; phlegm harassing the upper body manifests as dizziness; phlegm lodging in the chest and lateral costal region gives rise to fullness in the chest with dyspnea and cough causing pain in the chest; phlegm lodging in the limbs causes local numbness; phlegm lodging in the channels leads to scrofulous swellings and phlegm nodules. These different phlegm patterns are all associated with common general signs such as a moist, glossy, slimy tongue fur, and a wiry, slippery pulse.

The production of phlegm is mainly associated with impaired transformation, distribution, and discharge of fluid resulting from disorders of the lung, spleen, stomach, and kidney. Phlegm can form from fluid in the lung, when contraction of an exogenous pathogen impairs pulmonary depurative downbearing. It can form from gathering damp when habitual drinking or overconsumption of sweet, fatty foods causes impairment of splenic transformation. It can also form out of water that floods upward when kidney yang insufficiency leads to impairment of the transformative action of kidney qi. Finally, boiling of fluids can also result in the formation of phlegm. This occurs when, owing to affect damage, qi becomes depressed and transforms into fire, or when endogenous heat arises out of yin vacuity. Once formed, phlegm can lead to failure of pulmonary depurative downbearing, of splenic movement and transformation, and of the transformative action of kidney qi. It may also affect the normal flow of qi and blood and the distribution of fluids. Under such circumstances, phlegm acts as a pathogen harming the body.

Phlegm may take the form of damp phlegm, cold phlegm, heat phlegm, dryness phlegm, and wind phlegm. Phlegm patterns also include phlegm turbidity harassing the upper body, phlegm confounding the cardiac portals, and phlegm lodging in the channels. These are discussed below.

Damp phlegm

Pattern identification

Damp phlegm is a pattern characterized by copious, white phlegm, and attributable to splenic transformation failure. It may be accompanied by thoracic glomus, retching and nausea, and fatigued, cumbersome limbs.

The pulse is slippery, while the tongue fur is thick and slimy. This pattern is observed in diseases classified in Western medicine as chronic inflammatory disorders of the respiratory tract, such as chronic bronchitis.

Treatment

Drug therapy

Damp phlegm is treated by the method of eliminating damp and transforming phlegm. Commonly used agents include:

Damp Eliminators and Phlegm Transformers	
Rhizoma Pinelliae	bàn xià
Pericarpium Citri Reticulatae	chén pí
Sclerotium Poriae	fú líng
Rhizoma Atractylodis	cāng zhú
Cortex Magnoliae	hòu pò

Basic formulae for damp-eliminating and phlegm-transforming are Double Vintage Decoction (èr chén tāng) combined with Stomach-Calming Powder (píng wèi sǎn). The latter may be varied according to need.

Acumoxatherapy

Points such as ST-40 and CV-12 are used to transform phlegm. BL-20‡ strengthens splenic transformation, and BL-13‡ and BL-38‡ are added to support the lung. Points such as LU-7, LU-9, LI-4, SP-6, CV-17, and SP-9 may also be added according to the symptoms.

Cold phlegm

Pattern identification

Cold phlegm is characterized by cough and clear, thin, white phlegm, and a moist, white tongue fur. The pulse is generally slightly wiry. Patterns may also include cold form and frigidity of the limbs. Cold phlegm may also be observed in diseases classified by Western medicine as chronic inflammatory disorders of the respiratory tract such as chronic bronchitis and asthma.

Treatment

Drug therapy

Cold phlegm is treated by the method of warming the lung and transforming phlegm. Commonly used agents include:

Lung Warmers and Phlegm Transformers	
Herba Ephedrae	má huáng
Ramulus Cinnamomi	guì zhī
Rhizoma Zingiberis Exsiccatum	gān jiāng
Herba Asari	xì xīn
Rhizoma Pinelliae	bàn xià
Fructus Perillae Crispae	sū zǐ
Semen Sinapis Albae	bái jiè zǐ

The mostly commonly used formulae is Minor Cyan Dragon Decoction (xiǎo qīng lóng tāng).

Acumoxatherapy

Moxibustion at points such as BL-13, BL-38, CV-12, and LU-9 is used to warm the lung and transform phlegm. ST-40‡ is a major phlegm-transforming point. CV-17 clears the lung, transforms phlegm, and opens the chest. SP-9‡ drains damp, and SP-6‡ and BL-20‡ fortify the spleen. Other points used to treat cold-phlegm diseases include LI-4, BL-12‡, LU-7‡, PC-6, and SP-5‡.

Heat phlegm

Pattern identification

Heat phlegm is characterized by cough and rapid breathing. The phlegm is either thick and yellow, or white, gluey, and difficult to expectorate. General signs include fever, dry mouth, red tongue with yellow fur, and rapid, slippery pulse, all of which indicate heat. In Western medicine, heat phlegm corresponds roughly to acute inflammatory respiratory diseases (or acute attacks in chronic conditions).

In endogenous and miscellaneous diseases, repeated incidence of heat phlegm signs usually indicates phlegm fire. This occurs when phlegm heat, failing to clear, brews in the inner body and transforms into fire. When phlegm heat is characterized by extremely scant, gluey phlegm that is difficult to expectorate and possibly streaked with blood, as well as dry throat, lips and tongue, it is known as dryness phlegm. Both phlegm fire and dryness phlegm are variant forms of heat phlegm.

Treatment

Drug therapy

Heat phlegm is treated by the method of clearing heat and resolving toxins, and by the method of transforming phlegm. Commonly used agents include:

Heat Clearers and Toxin Resolvents	
Radix Scutellariae	huáng qín
Flos Lonicerae	yín huā
Herba et Radix Taraxaci	pú gōng yīng
Herba Houttuyniae	yú xīng cǎo
Cortex Radicis Mori	sāng bái pí
Semen T'ing Li Tzu	tíng lì zǐ
Bulbus Fritillariae Cirrhosae	chuān bèi mǔ
Fructus Trichosanthis	guā lóu
Succus Bambusae	zhú lì
Rhizoma Phragmitis Vivum	xiān lú gēn
Semen Benincasae	dōng guā rén

Formulae include Lonicera and Phragmites Combination *(yín wěi hé jì)* and its variants.

Acumoxatherapy

Points that clear heat, such as PC-7, LU-10, LU-7, and LU-5 can be combined with points that transform phlegm, such as CV-12, PC-6, and ST-40, depending on the location and nature of the pathogen. Other points used to treat heat-phlegm include SP-9, CV-17, BL-13, LU-11, and LU-9.

Wind phlegm

Pattern identification

Wind phlegm is characterized by the presence of both wind and phlegm signs. It manifests as seizures characterized by sudden collapse and loss of consciousness, foaming at the mouth, and convulsive spasms, and is mostly seen in epilepsy.

Treatment

Drug therapy

Dispelling wind phlegm employs agents such as:

Wind Phlegm Dispelling Agents	
Rhizoma Aconiti Coreani	bái fù zǐ
Rhizoma Arisaematis	nán xīng
Rhizoma Pinelliae	bàn xià
Bombyx Batryticatus	jiāng cán
Buthus	quán xiē
Succus Bambusae	zhú lì
Succus Zingiberis	jiāng zhī

A commonly used formula is Fit-Settling Pills *(dìng xián wán)*, which may be varied according to need.

Acumoxatherapy

Wind phlegm presenting as epilepsy is treated by opening the portals and transforming phlegm, and by calming the liver and extinguishing wind.

Points such as GV-26, M-BW-29 *(yao qi)*, HT-7, and BL-15 are used to open the portals and quiet the spirit, while GV-16 and GB-20 are used to extinguish wind. PC-6, CV-12, and ST-40 help transform phlegm, and LV-3 calms the liver. SP-6, GV-20, LI-15, PC-5, HT-5, KI-1, and GV-14 are used to resuscitate the patient, quiet the spirit, calm the liver, eliminate yang surfeits, and arrest seizures.

It is interesting to note that the master point of the yang motility vessel, BL-62, is used for diurnal seizures, while the master point of the yin motility vessel, KI-6, is used to treat nocturnal seizures.

Upper-body harassment by phlegm turbidity

Pattern identification

Dizziness is the essential feature of phlegm turbidity harassing the upper body. Hence it is said, "Where no phlegm is present, dizziness does not arise." Disturbance of vision may be so severe as to confine the patient to recumbency. Milder cases present as mental dizziness, pressure in the head, and heavy headedness. Other symptoms include insomnia, oppression in the chest, retching and nausea, little thought of food and drink, or non-transformation of ingested food. The tongue fur is slimy in texture and either white or yellow in color. The pulse is slippery, and may also be wiry. Where there is a heat complication, restlessness and bitter taste in the mouth may also be observed. These symptoms indicate disturbance of clear yang in the upper body due to thoracic phlegm turbidity obstruction. This may develop when damp gathers and transforms into phlegm as a result of splenic transformation failure. Phlegm turbidity harrassment of the upper body may be observed in diseases described in Western medicine as otogenic vertigo and hypertension.

Treatment

Drug therapy

Consideration is given not only to the splenic transformation failure from which the condition stems, but also to the connection between dizziness and liver wind. "Wind patterns characterized by shaking and visual dizziness are associated with the liver." Therefore, phlegm transformation, which forms the basis of treatment, is complemented on the one hand by fortifying the spleen, and on the other by calming the liver and extinguishing wind. The following agents transform phlegm and fortify the spleen:

Phlegm-Transforming and Spleen-Fortifying Agents	
Rhizoma Pinelliae	*bàn xià*
Pericarpium Citri Reticulatae	*chén pí*
Sclerotium Poriae	*fú líng*
Rhizoma Atractylodis Macrocephalae	*bái zhú*

Agents that calm the liver and extinguish wind include:

Liver-Calming Wind-Extinguishing Agents	
Rhizoma Gastrodiae	*tiān má*
Bombyx Batryticatus	*jiāng cán*
Buthus	*quán xiē*
Ramulus et Uncus Uncariae	*gōu téng*

Formulae such as Pinellia, Atractylodes and Gastrodia Decoction *(bàn-xià bái-zhú tiān-má tāng)* are mainly used for dizziness patterns attributed to phlegm. Coptis Gallbladder-Warming Decoction *(huáng-lián wēn dǎn tāng)* is chiefly used to treat phlegm turbidity and heat harassing clear yang in the upper body, characterized by dizziness, restlessness, bitter taste in the mouth, insomnia, red tongue, and slimy, yellow tongue fur.

Acumoxatherapy

Phlegm turbidity dizziness is treated by draining rising fire, using points such as GV-24. CV-12 and BL-21 calm the stomach and transform phlegm, and in combination with ST-40 clear fire and downbear turbidity. SI-7 and BL-58 are an ancient combination used to treat dizziness; together these points quiet the spirit and resuscitate the patient. Other points commonly used to treat this condition are GB-15, LV-3, TB-17, SI-19, GB-20, SP-4, and PC-6.

If there is heat harrassing clear yang in the upper body, bleeding the additional points GV-20, GV-14, and M-HN-9 *(tai-yang)* can drain yang surfeits from the upper body.

Phlegm confounding the cardiac portals

Pattern identification

Phlegm confounding the cardiac portals may also be described as phlegm turbidity clouding the pericardium. When the "heart" is obstructed by phlegm turbidity, the clear portals cease to function, a condition characterized by coma or essence-spirit derangement. At the same time, the tongue fur is thick and slimy and the pulse is slippery and wiry. Such patterns are seen in exogenous heat diseases, windstrike, and essence-spirit disorders.

Occurring in exogenous heat diseases, phlegm confounding the cardiac portals is characterized by coma or semiconsciousness, moderate or unsurfaced fever, and a slippery, rapid pulse. The tongue fur is either white and slimy, covering the tongue completely, or else yellow, slimy, and unclean. These signs differ from heat entering the pericardium which is characterized by coma, fright inversion, agitation, high fever, rapid pulse, and a dry, crimson tongue with scant fur. When windstrike takes the form of phlegm confounding the cardiac portals, signs include phlegm rattle in the throat, red complexion, rough breathing, slimy, yellow tongue fur, and slippery, wiry, rapid pulse. It may also present with pronounced lack of warmth in the extremities, slimy, glossy tongue fur, and deep, slippery pulse. Occurring in essence-spirit disorders, there may be such signs as essence-spirit derangement, feebleminded withdrawal, or manic agitation. The tongue fur is slimy in texture and either whte or yellow in color, and the pulse is slippery and wiry.

Treatment

Drug therapy

Phlegm confounding the cardiac portals is treated by sweeping phlegm and opening the portals. Commonly used are ready-prepared medicaments including:

Phlegm-Sweeping Portal-Opening Formulae	
Crown Jewel Elixir	*zhì bǎo dān*
Liquid Styrax Pills	*sū hé xiāng wán*

Cardiac phlegm agents used include:

Cardiac Phlegm Agents	
Rhizoma Acori Graminei	*chāng pú*
Tuber Curcumae	*yù jīn*
Radix Polygalae	*yuǎn zhì*
Rhizoma Pinelliae	*bàn xià*
Pulvis Arisaemae cum Felle Bovis	*dǎn nán xīng*
Sclerotium Poriae	*fú líng*
Succus Bambusae (with Succus Zingiberis)	*zhú lì*
Lapis Chloriti	*méng shí*

Acumoxatherapy

Points such as GV-26, KI-1, HT-7, and PC-8 are used to open the cardiac portals. Points such as PC-7, PC-6, and HT-5 are added to quiet the heart and spirit. Other useful points include SI-3, LV-3, SP-6, GV-20, LI-11, SP-9, and KI-4.

Phlegm lodging in the channels or limbs

Pattern identification

Phlegm lodging in the channels is mainly characterized by struma, phlegm nodules, and scrofulous swellings, all of which are relatively soft to the touch. Phlegm lodging in the limbs is characterized by numbness and pain in the upper or lower limbs, or in one limb. It is not accompanied by any signs of blood vacuity or wind-cold-damp obturation. The tongue fur is white and slimy, and the pulse is slippery.

Treatment

Drug therapy

Phlegm lodging in the channels or the limbs is treated by dispersing phlegm and softening hardness. Commonly used agents include:

Phlegm-Dispersing and Hardness-Softening Agents	
Herba Sargassii	hǎi zǎo
Thallus Algae	kūn bù
Spica Prunellae	xià kū cǎo
Semen Sinapis Albae	bái jiè zǐ
Mirabilitum	máng xiāo
Sclerotium Poriae	fú líng

Most formulae chosen to treat these patterns are ready-prepared medicaments such as:

Phlegm Dispersers and Hardness Softeners	
Prunella Paste	xià-kū-cǎo gāo
Scrofula-Dispersing Pills	nèi xiāo luǒ lì wán
Pathfinder Poria Pills	zhǐ mí fú-líng wán

The first two of these formulae treat struma, phlegm nodules, and scrofulous swellings. Pathfinder Poria Pills *(zhǐ mí fú-líng wán)* are used for pain and numbness in the limbs caused by the presence of phlegm.

Acumoxatherapy

Points such as LI-4 and ST-36 are used to supplement qi and stimulate channel flow. Moxibustion and needling with strong stimulation at local points is used to move qi and blood in the affected area and restore channel flow. Nodules and scrofulous swellings are often encircled by needles, this being known as the "turtle technique."

Phlegm lodging in the chest and lateral costal region

Pattern identification

Phlegm lodging in the chest and lateral costal region is composed of stubborn phlegm and accumulated rheum that form evasive masses. It is characterized by pain in the chest and lateral costal region, cough, labored breathing, and pain experienced when turning over in bed, as well as rapid breathing, and expectoration of white phlegm and drool. There may also be fullness and distention in the chest and lateral costal region, edematous swelling of the face, and a deep, wiry pulse.

Treatment

Drug therapy

The type of phlegm lodging in the chest and lateral costal region is generally a yin, congealing pathogen, which can only be transformed by warming, and eliminated by offensive treatment. Thus the method of treatment is transforming rheum and expelling phlegm. Commonly used rheum-transformers include:

Rheum Transformers	
Herba Ephedrae	má huáng
Ramulus Cinnamomi	guì zhī
Herba Asari	xì xīn
Rhizoma Zingiberis Exsiccatum	gān jiāng
Radix Aconiti Fu Tzu	fù zǐ
Semen Sinapis Albae	bái jiè zǐ

Phlegm expellants include:

Phlegm Expellants	
Semen T'ing Li Tzu	tíng lì zǐ
Radix Euphorbiae Kan Sui	gān suì
Radix Euphorbiae	dà jǐ
Semen Pharbitidis	qiān niú zǐ

A commonly used formula is Minor Cyan Dragon Decoction *(xiǎo qīng lóng tāng)*, which may be combined with T'ing Li Tzu and Jujube Lung-Draining Decoction *(tíng-lì dà-xǎo xiè fèi tāng)* or Drool-Controlling Elixir *(kòng xián dān)*.

Acumoxatherapy

TB-5 and TB-6 clear the triple burner. PC-6 and CV-17 transform phlegm and open the chest. GB-34 clears the foot shao yang gallbladder channel and is a major point for costal pain. ST-40 and SP-9 transform phlegm damp. CV-13 can move the center and dispel phlegm accumulations. Selection of points is determined by the presenting symptoms.

Identification and treatment of phlegm disease patterns

Color, quantity, and consistency of phlegm

The quantity, degree of yellowness, consistency, and presence of blood in expectorated phlegm is of importance in identifying cold, heat, dryness, and damp.

Variety of phlegm patterns

Phlegm patterns may involve any part of the body, and include a wide variety of different signs. Furthermore, some symptoms, such as dizziness, thoracic glomus, numbness of the limbs, and essence-spirit disturbances, are not exclusively associated with phlegm, so they must be correlated with the tongue fur and pulse. The presence of a slimy or glossy, moist tongue fur and slippery, wiry pulse is usually a clear indication of a phlegm pattern or complication. (See Table 10-8.)

The term phlegm-rheum in its wider meaning denotes accumulations of water-rheum resulting when fluids fail to be moved and transformed. Such accumulations are denoted by different terms, depending on the location in the body. The most important of these terms are phlegm-rheum (in a narrow sense), suspended rheum, spillage rheum, and column rheum. Nowadays, phlegm-rheum is generally used to denote column rheum. This is associated with expectoration of phlegm and drool that is clear and thin in appearance. Any thin phlegm is known as rheum. Despite the difference in name, there is no strict distinction between phlegm and rheum in practice. Phlegm-rheum (column rheum) usually appears as cold phlegm, which is discussed in the relevant section. Similarly, suspended rheum can be said to be synonymous with phlegm lodging in the chest and lateral costal region, discussed in the relevant section.

Phlegm-rheum

This denotes water in the intestines, characterized by general emaciation, and the gurgling of water in the intestines.

Suspended rheum

Suspended rheum describes water in the chest and lateral costal region, characterized by local pain, and cough with copious phlegm.

Spillage rheum

Spillage rheum denotes water in the limbs, characterized by heavy, painful, swollen limbs.

Column rheum

Column rheum denotes water in the infracardiac region (diaphragm and lungs), characterized by cough, copious phlegm, rapid breathing, inability to lie flat, and facial edema.

Table 10-1
Identification and Treatment of Wind Disease Patterns

	Pattern Type	Principal Signs	Treatment Method	Commonly Used Formulae	Acupoints
Contraction of Exogenous Wind	Wind Cold	Headache Aversion to cold Fever	Pronounced aversion to cold with headache and aching bones or fever and thirst; Moist, white tongue fur	Warm, pungent exterior resolution	Schizonepeta and Ledebouriella Detoxifying Powder	LI-4 GB-20 LU-7 TB-5
	Wind Heat	Itchy throat Floating pulse	Unpronounced aversion to cold Sore pharynx Dry mouth Red tongue	Cold, pungent exterior resolution	Lonicera and Forsythia Powder Mulberry and Chrysanthemum Cool Decoction Ephedra Decoction	LI-4 GV-14 LI-10 LV-11 LV-5
Invasion of the Channels and Vessels by the Wind Pathogen	Local Sinews and Vessels	Local palsy or paralysis	Dispelling wind and settling tetany	Anti-Contraction Powder	Local points LI-4 LV-3
	General Sinews and Vessels	Rigidity of the neck Tetanus Convulsive spasm	Dispelling wind and settling tetany	Five-Tigers-Chasing-the-Wind-Powder	GB-20 GV-16 GV-26 LI-11
	Wind Cold Damp Obturation	Muscular and articular pain	Dispelling wind, transforming damp, and dissipating cold	Anti-Obturation Decoction	LI-15 GB-30 ST-36 BL-54

Table 10-2 page 1

Identification and Treatment of Cold Disease Patterns

Pattern Type	Principal Signs	Treatment Method	Commonly Used Formulae	Acupoints
Contraction of the Cold Pathogen	Aversion to cold with: Fever, Headache, Aching bones, Floating, sometimes slightly tight pulse, Moist, white tongue fur	Warm pungent exterior resolution	Schizonepeta and Ledebouriella Detoxifying Powder, Ephedra Decoction	LI-4, GB-20‡, LU-7
Cold Obturation	Muscular or articular pain of relatively fixed location. Severe cases are characterized by hypertonicity	Warming the channels and dissipating cold	Wo T'ou Aconite Decoction	GB-20‡ Local points‡
Cold Pain	Abdominal pain exacerbated by cold. History of cold contraction	Dissipating cold and relieving pain	Alipina and Cyperus Pills	BL-25, ST-25, ST-36‡, SP-6

320

Table 10-2 page 2

Identification and Treatment of Cold Disease Patterns

Pattern Type	Principal Signs	Treatment Method	Commonly Used Formulae	Acupoints
Cold Diarrhea	Abdominal pain and diarrhea relieved by warmth Lack of warmth in the extremities Pale tongue with white fur	Warming the center and fortifying the spleen	Center-Rectifying Pills	BL-20‡ SP-6‡ SP-4‡ ST-36‡ CV-12‡ CV-4‡ CV-6‡
Cold Shan	Sagging testicles with pain reaching into the abdomen that is relieved by warmth Deep, wiry, tight pulse White, glossy, tongue fur	Warming the liver and dissipating cold Rectifying qi and relieving pain	Liver-Warming Decoction T'ien T'ai Lindera Powder	LV-1‡ KI-6 LV-14 ST-28 ST-33

Table 10-3 page 1

Identification and Treatment of Heat and Fire Disease Patterns

Pattern Type	Principal Signs	Treatment Method	Commonly Used Formulae	Acupoints
Repletion Heat	Vigorous fever, restlessness, and thirst In severe cases: manic delirium palpable heat and pain in the abdomen exacerbated by pressure; constipation or diarrhea with foul-smelling stool, possibly containing pus or blood maculopapular eruptions hematemesis epistaxis slippery, rapid pulse yellow tongue fur	Clearing heat and detoxifying and draining fire Draining fire	Coptis Detoxifying Decoction Heart-Draining Decoction	HT-5 HT-7 ST-44 LI-11 LU-5 GV-14 GB-34
Vacuity Heat	Tidal fever or inner-body fever Tidal flushing of the cheeks or upbearing fire, dry mouth and throat, steaming bone fever Night sweating Forceless, fine pulse Red tongue with little fur or completely peeled fur	Enriching yin and clearing heat	Great Yin Supplementation Pills Two-A Decoction	LV-3 LI-4 KI-3 TB-2 LU-10

Table 10-3 page 2

Identification and Treatment of Summerheat Disease Patterns

Pattern Type	Principal Signs	Treatment Method	Commonly Used Formulae	Acupoints
Summerheat Heat	Great heat Great thirst Profuse sweating or absence of sweating Agitation Large, surging pulse	Clearing summerheat	White Tiger Decoction	LI-4 BL-54 (bleed capillaries) GV-14 LI-11
Summerheat Damp	Persistent low fever Thick, slimy tongue fur Lack of strength Thoracic oppression Nausea and retching Thin stool with feeling of discomfort after defecation Short micturition with dark-colored urine	Clearing summerheat and transforming damp	Artemesia Apiacea and Scutellaria Gallbladder-Clearing Decoction	ST-40 SP-9 BL-54 GB-34

Table 10-4

Prominence of Pathogens in Damp-Heat Patterns		
Symptoms and Treatment	Pattern Type	
	Prominence of Damp	Prominence of Heat
Fever	Low, but generally persistent fever that is usually milder in the morning than in the evening	Higher fever
Chest and Abdomen	Discomfort, oppression	Pain, or painful distension and oppression
Thirst	No thirst, or thirst with no desire for fluid	Thirst and high fluid intake, or thirst with a desire for fluid and discomfort after drinking
Urine	Short micturition with scant, yellow urine	Short micturition with dark-colored urine
Pulse	Soggy, not too rapid	Slippery and rapid
Tongue	Slightly red tongue; slimy white or dry, slightly yellow fur	Red tongue with thick, slimy or rough yellow fur
Treatment	Transforming damp, assisted by clearing-heat	Clearing heat, assisted by transforming damp

Table 10-5 page 1

Identification and Treatment of Damp Disease Patterns

Pattern Type	Principal Signs	Treatment Method	Commonly Used Formulae	Acupoints
Damp Obstruction	Low fever Repeated summer recurrence pattern	Transforming damp with aromatics Drying damp Disinhibiting damp	Agastache, Magnolia, Pinellia, and Poria Decoction	SP-6 PC-6 SP-9 CV-12
Damp-Heat Lodged in the Qi Aspect (in triple burner)	Thoracic oppression Dyspeptic anorexia Upflow and nausea Sickly taste in mouth Abdominal distension with dark-colored urine Slimy tongue fur Shiny yellow tongue fur	Clearing heat and transforming damp	Sweet Dew Toxin-Dispersing Decoction Three Kernel Decoction	BL-21 TB-6 LI-4 BL-20
HEAT Splenogastric Damp Obstruction	General cumbersomeness and fatigue Fever Thirst with no desire to drink Short micturition Prominence of gastrosplenic signs Thick, slimy (possibly yellow) tongue Persistent fever is also possible	Pungent opening and bitter discharge	Coptis and Magnolia Cool Decoction	CV-12 SP-4 BL-20 BL-21 SP-9

325

Table 10-5 page 2

Identification and Treatment of Damp Disease Patterns

Pattern Type		Principal Signs	Treatment Method	Commonly Used Formulae	Acupoints
D A M P **H E A T**	Brewing Hepatocystic Damp-Heat	Jaundice, Bitter taste in mouth, Painful distention of chest and lateral costal region, possibly accompanied by abdominal pain, Rapid wiry pulse, Slimy (possibly yellow) tongue fur	Coursing hepatocystic damp-heat	Artemesia Capillaris Decoction	LV-3 BL-18 GB-34 GB-40
	Downpour of Damp-Heat into the Large Intestine	Thoracic oppression, Dyspeptic anorexia, Upflow and nausea, Sickly taste in mouth, Abdominal distention, Slimy tongue fur, General cumbersomeness and fatigue, Diarrhea with foul-smelling stool (possibly containing pus and blood), Tenesmus, abdominal pain (possibly with fever)	Clearing heat and disinhibiting damp, Detoxification	Minor Bupleurum Decoction, Pulsatilla Decoction	BL-25 ST-25 LI-9 BL-54
	Downpour of Damp-Heat into the Bladder	Urinary frequency and urgency, turbid urine	Clearing heat and disinhibiting water, Freeing strangury	Eight Corrections Powder, Pyrrosia Powder	BL-54 CV-3 KI-7

Table 10-6 page 1

Identification and Treatment of Dryness Patterns

Pattern Type	Principal Signs	Treatment Method	Commonly Used Formulae	Acupoints
Contraction of Exogenous Dryness	Dry cough Little phlegm Dry nose Epistaxis Blood in phlegm Dry mouth Dry lips	Clearing the lung and moistening dryness	Mulberry and Apricot Kernel Decoction Dryness-Clearing Lung-Restorative Decoction	KI-3 LI-10 TB-6 BL-13 LI-11
Damage to Liquid	or Dry, bound stool Caused by high fever and excessive sweating Dry tongue fur Tongue tends to be red	Engendering liquid and clearing heat	Humor-Increasing Decoction White Tiger Decoction	TB-2 LU-10 KI-7 KI-3 PC-7 TB-6

Table 10-6 page 2

Identification and Treatment of Dryness Patterns

Pattern Type	Principal Signs	Treatment Method	Commonly Used Formulae	Acupoints
Damage to Yin	Usually occurs in latter stages of heat diseases Generally poor physical state Clear tongue with little fur Fine, rapid pulse	Enriching yin humor	Pulse-Restorative Variant Decoction	TB-2 LU-10 KI-7 KI-3 PC-7 TB-6
Blood Dryness	Dry mouth Dry lips Dry, bound stool Occurs in old age after prolonged nutritional disturbance or when static blood binds in the inner body Signs include: general emaciation rough, dry itching skin thin, brittle nails mirror tongue	Nourishing the blood and moistening dryness	Dryness-Moistening Contruction-Nourishing Decoction	BL-20 BL-54 LV-8 SP-10 LV-3 SP-6

Table 10-7

Identification and Treatment of Digestate Accumulation Patterns

Pattern Type	Principal Signs	Treatment Method	Commonly Used Formulae	Acupoints
Ingesta Damage	Nausea Vomiting Eructation of sour, putrid gas Painful abdominal distention Diarrhea or constipation Flatulence Thoracic oppression	Abductive dispersion	Harmony-Preserving Pills	SP-6 CV-12 SP-4 PC-6 ST-36 CV-21
Gastrointestinal Accumulation	Hard abdominal glomus or abdominal pain exacerbated by pressure Old, yellow, or thick, slimy tongue fur Slimy or unclean tongue fur Little thought of food and bloating	Offensive precipitation	Minor Purgative Decoction Immature Citrus Stagnation-Abducting Pills Saussurea and Areca Pills	TB-6 ST-25 BL-20 BL-25
Splenic Vacuity with Ingesta Damage Complication	Non-transformation of ingested food Thin stool or diarrhea with undigested food in stool Generally no abdominal pain Tongue may be normal	Increasing appetite and fortifying the spleen Simultaneous dispersion and supplementation	Ginseng, Poria and Atractylodes Powder Great Calming Pills	SP-2 ST-44 ST-36 ST-25 TB-6

Table 10-8 page 1

Identification and Treatment of Phlegm Disease Patterns

Pattern Type	Principal Signs	Treatment Method	Commonly Used Formulae	Acupoints
Damp Phlegm	Copious, white, easily expectorated phlegm; Thick, slimy tongue fur; Thoracic oppression; Fatigued, cumbersome limbs and other signs of spleen vacuity damp encumbrance	Drying damp and transforming phlegm	Combination of Double Vintage Decoction and Stomach-Calming Powder and Variants	ST-40, CV-12, BL-20, BL-13
Cold Phlegm	Cough; Expectoration of phlegm; Thin, clear white phlegm; Moist white tongue fur; Cold form; Lack of warmth in the extremities; Slippery pulse (possibly wiry)	Warming transformation of cold phlegm	Minor Cyan Dragon Decoction	ST-40, LU-9, BL-13, CV-12
Heat Phlegm	Thick, yellow phlegm possibly containing blood or pus; Difficult expectoration; Fever; Red tongue with yellow fur	Clearing heat and transforming phlegm	Lonicera and Phragmites Combination	PC-6, ST-40, CV-22, PC-7, LU-5

Table 10-8 page 2

Identification and Treatment of Phlegm Disease Patterns

Pattern Type		Principal Signs	Treatment Method	Commonly Used Formulae	Acupoints
Wind Phlegm		Sudden onset Foaming at the mouth Convulsive spasms	Dispelling wind phlegm	Fit-Settling Pills	LV-3 PC-6 KI-1
Upper-Body Harrassment by Phlegm Turbidity	Slimy or unclean tongue fur Slippery pulse (possibly wiry)	Dizziness (the major sign) Thoracic oppression Nausea and vomiturition Restlessness Bitter taste in the mouth	Transforming phlegm and fortifying the spleen Calming the liver and extinguishing wind	Pinellia, Atractylodes and Gastrodia Decoction Coptis Gallbladder-Warming Decoction	GV-24 CV-12 ST-40 SI-7 BL-58
Phlegm Confounding the Cardiac Portals		Sudden stupor of spirit-disposition, or Essence-spirit derangement	Sweeping phlegm and opening the portals	Crown Jewel Elixir Liquid Styrax Pills	PC-8 PC-7 PC-6 GV-26

Table 10-8 page 3

Identification and Treatment of Phlegm Disease Patterns

Pattern Type	Principal Signs	Treatment Method	Commonly Used Formulae	Acupoints
Phlegm Lodging in the Channels or Limbs	Struma Phlegm nodules Scrofulous swellings or numbness of the limbs. Slimy or unclean tongue fur	Dispersing phlegm and softening hardness Freeing the connecting channels	Prunella Paste Scrofula-Dispersing Pills Secret Formulary Poria Pills	LI-4 ST-36 Local points
Phlegm Lodging in the Chest and Lateral Costal Region	Distention and fullness in the chest and lateral costal region Pain caused by breathing or coughing Dyspnea with distressed rapid breathing Possibly facial edema slippery pulse (possibly wiry)	Transforming rheum and Expelling phlegm	Minor Cyan Dragon Decoction T'ing Li Tzu and Jujube Lung-Draining Decoction Ten Jujubes Decoction Drool-Controlling Elixir	TB-6 TB-5 CV-17 GB-34 SP-9 LV-13 ST-40

Notes

[1] Tetanus refers to the disease also known as lockjaw. By contrast, (muscular) tetany is a term denoting certain forms of spasm. See Glossary for further elaboration.

Chapter 11
Exogenous Heat Disease

Pattern Identification

Exogenous heat diseases are caused by invasion of exogenous pathogens, and are characterized by fever in their early stages. They correspond in Western medicine to acute infectious diseases and include bacterial and viral infections and sunstroke.

The vast body of theory concerning the identification of exogenous heat disease patterns, forming a primary constituent of Chinese medicine, was built on millenia of experience. The earliest extant compilation dealing with exogenous heat diseases is *A Treatise on Cold Damage,* written in the Han Dynasty, which identifies and treats diseases according to their location within the six channels. Further accumulation of experience and developments in theory in the ages that followed culminated in the theory of thermic diseases. *A Treatise on Thermic Heat Diseases* and *Systematized Identification of Thermic Diseases* are two works of the Qing Dynasty that further synthesized the laws governing the origin and development of exogenous heat diseases into the system known as four-aspect pattern identification and treatment. As a result of these latter-day developments there have emerged two separate schools of thought, the "cold-damage" school and the "thermic diseases" school.

The major contention between the cold-damage school and the thermic diseases school concerns the definition and scope of the two systems. The cold-damage school claims that all heat diseases belong to the category of cold-damage, and that six-channel pattern identification is applicable to all exogenous heat diseases. By contrast, the thermic diseases school interprets the term cold-damage in a narrow sense, and considers six-channel pattern identification and treatment inapplicable to what it regards as thermic diseases. The most widely accepted view today is that thermic disease theory is based on and developed from cold-damage theory. Both represent a synthesis of experience, and may be used together in clinical practice.

Exogenous heat diseases bear two main characteristics: fever and stage-by-stage development. Fever results from the fierce struggle between correct qi and the pathogen, and is the essential characteristic of exogenous heat diseases. Its progress reflects the changing relationship between correct qi and pathogenic qi. For example, high fever reflects the strong reaction of an undamaged correct qi to a highly toxic pathogen. The fever will gradually subside as correct qi overcomes the pathogen. A remittent fever or persistent fever reflects a condition where the pathogen has weakened but has not been fully eradicated and correct qi has suffered damage. Absence of initial-stage fever, or even a sudden drop in body temperature, are signs of yang collapse as a result of the presence of a highly toxic pathogen and extreme vacuity of the correct.

Exogenous heat diseases usually develop through three stages: the initial stage, the exuberant fever stage, and the recovery stage. These three stages reflect the changing relationship between the pathogen and the correct. In the initial stage, the struggle between the pathogen and the correct has still not reached its height, so that the fever is less severe than in the exuberant fever stage. As the struggle becomes more intense, the disease moves into the exuberant fever stage; symptoms are most pronounced, indicating that the disease has reached its climax. It is at this crucial stage that deterioration or improvement is decided. If the correct defeats the pathogen, the disease passes into the recovery stage. If it fails to do so, the patient's condition deteriorates, leading to possible death. Of course, recovery may come about at any point during the progression of a disease if pathogenic qi weakens and correct qi strengthens, either spontaneously or by appropriate treatment. Similarly, deterioration or relapse may occur at any time if pathogenic qi strengthens and correct qi weakens, either spontaneously or by inappropriate treatment. Most incidences of exogenous heat diseases are characterized by the above-mentioned three stages.

In addition to describing six-channel and four-aspect pattern identification and treatment, this chapter offers some views about combining the two in clinical practice. We should also point out that another method, triple burner pattern identification, which also forms part of the thermic diseases theory, is omitted from this chapter since it largely corresponds to four-aspect pattern identification.

Six-Channel Pattern Identification

Six-channel pattern identification was first mentioned in *The Inner Canon* and subsequently refined in *A Treatise on Cold Damage*. The latter represents a systematic synthesis of pre—Han Dynasty experience and theory concerning exogenous heat diseases, and elaborated on the six-channel patterns discussed in *Essential Questions*,[1] in which observable signs and disease shifts are explained in terms of tai yang, yang ming, and shao yang diseases (collectively known as the three yang channel diseases), and tai yin, shao yin, and jue yin diseases (collectively known as the three yin channel diseases). It describes the principal patterns, the methods and formulae used to treat them, as well as combined and transmuted patterns and sequences of channel passage. *A Treatise on Cold Damage* is considered the basis of identification and treatment of exogenous heat disease patterns; the pathology, methods of treatment, formulae, and drugs it discusses are used as a guide for endogenous damage and miscellaneous disease as well.

In this section, only the principal patterns, methods of treatment, and formulae for the diseases of each of the six channels are discussed. Combined patterns and points relating to endogenous damage and miscellaneous diseases are beyond the scope of this book.

Tai yang disease

Pattern identification

Tai yang diseases are characterized by aversion to cold or wind, headache, and a floating pulse. *A Treatise on Cold Damage* states, "When the tai yang is diseased, there is a floating pulse, headache, stiffness in the neck, and aversion to cold." Usually there is fever. Generalized pain, and tension and stiffness in the neck and back are among the other possible signs.

This pattern is seen in many initial-stage exogenous heat diseases, and in terms of eight-parameter pattern identification it is a cold pattern. According to explanations of the cold-damage theory, exogenous heat diseases are mostly attributable to contraction of the wind-cold pathogen, which first affects the yang channels. Of the yang channels, the first to be affected is the tai yang; consequently it is said to govern the exterior of the body. The tai yang channel passes through the head and neck, so that when its qi is depressed by an invading wind-cold pathogen, stiffness and pain occur in this region. Aversion to cold or wind and fever is the pathological reaction of a body whose correct qi (construction and defense) is struggling to resist pathogenic qi. The floating pulse reflects that the disease is in the exterior. Although *A Treatise on Cold Damage* makes no reference to the tongue or its fur, it is important to note that in most cases the tongue fur is thin, white and moist.

Differentiation between vacuity and repletion of the exterior is of crucial importance in identification of tai yang diseases. Judgement rests largely on the following factors: the presence or absence of aversion to cold or wind; whether the floating pulse is tight or moderate; and most crucially, the presence or absence of perspiration. Exterior vacuity patterns are diaphoretic. They most commonly occur where, owing to construction-defense disharmony, the striations are unsound and allow sweat to flow, while resistance is inadequate to expel the pathogen. In exterior repletion patterns, which occur when the cold pathogen invades tai yang, sweating does not occur since the pathogen impedes construction qi, leading to blockage of the striations.

Treatment

The principal method used to treat tai yang diseases is diaphoresis, i.e., exterior resolution. Its effect is to free defense qi, open the striations, and expel the pathogen from the body through sweating.

Drug therapy

Tai yang diseases characterized by the cold pathogen present in the exterior are treated by resolving the exterior with warm, pungent agents. Tai yang exterior repletion patterns, pathomechanically explained as obstruction of defense qi by an exogenous pathogen leading to blockage of the striations, are treated by promoting diffusion and dissipating the pathogen using the diaphoretic Ephedra Decoction *(má-huáng tāng)*. Exterior vacuity patterns, pathomechanically explained as construction-defense disharmony preventing expulsion of the pathogen, are primarily treated by harmonizing construction and defense, using Cinnamon-Twig Decoction *(guì-zhī tāng)* which resolves the muscles. Ephedra Decoction, containing both Herba Ephedrae *(má huáng)* and Ramulus Cinnamomi *(guì zhī)*, dissipates the pathogen. Cinnamon-Twig Decoction, containing Ramulus Cinnamomi *(guì zhī)* and Radix Paeoniae Albae *(bái sháo)*, is mainly designed to harmonize construction and defense as a prerequisite for expulsion of the pathogen.

Both Ephedra Decoction and Cinnamon-Twig Decoction are formulae that are varied frequently. A number of important formulae are derived from Ephedra Decoction. For example, Major Cyan Dragon Decoction *(dà qīng lóng tāng)* treats patterns comprising signs such as agitation and absense of sweating, which arise when exterior cold, failing diaphoretic resolution, becomes depressed and transforms into heat. Minor Cyan Dragon Decoction *(xiǎo qīng lóng tāng)* is used for dual patterns of exterior cold and interior rheum, where exterior signs such as aversion to cold, fever, and absence of thirst are accompanied by pronounced cough and dyspnea. Ephedra, Apricot, Gypsum and Liquorice Decoction *(má xìng shí gān tāng)* treats heat gathering in the lung, characterized by heat, thirst, cough and dyspnea. Cinnamon-Twig Decoction *(guì-zhī tāng)* may be varied depending on the symptoms. For instance, Radix Puerariae *(gé gēn)* may be added when signs include stiffness in the neck and back, while Cortex Magnoliae *(hòu pò)* and Semen Pruni Armeniacae *(xìng rén)* may be added for the treatment of patterns that include dyspnea. Most patterns treated by Cinnamon-Twig Decoction, Ephedra Decoction, and their variants fall within the scope of tai yang disease.

Acumoxatherapy

A Treatise on Cold Damage identifies each stage of disease by its associated symptoms and appropriate formula. Essentially concerned with drug therapy, the book mentions few acupuncture points.[2] In general, points such as LI-4 and TB-5 are chosen to resolve the exterior, while GV-16, GB-20, and ST-8 may be used to dispel wind. Other points are chosen according to the presenting symptoms and the patient's constitution. Some examples are listed below:

Stiff neck, aversion to cold: GB-20‡, GV-12, BL-12‡, GV-16

Headache: LI-4, GB-20, ST-8, BL-62

Retching, aversion to wind: TB-5, LI-4

Aversion to cold: GV-14‡, CV-8 (moxa only)

Generalized itching; to promote perspiration: BL-67, LI-11

To stop perspiration: HT-6‡

Absence of sweating: LI-4, LU-8

Alternating fever and chills: GV-14, PC-5, LI-4

To clear heat: GV-14, LI-11, ST-44

Dry throat: KI-6, KI-7, CV-23

Agitation: KI-7, PC-5

Vomiting and counterflow: CV-13, ST-36

Delirious speech: HT-7, CV-13, ST-40

Hypertonicity in the leg: BL-60, BL-57

Lower back pain: SI-3, BL-54

Fullness in the chest with costal pain: PC-6, GB-34, GB-41

Cough and dyspnea: LU-9, CV-12, CV-22

To downbear phlegm: ST-40

Hiccough: PC-6

Thirst: LU-9, CV-12

Yang ming disease

Pattern identification

Yang ming diseases are characterized by generalized fever and sweating, aversion to heat, agitation, and thirst, or in more severe cases, abdominal fullness and pain, constipation, and even delirious mania. The tongue fur is usually dry and old yellow in color. The pulse is generally surging and large, slippery and rapid, or strong, deep, and replete.

Yang ming disease generally occurs in the exuberant fever stage of exogenous heat diseases, and presents, in terms of the eight parameters, as interior heat or interior repletion. It may be divided into two broad categories: yang ming channel patterns and yang ming bowel patterns. Yang ming channel patterns are associated with the four greatnesses: great heat, profuse sweating, pronounced agitation, and a large, surging pulse. Yang ming bowel patterns comprise tidal fever, delirious speech, a hard, full, distended abdomen with pain that is exacerbated by pressure, constipation, burnt yellow or old yellow tongue fur, and a strong, deep, replete pulse. In yang ming channel patterns, the gastric liquid is damaged by exuberant heat, although there is no heat-bind in the yang ming bowels (the stomach and large intestine). Yang ming bowel patterns are so named because they arise when a pathogen binds with digestate accumulation or dry waste in the stomach or intestines, giving rise to repletion heat.

Treatment

The main methods used for the treatment of yang ming disease are clearage and precipitation.

Drug therapy

Heat clearing applies to yang ming channel patterns, and involves the use of heat-clearing and fire-draining agents to safeguard liquid. White Tiger Decoction *(bái hǔ tāng)* is the basic formula, to which Radix Ginseng *(rén shēn)* may be added to boost qi and engender liquid in cases of damage to both qi and yin. Precipitation applies to yang ming bowel patterns, and involves the use of cold, bitter precipitants that flush the gastrointestinal heat accumulation. The principal formula is Major Purgative Decoction *(dà chéng qì tāng)*.

Classically, the pattern treated by Major Purgative Decoction *(dà chéng qì tāng)* is summed up in four signs: glomus, fullness, dryness, and repletion. Glomus refers to the painful glomus-bind in the abdomen. Fullness refers to abdominal fullness and distention. Dryness refers to dry waste in the intestines, as well as attendant symptoms such as restlessness and thirst, and dry tongue fur. Repletion refers to repletion of the bowels, characterized by constipation, and the presence of pathogenic heat and stagnation in the intestines. If dryness and repletion signs are not pronounced, Minor Purgative Decoction *(xiǎo chéng qì tāng)* is used. Where the glomus and fullness are not pronounced, Stomach-Regulating Purgative Decoction *(tiáo wèi chéng qì tāng)* may be used.

Acumoxatherapy

Yang ming channel patterns may be treated with points such as LI-15, LI-11, TB-5, and ST-44 to clear heat, together with PC-5, BL-11, ST-40, ST-36, and CV-12 which harmonize the center, clear gastrointestinal heat, and fortify center qi. Yang ming bowel patterns require points such as TB-2, BL-57, and TB-6, to moisten and harmonize the intestines, along with LI-11 and ST-44 to clear heat and harmonize the intestines. Other points are added according to the symptoms:

Constipation: BL-25, TB-6, BL-57, LU-6

Clear-food diarrhea: CV-8 (moxa only), ST-25, ST-36

Abdominal fullness: ST-36, BL-57, ST-44

Pain below the ribs: PC-7, GB-34

Jaundice: BL-67, BL-17, SI-4, SP-4

Inhibited urination: CV-3, SP-9

Tidal fever: GV-14, PC-5, TB-6, BL-57

Vomiting: PC-6, SP-4, CV-13, ST-36

Stasis heat: BL-17, SP-6, SP-4

Shao yang disease

Pattern identification

The essential symptoms characterizing shao yang disease are alternating fever and chills, pain and bitter fullness in the chest and lateral costal region, bitter taste in the mouth, and vomiting. Other patterns include no desire for food and drink, restlessness, desire to vomit, visual dizziness, and painful, hard, hypochondriac glomus. The pulse is usually wiry.

Shao yang disease occurs when, owing to debilitation of correct qi, a pathogen invades the body through the striations and binds the gallbladder, impeding qi dynamic and disrupting upbearing and downbearing. Bitter fullness in the chest and lateral costal region is explained by the shao yang gallbladder channel that traverses this area. Alternating fever and chills are explained by the struggle between the pathogen and the correct. Restlessness, bitter taste in the mouth, dry pharynx, visual dizziness, as well as vomiting and no desire for food and drink, are the result of gallbladder heat rising counterflow up the channel, disturbing the harmony and downbearing of gastric qi. A wiry pulse is classically associated with the gallbladder. Shao yang disease is different from tai yang and yang ming disease, lying midway between the two. Tai yang disease can pass to both yang ming and shao yang. Shao yang disease may resolve in an exterior pattern through a constant sweat, or may pass to the yang ming to form an interior pattern. It may pass to the yin channels, giving rise to vacuity patterns. Consequently, shao yang disease is commonly termed a midstage pattern. However, it may occur in combination with an exterior pattern characterized by fever, aversion to cold, and nagging pain in the joints of the limbs, or with a yang ming interior pattern characterized by fullness and distention in the abdomen and constipation.

Treatment

Shao yang disease is treated by the method of harmonization and resolution. This involves outthrusting the pathogen and clearing the interior, and regulating qi dynamic, in accordance with the principle of supporting the correct and dispelling the pathogen.

Drug therapy

The chief formula used is Minor Bupleurum Decoction *(xiǎo chái-hú tāng)*. However, where an exterior pattern is also present, giving rise to a tai yang and shao yang combination, diaphoretic action is needed. In such cases, Bupleurum and Cinnamon Decoction *(chái-hú guì-zhī tāng)* may be used. Concurrence of an interior repletion pattern, forming a shao yang and yang ming combination, may be treated with Major Bupleurum Decoction *(dà chái-hú tāng)* which possesses an additional precipitant effect.

Acumoxatherapy

Shao yang disease may be treated with PC-5, CV-13, GB-41, and GB-34, to clear heat from the liver, gallbladder, and pericardium, open the chest, and resolve depressed heat. Tai yang and shao yang combinations may require the addition of GB-20, TB-5, and LI-4 to help expel the pathogen. Other points are added according to the symptoms:

Pain in the chest and lateral costal region: TB-6, GB-34

Nausea: PC-6

Vomiting: PC-6, SP-4, ST-36

Dry pharynx: TB-2, TB-3

Visual dizziness: GB-15

Hard stool: TB-6

Diarrhea with discomfort unrelieved by evacuation: LI-11, ST-36

Fever: TB-10, GB-34

Alternating fever and chills: TB-10, GB-34, GV-14, PC-5

It is interesting to note that the majority of points used are on the hand and foot shao yang channels. Also prominent are points on the jue yin channels (pericardium and liver), which have an interior-exterior correspondence with the shao yang.

Tai yin disease

Pattern identification

Tai yin disease is characterized by abdominal fullness with periodic pain, vomiting, diarrhea, non-movement of ingested food, absence of thirst, and a weak, moderate pulse.

The pathomechanism of tai yin disease is failure of movement and transformation of the digestate, resulting from devitalization of splenic yang, and manifesting as vomiting and diarrhea. The abdominal distention is explained by splenic vacuity qi stagnation, while the abdominal pain results from vacuity cold. Although it rarely occurs naturally in the progression of exogenous heat diseases, it may arise when incorrect treatment of yang diseases, such as inappropriate precipitation in tai yang and shao yang disease, or excessive use of cold and cool flow-restorative precipitants in yang ming disease, damages splenic yang. It may also occur when, owing to a regular spleen qi vacuity, the cold pathogen enters the tai yin directly. This is known as a direct strike on tai yin. Like the yang ming bowel pattern, tai yin disease is a digestive tract disorder, but presents as vacuity rather than as repletion. It is characterized by vomiting, diarrhea, absence of thirst, vacuity fullness and pain, and a weak, moderate pulse, whereas yang ming bowel patterns are identified by the presence of constipation, thirst, great repletion and fullness, and a deep, replete pulse. It is said, "Tai yin disease is associated with vacuity, and yang ming disease is associated with repletion."

Treatment

Since tai yin disease is attributable to damage to splenic yang by cold, it is treated by warming the center and dissipating cold, and by restoring the correct and fortifying the spleen.

Drug therapy

The principal formula is Center-Rectifying Pills (lǐ zhōng wán). Where interior cold is pronounced, Aconite Center-Rectifying Decoction (fù-zǐ lǐ zhōng tāng) is used, which is the same formula with the addition of Radix Aconiti Fu Tzu (fù zǐ).

Acumoxatherapy

Tai yin diseases with vacuity cold symptoms such as vomiting, diarrhea, and abdominal fullness can be treated with points such as LI-4, ST-25‡, GB-20, and ST-36‡, which supplement and move qi, particularly in the middle burner.

If there is hard binding below the chest, PC-6 and SP-4 may be added. If there is abdominal fullness, such points as SP-6‡, LI-4, TB-5, ST-25‡, ST-36‡, and CV-6‡ may be used.

If there is accumulation and pain in the lower abdomen, which may be described as a condition of repletion due to vacuity, points such as LI-4, ST-36, TB-6, ST-25, and BL-57 are added.

Shao yin disease

Pattern identification

Shao yin disease may take two different forms. The main form manifests as aversion to cold, curled recumbent posture, somnolence, inversion frigidity of the limbs, and a fine, faint pulse. Clear-food diarrhea may occur in some cases. Generally there is no fever, and in severe cases the limbs may suffer a drop in temperature, indicating yang collapse vacuity desertion. The other form is a vacuity heat pattern comprising restlessness, insomnia, and dry pharynx and mouth. *A Treatise on Cold Damage* provides little detail concerning the latter pattern, although clinical observation shows that a red or crimson tongue, and a fine, rapid, or vacuous, rapid pulse are determining symptoms.

Shao yin disease arises when the heart and kidney are vacuous, and there is a marked drop in resistance to disease. It is clearly distinguished from the devitalization of splenic yang associated with tai yin disease. In *A Treatise on Cold Damage,* the section on shao yin disease is headed with the statement, "The patient has a fine, faint pulse, and desires only to sleep." A fine, faint pulse indicates vacuity of the qi and blood, and desire only for sleep indicates debilitation of the spirit. These are both signs of general vacuity. Wherever a fine, faint pulse occurs, whether in disease of recent onset or enduring disease, thought should be given to the possibility of shao yin disease. Absence of fever and aversion to cold, curled recumbent posture, and inversion frigidity of the limbs occurring with this pulse indicate inner-body exuberance of yin cold and inability of debilitated yang qi to warm and nourish the skin and muscle and fully permeate the limbs, and provide confirmation of shao yin vacuity cold. Clear-food diarrhea is explained by kidney vacuity affecting the spleen (splenorenal yang vacuity), causing failure to move and transform the digestate. Profuse sweating, inversion frigidity of the limbs, and a faint pulse verging on expiry indicate fulminant desertion of yang qi.

Cardiorenal vacuity may be primarily a vacuity either of yin or of yang. Therefore, shao yin disease may manifest as restlessness, insomnia, dry pharynx, dry mouth, red to crimson tongue, and a fine, rapid pulse, indicating insufficiency of kidney yin and upflaming of heart fire. However, since the cold pathogen readily damages yang, vacuity cold is the essential and most commonly encountered shao yin disease pattern. The vacuity heat pattern is a transmuted shao yin pattern, and is much rarer.

Treatment

Shao yin vacuity cold patterns are treated by the method of salvaging yang and checking counterflow.

Drug therapy

The most appropriate formula is Counterflow Cold Decoction *(sì nì tāng)*. Vacuity heat patterns are chiefly treated by enriching yin and clearing heat. The principal formula is Coptis and Ass-Hide Glue Decoction *(huáng-lián ē-jiāo tāng)*.

Counterflow Cold Decoction may be varied to suit different patterns. Radix Ginseng *(rén shēn)* may be added where vacuity is prominent, while

Rhizoma Zingiberis Exsiccatum *(gān jiāng)* may be increased in quantity where cold is prominent. Where exuberant yin repels yang, pig's bile may be added. Patterns that include signs of water qi may be treated with True Warrior Decoction *(zhēn wǔ tāng)*, a variant of Counterflow Cold Decoction *(sì nì tāng)*.

Acumoxatherapy

General points for the treatment of shao yin disease include GV-4‡, CV-8 (moxa only), KI-3‡, CV-6‡, and ST-36‡. Accompanying symptoms may be treated with the points listed below:

> Desire only for sleep: GV-5
>
> Ungratified desire to vomit: PC-6
>
> Irritability: PC-6, HT-7
>
> Thirst: KI-3
>
> Lower-burner vacuity cold: CV-3‡, LI-4‡
>
> Shao yin vacuity fire sore throat: KI-6, LU-10, LU-7
>
> Cough and diarrhea: LU-9, LU-7, CV-6, BL-62, BL-25
>
> Inhibited urination: CV-3, BL-28, BL-22, BL-53
>
> Articular pain: KI-3, HT-7
>
> Generalized aching: LI-4, LI-3
>
> Hand and foot pain: moxa at CV-4
>
> Hemafecia: GV-4‡, BL-22, BL-29, GV-1
>
> Water qi: moxa at CV-6 and BL-20
>
> Diarrhea: CV-8 (moxa only), ST-25‡, CV-6‡, ST-36‡
>
> Counterflow frigidity: TB-5
>
> Vomiting with cough: PC-5, PC-6
>
> Vomiting with diarrhea: moxa CV-12

Jue yin disease

In the classical sequence, the jue yin is the last of the three yin channels. Hence, in theory it should be associated with the most severe pathologies. *Essential Questions,* states, "The jue yin channel skirts round the genitals and connects with the liver, so that pathologies include restlessness and fullness, and retraction of the scrotum." The same chapter also mentions, among the symptoms of jue yin disease, "deafness, retraction of the scrotum, inability to ingest {even} liquid foods, and failure to recognize people." *Essential Questions* enumerates symptoms but prescribes no formulae. Because the jue yin patterns described in *A Treatise on Cold*

Damage are less severe, the real nature of jue yin disease is still in question. Further research is required to clarify the matter fully.

Pattern identification

Jue yin disease as described in *A Treatise on Cold Damage* is characterized by upper-body heat and lower-body cold, and may take the form of diabetic disease, qi surging up into the cardiac region, pain and heat in the cardiac region, hunger with no desire to eat, or vomiting of roundworms. Inversion frigidity of the limbs is also observed in some cases.

Pathomechanically, upper-body heat and lower-body cold is explained as a cold-heat complex resulting from interior vacuity. Diabetic disease, qi surging up into the cardiac region, pain and heat in the cardiac region, and clamoring stomach discomfort are the manifestations of upper-body heat (heat in the area just above the diaphragm). No desire for food and vomiting of roundworms reflect lower-body cold (in the intestines). This impairs movement and transformation of the digestate, which disquiets the roundworm and causes it to rise counterflow. The inversion frigidity of the limbs indicates failure of yang qi to reach the periphery of the body, arising when a cold-heat complex disrupts qi dynamic.

Treatment

Jue yin upper-body heat and lower-body cold patterns are treated by addressing the cold-heat complex resulting from interior vacuity. Thus, the basic treatment is supplementation to eliminate vacuity, complemented by simultaneous warming and clearing to eliminate cold and heat.

Drug therapy

The classical formula devised for this pattern is Mume Pills *(wū méi wán)*. The same formula, by dint of its additional roundworm-quieting effect, is currently used to treat biliary tract ascariasis. Since this disease falls within the category of miscellaneous diseases and is not necessarily a result of interior vacuity, the application of Mume Pills is now broader than originally intended.

In the chapter relating to jue yin disease, *A Treatise on Cold Damage* cites alternating fever and inversion frigidity of the limbs and various other patterns of inversion frigidity of the limbs, diarrhea, vomiting, and hiccough. Although alternating fever and inversion frigidity of the limbs in theory indicates a cold-heat complex resulting from interior vacuity, it is rare in clinical practice. Patterns comprised of inversion frigidity of the limbs, diarrhea, vomiting, and hiccough may occur in both exogenous heat diseases and endogenous and miscellaneous diseases. Since they are not essentially associated with jue yin disease, they are omitted from this section.

Acumoxatherapy

Cheng Dan-An suggests that BL-18 and LV-14 be needled to course the liver and prevent stagnation of liver blood. Moxibustion at CV-12 and ST-36 can downbear stomach qi. Moxa at CV-6 is suggested to course the lower burner qi and blood. Cheng also suggests moxa at SI-5 and needling of LI-4 to course the qi and blood of the limbs. Other points may be added according to the symptoms:

Parasites: ST-4

Qi surging up into the heart: LV-3, PC-6

Interior heat, exterior cold: LI-11, LI-4, TB-2, ST-36, GB-41

Interior cold: CV-12‡, ST-36‡, CV-8 (moxa only), ST-25‡, CV-4‡

(Any) pathogen in the chest: PC-6

Racing of the heart: CV-14, CV-9, SP-9

Vacuity irritability and insomnia: PC-5, ST-45

Heat diarrhea: LI-11, LI-4, BL-25, BL-29, BL-30, ST-36

The pathomechanisms and principal signs of six-channel diseases, together with methods of treatment and formulae are presented schematically in the tables at the end of this chapter.

The system of six-channel pattern identification and treatment posited in *A Treatise on Cold Damage* emphasizes the yin-yang, interior-exterior, vacuity-repletion, and cold-heat parameters in identifying exogenous heat disease patterns. The diseases associated with each of the channels have different eight-parameter characteristics:

Eight-parameter Characteristics	
Tai yang	exterior cold
Yang ming	interior heat, interior repletion
Shao yang	midstage complex resulting from interior vacuity
Tai yin	damage to spleen by cold
Shao yin	cardiorenal vacuity and general debilitation
Jue yin	interior vacuity

However, the six-channel patterns are interrelated, and disease may shift from one to another. As a rule, the initial and middle stages of exogenous heat diseases — while the strength of correct qi can match that of the invading pathogen — are associated with disease in the yang channels characterized by heat and repletion. If correct qi is gradually debilitated, yin channel patterns occur as the disease progresses. These are associated mainly with repletion and cold, and less commonly with vacuity heat patterns and cold-heat complexes. Pre-febrile yang channel diseases generally start in tai yang, from where they may pass to other channels. The order of disease passage through the yang channels may be schematically presented as follows:

tai yang → shao yang / yang ming ↑

Yin channel patterns usually occur in the advanced stages of disease. However, resistance and strength of pathogen varies with the individual; thus passage from channel to channel is subject to no absolutely rigid sequence. Sometimes disease may be present in more than one channel at one time. The simultaneous affection of two yang channels is generally referred to as a combination disease. For example, combination disease of shao yang and yang ming is characterized by shao yang signs such as alternating fever and chills, and pain and distress in the chest and lateral costal region, as well as yang ming signs such fullness and pain in the abdomen, constipation, and yellow tongue fur. Disease simultaneously present in yang and yin channels is known as a dual affection. An example of this is dual affection of the tai yang and shao yin, which in the initial stages is characterized by fever and deep pulse. Yang ming and shao yang diseases generally develop from tai yang disease. However, yang ming and shao yang patterns may appear at onset, in which case the the disease is said to originate in channel.

Yin channel patterns generally develop out of yang channel patterns, but the appearance of a yin pattern at onset, known as a direct strike, is not excluded. Thus six-channel diseases may be regarded both as six stages in the progression of a disease, or as six different diseases. Shift from exterior to interior and from yang to yin reflects the advance of disease and debilitation of correct qi, while progression from interior to exterior and from yin to yang indicates the defeat of the pathogen and improvement in the patient's condition. Each channel disease cannot therefore be considered in isolation. Successful identification and treatment of exogenous heat diseases is dependent on understanding the interrelationship of six-channel diseases and the struggle between correct and pathogenic qi.

Four-Aspect Pattern Identification and Treatment

The theory of thermic diseases, which appeared relatively late in the history of Chinese medicine, has it own system of classifying diseases and disease factors, and explaining pathomechanisms. Accordingly, it has its own system of pattern identification and treatment.

Proponents of the theory state that thermic disease is a term embracing all exogenous heat diseases. The common denominator of all such diseases is heat rather than cold, and consequently they show a tendency toward dryness formation and resultant damage to yin. Although the theory identifies many different diseases, the major classifications are wind thermia, damp thermia, and thermic heat. Generally, diseases characterized by fever, and signs of exuberant lung or stomach heat such as cough, rapid breathing, flaring of the nostrils, and thirst, fall into the category of wind thermia. Diseases characterized by persistent fever and signs of obstruction and stagnation caused by damp, such as oppression in the chest, nausea, diminished appetite, abdominal distention, constipation or diarrhea, and slimy tongue fur, fall into the category of damp thermia. Diseases characterized by high fever, red complexion, thirst, maculopapular eruptions, restlessness and, in severe cases, clouding of the spirit, fall within the category of thermic heat. The development of such diseases is subject to specific laws, and in most cases the system of four-aspect pattern identification and treatment may be used.

Defense, qi, construction, and blood are the four aspects used for identification and treatment of thermic disease patterns.[3] They are used to explain the origin and development of exogenous heat diseases; like the six channels of the cold-damage theory, they explain the degree of penetration, severity, and acuteness of diseases. In *A Treatise on Thermic Heat Diseases*, Ye Tian-shi states:

> The general conception {of the theory of thermic diseases} is that qi is subjacent to defense and that blood is subjacent to construction. When disease affects defense, diaphoretic treatment may be given. Only when it reaches the qi aspect can qi-clearing treatment be prescribed. When it enters construction, treatment involves outthrust of heat to the qi aspect. Finally, when it reaches blood and causes depletion and frenetic movement, blood cooling and dissipation is prescribed.

These lines represent the general outline of the four-aspect pattern identification and treatment system of the theory of thermic diseases.

Although the four-aspect system originated in *A Treatise on Thermic Heat Diseases*, it is derived from the practical experience and theoretical knowledge accumulated over generations. Because *A Treatise on Thermic Heat Diseases* is largely a theoretical work and devotes only scant attention to actual formulae and drugs, this chapter draws on other relevant works as well as practical clinical experience.

Defense-aspect patterns

Pattern identification

Defense-aspect patterns principally include fever, slight aversion to cold, presence or absence of sweating, and dry mouth. The tongue is distinctly red and the pulse is floating and rapid. In some cases there may also be headache, cough, and sore, red pharynx, and in others, pressure in the head, clouded head, oppression in the chest, and upflow and nausea.

Defense-aspect patterns include signs common to the initial stage of all exogenous heat diseases. Of these signs, fever and slight aversion to wind and cold are the essential indicators of defense-aspect disease. Like tai yang disease of the cold-damage theory, defense-aspect disease is seen as an exterior pattern in terms of the eight parameters. However, while tai yang disease may generally be classified as caused by cold, defense-aspect disease is classified as caused by heat.

Thermic pathogens enter the body through the nose and mouth, invariably invading the lung first. The lung is connected with the surface skin and body hair and governs the exterior and defense. Thus, when it is invaded by an exogenous pathogen, the defensive exterior is depressed and obstructed, giving rise to fever and slight aversion to cold. This is the fundamental law applied to defense-aspect disease. Thermic pathogens are hot in nature, so that defense-aspect patterns include heat signs, and as such differ from tai yang exterior patterns, which tend to be marked by cold signs.

Once a defense-aspect pattern has been identified, it is usually necessary to determine whether the thermic pathogen is accompanied by wind or damp. Wind thermia patterns are generally characterized by signs of lung heat such as cough, sore pharynx, and distinctly red tongue. Damp thermia patterns are characterized by signs of damp turbidity obstructing the center such as general sensations of heaviness, oppression in the chest, upflow and nausea, dry throat with no desire for fluid, and a distinctly slimy tongue.

Treatment

Defense-aspect patterns are chiefly treated by the method of resolving the exterior with cool and pungent agents that discharge the thermic pathogens from the defense aspect.

Drug therapy

A commonly used formula is Lonicera and Forsythia Powder *(yín qiào sǎn)*, which not only resolves the exterior but also clears heat and resolves toxins. Mild patterns that include wind signs may be treated with Mulberry and Chrysanthemum Cool Decoction *(sāng jú yǐn)*. Damp complexes may be treated with such agents as:

Damp-Resolving Agents	
Talcum	*huá shí*
Sclerotium Poriae	*fú líng*
Herba Agastaches	*huò xiāng*
Rhizoma Atractylodis	*cāng zhú*
Semen Glycenes Germinatum	*dà dòu juǎn*

A commonly used formula is Agastache, Magnolia, Pinellia, and Poria Decoction *(huò pò xià líng tāng)*, which promotes qi diffusion and transforms damp with aromatic agents.

Acumoxatherapy

Defense-aspect patterns are treated by resolving the exterior and expelling wind by needling points such as LI-4 and BL-13. SI-3 secures the exterior and expels heat. LU-10 and LI-11 are used to clear heat. PC-6, SP-9, and CV-12 are used for damp causing such signs as oppression in the chest and a slimy tongue fur.

Qi-aspect patterns

Pattern identification

Qi-aspect patterns are generally characterized by fever, aversion to heat rather than cold, thirst, bitter taste in the mouth, and yellow or dark-colored urine. The pulse is rapid and the tongue fur is yellow or yellow and white. There may be impeded or copious perspiration, and unabating fever. Qi-aspect disease is broad in scope, including a large variety of exuberant fever stage exogenous heat diseases. These may be divided as follows:

First-stage qi-aspect heat:

Principal signs include general fever, thirst, restlessness, upper ventral vexation, and mixed yellow and white tongue fur.

Exuberant pulmogastric heat:

Exuberant pulmogastric heat presents the classical signs of wind thermia: high fever, cough, rapid breathing, thirst, and yellow tongue fur.

Great heat in the qi aspect:

Equivalent to yang ming channel disease (see previous section).

Gastrointestinal heat-bind:

Equivalent to the yang ming bowel pattern (see previous section).

Damp-heat lodging in the triple burner:

Damp-heat lodging in the triple burner presents the classical signs of damp thermia: persistent remittent fever, oppression in the chest, thirst without great intake of fluids, upflow nausea, abdominal distention, and short micturition with scant urine. The tongue fur is slimy in nature and either white or slightly yellow in color. The pulse is soggy and rapid. Also observable at this stage is brewing damp-heat steaming the intestines and stomach, characterized either by oppression in the chest and hard stool or by foul-smelling diarrhea. The tongue fur is yellow and slimy and the pulse deep, slippery, and rapid.

Despite the multiplicity of qi-aspect patterns, they have in common signs of exuberant heat, indicating that although the pathogen is advancing, correct qi is still offering firm resistance. First-stage qi-aspect disease is marked by restlessness and upper ventral vexation, indicating that the pathogen is in the area immediately above the diaphragm. The mixed yellow and white tongue fur shows that the pathogen has not fully entered the interior, and that resolution can be brought about by outthrusting the pathogen. If the disease advances further, the pathogen penetrates into the interior, giving rise either to great heat in the qi aspect, which is an interior heat pattern characterized by damage to liquid by exuberant heat, or to gastrointestinal heat-bind, which is an interior repletion pattern. These two patterns are equivalent to the yang ming channel and yang ming bowel patterns of the cold-damage theory. The only difference is the rapidity of development. The thermic pathogen falls inward and transforms into heat faster than it takes a pathogen to pass from the tai yang to the yang ming. Thus, *A Treatise on Thermic Heat* states:

> Cold-damage pathogens first lodge in the exterior, before transforming into heat and entering the interior. Thermic pathogens change into heat far more quickly.

Marked differences are observed between wind and damp thermia in the qi aspect. Wind thermia may take the form of first-stage qi-aspect heat, great heat in the qi aspect, gastrointestinal heat-bind, or exuberant pulmogastric heat. This latter pattern is characterized by pronounced signs of exuberant heat and of heat brewing in the lung and stomach. The four major signs are heat, thirst, cough, and dyspnea. Damp thermia presents differently. It is marked by unsurfaced fever and steaming of the stomach by brewing damp-heat. It develops slowly over a relatively long period of time; hence the term lingering damp-heat.

Treatment

Qi-aspect patterns are treated by the method of clearing heat.

Drug therapy

First-stage qi-aspect heat is treated with Gardenia and Fermented Soybean Decoction *(zhī-zǐ shì tāng)* to clear heat and outthrust pathogens. The main formula treating exuberant pulmogastric heat is Ephedra, Apricot, Gypsum, and Liquorice Decoction *(má xìng shí gān tāng)* which clears heat and diffuses the lung. This formula may be combined with heat-clearing phlegm-transforming formulae such as Minor Chest-Bind Decoction *(xiǎo xiàn xiōng tāng)*, and further supplemented with heat-clearing toxin-resolving agents such as:

Heat-Clearing and Toxin-Resolving Agents	
Flos Lonicerae	yín huā
Fructus Forsythiae	lián qiào
Radix Scutellariae	huáng qín
Fructus Gardeniae	zhī zǐ

Great heat in the qi aspect is mainly treated by cold pungent qi clearage, using agents such as White Tiger Decoction *(bái hǔ tāng)*. Gastrointestinal heat-bind apppearing as bowel repletion may be treated with the Major and Minor Purgative Decoctions, which flush fire. Damp-heat lingering in the triple burner is treated by transforming damp and clearing heat, using such formulae as Artemisia Apiacea and Scutellaria Gallbladder-Clearing Decoction *(hāo qín qīng dǎn tāng)*. Patterns characterized by prominence of heat may be treated with Coptis and Magnolia Cool Decoction *(lián pò yǐn)* which is a pungent opening and bitter downbearing formula. In some cases, this may by supplemented with heat-clearing and damp-disinhibiting formulae such as Sweet Dew Toxin-Dispersing Elixir *(gān lù xiāo dú dān)*. Patterns characterized by prominence of damp may be treated with formulae such as Three Kernel Decoction *(sān rén tāng)* which transform damp with aromatic agents, drain qi heat, and promote qi dynamic. Brewing damp-heat steaming the intestines and stomach characterized by prominence of heat may be treated with formulae such as Heart-Draining Decoction *(xiè xīn tāng)* and Coptis Detoxifying Decoction *(huáng-lián jiě dú tāng)*, which dry damp and drain heat with cold, bitter agents.

Treatment of all qi-aspect heat patterns is based on heat clearage. This is combined with other methods, according to the nature of the pattern. Qi-aspect heat patterns caused by a simple thermic heat pathogen may be treated by the method of clearing qi, which in severe cases may be supplemented by that of draining fire or resolving toxin. If the qi-aspect pathogen is thermic heat combined with wind, heat clearage is coupled with pungent, dissipating lung diffusion. If combined with damp, heat clearage is coupled with aromatic damp transformation, pungent opening and bitter downbearing, or the method of separation, dispersion, and discharge. These methods prevent the accompanying pathogen from binding with the thermic heat. Qi-aspect patterns are more varied than those of any other aspect, and a full understanding of these main points is required before they can be identified and treated in clinical practice.

Acumoxatherapy

Qi-aspect heat patterns are treated by needling heat-clearing points. PC-7, HT-6, BL-67, and ST-36 are among the points often chosen to treat heat symptoms such as thirst, fever, restlessness, and yellow tongue fur. If damp-heat is present, SP-9, SP-6, and PC-6 can be used to aid the spleen to transform damp and relieve oppression in the chest. CV-3 and BL-53 clear damp heat from the lower burner and regulate urination. ST-36, CV-12, ST-25, and SP-4 are often added to treat gastrointestinal symptoms. Points mentioned above in the section on yang ming diseases are appropriate, depending on the nature and location of the heat symptoms.

Construction-aspect patterns

Pattern identification

Construction-aspect patterns are characterized by red or crimson tongue, a rapid pulse, general fever, restlessness, and restless sleep. In severe cases there may be delirium and mania, and clouding of the spirit-disposition (discussed in a following section, "Pericardiac Patterns"), or maculopapular eruptions. Where extreme heat engenders wind, tetanic inversion and convulsive spasms may also occur.

Construction-aspect patterns represent a more advanced stage of exuberant heat than qi-aspect patterns, and thus a more serious condition. Their essential characteristic is a red or crimson tongue, which indicates that pathogenic heat has entered the construction aspect. Identification of construction-aspect patterns poses two requirements. First, it is important to determine whether the pathogen entering the construction aspect is thermic heat, wind-heat, or damp-heat. Thermic heat and wind-heat pathogens entering the construction aspect are characterized by a red or crimson tongue with either no fur, or a very thin one. A damp-heat pathogen entering construction is characterized by a red or crimson tongue with a thick, slimy, or turbid tongue fur (indicating that the damp pathogen has not transformed dryness), or a parched, black tongue fur (indicating that dryness formation has occurred). Secondly, it is essential to determine the degree to which the construction aspect has been penetrated. First-stage construction-aspect patterns invariably include qi-aspect signs, such as red to deep red tongue, with a yellow, or mixed yellow-and-white tongue fur. Deep penetration of construction aspect is characterized by a dry, deep red tongue, as well as such signs as stupor of the spirit-disposition (see the section,"Pericardiac Patterns") and stirring wind and tetanic inversion.

Treatment

Construction-aspect patterns are mainly treated by clearing construction, clearing the heart, and resolving toxin.

Drug therapy

The main formula is Construction-Clearing Decoction *(qīng yíng tāng)*. Where there are pericardium signs such as clouding of the spirit, this formula may be combined with one that opens the portals, such as Peaceful Palace Bovine Bezoar Pills *(ān gōng niú-huáng wán)*, Divine Rhinoceros Elixir *(shēn xī dān)*, or Purple Snow Elixir *(zǐ xuě dān)*.

Where the pattern comprises stirring wind, Construction-Clearing Decoction may be combined with the liver-clearing and wind-extinguishing method, by the admixture of agents such as Cornu Antelopis *(líng yáng jiǎo)* and Ramulus et Uncus Uncariae *(gōu téng)*. If the pathogen entering the construction aspect is damp-heat, the basic methods must be combined with that of drying damp and clearing heat with cold, bitter agents such as Radix Scutellariae *(huáng qín)* and Rhizoma Coptidis *(huáng lián)*. First-stage construction-aspect heat patterns, where qi-aspect signs are still present, may be treated by combining the method of clearing construction and engendering liquid with that of promoting diffusion and outthrust with pungent dissipators, to outthrust heat to the qi aspect. The basic formula used for such cases is Black Paste Formula *(hēi gāo fāng)*.

Broadly speaking, construction-aspect patterns are treated with cold, bitter agents combined with cold, sweet agents, to drain heat and resolve toxin as well as to nourish yin and engender liquid. Construction-Clearing Decoction *(qīng yíng tāng)* has both these effects. Cold, sweet agents engender liquids. They enrich yin and increase humor. But if used alone, they not only fail to produce this effect, but may prevent elimination of the pathogen. Similarly, cold, bitter agents used alone may give rise to dryness formation and damage to yin, thus affecting their fire-draining and toxin-resolving effect.

Acumoxatherapy

Points such as LI-4, LI-11, GV-14, TB-2, and SI-3 are used to clear construction-aspect heat. PC-6, HT-7, HT-6, and PC-7 are added to clear the heart. If there is damp, SP-9 and CV-12 may be used. If there is extreme heat, GV-14 may be bled. If the fluids have been damaged, TB-2 is particularly useful.

Blood-aspect patterns

Pattern identification

Blood-aspect patterns represent penetration of the pathogen to an even deeper level than the construction aspect. They are characterized by a deep crimson tongue coloring and purple maculopapular eruptions. Signs of depletion or frenetic movement of blood are also observed. In addition to being crimson, the tongue is mirror clear, indicating damage to yin and fluid desertion that is often accompanied by signs of vacuity stirring endogenous wind, such as convulsion of the limbs or tetanic inversion. These latter signs are nevertheless differentiated from the tetanic inversion and convulsive spasms associated with extreme heat engendering wind.

There are two basic types of blood-aspect patterns. One is marked by heat entering the blood aspect, giving rise to repletion heat signs such as blood depletion and frenetic blood movement. This pattern is similar in nature to the construction-aspect pattern, but is more severe in degree. The other pattern is one of chronic pathogenic heat damaging yin humor. The difference between the two patterns lies in the the severity of the heat and the presence or absence of damage to yin. Severe heat without severe damage to yin appears, in most cases, as repletion heat. Patterns where the heat has subsided somewhat, though still with signs of damage to yin such as desiccated tongue and teeth, dry pharynx and mouth, feverishness, and a fine, rapid pulse, usually indicate vacuity of the correct and the presence of a lodged pathogen.

Treatment

The basic methods for treating blood-aspect patterns are blood cooling and blood dissipation.

Drug therapy

The principal formula used is Rhinoceros Horn and Rehmannia Decoction *(xī-jiǎo dì-huáng tāng)*. Conditions of vacuous correct qi and a lodged pathogen, marked by yin vacuity and humor dessication without great general fever, may be treated by enriching yin and nourishing the blood, using Pulse-Restorative Decoction *(fù mài tāng)* and its variants. Double-Armored or Triple-Armored Pulse-Restorative Decoction *(èr jiǎ, sān jiǎ fù mài tāng)* may also be prescribed in forms judiciously varied according to the patient's condition.

Acumoxatherapy

Points such as SP-6, SP-10, BL-17, LI-11, and BL-54 (bleed capillaries) are used to cool the blood, the choice of points being dependent on the nature and location of the heat. Other points, such as LV-3, LV-8, and PC-5 are added to cool and course the hand and foot jue yin channels that, because of their relationship with the pericardium and liver respectively, have a direct effect on blood circulation and storage. If the heat pathogen has damaged yin, KI-3 may be added.

Pericardiac patterns

Pattern identification

Pericardiac patterns are usually characterized by disorientation of the spirit-disposition, delirium and manic agitation, and in serious cases, by coma. The appearance of such signs as agitation, somnolence, and trembling of the tip of the tongue during the progression of exogenous heat diseases invariably portends entry of the pathogen into the pericardium. Special attention should be paid to such signs.

Thermic pathogens usually, though not invariably, pass to the construction aspect before gradually falling inwards to the pericardium. In some cases, such as that of infectious encephalitis B, the pathogen falls inward directly from the defense aspect without passing through the construction aspect. This is known as anticipated passage to the pericardium.

Thus, pericardiac patterns are characterized by coma or obtundation of the spirit-disposition, and are the result of direct inward fall of pathogens from the defense, qi, construction, or blood aspects. Two main forms are identified. One is known as heat entering the pericardium, and characterized by such heat signs as red to crimson tongue, and in most cases a burnt-yellow tongue. The other is a phlegm-damp pattern referred to as clouding of the pericardium by damp turbidity, characterized by an unclean, sticky, slimy fur covering what may or may not be a red or crimson tongue.

Treatment

The principal method of treating pericardic patterns is portal opening. Generally, essence-spirit agitation or somnolence are portending signs.

Drug therapy

At this stage, formulae containing agents such as Rhizoma Acori Graminei *(chāng pú)* and Tuber Curcumae *(yù jīn)* may be used to drain turbidity and open the portals. When the patient is about to fall into a coma, aromatic openers may be prescribed. The same drugs, with the addition of heat-clearing toxin resolvers, treat heat entering the pericardium, characterized by coma. This method is known as cool opening, and is represented by formulae such as:

Cool-Opening Formulae	
Peaceful Palace Bovine Bezoar Pills	*ān gōng niú-huáng wán*
Purple Snow Elixir	*zǐ xuě dān*
Divine Rhinoceros Elixir	*shēn xī dān*

Clouding of the pericardium by phlegm turbidity, characterized by unsurfaced fever and coma, is treated by warm opening, which represents a combination of portal opening with repelling foulness and transforming turbidity. Representative formulae include:

Warm-Opening Formulae	
Liquid Styrax Pills	sū hé xiāng wán
Jade Axis Elixir	yù shū dān

Gastrointestinal heat-bind (equivalent to the yang ming bowel pattern) occurring in exogenous heat diseases that present with such symptoms as delirious speech and clouding mania is referred to in the theory of thermic diseases as stomach heat overwhelming the heart, which also falls within the scope of heat entering the pericardium. The basic method of treating such patterns is restoring bowel flow and draining heat, assisted by portal opening.

Acumoxatherapy

Pericardiac patterns are treated with points on the heart and pericardium channels, using strong stimulation. PC-6, PC-7, PC-8, and HT-7 are commonly used. GV-26 and GV-20 may be added to open the portals and clear heat from the governing vessel.

The normal passage of thermic disease through the four aspects is: defense ⟶ qi ⟶ construction ⟶ blood. However, not all exogenous heat diseases follow this order strictly. The particular nature of the pathogen and the degree of strength of the correct may in some cases cause overpassing of one or more of the normal stages, known as irregular passage. An example of this is a disease passing from the defense aspect directly to construction. Also, the normal sequence of passage may be interrupted by treatment. In such cases the pathogen may retreat outwards before final termination. For example, a pathogen having just entered construction may be treated by the method of outthrusting heat to the qi aspect, causing the pathogen to retreat to the qi aspect and terminate. Damp-heat lingering in the qi aspect can be treated by the method of clearing heat and transforming damp, which conducts the pathogen outward.

Finally, in identifying and treating four-aspect patterns, attention must be paid to the differences and interrelationship of the four aspects. Each aspect has its own clinically observable differential characteristics. On the other hand, the pathomechanic relationship between adjacent aspects is close, so that dual defense-qi disease and qi-construction blaze represent commonly observed patterns. Pathomechanically, the four aspects exist as separate entities, but qi may be considered to embrace defense, and blood to embrace construction.

The Relationship Between Six-Channel and Four-Aspect Pattern Identification

Four-aspect pattern identification developed from and completes six-aspect pattern identification. Although theoretically the systems are different, in practice they have much in common. For example, qi-aspect patterns of the theory of thermic diseases correspond partly to yang ming disease of the cold-damage theory. The differences lie largely in emphasis and detail. The parts of the cold-damage theory dealing with initial stage exogenous heat diseases provide less detail about heat patterns than about cold patterns. This lack was compensated by the theory of thermic diseases. The cold-damage theory also contained little detail about construction and blood patterns, which were more comprehensively discussed in the theory of thermic diseases. The theory of thermic diseases also synthesized much experience in tongue diagnosis.

Nevertheless, thermic disease theory also has its weak points. It attributes disease to thermia, a yang pathogen that readily damages yin. Thus, it places far greater emphasis on damage to yin than damage to yang, and overlooks the principle of conversion spoken of in the cold-damage theory, whereby, for example, yang pathogens may under certain circumstances lead to yang collapse.

Both approaches are founded on clinical practice, and each reflects only one aspect of it. Ideally, a global approach needs to be adopted that acknowledges the strong points of each system and compensates for the weak points. Practical medicine will only be served by synthesizing what is useful in each system.

At the present time, major developments are taking place in the way Chinese medicine treats exogenous heat diseases. For example, the heat-clearing and toxin-resolving method of the theory of thermic diseases is now universally used to great effect in the treatment of initial-stage exogenous heat diseases. This has destroyed the cold-damage school prejudice of "first exterior followed by interior," and has also affected the thermic disease school theory that "cold, bitter agents should not be used too early." Such formulae as Major Purgative Decoction (dà chéng qì tāng), Major Bupleurum Decoction (dà chái-hú tāng), and Mume Pills (wū-méi wán) which are listed in *A Treatise on Cold Damage*, are now universally used to treat certain forms of acute abdomen such as cholecystitis, cholelithiasis, and ascariasis of the biliary tract. These formulae have not only proven effective, but scientific research relating to their use has led to new developments in theory, proving that both the cold-damage theory and the theory of thermic diseases represent a great mine of information, needing only further investigation and refinement. At the same time, they remind us that clinical practice is the correct point of departure. Both theories are of value and should be used together.

We believe that the eight parameters should form the basis of exogenous heat disease pattern identification. Thus, in the initial stages, exterior cold patterns may be treated as tai yang disease while exterior heat patterns may be treated as defense-aspect patterns. Interiorization implies passage to the exuberant heat stage, where different patterns may be observed: the yang ming channel and bowel patterns, shao yang disease of the six-channel system, and the qi-aspect patterns of the four-aspect system (great heat at the qi aspect and gastrointestinal heat-bind being essentially the same as the yang ming channel and bowel patterns). More advanced conditions may appear as construction aspect, blood aspect, and pericardiac patterns, and damage to yin humor may appear as blood-aspect vacuity-heat patterns.

Exogenous heat disease patterns are caused mainly by heat. Liu He-Jian (Wan Su), the father of the thermic disease theory, said, "Diseases passing through the six channels are all heat patterns." However, conversion to cold, or in serious cases yang collapse vacuity desertion, is not uncommon. This may occur in patients with weak constitutions, in infants or the aged, or as a result of inappropriate treatment. The nature of the invading pathogen may also be a determining factor. Yang collapse patterns occurring during the progression of a heat disease usually arise swiftly, but this is not to say that there are no warning signs. For example, a weak, vacuous pulse, pale tongue, and subduing and clouding of essence-spirit, occurring at the onset of disease, indicate insufficiency of original qi, which calls for prevention of damage to yang and yang collapse. Cold skin and sweating, and sudden appearance of a faint, fine or agitated, racing pulse, represent an even stronger indication of yang collapse vacuity desertion. Such eventualities represent an important part of shao yin disease of the six-channel system. These are yin patterns, vacuity patterns, and cold patterns, treated by salvaging yang and securing against desertion. The differentiation of heat diseases into three yang channel diseases and three yin channel diseases as set forth in *A Treatise on Cold Damage* is grounded in clinical practice. The phrase, "diseases passing through the six channels are all heat patterns," only points to common occurrences in heat diseases. Only by recognizing that under certain circumstances cold patterns may occur can mutations of heat diseases be fully understood. Exogenous heat diseases usually occur as exterior patterns in their initial stages, and as interior, heat and repletion patterns in their exuberant fever stage. However, under certain circumstances, they may convert into vacuity cold. The six-channel and four-aspect pattern identification systems represent permutations of the eight-parameter pattern identification, and must be synthesized to form a complete system.

Table 11-1 Six-Channel Patterns, Tai Yang and Yang Ming

Identification and Treatment of Tai Yang Disease Patterns

Pathomechanism	Principal Signs	Remarks Concerning Pattern Identification		Treatment Method	Principal Formulae	Acupoints
Assailment of the Exterior by Wind-Cold	Aversion to cold or wind General pain Floating pulse Fever	Exterior Repletion	Absence of Sweating Aversion to cold Tight pulse	Warm, pungent exterior resolution	Ephedra Decoction	LI-4 TB-5 GV-16 GB-20 ST-8
		Exterior Vacuity	Sweating Aversion to wind Moderate pulse		Cinnamon-Twig Decoction	

Identification and Treatment of Yang Ming Disease Patterns

Pathomechanism	Principal Signs	Remarks Concerning Pattern Identification		Treatment Method	Principal Formulae	Acupoints
Gastrointestinal Repletion Heat	General fever Sweating Aversion to heat Restlessness Thirst	Channel Pattern	Great Fever Profuse sweating Great thirst Large, surging pulse	Heat Clearage	White Tiger Decoction	LI-15 LI-11 TB-5 ST-44
		Bowel Pattern	Tidal fever Delirious speech Abdominal fullness and distention with palpitation Tenderness Constipation Deep, replete, forceful pulse	Offensive precipitation	Major Purgative Decoction	TB-2 BL-57 TB-6

Table 11-1 Six-Channel Patterns, Shao Yang and Tai Yin

Identification and Treatment of Shao Yang Disease Patterns

Pathomechanism	Principal Signs	Remarks Concerning Pattern Identification	Treatment Method	Principal Formulae	Acupoints
Pathogen at midstage between exterior and interior	Alternating fever and chills, bitter fullness in chest and lateral costal region	Exterior Pattern: Pain in the limb joints	Harmonization	Minor Bupleurum Decoction	PC-5 CV-13 GB-41 GB-34
	Vomiting	Interior Pattern: Abdominal fullness and pain Constipation		Bupleurum and Cinnamon Decoction	
	Wiry pulse			Major Bupleurum Decoction	

Identification and Treatment of Tai Yin Disease Patterns

Pathomechanism	Principal Signs	Remarks Concerning Pattern Identification	Treatment Method	Principal Formulae	Acupoints
Gastrosplenic Vacuity Cold	Abdominal fullness with intermittent pain	Tai yin disease is characterized by vacuity, whereas yang ming disease is characterized by repletion	Warming the center and fortifying the spleen	Center-Rectifying Pills	LI-4 ST-25‡ SP-6‡ ST-36‡
	Vomiting				
	Diarrhea				
	No desire for food or drink				
	Moderate, weak pulse				

Table 11-1 Six-Channel Patterns, *Shao Yin*

Identification and Treatment of Shao Yin Disease Patterns

Pathomechanism	Principal Signs	Remarks Concerning Pattern Identification	Treatment Method	Principal Formulae	Acupoints
Cardiorenal Debilitation	**Vacuity cold** Aversion to cold Curled, recumbent posture Somnolence Inversion frigidity of the limbs Diarrhea Fine, faint pulse In serious cases: yang collapse vacuity desertion	Vacuity cold is most common, but attention must be paid to the possibility of vacuity heat	Salvaging yang and checking counterflow	Counterflow Cold Decoction	GV-4‡ KI-3‡ CV-6‡ ST-36‡ CV-8‡
	Vacuity heat Restlessness and insomnia Dry pharynx and mouth Fine, rapid pulse		Enriching yin and clearing heat	Coptis and Ass-Hide Glue Decoction	

Table 11-1 Six-Channel Patterns, Jue Yin

Identification and Treatment of Jue Yin Disease Patterns

Pathomechanism	Principal Signs	Remarks Concerning Pattern Identification	Treatment Method	Principal Formulae	Acupoints
Interior Vacuity and Cold-Heat Complex	Upper-body heat and lower-body cold; Diabetic diseases; Qi surging upward into the cardiac region; Hunger with no desire for food; Vomiting of roundworm; (Occasionally) inversion frigidity of the limbs	It is important to determine the prominence of cold and heat	Simultaneous warming and clearing	Mume Pills	BL-18 LV-14 CV-12‡ ST-36‡ CV-10‡ LI-4 TB-5‡

Table 11-2 Four-Aspect Patterns, *Defense Aspect*

Identification and Treatment of Defense-Aspect Disease Patterns

Pathomechanism	Principal Signs	Remarks Concerning Pattern Identification	Treatment Method	Principal Formulae	Acupoints
Pathogen in the Defensive Exterior	Fever Slight aversion to cold or wind Headache Dry mouth Fast, floating pulse	**Wind Thermia** Cough Sore, red pharynx Tongue tends to be red	Cool, pungent exterior resolution	Lonicera and Forsythia Powder Mulberry and Chrysanthemum Cool Decoction	LI-4 BL-13 SI-3 LU-10 LU-11 PC-6
		Damp Thermia Thoracic oppression Upflow and nausea Dry mouth with no desire to drink General sensation of heaviness Tongue fur tends to be slimy	Promoting diffusion and transformation with aromatics	Agastache, Magnolia Pinellia and Poria Decoction	

Table 11-2 Four-Aspect Patterns, Qi Aspect

Identification and Treatment of Qi-Aspect Disease Patterns

Pathomechanism	Principal Signs	Remarks Concerning Pattern Identification	Treatment Method	Principal Formulae	Acupoints
Exuberant Heat in the Qi Aspect	Fever Aversion to heat rather than cold Thirst Bitter taste in the mouth Yellow or dark-colored urine Rapid pulse Yellow or mixed white-and-yellow tongue fur	First Stage Qi-Aspect Heat Thirst Restlessness Mixed yellow and white tongue fur	Clearing and outthrusting pathogenic heat	Gardenia and Fermented Soybean Decoction	TW-2 HT-5 BL-67 ST-36 PC-7
		Exuberant Pulmo-Gastric Heat High fever Cough Rapid breathing Thirst Yellow tongue fur	Clearing Heat and Diffusing the Lung	Ephedra, Apricot, Gypsum and Liquorice Decoction	
		Great Heat in the Qi Aspect Great heat Great thirst Profuse sweating Large, surging pulse	Clearing qi with cold, pungent agents	White Tiger Decoction	

Table 11-2 Four-Aspect Patterns, Qi Aspect, page 2

Identification and Treatment of Qi-Aspect Disease Patterns

Pathomechanism	Principal Signs	Remarks Concerning Pattern Identification	Treatment Method	Principle Formulae	Acupoints
Exuberant Heat in the Qi Aspect	Fever	Aversion to heat rather than cold			
	Thirst				
	Bitter taste in the mouth				
	Yellow or dark-colored urine				
	Rapid pulse				
	Yellow or mixed white-and-yellow tongue fur				
		Gastro-Intestinal Heat Bind: Abdominal distention and oppression with pain exacerbated by pressure	Flushing accumulated heat	Major Purgative Decoction	TW-2
		Heat Lodging in the Triple Burner: Persistent, remittent general fever; Thoracic oppression; Upflow and nausea; Thirst with no desire to drink; Short micturition with scant urine; Slimy, white or yellow tongue fur; Soggy, rapid pulse	Transforming phlegm and clearing heat	Artemisia Apeacea and Scutellaria Gallbladder-Clearing Decoction	HT-5
				Coptis and Magnolia Cool Decoction	BL-67
				Three Kernel Decoction	ST-36
				Sweet Dew Toxin-Dispersing Elixir	PC-7
		Brewing Damp-Heat Steaming the Intestine & Stomach: The preceding symptoms plus: Abdominal distention and oppression; Hard, bound stool or diarrhea with foul-smelling stool; Slimy yellow tongue fur; Deep, slippery, rapid pulse	Drying damp and draining heat with cold, bitter agents	Heart Draining Decoction	
				Coptis Detoxifying Decoction	

Table 11-2 Four-Aspect Patterns, Construction & Blood Aspects

Identification and Treatment of Construction-Aspect Disease Patterns

Pathomechanism	Principal Signs	Remarks Concerning Pattern Identification	Treatment Method	Principal Formulae	Acupoints
Inward Fall of Pathogenic Heat to the Construction Aspect	Red or crimson tongue, Rapid pulse, General fever, Restlessness, Restless sleep. In serious cases: Clouding of the spirit and tetanic inversion, or maculopapular erruptions	Inward Fall of Thermia Heat or Wind Thermia		Construction-Clearing Decoction	LI-4, HT-5, TB-2, GV-14, LI-11, PC-7, SI-3
		Inward Fall of Damp Thermia	Clearing Construction		

Identification and Treatment of Blood-Aspect Disease Patterns

Pathomechanism	Principal Signs	Remarks Concerning Pattern Identification	Treatment Method	Principal Formulae	Acupoints
Penetration of Pathogenic Heat to Blood Aspect Causing Depletion or Frenetic Movement of the Blood	Deep crimson tongue, Maculopapular erruptions, Hemorrhage, Clouding of the spirit, Convulsive spasm of the limbs, Tetanic inversion	Repletion Heat at Blood Aspect	Cooling the blood and resolving toxin	Rhinocerous Horn and Rehmania Decoction	SP-10, SP-6, BL-54, PC-5, LV-3, LI-11, LV-8
		Vacuity Heat at Blood Aspect	Enriching yin and nourishing the blood	Pulse-Restorative Decoction (and variants)	

Remarks Concerning Pattern Identification for Vacuity Heat at Blood Aspect: Pronounced signs of damage to yin

Remarks Concerning Pattern Identification for Repletion Heat at Blood Aspect: Prominence of heat signs

Remarks Concerning Pattern Identification for Inward Fall of Thermia Heat or Wind Thermia: Red or crimson tongue with little or no fur

Remarks Concerning Pattern Identification for Inward Fall of Damp Thermia: Crimson tongue with turbid or burnt black fur

Exogenous Heat Diseases

Table 11-3 Pericardiac Patterns

Identification and Treatment of Pericardiac Patterns

Aspects	Pathomechanism		
	Inward Fall of Thermic Pathogens to the Pericardium	*Clouding of the Pericardium by Phlegm Turbidity*	*Stomach Heat Sweltering the Pericardium*
Spirit-Disposition	Coma or tetanic inversion	Coma or semiconciousness	Delerious speech or manic agitation
Heat Signs	High fever	Absence of high fever or non-vigorous surface fever	Late afternoon tidal fever or high fever
Stool	No pronounced changes	Thin-stool diarrhea is sometimes observed	Usually hard and bound, or diarrhea with foul-smelling stool
Abdomen	No pronounced signs	No pronounced signs	Painful glomus and fullness
Pulse	Rapid, and either fine or wiry	Rapid, and either soggy or slippery	Deep, slippery and forceful
Tongue and Fur	Pure crimson with a fresh sheen Dry crimson with white fur or crimson with yellow-white fur	Slimy white fur covering the whole of the tongue or a turbid, slimy, yellow fur Tongue body is not necessarily crimson	Thick, slimy, or yellow tongue fur
Method of Treatment	Portal opening (cool opening)	Portal opening (warm opening)	Precipitation (sometimes together with portal opening)
Formulae	Peaceful Palace Bovine Bezoar Pills Purple Snow Elixir Divine Rhinoceros Elixir	Liquid Stryax Pills Jade Axis Elixir	Major Purgative Decoction Purple Snow Elixir (where portal opening also required)
Acupoints	PC-6 PC-7 PC-8 HT-7 GV-26 GV-20		

369

Notes

[1] The passage in *Essential Questions* discussing six-channel patterns is considered to be the basis of six-channel pattern identification and treatment on which *A Treatise on Cold Damage* is founded. It reads as follows:

> On the first day of cold-damage, tai yang is affected, and signs include headache and pain in the neck, and stiffness in the lower back. On the second day, yang ming is affected. Since the yang ming governs the flesh, and its channel passes up the side of the nose to connect with the eyes, there is generalized fever, eye pain and dry nose. On the third day, the shao yang is affected. Since the shao yang governs the gallbladder, and its channel passes through the lateral costal region and connects with the ears, symptoms include pain in the chest and lateral costal region and tinnitus. On the fourth day, the tai yin is affected. Since the tai yin channel passes through the stomach and connects with the throat, symptoms include fullness in the stomach and dry throat. On the fifth day, the shao yin is affected. Since the shao yin channel passes through the kidney, connects with the lung, and penetrates through to the root of the the tongue, symptoms include dry mouth and tongue, and thirst. On the sixth day, the jue yin is affected. Since the jue yin channel passes through the genitals and connects with the liver, symptoms include agitation and retraction of the scrotum.

[2] The points appearing in this section are almost entirely chosen from Cheng Dan-an's *Newly Annotated Treatise on Cold Damage* (Taipei, 1979), where the author states in his introduction that he has added acumoxa points to make the book more useful, drawing from his own experience and from various acupuncture texts.

[3] The four terms, construction, defense, qi, and blood, are discussed in Chapter 2. In thermic disease theory, the altered order of enumeration reflects the sequence of pathogen penetration.

Chapter 12
Principles and Methods of Treatment

This chapter is confined to oral medication and acumoxatherapy, the most commonly used forms of treatment in the practice of internal medicine.

Principles of Treatment

Treating disease from the root

The phrase, "disease should be treated from the root" has been the major guiding principle of pattern identification and treatment for millenia. The word "root" is used in opposition to "branches," the two terms being of varying significance depending on the context. For example, root frequently refers to the essential nature of the disease, while branches refer to symptoms; root can also refer to the factors of disease, while branches would refer to the clinically observable changes in the human body. When root denotes correct qi, branches would refer to the pathogen. Finally, in other contexts, the primary condition may be described as the root in contradistinction to resulting secondary conditions that are the branches.

The principle of treating disease from the root, or radical treatment, applies to most diseases and is divided into two forms: direct treatment and indirect treatment. Symptomatic treatment, treating a disease by the branches, represents an exception to this principle that applies under clearly defined conditions.

Direct and indirect treatment

The aim of treatment is to eradicate cold or heat, vacuity or repletion, after these have been identified through careful analysis of symptoms (see Chapter 7). Thus, as the *Inner Canon* states:

> Cold is treated with heat, heat is treated with cold, vacuity is treated by supplementation, and repletion is treated by drainage.

This approach is used where the manifestations of disease correspond to its essential nature, i.e., where cold diseases present cold signs, heat diseases present heat signs, vacuity disorders manifest in signs of vacuity, and repletion disorders manifest in signs of repletion. This straightforward correspondence between the essential nature of the disease and its clinically observable manifestations exists in most diseases.

Some diseases, however, present false signs, and in such cases the direct approach cannot be applied. For instance, exuberant heat in exogenous heat diseases may present false signs of cold such as aversion to cold or shivering, and frigidity of the limbs. When correctly identified as heat falsely presenting as cold, the pattern can be treated with heavy doses of heat-clearing and toxin-resolving agents. The principle of treating a heat disorder falsely presenting as cold with cold agents is known as treating cold with cold. Fundamentally, yang-collapse vacuity desertion is considered endogenous cold from yang debilitation, but may present such false heat symptoms as agitation and flushing of the face. Correctly identified as cold falsely presenting as heat, the pattern can be treated with Radix Ginseng *(rén shēn)* and Radix Aconiti Fu Tzu *(fŭ zĭ)* to restore yang and secure against counterflow frigidity.

Treating cold falsely presenting as heat with hot agents is known as treating heat with heat. Patients suffering from splenic or qi vacuities often display such symptoms as distention and oppression in the chest and abdomen, which indicate false repletion. Once stagnations of phlegm, water, digestate, and blood have been ruled out, the pattern may be identified as vacuity falsely presenting as repletion. In such cases, spleen fortifiers and qi boosters can be used to eradicate the vacuity distention and fullness, according to the principle of "treating the stopped by stopping." Diarrhea that occurs in dysentery or acute enteritis, if diagnosed as stagnation of damp-heat in the intestines, cannot be treated with antidiarrheic agents, irrespective of evacuation frequency. Instead, it should be treated with draining precipitants to eliminate stagnation, according to the principle of "treating flow by promoting flow."

Treating heat with heat, cold with cold, the stopped by stopping, and the loose by loosening are all forms of indirect treatment. Since in these cases, the nature of the treatment given is opposed to that of the disorder, the principle of indirect treatment is essentially the same as that of direct treatment; both are in accord with the fundamental principle of radical treatment.

Before prescribing direct or indirect treatment, information from all four examinations should be carefully correlated and a thorough assessment should be made of such factors as the causes and duration of the disease, the strength of the patient's constitution, and his mental state. Utmost care must be taken to distinguish signs that are true and signs that are false; only then can a disease be correctly identified and treated by the root.

Radical and symptomatic treatment

Symptomatic treatment refers to treatment of the branches (the clinical manifestations of a disease) as opposed to the root (the essential nature of the disease). Although the radical approach represents the central principle of treatment, it is not immutable. "Acute conditions are treated symptomatically, and non-acute conditions are treated radically," i.e., chronic and relatively mild acute conditions are treated radically, severe acute conditions call for palliative relief of the symptoms before radical treatment can be given. For example, in the case of massive bleeding, blood loss represents the branches of the disorder, while the cause of the bleeding is the root. While the ultimate aim is to eradicate the cause of the bleeding, the prime concern is to check blood loss. Ascites is another example of an acute condition requiring symptomatic relief. Though never the cause of disease, excessive accumulation of water in the abdomen may cause constipation and urine retention, and inhibit respiration. These symptoms must first be relieved by expelling the water before radical treatment can be prescribed.

Although symptomatic treatment should be applied as rarely as possible, many diseases call for simultaneous radical and symptomatic treatment, the approach whereby root and branches are treated at the same time. For example, spleen-vacuity qi stagnation, presenting as distention and fullness in the chest and abdomen, is frequently treated with Four Nobles Decoction *(sì jūn zǐ tāng)* to eradicate the underlying splenic vacuity, with the addition of qi rectifiers such as the following to alleviate the symptoms:

Qi Rectifiers	
Radix Saussureae	*mù xiāng*
Fructus Amomi	*shā rén*
Fructus Citri	*zhǐ ké*
Pericarpium Citri Reticulatae	*chén pí*

Dispelling pathogens and supporting the correct

Dispelling pathogens mainly involves the offensive method, also referred to as "attack," while restoring the correct mainly involves the method of supplementation. Usually, repletion patterns are treated offensively, while vacuity patterns are treated by supplementation. Most diseases attributable to exogenous pathogens are excessive in nature, so that treatment centers on dispelling the pathogen. Exterior resolution, heat clearage, toxin resolution, precipitation, phlegm dispersion, damp transformation, water disinhibition, and blood breaking are all designed to dispel pathogens and are all within the scope of the offensive method.

Pathogen dispelling can be used only in cases of repletion. Since pathogen dispellants rely on the strength of correct qi to produce their effect, this method is applicable to cases where pathogenic qi is strong but correct qi is unaffected. Where a strong pathogen is present and the correct is already weakened, exclusive application of the offensive method will fail to dispel the pathogen, and may even cause further damage to the correct by dint of drug side-effects. In these cases, the methods of attack followed by supplementation (first dispelling the pathogen and then

Attack followed by supplementation

This approach is used where an extremely strong pathogen has to be dispelled urgently, and correct qi, though markedly weakened, can still withstand offensive treatment. That the weakness of the correct is attributable to the strength of the pathogen is a further reason for using the principle of attack followed by supplementation. This principle may apply in the treatment of gastrointestinal heat-bind, an exogenous heat disease pattern characterized by constipation and painful distention and fullness in the abdomen. Such conditions may be treated with Major Purgative Decoction (dà chéng qì tāng) even though yin may have been damaged as a result of dryness formation; indeed, failure to precipitate the heat-bind would cause further damage to yin. Current treatment of acute abdominal conditions makes use of this principle.

Supplementation followed by attack

The principle of supplementation followed by attack is applied in cases where the pathogen is strong and the correct is vacuous to the point of debilitation of yang or depletion of yin, and is incapable of withstanding offensive treatment. *Essential Prescriptions of the Golden Coffer* states:

> If a disease is treated by precipitation, and the result is constant clear-food diarrhea and generalized pain, the immediate concern is to treat the interior. When this has been done, the bowels will return to normal, but there will still be generalized pain. This is then eradicated by treating the exterior.

These lines describe a condition following inappropriate splenogastric precipitation, where the patient displays an interior pattern characterized by persistent clear-food diarrhea and an exterior pattern characterized by generalized pain. These symptoms mean that a strong pathogen is located in the exterior and a vacuity of correct qi is in the interior. Persistent clear-food diarrhea indicates that correct qi is seriously weakened and is unable to expel the pathogen, and is also susceptible to yang-collapse vacuity desertion. Thus, the first concern is to support correct qi. When the interior pattern has been treated and the bowels have returned to normal, further treatment may be directed toward resolving the exterior by expelling the pathogen before it interiorizes causing new complications.

Simultaneous supplementation and attack

The principle of simultaneous supplementation and attack applies to patterns where the pathogen is strong but the correct is not too seriously weakened, or where pathogenic qi is strong and the first consideration is to expel it, while correct qi is weak and cannot withstand offensive treatment.

The first case is exemplified in the preceding quotation from *Essential Prescriptions of the Golden Coffer*. Consider a condition where the interior vacuity is not serious and the diarrhea is only the normal diarrhea of an interior cold pattern (less serious than persistent clear-food diarrhea). Such conditions may be treated by simultaneously resolving the exterior and warming the interior, using a formula such as Cinnamon Twig and Ginseng Decoction *(guì-zhī rén-shēn tāng)* as prescribed in *A Treatise on Cold Damage,* for dual resolution of interior and exterior. An example of the second case is a condition requiring swift precipitation to preserve yin, for which the normally prescribed Major Purgative Decoction *(dà chéng qì tāng)* is contraindicated because of the presence of a weak, soft pulse. Instead, Yellow Dragon Decoction *(huáng lóng tāng)* or Humor-Increasing Purgative Decoction *(zēng yè chéng qì tāng)* is used, to prevent sudden desertion following precipitation.

The principle of simultaneous supplementation and attack is frequently applied in clinical practice. Formulae may be adjusted to place the emphasis on supporting the correct or dispelling the pathogen, depending on the patient's particular condition.

Restoration of the yin-yang balance

Distinction is made of two basic forms of imbalance between yin and yang: a deficit of one or the other complement or a surfeit of one or the other complement. In pattern identification it is important to determine whether the condition is characterized by a surfeit of one complement or by a deficit of the other.

Correction of yin and yang surfeits

A surfeit of one or the other complement refers to a situation where a pathogen is relatively strong and causes a surfeit of the same complement in the organism. Here, it must be remembered that a strong yin pathogen readily damages yang qi: "If yin abounds yang ails." If a patient's constitution is characterized by vacuous yang qi, he will be particularly vulnerable to yin pathogens. Similarly, a patient with a yin vacuity constitution will be vulnerable to yang pathogens. Therefore, when evaluating surfeits, determine if there is a vacuity of the complement. If the other complement shows no deficit, the principle of eliminating surfeits may be applied, and treatment accordingly designed to drain the yin or yang pathogen.

Ephedra Decoction *(má-huáng tāng)* dissipates cold pathogens and so is used to treat exterior cold patterns, and White Tiger Decoction *(bái hǔ tāng)* clears interior heat and so is used for interior heat patterns. Both these formulae are designed to eliminate surfeits, to correct an imbalance of yin and yang characterized by a surfeit of one complement. However, if the surfeit of either yin or yang is accompanied by a deficit of its complement, the correct must be supported by supplying the insufficiency. For instance, True Warrior Decoction *(zhēn wǔ tāng)* warms kidney yang and dissipates cold-water. It is used to treat patterns characterized by flooding yin water and vacuous kidney yang. Jade Lady Decoction *(yù nǚ jiān)* supplements kidney yin and clears stomach heat thus treating patterns involving vacuous kidney yin and intense stomach fire. These formulae are designed to eliminate surfeits while supplying secondary insufficiencies, and are used to treat conditions characterized by a surfeit of yin or yang where its complement is in deficit.

Correction of yin and yang deficits

In pathology, yin and yang deficits are referred to as insufficiencies or vacuities. If a condition is identified as being one of yin vacuity, cold, bitter agents should not normally be used to treat any attendant heat signs. Instead, the principle of "invigorating the governor of water to counteract the brilliance of yang" is applied.

Formulae such as Rehmannia Six Pills *(liù wèi dì-huáng wán)* are used in accordance with this principle. It should be noted that a yang vacuity with cold signs, where the yang vacuity is the essential characteristic, cannot be treated with warm, pungent agents to disperse the yin cold. It should rather be treated with formulae such as Cinnamon Eight Pills *(guì-zhī bā wèi wán)* in accord with the principle of "boosting the source of fire to eliminate the entrenched surfeit of yin."

In correcting imbalances between yin and yang, the principles of "seeking yang in yin" and "seeking yin in yang," which are derived from the interdependence of yin and yang, are commonly applied. In practice, when supplementing yang, yin-supplementing drugs are added to the formula; when supplementing yin, yang-supplementing agents are included:

> Yang, when requiring supplementation, should be sought in yin, since with the help of yin, it can arise infinitely; yin, when requiring supplementation, must be sought in yang, since with the help of yang, its source is never ending.

Thus, Kidney Pills *(zuǒ guī wán)*, used to treat insufficiency of true yin, include Cornu Cervi *(lù jiǎo)*, Semen Cuscutae *(tù sī zǐ)*, and other yang supplementers. Vital Gate Pills *(yòu guī wán)* which treat insufficiency of true yang, contain Radix Rehmanniae Conquita *(shóu dì)*, Fructus Lycii *(qǐ zǐ)*, and other agents that supplement yin. However, the principles of seeking yang in yin and yin in yang are always secondary to that of supplying the yin or yang insufficiency.

Methods of Treatment

Diaphoresis

Diaphoresis refers to the method of exterior resolution. It involves the use of pungent, dissipating outthrust and effusion promoters[1] to open and discharge the striations and expel the pathogen from the body. Diaphoresis is used to eliminate a pathogen from the surface skin and body hair before it interiorizes. This is the meaning of the line in Chapter 5 of the *Essential Questions* that states, "when it {a pathogen} is in the skin, it is made to effuse."

Diaphoresis is mainly used in exterior patterns such as the onset of exogenous diseases and wind-damp and water-swelling disorders, as well as in measles immediately preceding papular outthrust. Warm, pungent exterior resolution treats cold patterns, while cool, pungent exterior resolution treats heat patterns.

The main difference between these two methods is the use of warm and cool agents. Warm, pungent, exterior-resolving formulae dissipate cold and have a relatively strong diaphoretic effect, while cold, pungent, exterior-resolving formulae clear heat but have a weaker diaphoretic effect. In recent clinical practice, the use of agents having a relatively strong diaphoretic and exterior-resolving action in combination with heat-clearing and toxin-resolving agents has proven particularly successful in the treatment of early-stage exogenous heat diseases.

Warm, pungent exterior resolution

Indications

Exterior cold patterns with strong aversion to cold, pronounced headache and aching bones, high or low fever, moist, white tongue fur, floating, tight pulse, and absence of any heat symptoms such as red tongue, dry mouth, or painful, red and swollen tongue.

Agents used

Warm, Pungent, Exterior Resolvents	
Herba Schizonepetae	*jīng jiè*
Radix Ledebouriellae	*fáng fēng*
Rhizoma et Radix Notopterygii	*qiāng huó*
Folium Perillae	*sū yè*
Rhizoma Zingiberis Recens	*shēng jiāng*

Warm, Pungent, Exterior Resolvents (continued)	
Herba Allii Fistulosi	*cōng bái*
Herba Ephedrae	*má huáng*
Ramulus Cinnamomi	*guì zhī*

Herba Schizonepetae and Radix Ledebouriellae are the most commonly used. Rhizoma et Radix Notopterygii possesses a much stronger diaphoretic, fever-abating and pain-relieving effect than either of these. It is mainly prescribed for severe pain in the joints. Rhizoma Zingiberis Recens and Herba Allii Fistulosi are often administered in combination with other warm, pungent exterior resolvents, but may also be used alone. Folium Perillae *(sū yè)* warms and dissipates, and can also harmonize the center. It is mainly used in exterior cold patterns where gastrointestinal symptoms are also present. Herba Ephedrae *(má huáng)* is mainly used in exterior cold patterns where cough, dyspnea, or water swelling are also present. Ramulus Cinnamomi *(guì zhī)* and Radix Paeoniae Albae *(bái shǎo)* are used in exterior cold patterns involving construction-defense disharmony.

Representative formulae

Exterior Cold Formulae	
Ephedra Decoction	*má-huáng tāng*
Cinnamon-Twig Decoction	*guì-zhī tāng*
Schizonepeta and Ledebouriella Detoxifying Powder	*jīng fáng bài dú sǎn*

Schizonepeta and Ledebouriella Detoxifying Powder is used to treat colds and influenza caused by wind-cold. Ephedra Decoction is best suited for adiaphoretic exterior repletion patterns with cough and dyspnea. Cinnamon-Twig Decoction is prescribed for patterns characterized by construction-defense disharmony, exterior vacuity, and fever unabated by sweating.

Acumoxatherapy

The main points used to promote diaphoresis are KI-7 and LI-4. Strong stimulation is necessary to achieve effective results. This aspect of treatment is the same whether the pattern is one of exterior cold or exterior heat. However, the accompanying points and treatment methods differ according to the nature of the disease and the strength of the patient's resistance.

In exterior cold patterns, points such as GV-14‡, GV-15, GB-20‡, SP-6‡, BL-12‡, and BL-13‡ are commonly used. In exterior heat patterns, points such as SI-3, TB-5, LU-10, GV-14, LI-11, and LU-5 may be added.

Cool, pungent exterior resolution

Indications

Exterior heat patterns with mild aversion to cold and pronounced heat symptoms, thirst, red or sore pharynx, red tongue, dry, thin, white tongue fur, and rapid, floating pulse.

Agents used

Cool, Pungent Exterior Resolvents	
Herba Menthae	bò hé
Folium Mori	sāng yè
Semen Sojae Praeparatum	dòu shǐ
Fructus Arctii	niú bàng zǐ
Radix Puerariae	gé gēn
Ramulus et Folium Tamaricis	xī hé liǔ

The first four agents listed are the most commonly used. Of the cool exterior resolvents, Herba Menthae has the strongest diaphoretic and heat-abating effect. Folium Mori can also clear lung and liver heat and is thus particularly suitable for patterns involving headache, ocular rubor and cough. Semen Sojae Praeparatum is effective in outthrusting pathogens and abating heat. Fructus Arctii has the additional effect of clearing the throat, promoting lung qi diffusion, and clearing phlegm-heat. Radix Puerariae Lobatae is suitable for patterns also involving diarrhea and stiffness in the neck and back. Ramulus et Folium Tamaricis may be used for inducing outthrust of papules in treating measles and can also dispel wind-damp. In cool, pungent exterior resolution, the emphasis is on cool rather than pungent.

For intense heat patterns, agents that clear heat and resolve toxin may also be used:

Heat-Clearing and Toxin-Resolving Agents	
Radix Scutellariae	huáng qín
Fructus Gardeniae	zhī zǐ
Flos Lonicerae	yín huā
Fructus Forsythiae	lián qiào
Radix Isatidis	bǎn lán gēn
Herba et Radix Taraxaci	pú gōng yīng

The use of certain warm exterior resolvents is not excluded in the treatment of exterior heat patterns:

Principles and Methods of Treatment

Warm Exterior Resolvents	
Herba Schizonepetae	*jīng jiè*
Radix Ledebouriellae	*fáng fēng*
Rhizoma et Radix Notopterygii	*qiāng huó*
Herba Ephedrae	*má huáng*

These are used with large quantities of heat clearers. For example, Lonicera and Forsythia Powder *(yín qiào sǎn)* includes Herba Schizonepetae. Notopterygium, Arctium, Taraxacum, and Mentha Decoction *(qiāng bàng pú bò tāng)* includes Rhizoma et Radix Notopterygii, although both are cool, pungent exterior-resolving formulae.

Representative formulae

Exterior Heat Formulae	
Lonicera and Forsythia Powder	*yín qiào sǎn*
Mulberry and Chrysanthemum Cool Decoction	*sāng jú yǐn*
Notopterygium, Arctium, Taraxacum, & Mentha Dec.	*qiāng bàng pú bò tāng*

These three formulae constitute effective cool, pungent exterior-resolving formulae, which may be used for the purposes of clearing heat and resolving toxin. The most commonly used is Lonicera and Forsythia Powder *(yín qiào sǎn)*. Notopterygium, Arctium, Taraxacum, and Mentha Decoction, a formula proven in modern clinical practice, contains cool and warm pungent agents, with the addition of heat clearers and toxin resolvents.

Variants of exterior resolution

Where exterior patterns are accompanied by qi or yin vacuities, qi boosting or yin enrichment may be combined with exterior resolution. Boosting qi and resolving the exterior is used for continual colds and heavy sweating where a qi vacuity is present. Qi vacuity increases vulnerability to exogenous pathogens and reduces the body's ability to expel a pathogen once it has entered.

In such cases, qi boosters may be added to exterior-resolving formulae. An example of such a formula is Ginseng and Perilla Leaf Cool Decoction *(shēn sū yǐn)*.

Enriching yin and resolving the exterior is used for yin vacuity patients displaying an exterior pattern due to the contraction of an exogenous pathogen. In such cases diaphoretic treatment is contraindicated since yin vacuity implies depletion of the blood and fluids from which sweat is produced. Yin enrichers must be used with exterior resolvents to increase perspiration and to expel the pathogen.

Agents used

Commonly used yin-enriching and humor-increasing agents include:

Yin Enrichers	
Radix Rehmanniae Cruda	*shēng dì*
Rhizoma Polygonati Odorati	*yù zhú*
Tuber Ophiopogonis	*mài dōng*

These are used with exterior resolvents such as:

Exterior Resolvents	
Semen Sojae Praeparatum	*dòu shì*
Radix Puerariae Lobatae	*ge gen*
Folium Perillae	*sū yè*
Herba Allii Fistulosi	*cōng bái*
Herba Menthae	*bò hé*

Representative Formulae

A commonly used formula is Polygonatum Odoratum Decoction (*wěi ruǐ tāng*).

Acumoxatherapy

When an exterior pattern simultaneously exists with qi vacuity, points that supplement qi are added to the combinations previously discussed. These include: ST-36‡, SP-6‡, CV-6‡, CV-4‡, and LI-4. Strong stimulation is contraindicated in qi vacuity patterns, and the degree of stimulation as well as the number of points chosen are thus dependent on the respective strengths of the pathogen and the correct. These factors must always be carefully considered in acumoxatherapy.

One method is to combine mild needle stimulation with moxibustion at such points as ST-36, SP-6, and CV-4 (as well as moxibustion on salt at CV-8), to supplement qi. At the same time use moderate stimulus at LI-4 and GB-20 to expel the pathogen.

To nourish yin, points related to the organs affected are usually chosen. Since kidney yin is considered to be the root of the yin of the entire body, KI-3 is often added in any yin vacuity condition because of its ability to nourish kidney yin.

Remarks concerning the use of diaphoresis

Diaphoresis is used in the treatment of exterior patterns, but if the condition progresses to an interior pattern, other methods of treatment must be used. In hot weather, perspiration naturally increases, so that warm and pungent agents must be used judiciously. For more particulars regarding treatment of exterior patterns, refer to the tai yang disease section in Chapter 11.

Clearage

The method of clearage involves the use of cool and cold agents to clear and drain pathogenic heat. *Essential Questions* refers to this method when it states, "Heat is treated with cold." It includes heat clearage, fire drainage, blood cooling, and detoxification. These are the main methods for treating heat patterns.

Clearage is used in the treatment of interior heat patterns such as qi-aspect heat, blood-aspect heat, damp-heat, and yang lesion patterns. Vacuity heat and exterior heat patterns may be treated by combining heat clearage with supplementation and exterior resolution.

Clearing heat and resolving toxin

All repletion patterns caused by heat toxin, such as intense heat toxin in exogenous heat diseases, yang lesion patterns, erysipelas, maculopapular eruptions, pulmonary abscesses, dysentery with blood and pus in the stool, heat strangury, painful urination, and dark-colored urine, are treated by clearing heat and resolving toxin. Such patterns are characterized by palpable heat, fever, swelling and distention, pain, suppuration, and putrefaction.

Agents used

Most agents that clear heat and resolve toxin are cool or cold in nature. Among the most common are:

Heat-Clearing and Toxin-Resolving Agents	
Folium Ta Ch'ing Yeh	*dà qīng yè*
Radix Isatidis	*bǎn lán gēn*
Herba et Radix Taraxaci	*pú gōng yīng*
Radix Scutellariae	*huáng qín*
Rhizoma Coptidis	*huáng lián*
Cortex Phellodendri	*huáng bó*
Cortex Radicis Mu Tan	*mǔ dān pí*
Radix Paeoniae Rubrae	*chì sháo*
Flos Lonicerae	*yín huā*
Fructus Forsythiae	*lián qiào*
Rhizoma Zingiberis Recens	*shēng jiāng*
Fructus Gardeniae	*zhī zǐ*

Other agents in this category have specialized applications: Herba Portulacae *(mǎ chǐ xiàn)* and Radix Pulsatillae *(bái tóu wēng)* are mainly used for dysentery. Radix Fagopyri Vulgaris *(yě qiáo)* is mostly used to treat pulmonary abscesses, and Caulis Sargentodoxae *(hóng téng)*, is mainly used for intestinal abscesses.

Representative formula

Coptis Detoxifying Powder *(huáng-lián jiě dú sǎn)*.

Acumoxatherapy

Like medicinal agents, acupuncture points are chosen according to the location and nature of the heat pathogen. Generally, a strong stimulus is desired since heat toxin produces a condition of repletion. This is not the case with vacuity heat, discussed later in this chapter. Points that clear heat toxin include:

TB-3: triple burner heat

SI-3: malarial heat, ocular rubor, yellow to dark-colored urine

ST-45: stomach heat

BL-54: heat toxicity from the blood (bleed capillaries around point)

GV-20: exuberant heat in the yang channels

LI-11: pathogenic heat

If heat is extreme, points are often bled to drain pathogenic heat.

Clearing Qi Heat

Indications

Qi-aspect heat patterns with vigorous (surfaced) fever, thirst, dry tongue, and surging pulse.

Agents used

Most commonly used are cold agents that are either pungent or bitter in sapor, such as Gypsum *(shí gāo)*, Rhizoma Anemarrhenae *(zhī mǔ)*, and Fructus Gardeniae *(zhī zǐ)*.

Two points should be remembered when clearing qi heat. First, the goal is to induce diffusion and outthrust, so that the pathogen is expelled from the body rather than entering construction-blood; second, the liquid must be safeguarded against damage by intense heat.

Principles and Methods of Treatment

Diffusing outthrusters include:

Diffusing Outthrusters	
Gypsum	*shí gāo*
Semen Sojae Praeparatum	*dòu shǐ*
Fructus Gardeniae	*zhī zǐ*
Radix Puerariae	*gé gēn*
Herba Artemisiae Apiaceae	*qīng hāo*

Agents that promote lung qi diffusion may also be used. Liquid safeguarders include:

Liquid Safeguarders	
Rhizoma Anemarrhenae	*zhī mǔ*
Radix Trichosanthis	*tiān huā fěn*
Rhizoma Phragmitis	*lú gēn*
Radix Adenophorae Viva	*xiān shā shēn*
Herba Dendrobii Viva	*xiān shí hú*

Radix Pueriariae *(gé gēn)* and Herba Artemisiae Apiaceae *(qīng hāo)* are liquid engenderers that may also be used.

Representative formulae

Qi Heat Clearage Formulae	
White Tiger Decoction	*bái hǔ tāng*
Gardenia and Fermented Soybean Decoction	*zhī-zǐ shǐ tāng*

White Tiger Decoction clears heat to safeguard liquid, and is used in major qi-aspect heat patterns. Gardenia and Fermented Soybean Decoction, which induces diffusion and outthrust while also clearing heat, is used to treat the initial penetration of pathogenic heat to the qi aspect and eradicate thoracic vexation.

Acumoxatherapy

Points commonly used to clear qi-aspect heat include LI-11, GV-14, LI-4, GB-34, and LU-5.

Clearing blood heat

Indications

Heat penetrating construction-blood in heat diseases (high fever, clouding of the spirit, crimson tongue), and hemorrhage and maculopapular eruptions due to blood heat, are common indications of blood heat.

Agents used

The agents most commonly used in clearing blood heat are blood-cooling and toxin-resolving agents such as:

Blood-Cooling and Toxin-Resolving Agents	
Radix Rehmanniae Viva	xiān shēng dì
Radix Scrophulariae	xuán shēn
Radix Lithospermi	zǐ cǎo
Folium Ta Ch'ing Yeh	dà qīng yè
Radix Isatidis	bǎn lán gēn
Flos Lonicerae	yín huā
Radix Paeoniae Rubrae	chì sháo
Cortex Radicis Mu Tan	mǔ dān pí
Cornu Rhinoceri	xī jiǎo

Some blood-heat patterns, particularly construction-blood patterns occurring in heat diseases, cannot, because of the complexity of their nature, be treated by blood-cooling and toxin-resolving agents alone. Formulae must often include heart clearers, portal openers, and liver-clearing wind-extinguishing agents.

Representative formulae

Blood-Cooling and Toxin-Resolving Formulae	
Minor Cyan Dragon Decoction	xiǎo qīng lóng tāng
Construction-Clearing Decoction	qīng yíng tāng

Minor Cyan Dragon Decoction cools the blood and resolves toxins, and represents a basic formula for clearing blood heat. Construction-Clearing Decoction has the same basic blood-cooling toxin-resolving action, but also contains heat clearers and yin enrichers, and mainly treats heat penetrating construction-blood. In clinical practice, qi-aspect heat clearers, blood-aspect heat clearers, and heat-clearing, toxin-resolving agents may be added. An example of such a formula is Scourge-Clearing Detoxifying Cool Decoction *(qīng wēn bài dú yǐn)* which is used to treat such diseases as encephalitis B (Japanese encephalitis). This formula is a combination of White Tiger Decoction *(bái hǔ tāng)*, Rhinoceros Horn and Rehmannia Decoction *(xī-jiǎo dì-huáng tāng)*, and Coptis Detoxifying Decoction *(huáng-lián jiě dú tāng)*.

Acumoxatherapy

Points used to clear blood-aspect heat include LU-10, BL-17, BL-54, SP-10, and LI-11. The selection of points depends on the location and nature of the heat pathogen.

Damp-heat clearage

Indications

Damp-heat conditions such as liver channel damp-heat, damp-heat jaundice, and persistent damp-heat in exogenous heat diseases may be observed. General damp-heat symptoms include oppression in the chest, nausea, poor appetite, short micturition with dark-colored urine, thin or sometimes hard stool, and slimy, yellow tongue fur. Fever, if present, is persistent and usually unsurfaced. Damp-heat skin diseases are characterized by heavy serous discharge.

Agents used

Clearage of damp-heat involves the use of cold, bitter, heat-clearing damp driers such as:

Cold, Bitter, Heat-Clearing Damp Driers	
Rhizoma Coptidis	*huáng lián*
Cortex Phellodendri	*huáng bó*
Radix Scutellariae	*huáng qín*
Radix Gentianae	*lóng dǎn cǎo*

As well, warm, bitter damp dryers are used:

Warm, Bitter Damp Driers	
Rhizoma Atractylodis	*cāng zhú*
Cortex Magnoliae	*hòu pò*
Rhizoma Pinelliae	*bàn xià*

Aromatic damp transformers may be added to these, such as:

Aromatic Damp Transformers	
Herba Agastaches	*huò xiāng*
Herba Eupatorii	*pèi lán*
Fructus Amomi Cardamomi	*kòu rén*

Bland percolating water-disinhibitors may also be used:

Water Disinhibitors	
Talcum	*huá shí*
Medulla Tetrapanacis	*tōng cǎo*
Sclerotium Poriae	*fú líng*
Herba Lophatheri	*dàn zhú yè*

Where damp-heat is severe or leads to fire formation, it is treated with formulae comprising cold, bitter agents that not only clear heat and transform damp, but also drain fire and resolve toxin. In cases of persistent damp-heat characterized by oppression in the chest, abdominal distention, upflow and nausea, dyspeptic anorexia, thin stool, slimy tongue fur, and remittent fever, warm, bitter damp-dryers or aromatic damp-transformers are generally used if the damp symptoms are more pronounced. If the heat symptoms are more pronounced, cold, bitter, heat-clearing, damp-drying agents are used. "Pungent opening and bitter discharging," opening with pungent agents and discharging with bitter agents, is a commonly used method of clearing damp-heat. Such combinations include Rhizoma Pinelliae *(bàn xià)* with Radix Scutellariae *(huáng qín)*, and Cortex Magnoliae *(hòu pò)* with Rhizoma Coptidis *(huáng lián)*. Damp-heat skin diseases are frequently treated with Radix Sophorae Flavescentis *(kǔ shēn)*, Rhizoma Smilacis Glabrae *(tǔ fú líng)*, and Cortex Perillae *(bái sū pí)*.

Representative formulae

Damp-Heat Formulae	
Gentian Liver-Draining Decoction	*lóng dǎn xiè gān tāng*
Artemisia Capillaris Decoction	*yīn-chén-hāo tāng*
Three Kernel Decoction	*sān rén tāng*
Sweet Dew Toxin-Dispersing Elixir	*gān lù xiāo dú dān*
Coptis and Magnolia Cool Decoction	*lián pò yǐn*

Gentian Liver-Draining Decoction is used to treat damp-heat in the liver channel. Artemesia Capillaris Decoction treats damp-heat jaundice. Three Kernel Decoction may be used to treat persistent damp-heat where the damp symptoms are more pronounced than the heat symptoms. Sweet Dew Toxin-Dispersing Elixir treats persistent damp-heat patterns where the heat symptoms are more pronounced. Coptis and Magnolia Cool Decoction is used for "pungent opening and bitter discharging."

Acumoxatherapy

Damp-heat is treated by combining points that transform or drain damp with points that drain fire or clear heat. Also included are points that course and abduct or drain damp-heat. For example, damp-heat jaundice might be treated with the following points:

LV-3: drain liver fire

BL-43, BL-19: course and abduct damp-heat; clear gallbladder fire

GB-34: drain gallbladder fire

CV-11: harmonize stomach, promote center flow; transform damp.

BL-53: promote diaphoresis and thereby drain damp-heat

Similar treatments are used for other damp-heat disorders. Red dysentery (dysentery with blood in the stool) is treated with BL-25, BL-27, SP-15, ST-44, ST-25, and PC-6. In this formula, BL-25, ST-25, and SP-15 are used to drain large intestine damp-heat; BL-27 clears turbidity, and by acting as a diaphoretic transforms damp. PC-6 is an effective point for draining blood-aspect heat because it is the connecting point of the pericardium channel and the master point of the yin linking vessel, both of which are intimately related to blood and blood circulation. It also has a calming effect on the stomach and may be used for any accompanying nausea. ST-44 clears yang ming heat.

Other points commonly used to treat damp-heat diseases include ST-40, SP-9, LV-8, GB-39, and LU-9, to transform or drain damp, and points such as LU-5, LI-11, and BL-54, to clear heat.

Because damp-heat is a repletion condition, a strong stimulation is usually preferable.

Clearing vacuity heat

Indications

In advanced stages of exogenous heat diseases or chronic diseases such as tuberculosis, the yin humor is damaged and pathogenic heat is lodged at the yin levels. Symptoms include steaming bone or tidal fever, persistent low fever, flushing of the cheeks, emaciation, and red or crimson tongue with little fur.

Agents used

Vacuity Heat Clearers	
Carapax Amydae	*biē jiǎ*
Herba Artemisiae Apiaceae	*qīng hāo*
Cortex Radicis Lycii	*dì gǔ pí*
Radix Stellariae Dichotomae	*yín chái hú*
Herba Gentianae Macrophyllae	*qín jiāo*
Radix Cynanchi Atrati	*bái wéi*

Emphasis may be on either enriching yin or clearing heat, depending on the degree of yin vacuity and the strength of the pathogenic heat.

Representative formulae

Damp-Heat Resolving Formulae	
Two-A Decoction	*qīng-hāo biē-jiǎ tāng*
Bone-clearing Powder	*qīng gǔ sǎn*

Two-A Decoction primarily nourishes yin, whereas Steaming Bone Fever Powder primarily clears heat.

Acumoxatherapy

Treatment is based on supplementing yin while downbearing counterflow and draining fire. For example, a vacuity-fire toothache may be treated with mild stimulus at KI-3 to enrich water, with strong stimulus at LI-4 and LV-3, to clear yang ming heat and liver heat respectively.

Points previously indicated for clearing repletion heat are also often used to clear vacuity heat.

Remarks concerning the use of clearage

Clearage is based on the use of cool and cold agents, which if used in excessively large quantities or over extended periods of time, may affect splenogastric function, precipitating loss of appetite. Clearage is contraindicated in patients regularly suffering from organic vacuity cold.

Ejection

Ejection denotes the expulsion of pathogens or potentially harmful substances through the mouth. It is used in acute conditions where the pathogen is in the upper or middle burner.

Emesis

Indications

Conditions resulting from voracious eating characterized by gastric congestion inhibiting digestion and causing painful fullness and distention call for emesis. This method may also be used to treat poisoning, provided treatment is administered swiftly after ingestion of the toxic substance.

Representative formulae

Emetic Formulae	
Pedicellus Cucumeris Powder	*guā-dì sǎn*
Cervix Ginseng Powder	*shēn lǜ sǎn*

Acumoxatherapy

Regarding emesis, the *Gateway to Medicine* says:

> To promote vomiting, needle *nei-guan* {PC-6} to a depth of 0.3 body inches; first supplement six times, then drain three times.... Direct the qi upward. The patient will often vomit.

... If the vomiting does not cease, a supplementing stimulus should be applied at *zu-san-li* {ST-36}.

In modern clinical practice, vomiting is often induced by applying strong stimulus to CV-12 and CV-22.

Phlegm-drool ejection

Indications

This method of ejection is called for in conditions of laryngeal wind, swollen tonsils, or laryngeal obturation patterns, caused by exuberant phlegm obstructing the throat; or windstrike phlegm inversion characterized by phlegm-drool congesting the diaphragm and throat, causing a rasping sound, and comatose states.

Representative formulae

Phlegm Ejection Formulae	
Realgar Detoxifying Pills	*xióng-huáng jiě dú wán*
Thin Drool Powder	*xī xián sǎn*

Realgar Detoxifying Pills are used for laryngeal disorders, while Thin Drool Powder treats windstrike patterns.

Acumoxatherapy

Major points used to promote phlegm-drool ejection include CV-22, CV-12, ST-40, and PC-6. CV-22 helps clear phlegm and turbidity in the throat. CV-12 and ST-40 are useful points for eliminating phlegm. PC-6 moves the yin linking vessel, clears the heart, frees the chest, and benefits the diaphragm. These points are most effective when combined with points that treat the underlying condition.

Remarks concerning the use of ejection

Ejection is a potent method of treatment and can damage original qi and deplete the stomach juices, especially if used when inappropriate. It is contraindicated in pregnancy, for infants or the elderly, for patients suffering from tuberculosis, stomach complaints, or severe foot-qi disease, patients in weak health, or those with a history of blood ejection or hematemesis.

Precipitation

Precipitation (purgation) denotes stimulating fecal flow for the purposes of expelling repletion pathogens and removing accumulation and stagnation. The *Inner Canon* states, "Precipitation involves the drawing out {of pathogens}," and "lodging {accumulation and stagnation} is treated by attack."

There are four aspects to precipitation:

Fire drainage, which can be subdivided into three aspects:

precipitation of gastrointestinal heat-bind (used in yang ming bowel patterns);

precipitation of heat toxin (used to expel pathogenic fire and heat toxin through the bowels);

precipitation of depressed upper-body fire (used to treat upflaming of liver fire and depressed pulmogastric heat).

Expulsion of cold accumulations.

Expulsion of water-rheum.

Lubricating the intestines and freeing the stool.

In addition, precipitation may be combined with other methods of treatment such as transforming phlegm, transforming blood-stasis, dispersing digestate accumulations, and expelling parasites. An important method of expelling pathogens, precipitation may be used when concentration of pathogens in the interior precipitates interior repletion patterns. In clinical practice, careful evaluation of the relative strength of correct qi and the pathogen is necessary to ensure that a formula appropriate for the patient's condition is chosen.

Precipitation is currently used with satisfactory results for a wide variety of acute abdomen patterns such as intestinal obstruction, acute cholecystitis, and acute pancreatitis.

Precipitation of gastrointestinal heat-bind

Indications

This method would be used for patterns of yang ming bowel repletion, characterized by tidal fever, abdominal distention and palpatory tenderness, constipation, old yellow or burnt-yellow tongue fur, or a dry fissured tongue with black, parched fur and prickles at the tip and edges, and a strong, deep, slippery pulse. These symptoms are classically summarized with the words glomus, fullness, dryness, and repletion. In severe cases there may be delirious speech and manic agitation, or diarrhea characterized by foul-smelling stool and burning sensations, together with fecal impaction (classically referred to as "heat-bind with circumfluence").

Agents used

The principal drug used in precipitating gastrointestinal heat-bind is Rhizoma Rhei *(dà huáng)*, which frees the stool, drains fire, resolves toxin, and flushes the heat-bind. It is often used with Mirabilitum *(máng xiāo)* which is salty and cold, and which softens hardness and drains heat. Patients with pronounced abdominal pain and distention should be prescribed formulae that also contain Fructus Citri Immaturus *(zhǐ shí)* and Cortex Magnoliae *(hòu pò)* which loosen the center and break qi, thereby eliminating glomus and fullness. These three agents enhance the precipitant effect of Rhizoma Rhei.

Representative formulae

Gastrointestinal Heat-Bind Formulae	
Major Purgative Decoction	*dà chéng qì tāng*
Minor Purgative Decoction	*xiǎo chéng qì tāng*
Stomach-Regulating Purgative Decoction	*tiáo wèi chéng qì tāng*

For elaboration of the difference between these three purgative decoctions, see in the previous chapter, under "Exogenous Heat Disease Pattern Identification."

Acumoxatherapy

Precipitation is not a major technique employed in acumoxatherapy. However, there are points known to free the stool, such as ST-25, TB-6, ST-36, LI-4, and BL-25.[2]

Precipitation of heat toxin

Indications

Precipitation of heat toxin would be called for in patterns of exogenous heat disease of either high fever, agitation, clouding of the spirit, or of heat toxin penetrating the construction aspect with such symptoms as frenetic blood movement, maculopapular eruptions, bleeding, and intestinal abscesses.

Agents used

The principal agent used to precipitate heat toxin is Rhizoma Rhei *(dà huáng)*, which is combined with large quantities of heat-clearing, toxin-resolving, and blood-cooling agents such as:

Heat-Clearing, Blood-Cooling, & Toxin-Resolving Agents	
Rhizoma Coptidis	*huáng lián*
Radix Scutellariae	*huáng qín*
Radix Lithospermi	*zǐ cǎo*
Cortex Radicis Mu Tan	*mǔ dān pí*
Radix Rehmanniae Conquita	*shóu dì*
Folium Ta Ch'ing Yeh	*dà qīng yè*
Flos Lonicerae	*yín huā*
Herba et Radix Taraxaci	*pú gōng yīng*

Representative formulae

Heat Toxin Precipitation Formulae	
Heart-Draining Decoction	xiè xīn tāng
Rhizoma Rhei and Mu Tan Decoction	dà-huáng mǔ-dān tāng

Heart-Draining Decoction primarily drains heat. Rhizoma Rhei and Mu Tan Decoction, which includes pus-expelling and toxin-resolving agents, is used mostly in the treatment of intestinal abscesses.

Acumoxatherapy

Toxic heat may be treated with GV-14 (bleed), GV-12 (bleed), M-UE-1 *(shi xuan)* (bleed), LI-4, BL-54, LI-11, and GB-34. In general, a strong stimulation is desirable.

Precipitation of depressed upper-body fire

Indications

Precipitation of depressed upper-body fire would be appropriate treatment in two instances. The first is depressed pulmogastric heat characterized by sore, swollen throat, lesions of the mouth and tongue, painful, swollen gums, periodontal *xuan*, nosebleed, feverish agitation in the chest and diaphragm, constipation, and halitosis. The second instance is upflaming of liver fire characterized by headache, red face and ocular rubor, yellow tongue fur, constipation, loss of hearing and tinnitus, restlessness and irascibility.

Agents used

The chief agent is Rhizoma Rhei *(dà huáng)*. In the treatment of depressed pulmogastric heat it is combined with heat-clearing and toxin-resolving agents such as:

Heat-Clearing and Toxin-Resolving Agents	
Fructus Gardeniae	zhī zǐ
Cortex Radicis Mu Tan	mǔ dān pí
Radix Scrophulariae	xuán shēn
Fructus Arctii	niú bàng zǐ
Radix Achyranthis	tǔ niú xī

To treat upflaming of liver fire, Rhizoma Rhei *(dà huáng)* is combined with liver drainers such as:

Liver Drainers	
Herba Aloes	lú huì
Semen Cassiae	jué míng zǐ
Spica Prunellae	xià kū cǎo
Radix Gentianae	lóng dǎn cǎo

Representative formulae

Depressed Upper-Body Fire Formulae	
Diaphragm-Cooling Powder	liáng gé sǎn
Angelica, Gentiana, and Aloe Pills	dāng-guī lóng huì wán
Toilette Pills	gēng yī wán

Diaphragm-Cooling Powder drains upper- and middle-burner heat, and is used to treat depressed pulmogastric heat. Both Angelica, Gentiana, and Aloe Pills and Toilette Pills drain the liver.

Acumoxatherapy

Depressed pulmogastric heat is treated with strong stimulation at ST-44, LI-4, TB-2, PC-6, PC-7, and LU-10. Upflaming liver fire is treated by supplementing kidney yin (which in turn supplements liver yin) through such points as LV-2 and KI-3. ST-44 may be included as well. In addition, head points such as GV-20 and M-HN-9 *(tai-yang)* are often added to disperse repletion and relieve local symptoms.

Expulsion of cold accumulations

Indications

Stagnation and accumulation patterns characterized by abdominal distention, abdominal pain, constipation, thick, slimy tongue fur, or moist tongue with white fur and absence of thirst, call for this method of treatment. Other patterns may be characterized by aversion to cold, frigidity of the limbs, and thirst with a desire for warm fluids. In clinical practice, the method of expelling cold accumulations treats exogenous cold contractions with pre-existing digestate accumulations as well as chronic bacillary dysentery and nephritic uremia.

Agents used

The basic drug is generally Rhizoma Rhei *(dà huáng)*, which is used with warm and hot agents such as Radix Aconiti Fu Tzu *(fù zǐ)*, Rhizoma Zingiberis Exsiccatum *(gān jiāng)*, and Cortex Cinnamomi *(ròu gùi)*. Warm agents with a powerful draining precipitant action such as Pulvis Seminis Crotonis *(bā dòu shuāng)* may be prescribed, but in clinical practice few cases warrant their use.

Representative formula

Spleen-Warming Decoction *(wēn pí tāng)*.

Acumoxatherapy

Cold accumulations may be expelled by needling CV-12‡, ST-36‡, SP-4‡, BL-25, and moxa on salt at CV-8.

Water Expulsion

Indications

Yang water repletion patterns such as severe thoracic water accumulations and ascites, characterized by constipation and urine retention, abdominothoracic distention and fullness inhibiting respiration, and a strong, full pulse, call for this type of treatment. The method of expelling water may be used where the pathogen is strong yet correct qi is still resilient enough to withstand offensive treatment. In clinical practice, this method is mainly used to treat ascites due to liver cirrhosis.

Agents used

Water Expellants	
Radix Euphorbiae Kan Sui	*gān suì*
Flos Daphnes Genkwa	*yuán huā*
Radix Euphorbiae	*dà jǐ*
Semen Pharbitidis	*qiān niú zǐ*

Rhizoma Rhei *(dà huáng)* might also be included in some formulae.

Representative formulae

Water Expulsion Formulae	
Ten Jujubes Pills	*shí zǎo wán*
Boats and Carts Pills	*zhōu chē wán*
Drool-Controlling Elixir	*kòng xián dān*

These three formulae are all supplied in prepared form. The first two are used to drain ascites, while the latter is used to drain thoracic water accumulations. The daily dose of each is 3 fen to 1 qian. Prepared freshly by pulverizing the constituents, and swallowed in powder form, these formulae have a stronger effect per dose than commercial preparations. All three are most effective when taken three hours after eating. In rare cases, they may cause gastroenteritis or reduce the potassium content of the blood.

Water expelling is often combined with supplementation, either by simultaneous supplementation and attack, or by attack followed by supplementation. The method is contraindicated for patients whose correct qi is too weak to withstand offensive treatment, those suffering from seriously damaged hepatic or renal functions, and those with hemorrhagic tendencies.

Acumoxatherapy

Yang water accumulations are treated with points that promote urination, such as SP-9 and CV-9, as well as SP-6‡, SP-4‡, and LU-7 which diffuse the lung and fortify the spleen. GV-26, KI-7, and BL-23‡ may also be added, depending on the location and severity of the accumulation.

Intestinal Lubrication

Indications

Constipation due to habit, senile or constitutional vacuity, or postpartum insufficiency of liquid and blood require intestinal lubrication.

Agents used

Intestinal lubricant formulae are based on high fat-content seeds such as:

Intestinal Lubricants	
Semen Cannabis	*má rén*
Fructus Trichosanthis	*guā lóu*
Semen Pruni Armeniacae	*xìng rén*

Patients with particularly weak constitutions may be given formulae that also contain agents with an enriching and intestine-lubricating action such as:

Enriching Intestinal Lubricants	
Radix Angelicae Sinensis Pinguis	*yóu dāng guī*
Radix Polygoni Multiflori Viva	*xiān shǒu wū*
Herba Cistanches	*cōng róng*

Formula prescribed for elderly patients with pronounced yang vacuities may include Sulfur Praeparatum *(zhì liú huáng)*. Constipation occurring in exogenous heat diseases other than yang ming heat-bind patterns may be treated with agents possessing both heat-clearing and intestine-moistening action, such as Fructus Trichosanthis *(guā lóu)* and Radix Scrophulariae *(xuán shēn)*.

Representative formulae

Intestinal Lubricant Formulae	
Cannabis Pills	má-zǐ-rén wán
Pinellia and Sulfur Pills	bàn liú wán

Cannabis Pills treat habitual diarrhea and Pinellia and Sulfur Pills treat vacuity cold diarrhea in the elderly.

Acumoxatherapy

TB-6, ST-25, ST-37, and ST-24 are useful for moistening the intestines. LI-4, ST-36, and BL-25 are often added, as are SP-15, ST-44, LI-11, and KI-6.

TB-6 drains depressed fire; LI-11 and ST-44 clear yang ming heat; KI-6 nourishes yin and drains fire; and SP-15 frees the stool.

Offensive elimination of phlegm

Indications

The method of offensive elimination of phlegm is used in binding of stagnant phlegm such as occurs in epilepsy, and mania and withdrawal; or in child fright wind characterized by gurgling phlegm and drool congesting the throat, with convulsive spasm of the limbs in serious cases.

Agents used

The main agents used are:

Offensive Phlegm Eliminators	
Lapis Chloriti	méng shí
Semen T'ing Li Tzu	tíng lì zǐ

Rhizoma Rhei may be added if necessary. Potent agents such as Pulvis Seminis Crotonis *(bā dòu shuāng)* are generally used in preprepared medicines rather than in fresh decoctions.

Representative formulae

Chlorite Phlegm-Expelling Pills *(méng-shí gǔn tán wán)*.

Acumoxatherapy

General points to transform phlegm and downbear turbidity, such as ST-40, are combined with points that lift depression, such as PC-6 and CV-11, and points the clear the heart and spirit, such as HT-7 and BL-15.

Other points useful for epilepsy and child fright wind include: GV-26, PC-8, CV-14, GB-20, CV-12, GV-15, SI-3, and ST-42.

Expulsion of static blood

Indications

The method of expulsion of static blood may be called for in various forms of blood amassment and inner-body static blood bind, including: a) inner-body static blood bind characterized by abdominal pain and distention, or lumps, black stool, oligomenorrhea, black menstrual discharge, fever, and in serious cases, manic states, and constipation; b) amenorrhea or oligomenorrhea, black menstrual discharge and irregular menses resulting from the presence of static blood; c) uterine concretions and gatherings; d) extra-uterine pregnancy.

Agents used

The principal agents used are blood breakers and draining precipitants such as:

Blood Breakers and Draining Precipitants	
Rhizoma Rhei	dà huáng
Mirabilitum	máng xiāo
Eupolyphaga	dì biē chóng
Semen Persicae	táo rén
Flos Carthami	hóng huā
Rhizoma Sparganii	sān léng
Rhizoma Curcumae Zedoariae	é zhú
Squama Manitis	shān jiǎ

Representative formulae

Static Blood Expulsion Formulae	
Peach Pit Purgative Decoction	táo-rén chéng qì tāng
Dead-On Pills	dǐ-dāng wán

Peach Pit Purgative Decoction is used for recent static blood formations, and Dead-On Pills are used for old formations. Recent reports discuss the treatment of extra-uterine pregnancy by the method of expelling static blood, using Gynecological Decoction *(shēng huà tāng)* with the addition of Rhizoma Rhei *(da huang)* and Mirabilitum *(mang xiao)*, or combined with Nine Pains Pills *(jiǔ tòng wán)*.

Acumoxatherapy

Inner body static blood-bind calls for points such as KI-14 to move the blood and qi in the abdomen[3] and SP-6 to move the blood and qi of the three yin channels of the foot and dispel static blood-bind. Strong stimulation of local points such as ST-25 and CV-10, in combination with the back-associated and lower-uniting points of the large intestine, BL-25 and ST-37 respectively, can aid the elimination of intestinal stagnations.

Menstrual disorders due to static blood are treated using liver channel points, notably LV-8 and LV-3, which course and drain liver qi, combined with SP-8, which moves liver blood. Often added are ST-30, CV-4, SP-6, and M-CA-18 *(zi gong)*. Because stagnation represents a repletion condition, a strong stimulus is usually employed. LI-4 may be added with mild stimulation, to supplement and move qi, thereby moving the blood.

Variations of precipitation

Simultaneous supplementation and attack

This principle is used to treat conditions characterized by a strong pathogen and weak correct qi, where it is necessary to ensure that the correct will withstand offensive treatment.

Representative formulae

Among the formulae used are Newly Supplemented Yellow Dragon Decoction *(xīn jiā huáng lóng tāng)* and its variants. This formula is a combination of Stomach-Regulating Purgative Decoction *(tiáo wèi chéng qì tāng)* which drains heat, and Humor-Increasing Decoction *(zēng yè tāng)* which enriches the fluids, with the admixture of Radix Salviae Miltiorrhizae *(dān shēn)*, to supplement qi, Radix Angelicae Sinensis *(dāng guī)*, to supplement the blood, and Succus Zingiberis *(jiāng zhī)*, to ensure perfusion of gastrointestinal qi, thereby promoting the flow of the digestate.

Acumoxatherapy

Since it is possible to either supplement or drain by varying the needle stimulus during treatment, simultaneous supplementation and attack is a commonly used method in acumoxatherapy. Points used include ST-36, LI-4, ST-41, CV-10, and ST-25.

Refloating the grounded ship

The Chinese term literally translated means "increasing water to move the boat." This method is used to treat heat patterns characterized by fluid depletion, and constipation due to dryness in the intestines.

Representative Formulae

The appropriate medication is heavy doses of Humor-Increasing Decoction *(zēng yè tāng)* which in cases of pronounced repletion heat may be supplemented with Rhizoma Rhei *(da huang)* and Mirabilitum *(máng xiāo)*, thus forming Humor-Increasing Purgative Decoction *(zēng yè chéng qì tāng)*.

Draining precipitants such as Mirabilitum and Rhizoma Rhei are frequently used in other methods that expel parasites and digestate accumulations. Further elaboration of these methods is discussed later in this chapter.

Acumoxatherapy

Points stimulating fluid formation include TB-6, ST-25, GB-34, and ST-40. BL-25, ST-36, and LI-4 may also be needled.

Remarks concerning the use of precipitation

Precipitation is contraindicated for elderly, weak, and postpartum patients, and those suffering from damage to liquid after illness or blood collapse, even where stool is hard. Exceptions may be made, but extreme caution is indicated. Precipitation should be used cautiously during pregnancy and menstruation.

The aim of precipitant treatment is to eliminate pathogens. Treatment should cease as soon as this purpose is achieved. Used to excess, it may damage correct qi. Since draining precipitants readily deplete stomach qi, diet should exclude foods that are fatty or difficult to digest.

Harmonization

Harmonization refers to the adjustment of functions within the human body. Where a pathogen is at midstage penetration, there is disharmony between qi and bood, or between the organs, and the methods of diaphoresis, ejection, precipitation, warming, clearage, dispersion, and supplementation cannot be used. Instead, harmonization methods, such as resolving the exterior and harmonizing the interior, rectifying qi and harmonizing construction, and harmonizing the organs, are used.

Midstage harmonization

Indications

Midstage harmonization would be appropriate in exogenous heat diseases characterized by alternating fever and chills, oppression and fullness in the chest and lateral costal region, bitter taste in the mouth and dry pharynx, and nausea and vomiting — shao yang midstage patterns (q.v. Chapter 11).

Agents used

The main agents used are:

Midstage Harmonizers	
Radix Bupleuri	*chái hú*
(or) Herba Artemisiae Apiaceae	*qīng hāo*
(combined with) Radix Scutellariae	*huáng qín*

The first two of these agents promote outthrust of exterior pathogens, while the third clears interior heat. Formulae also include center harmonizers such as:

Center Harmonizers	
Rhizoma Pinelliae	*bàn xià*
Rhizoma Zingiberis Recens	*shēng jiāng*
Radix Glycyrrhizae	*gān cǎo*
Fructus Zizyphi Jujubae	*dà zǎo*

Vacuity of correct qi may justify the judicious addition of correct-restorative agents such as Radix Codonopsis Pilosulae *(dang shen)*.

Representative formula

Minor Bupleurum Decoction *(xiǎo chái-hú tāng)*, which in modern clinical practice is usually prescribed without Radix Ginseng *(rén shēn)*, Radix Glycyrrhizae *(gān cǎo)*, and Fructus Zizyphi Jujubae *(dà zǎo)*, is the standard decoction for clearing shao yang liver and gallbladder heat. Midstage patterns involving abdominal pain and distention and other yang ming bowel repletion symptoms may be treated with Major Bupleurum Decoction *(dà chái-hú tāng)* or other formulae containing draining precipitants such as:

Draining Precipitant Agents	
Rhizoma Rhei	*dà huáng*
Mirabilitum	*máng xiāo*
Fructus Citri Immaturus	*zhǐ shí*

Acumoxatherapy

Commonly used points include PC-6, TB-5, TB-6, GB-34, and TB-2. Most of these are located on the shao yang gallbladder and triple burner channels. PC-6, which connects the primary channel of the pericardium with the divergent channel of the triple burner, calms the chest and relieves nausea.

Rectifying qi and harmonizing construction

Indications

Binding depression of liver qi with construction-blood disharmony, characterized by depression, agitation, pain in the lateral costal region, qi stagnation in the chest and lateral costal region causing local distention, or swollen breasts, menstrual disorders, and menorrhalgia, calls for treatment using the methods of rectifying qi and harmonizing construction.

Agents used

Treatment is based on liver-coursing and qi-rectifying agents such as:

Liver-Coursing and Qi-Rectifying Agents	
Radix Bupleuri	*chái hú*
Pericarpium Citri Reticulatae Viride	*qīng pí*
Rhizoma Cyperi	*xiāng fù*
Fructus Meliae Toosendan	*chuān liàn zǐ*

These are combined with blood-nourishing construction-harmonizing agents.

Blood-Nourishing and Construction-Harmonizing Agents	
Radix Angelicae Sinensis	*dāng guī*
Radix Paeoniae	*sháo yào*
Radix Salviae Miltiorrhizae	*dān shēn*

Agents that quicken the blood and transform stasis may be added where pain is particularly pronounced or static blood symptoms are present.

Blood-Quickening and Stasis-Transforming Agents	
Rhizoma Corydalis	*yán hú suǒ*
Flos Carthami	*hóng huā*
Radix Rubiae	*qiàn cǎo*
Tuber Curcumae	*yù jīn*

Patterns involving liver fire may call for the admixture of agents such as Fructus Gardeniae *(zhī zǐ)* and Cortex Radicis Mu Tan *(mǔ dān pí)*.

Representative formula

Free Wanderer Powder *(xiāo yáo sǎn)*.

Acumoxatherapy

Points such as LV-2 and LV-14 are used to course liver qi and drain liver fire. GB-40 and GB-34 are often used to course the gallbladder channel, and PC-6 is added to open the chest, relieve pain, and quiet the spirit.

SP-4 is an especially useful point for this type of condition. The meeting point of the penetrating vessel channel, it rectifies the qi and blood of the lower abdomen, has a rectifying effect on qi dynamic, and rectifies the "sea of blood," i.e., menstruation and reproduction. SP-6 is another point that specifically harmonizes qi and blood; a point of intersection of the three yin channels of the leg, it also has a strong effect on lower abdominal and menstrual disorders. To quiet the spirit, HT-7 may also be added.

Hepatogastric harmonization

Indications

Disharmony between the liver and stomach from impairment of the hepatic governance of free-coursing and impaired downbearing of stomach qi shows symptoms including painful distention in the chest and lateral costal region, pain, fullness, and distention in the stomach, loss of appetite, eructation, vomiting of sour matter, or retching and nausea.

Agents used

Liver coursers such as Fructus Evodiae *(wú zhū yú)* and Herba Perillae Crispae *(zǐ sū)*, in combination with stomach harmonizers such as Rhizoma Pinelliae *(bàn xià)* or Rhizoma Zingiberis Recens *(shēng jiāng)*, or with stomach heat clearers such as Rhizoma Coptidis *(huáng lián)* and Caulis Bambusae in Taenis *(zhú rú)* are used. The emphasis may be variously placed on coursing the liver, harmonizing the stomach, or clearing the stomach, depending on the nature of the pattern.

Representative formulae

Hepatogastric Harmonization Formulae	
Four-Seven Decoction	*sì qī tāng*
Kidney Pills	*zuǒ guī wán*

Four-Seven Decoction is prescribed primarily for conditions with prominent liver qi depression. Kidney Pills are used primarily to treat disruption of stomach harmony and downflow.

Acumoxatherapy

Liver-coursing points such as LV-3 are combined with points that benefit the stomach, such as ST-36 and CV-12. PC-6 helps relieve nausea and regurgitation. SP-4 harmonizes and rectifies the spleen and stomach. GB-34 is often added to course the gallbladder channel.

Hepatosplenic harmonization

Indications

Hepatosplenic disharmony arises when liver qi is depressed and the movement and transformation functions of the spleen are disrupted. Symptoms include abdominal distention, abdominal pain, borborygmus, and diarrhea. Paroxysms are usually associated with emotional factors.

Agents used

Liver-coursers such as Radix Bupleuri *(chái hú)* and Radix Paeoniae Albae *(bái sháo),* are combined with spleen fortifiers such as Rhizoma Atractylodis Macrocephalae *(bái zhú),* Sclerotium Poriae *(fú líng),* and Pericarpium Citri Tangerinae *(chén pí).*

Representative formulae

Hepatosplenic Harmonizing Formulae	
Pain and Diarrhea Formula	*tòng xiè yào fāng*
Free Wanderer Powder	*xiāo yáo sǎn*

Free Wanderer Powder includes Radix Bupleuri *(chái hú)* and Radix Paeoniae Albae *(bái sháo)* combined with Rhizoma Atractylodis Macrocephalae *(bái zhú)* and Sclerotium Poriae *(fú líng).* It is essentially a qi-rectifying and construction-harmonizing formula. However, these agents are equally effective in treating hepatosplenic disharmony.

Acumoxatherapy

LV-5 and LV-3, both of which course and harmonize, are combined with points such as SP-6‡, SP-4‡, and BL-20‡, which recify spleen qi and fortify splenic function, and BL-18, which quiets the spirit and disperses congealing static blood. Other points may be added, depending on the symptoms. For example, ST-25‡ is used to treat diarrhea, and CV-10‡ is frequently used for abdominal pain and/or distention.

Gastrointestinal harmonization

Indications

Gastrointestinal disharmony exhibits symptoms including disruption of normal upbearing and downbearing and cold-heat complexes precipitating infracardiac glomus and fullness, vomiting, borborygmi, and diarrhea. Gastrointentinal harmonization is the prescribed treatment.

Agents used

Cold, bitter agents, Rhizoma Coptidis *(huáng lián)* and Radix Scutellariae *(huáng qín)*, are used with warm, pungent agents such as Rhizoma Zingiberis Exsiccatum *(gān jiāng)* and Rhizoma Pinelliae *(bàn xià)*. The cold, bitter agents drain heat, while the pungent agents dissipate glomus, and together have the effect of harmonizing the middle burner and restoring normal upbearing and downbearing.

Representative formula

Pinellia Heart-Draining Decoction *(bàn-xià xiè xīn tāng)*.

Acumoxatherapy

Normal upbearing and downbearing of qi is promoted by needling points that harmonize the stomach and intestines, such as CV-12, ST-36, ST-37, and ST-25, as well as points that benefit the large intestine, such as BL-25 and LI-4. PC-6 can also be used to harmonize the stomach and downbear counterflow.

Warming

Essential Questions states, "Cold is treated with heat." Thus, warming, which is applied in interior cold patterns, involves the use of warm or hot agents to supplement yang qi and expel the cold pathogen.

Interior cold patterns include the following:

> Invasion of the interior by the cold pathogen inhibiting yang qi, precipitating vomiturition and diarrhea, cold and pain in the stomach and abdomen, frigid limbs and aversion to cold, and other signs of splenogastric vacuity and interior cold, all of which are treated by warming the center and dissipating cold.

> Debilitation of original qi, precipitating endogenous yin cold, sweating, aversion to cold, clear-food diarrhea, counterflow frigidity of the limbs, faint pulse, and other signs of yang collapse, treated by moistening the kidney and restoring yang.

> Water-damp flood from yang qi vacuity, characterized by water swelling and treated by warming yang and disinhibiting water.

> Invasion of the channels by the cold pathogen, causing pain in the sinews and bones, hypertonicity, and impeded movement, treated by freeing and warming the channels.

In acumoxatherapy, warming is achieved through moxibustion. There is a growing tendency among modern physicians to regard direct, scarring moxibustion as unnecessarily painful and uncosmetic. Consequently, indirect moxibustion has become the primary mode of application. Some

Principles and Methods of Treatment

physicians continue to use the direct techniques, claiming the effects are superior. The warnings concerning the use of the warming method cited at the end of this chapter are all applicable to moxibustion, although moxibustion on points such as SP-1 and LV-1, used to stop bleeding, is an exception to the rule. Though some repletion heat patterns warrant the use of moxibustion, in general it is contraindicated in heat conditions.

Warming the center and dissipating cold

Indications

Constitutional yang vacuity, splenogastric vacuity cold, and interiorization of exogenous cold call for warming the center and dissipating cold. Signs include white, moist tongue fur, moderate, soggy pulse or deep, slow pulse, physical debilitation and spiritual fatigue; or aversion to cold, diarrhea, pain in the abdomen relieved by palpation and by heat, and stomachache and vomiting of clear fluid.

Agents used

Treatment is based on center warmers:

Center Warmers	
Rhizoma Zingiberis Exsiccatum	*gān jiāng*
Rhizoma Zingiberis blast-fried	*pāo jiāng*
Rhizoma Alpiniae Officinari	*liáng jiāng*
Fructus Zanthoxyli Szechuanensis	*chuān jiāo*

These are combined with spleen fortifiers and stomach boosters:

Spleen-Fortifying and Stomach-Boosting Agents	
Rhizoma Atractylodis Macrocephalae	*bái zhú*
Sclerotium Poriae	*fú líng*
Radix Glycyrrhizae mix-fried	*zhì gān cǎo*

Where cold signs are particularly pronounced, yang warming agents may be added:

Yang Warmers	
Radix Aconiti Fu Tzu	*fù zǐ*
Cortex Cinnamomi	*ròu guì*

Representative formulae

Center-Warming and Cold-Dissipating Formulae	
Winning Streak Powder	*dà shùn sǎn*
Center-Rectifying Pills	*lǐ zhōng wán*
Evodia Decoction	*wú-zhū-yú tāng*

Winning-Streak Powder dissipates cold and relieves pain. Center-Rectifying Pills warm the spleen and stop diarrhea. Evodia Decoction warms the stomach and checks vomiting.

Acumoxatherapy

Points that warm the center, such as CV-12‡ and ST-25‡, are combined with points that fortify the spleen, such as SP-6‡, BL-20‡, and SP-4‡. ST-36‡ is also commonly used in the treatment of splenogastric vacuity.

Salvaging yang and eliminating counterflow frigidity

Indications

Yang collapse vacuity desertion, characterized by aversion to cold, curled, recumbent posture, counterflow frigidity of the limbs, drop in body temperature and blood pressure, cold sweats, somber white complexion, and a faint, fine pulse, or vacuous, rapid pulse, calls for treatment by salvaging yang and eliminating counterflow frigidity.

Agents used

Treatment is based on yang warmers:

Yang Warmers	
Radix Aconiti Fu Tzu	*fù zǐ*
Rhizoma Zingiberis Exsiccatum	*gān jiāng*
Cortex Cinnamomi	*ròu guì*

These are used together with qi boosters:

Qi Boosters	
Radix Glycyrrhizae	*gān cǎo*
Radix Codonopsis Pilosulae	*dǎng shēn*

In severe cases, Radix Ginseng *(rén shēn)* may be added. If copious perspiration indicates a desertion trend, formulae may contain agents such as Os Draconis *(lóng gǔ)* and Concha Ostreae *(mǔ lì)*, which constrain perspiration and secure against desertion. For yin humor depletion, yin-

Principles and Methods of Treatment

constraining and humor-nourishing agents may be used, such as Fructus Schisandrae *(wŭ wèi zĭ)* and Radix Rehmanniae Conquita *(shóu dì)*.

Representative Formula

Counterflow Cold Decoction *(sì nì tāng)*.

Acumoxatherapy

Moxibustion is used at GV-4 and ST-36 to supplement yang and qi, and at GV-20 to raise yang. Needling LI-4 can supplement and move qi, while in extreme cases KI-1 may also be needled. BL-38‡ is also combined with ST-36‡ to warm the triple burner.

Warming yang and disinhibiting water

Indications

Yang vacuity reducing the transformative action of qi, characterized by water swelling confined to the legs, or disposition to generalized, short micturition; somber white complexion, frigid limbs and aversion to cold; pale tongue, and a weak, deep, fine pulse, are symptoms that call for treatment using the method of warming yang and disinhibiting water.

Agents used

Treatment is based on yang warmers:

Yang Warmers	
Radix Aconiti Fu Tzu	*fù zĭ*
Rhizoma Zingiberis Exsiccatum	*gān jiāng*
Ramulus Cinnamomi	*guì zhī*

These are used with water disinhibitors:

Water Disinhibitors	
Sclerotium Poriae	*fú líng*
Semen Plantaginis	*chē qián zĭ*
Rhizoma Alismatis	*zé xiè*

Representative formulae

Yang-Warming Water-Disinhibiting Formulae	
Life-Saver Kidney Qi Pills	*jì shēng shèn qì wán*
True Warrior Decoction	*zhēn wŭ tāng*

Life-Saver Kidney Qi Pills warm and supplement kidney yang. By stimulating the transformative action of qi, they promote water disinhibition. True Warrior Decoction warms the kidney and fortifies the spleen, and by dissipating cold, eliminates water qi.

Acumoxatherapy

BL-23‡ and BL-28‡, the back-associated points of the kidney and bladder respectively, are combined with CV-3‡, the front-alarm point of the bladder, to warm kidney and bladder yang. SP-9‡ disinhibits water by promoting diuresis, and moxibustion at BL-67 can free lower burner qi dynamic. SP-6‡ is often added when treating cold patterns.

Warming the channels and dissipating cold

Indications

Wind-cold-damp obturation with pronounced cold signs, such as articular pain relieved by warmth, and inhibited bending and stretching, may be treated using the method of warming the channels and dissipating cold.

Agents used

Treatment is based primarily on channel warmers such as:

Channel Warmers	
Radix Aconiti Wu T'ou Szechuanensis	*chuān wū*
Ramulus Cinnamomi	*guì zhī*
Buthus	*quán xiē*
Radix Tu Huo	*dú huó*
Herba Asari	*xì xīn*

In cases with longer history, combinations include blood-quickening stasis transformers as well as bone and sinew strengtheners. Patients with weak constitutions may be given combinations including blood-nourishing and qi-boosting agents such as:

Blood Nourishers and Qi Boosters	
Radix Angelicae Sinensis	*dāng guī*
Radix Paeoniae Albae	*bái sháo*
Radix Astragali	*huáng qí*
Radix Codonopsis Pilosulae	*dǎng shēn*

Representative formula

Wu T'ou Aconite Decoction *(wū-tóu tāng)*.

Acumoxatherapy

Combining local points with related distal points on the extremities is especially effective in dispersing wind-cold-damp obturation in the channels. Distal points include:

BL-60‡ (knee and lower back);
LI-4‡ (elbow and shoulder);
SI-3‡ (neck and lower back);
GB-34‡ (neck, knee, leg, and lower back);
BL-57‡ (leg and lower back); and
TB-3‡ (shoulder, elbow, and back).

Remarks concerning the use of warming

Warming is contraindicated in the presence of hematemesis, hematuria, or hemafecia, since these symptoms indicate frenetic blood heat. Also, most warm agents are dry in nature, and if administered over extended periods, may cause damage to yin. It should be noted that the warming method should be applied with caution in patients with yin vacuity constitutions, characterized by such symptoms as a red tongue and dry throat.

Supplementation

The method of supplementation, also known as the method of supplementation and boosting, is derived from the principles, "vacuity is treated by supplemention," and "detriment is treated by boosting." Supplementation is the method that supplies insufficiencies of yin and yang, blood and qi, and organic functions. When correct qi is too weak to expel a pathogen, the method of supplementation can restore correct qi to normal strength, helping it to eliminate the pathogen; hence the principle, "By supporting the correct, pathogens are dispelled." There are four fundamental objects of supplementation: qi, blood, yin, and yang.

Supplementation of qi

Indications

Qi vacuity with general physical weakness, shortness of breath, lassitude, spontaneous sweating, weak, soggy, soft pulse, prolapse of the rectum or uterus; general physical debilitation following illness; and sequential blood and qi desertion in cases of massive bleeding, may be treated using the method of supplementation of qi.

Agents used

Mainly used are qi supplementers:

Qi Supplementers	
Radix Astragali	*huáng qí*
Radix Codonopsis Pilosulae	*dǎng shēn*
Radix Glycyrrhizae	*gān cǎo*

These are often combined with spleen fortifiers. Uplifters, blood nourishers, damp transformers, and qi movers may also be used.

Representative formulae

Qi-Supplementing Formulae	
Four Nobles Decoction	*sì jūn zǐ tāng*
Center-Supplementing Qi-Boosting Decoction	*bǔ zhōng yì qì tāng*
Ginseng Solo Decoction	*dú shēn tāng*

Four Nobles Decoction is a general qi-supplementing formula. Center-Supplementing Qi-Boosting Decoction counters center qi fall. Ginseng Solo Decoction treats massive bleeding where the primary concern is to secure original qi and contain the blood.

Acumoxatherapy

Points on the conception vessel, such as CV-4‡, CV-6‡, and CV-12‡, are used to supplement qi. The three yin channels of the leg can be supplemented through SP-6‡, lung qi through GV-12‡, kidney qi through BL-23‡ and KI-3‡, and the qi of the entire body through ST-36‡ and BL-24‡. GV-20‡ is used for prolapse, and BL-38‡ is frequently used together with ST-36‡ to treat debilitation after prolonged illness. KI-7 combined with LI-4 is a well known formula for treating spontaneous sweating.

Supplementation of the blood

Indications

This method of treatment should be applied for conditions of blood vacuity characterized by a drawn, withered yellow or pale white complexion, mental dizziness, tinnitus, palpitations, oligomenorrhea with pale discharge, fine pulse and pale tongue. Blood vacuity may occur in acute bleeding, in chronic diseases, or postpartum.

Agents used

Treatment is mainly based on blood supplementers:

Principles and Methods of Treatment

Blood Supplementers	
Radix Rehmanniae Cruda	*shēng dì*
Radix Angelicae Sinensis	*dāng guī*
Radix Polygoni Multiflori	*shǒu wū*
Fructus Lycii	*qǐ zǐ*
Gelatinum Corii Asini	*lǘ pí jiāo*
Arillus Euphoriae Longanae	*lóng yǎn*

These are often combined with qi supplementers and, depending on the condition of the patient, with blood quickeners, antihemorrhagics, and spirit quietants.

Representative formulae

Blood-Supplementing Formulae	
Four Agents Decoction	*sì wù tāng*
Eight Jewel Decoction	*bā zhēn tāng*
Angelica Splenic Decoction	*guī pí tāng*

Four Agents Decoction is a basic formula for supplementing the blood, regulating menstruation and quickening the blood. Eight Jewel Decoction treats dual vacuities of qi and blood. Angelica Splenic Decoction treats dual vacuities of heart and spleen blood characterized by palpitations, restlessness, insomnia, and excessive dreaming.

Acumoxatherapy

SP-10‡ and BL-17 are major points used in treating blood vacuity, but other points must be added according to the symptoms. For example, postpartum blood vacuity dizziness can be treated with SP-9, KI-3, BL-17‡, BL-18‡, CV-4‡, and ST-36‡. Here, CV-4‡ and ST-36‡ are used to supplement qi, which in turn supplements the blood. BL-17‡ and BL-18‡ supplement and regulate the blood. SP-6 and KI-3 are added to supplement and nourish yin and essence.

"Qi is the commander of the blood," and "Qi engenders blood." It is evident from the sample treatment above that acumoxatherapy utilizes these principles to treat blood vacuities. For further elaboration, see Chapter 8.

Supplementation of yin

Indications

Yin vacuity is characterized by emaciation, vacuity heat, upbearing fire, night sweating, dry mouth, dry pharynx, expectoration of blood, insomnia, restlessness, hot palms and soles, red tongue with scant or peeling fur, and a thin, fast pulse. Agents commonly used to treat lung or stomach yin vacuity include:

Agents used

Pulmogastric Yin Supplementers	
Radix Adenophorae	shā shēn
Tuber Ophiopogonis	mài dōng
Herba Dendrobii	shí hú
Rhizoma Polygonati Odorati	yù zhú

The following agents clear heat as well as supplement yin, and treat yin vacuity in the recovery stage of exogenous heat disease:

Heat-Clearing and Yin-Supplementing Agents	
Radix Rehmanniae Cruda	shēng dì
Herba Dendrobii	shí hú
Radix Scrophulariae	xuán shēn

The following agents have a stronger enriching effect, and are generally used to treat hepatorenal yin vacuities:

Potent Hepatorenal Yin Enrichers	
Radix Rehmanniae Cruda	shēng dì
Gelatinum Corii Asini	lǘ pí jiāo
Tuber Asparagi	tiān dōng
Plastrum Testudinis	guī bǎn
Carapax Amydae	biē jiǎ

The following agents, used to treat hepatorenal yin vacuities, have a lesser enriching effect, but have the advantage of supplementing without being glutinous:

Non-Glutinous Heptorenal Yin Enrichers	
Fructus Ligustri Lucidi	nǚ zhēn zǐ
Herba Ecliptae	hàn lián cǎo
Fructus Mori	sāng shēn zǐ

The following are used to nourish heart, lung, and kidney yin:

Heart, Lung, and Kidney Yin Enrichers	
Tuber Ophiopogonis	mài dōng
Bulbus Lilii	bǎi hé
Radix Scrophulariae	xuán shēn
Semen Biotae	bó zǐ rén

Representative formulae

Yin-Supplementing Formulae	
Rehmannia Six Pills	liù wèi dì-huáng wán
Anemarrhena, Phellodendron and Rehmannia Pills	zhī bó dì-huáng wán
Great Yin Supplementation Pills	dà bǔ yīn wán
Humor-Increasing Decoction	zēng yè tāng
Stomach-Nourishing Decoction	yǎng wèi tāng

Anemarrhena, Phellodendron, and Rehmannia Pills and Great Yin Supplementation Pills treat yin vacuity with pronounced fire effulgence. Humor-Increasing Decoction is mostly used in heat diseases where the heat pathogen is still present and yin humor is already showing signs of vacuity. Stomach-Nourishing Decoction engenders liquid and nourishes the stomach, and is mostly used in the treatment of stomach yin vacuity after illness.

Acumoxatherapy

KI-3 and LV-8 are used to nourish the yin of the kidney and liver respectively. They may be combined with points that clear heat or drain fire, such as LU-10, ST-45, LI-2, or GV-14. If the spirit is affected, HT-7, PC-6, or PC-7 may be added.

Supplementation of yang

Indications

Yang vacuity is characterized by aversion to cold, frigid extremities, aching and weakness in the knees and lumbar region, impotence, spermatorrhea, long micturition with copious, clear urine, pale tongue, and a deep, weak pulse.

Agents used

Treatment is based primarily on agents that warm and supplement kidney yang, such as:

Warming Kidney Yang Supplementers	
Rhizoma Curculiginis	xiān máo
Herba Epimedii	xiān líng pí
Cornu Cervi	lù jiǎo
Herba Cistanches	cōng róng

Fire invigorators such as Radix Aconiti Fu Tzu (fù zǐ) and Cortex Cinnamomi (ròu guì) may be added where cold signs are especially pronounced, but if used over extended periods, must be complemented by kidney essence nourishers.

Representative formulae

Warming Kidney Yang Supplementation Formulae	
Aconite and Cinnamon Eight Pills	fù guì bā wèi wán
Vital Gate Pills	yòu guì wán

Both these formulae supplement yang and invigorate the body fire. With the addition of kidney essence nourishers, Vital Gate Pills supplement yang while supporting yin.

Acumoxatherapy

Moxibustion at GV-20, CV-4, GV-4, CV-6, and CV-12 is used to supplement the yang of the entire body. Organic yang vacuity is treated according to the organ involved, with the addition of the above points. For example, spermatorrhea could be treated by moxibustion at CV-12, CV-6, BL-23, and GV-20. Here, BL-23 is included to enhance the kidney's ability to contain essence.

The interrelationship of qi, blood, yin, and yang supplementation

Each of the four forms of supplementation may be used individually if the patient's condition is attributable to a simple vacuity of one element or complement. In more complex conditions, however, they invariably must be combined. For example, frequently blood and qi are supplemented simultaneously, as are yin and yang. Dual vacuity of qi and yin may also occur. It is most commonly seen during the recovery stage of exogenous heat diseases, where often it is treated with Pulse-Engendering Powder (shēng mài sǎn) and occurs in pulmonary tuberculosis, where it may be treated with Nectar Paste (qióng yù gāo). Since "qi and blood are of the same source" and "yin and yang are rooted in each other," in treating yang vacuities, yin supplementing agents may sometimes enhance the effect of yang supplementers, and when treating yin vacuities, yang supplementers may be added to enhance the effect of yin supplementers.

Dual yin-yang vacuities are treated by dual supplementation of yin and yang. It is important to determine in which complement the vacuity is most severe. Dual vacuities, where yin vacuity is prominent, are treated by the method of "fostering yin and supporting yang," using Kidney Pills *(zuǒ guī wán)*. Where yang vacuity is more pronounced, the method of "restoring yang while supporting yin" is used, and Vital Gate Pills *(yòu guī wán)* are prescribed.

Fire effulgence frequently occurs in yin vacuities, and is treated with Anemarrhena, Phellodendron and Rehmannia Pills *(zhī bó dì-huáng wán)* or Great Yin Supplementation Pills *(dà bǔ yīn wán)* to enrich yin and downbear fire. However, it may be associated with yang vacuities, in which case symptoms include aversion to cold, frigid extremities, exhaustion, low back pain, and limpness of the legs. At the same time, there is insomnia, seminal emission, steady fever, or restlessness. Hypertension in the elderly, chronic nephritis, and neurasthenia may appear as yin vacuity fire effulgence, and hence are treated with formulae such as Two Immortals Decoction *(èr xiān tāng)* which combines yang supplementers with yin-enriching and fire-draining agents.

"When form is insufficient, it should be warmed with qi {supplementing} drugs; when essence is insufficient, it should be supplemented with sapor." Insufficiency of form generally refers to qi or yang vacuity, and may be treated by warm agents that are either sweet or pungent in sapor, such as:

Form Insufficiency Agents	
Radix Ginseng	*rén shēn*
Radix Astragali	*huáng qí*
Ramulus Cinnamomi	*guì zhī*
Radix Aconiti Fu Tzu	*fù zǐ*

Insufficiency of essence mainly refers to kidney essence vacuity, or kidney yin vacuity, and is treated with glutinous drugs of heavy sapor such as:

Essence Insufficiency Agents	
Radix Rehmanniae Conquita	*shóu dì*
Mesocarpium Corni	*yú ròu*
Fructus Lycii	*qǐ zǐ*
Placenta Hominis	*zǐ hé jū*
Plastrum Testudinis	*guī bǎn*
Gelatinum Corii Asini	*lǘ pí jiāo*

Attention should be paid to the scope of action of supplementers. For example, Radix Angelicae Sinensis *(dāng guī)* supplements the blood, but not yin. Radix Adenophorae *(shā shēn)*, Tuber Ophiopogonis *(mài dōng)*, Herba Dendrobii *(shí hú)*, and Radix Scrophulariae *(xuán shēn)*, supplement yin but not blood. Radix Rehmanniae Cruda *(shēng dì)* and Gelatinum Corii Asini *(lǘ pí jiāo)* supplement yin, but not yang; whereas Rhizoma Curculiginis *(xiān máo)*, Herba Epimedii *(xiān líng pí)*, Semen Trigonellae *(hú lú bā)*, and Herba Cynomorii *(suǒ yáng)* supplement yang, but not yin. Some drugs are broader in their effect. Radix Rehmanniae Conquita *(shóu dì)*, Gelatinum Corii Asini *(lǘ pí jiāo)*, Radix Polygoni Multiflori *(shóu wū)*, and Herba Ecliptae *(hàn lián cǎo)* supplement the blood as well as yin, while Placenta Hominis *(zǐ hé jū)* and Mesocarpium Corni *(shān yú ròu)* supplement both yin and yang.

Remarks concerning the use of supplementation

When using the method of supplementation, care must be taken to ensure that the stomach and spleen are capable of assimilating the drugs, otherwise medication will not produce its full effect. Supplementing and boosting formulae are glutinous and it may be necessary to add qi rectifiers and gastrosplenic fortifiers such as:

Qi Rectifiers and Gastrosplenic Fortifiers	
Rhizoma Atractylodis Macrocephalae	*bái zhú*
Pericarpium Citri Reticulatae	*chén pí*
Fructus Amomi	*shā rén*
Fructus Citri	*zhǐ ké*

The method of supplementation should be used with care. Where there is a strong pathogen, but the correct shows no pronounced weakening, treatment should be directed at dispelling the pathogen. The use of supplementation in such cases might cause the pathogen to lodge more firmly in the body.

Dispersion

The method of dispersion involves the dispersion or disintegration of accumulations of noxious substances in the body, using dispersers, abducting dispersers, hardness softeners, and accumulation transformers. *Essential Questions* states, "Hardness is disintegrated," and "Binds are dispersed." In practice, the dispersion method possesses a broad field of application. It may be used for concretions and conglomerations, lump glomus, digestate accumulations, water amassment, calculi, scrofulous swellings, and phlegm nodules.

Principles and Methods of Treatment

The essence of the notion of dispersion is expressed in the principle, "hardness is disintegrated." Dispersion refers to the *gradual* breakup of accumulations and differs from emergency offensive treatment with highly potent drugs in that it safeguards correct qi. It is therefore particularly appropriate for treating concretions and conglomerations, glomus lumps, calculi, scrofulous swellings, and phlegm nodules. Precipitation differs from dispersion in that it is used to treat dry stool, static blood, and lodged phlegm-rheum where there is a substantial pathogen whose elimination requires swift administration of offensive treatment using highly potent precipitants. Dispersion, by contrast, treats chronic accumulations that cannot be treated by emergency offensive treatment with highly potent precipitants.

The main forms of the dispersion method are dispersion of digestate accumulations, transformation of static blood (stasis transformation), softening, transformation of phlegm, transformation of damp, and disinhibition of water.

Dispersion of digestate accumulations

Indications

Indigestion causing oppression in the venter and abdominal distention, loss of appetite, eructation of putrid-smelling gas, acid regurgitation, and nausea and regurgitation; or abdominal pain, constipation; or diarrhea with discomfort unrelieved by evacuation, call for treatment using the method of dispersion of digestate accumulations.

Agents used

Agents commonly used to disperse digestate of high cereal content are:

Cereal Digestate Dispersers	
Massa Fermentata	*liù qū*
Fructus Oryzae Sativae Germinatus	*gǔ yá*
Fructus Hordei Germinatus	*mài yá*

Agents commonly used to disperse digestate of high meat content are:

Meat Digestate Dispersers	
Fructus Crataegi	*shān zhā*
Endothelium Gigeriae Galli	*jī nèi jīn*

The following agents break qi, precipitate phlegm, and restore stool flow:

Qi Breakers, Phlegm Precipitants, and Laxatives	
Semen Raphani	lái fú zǐ
Fructus Citri Immaturus	zhǐ shí
Semen Arecae	bīn láng

Fructus Crataegi Carbonisatus *(shān zhā tàn)*, and Massa Fermentata Ustulata *(jiāo liù qū)* are antidiarrheic. Fructus Oryzae Sativae Germinatus *(gǔ yá)* increases the appetite.

These drugs may be included in formulae according to the patient's condition, since digestate accumulations are frequently accompanied by phlegm-damp and qi stagnation. For stubborn digestate accumulations engendering heat, heat-clearing agents such as Radix Scutellariae *(huáng qín)* and Flos Lonicerae *(yín huā)* may be used. In severe cases of digestate accumulation, draining precipitants may be combined with dispersers. Splenogastric vacuity may warrant the addition of spleen fortifiers and stomach harmonizers.

Representative formulae

Digestate Dispersion Formulae	
Harmony-Preserving Pills	bǎo hé wán
Citrus Stagnation-Abducting Pills	zhi-shi dao zhi wan
Great Quieting Pills	dà ān wán

Harmony-Preserving Pills are primarily a dispersive formula. Citrus Stagnation-Abducting Pills have an additional mild precipitant action. Great Quieting Pills disperse and fortify the spleen and harmonize the stomach.

Acumoxatherapy

Points such as ST-25, CV-10, ST-36, ST-37, and BL-25 are drained to disperse repletion, while a supplementing stimulus is given through points such as SP-4, ST-44, and BL-20 to aid splenic movement and thereby disperse accumulations. PC-6 may be added to relieve nausea. CV-21 can be needled in combination with ST-36 to disperse digestate accumulations.

Transformation of static blood

Indications

This method of treatment may be used in traumatology for painful swellings and bruises, often in combination with qi-rectifying and pain-relieving agents; to treat menstrual disorders such as metrorrhagia and menorrhalgia where signs of blood stasis are present; for hemorrhagic diseases with signs of blood stasis; for internal masses, and cardiovascular diseases with blood stagnation signs; or for stubborn wind-cold-damp obturation, known as persistent pain penetrating the connecting channels (treated by the method of dispelling stasis and freeing the channels).

Agents used

Depending on the severity of the condition, blood stasis patterns may be treated by one or combinations of three methods: blood quickening, stasis transformation, and blood breaking. Blood quickeners include:

Blood Quickeners	
Radix Salviae Miltiorrhizae	dān shēn
Radix Paeoniae Rubrae	chì sháo
Rhizoma Ligustici Wallichii Szechuanensis	chuān xiōng
Cortex Radicis Mu Tan	mǔ dān pí
Radix et Caulis Chi Hsëh T'eng	jī xuè téng

These are mild and can be used for most cases of blood stasis. Stasis transformers, which are stronger agents used in more pronounced cases, include:

Stasis Transformers	
Semen Persicae	táo rén
Flos Carthami	hóng huā
Rhizoma Rhei	dà huáng

Other agents especially effective in the treatment of gynecologic disorders include:

Gynecologic Stasis Transformers	
Herba Lycopi	zé lán
Herba Leonuri	yì mǔ cǎo
Pollen Typhae	pú huáng
Excrementum Trogopteri	wǔ líng zhī

The following agents have a pronounced analgesic effect:

Analgesic Stasis Transformers	
Rhizoma Corydalis	yán hú suǒ
Gummi Olibanum	rǔ xiāng
Myrrha	mò yào
Radix Pseudoginseng	sān qī

Radix Pseudoginseng is both an analgesic and an antihemorrhagic. The most potent agents of all are blood breakers, mostly used to treat prolonged amenorrhea and pronounced masses. They include:

Blood Breakers	
Hirudo	*shuǐ zhì*
Tabanus	*méng chóng*
Eupolyphaga	*dì biē chóng*
Rhizoma Sparganii	*sān léng*
Rhizoma Curcumae Zedoariae	*é zhú*
Catharsius	*qiāng láng*

These agents are contraindicated in the presence of hemorrhage and pregnancy. The stasis transformers and blood quickeners belonging to the category of *chong* products are often used for persistent pain penetrating the connecting channels.

Representative formulae

Stasis-Transforming Formulae	
Origin-Restorative Blood-Quickening Decoction	*fù yuán huó xuè tāng*
Four Agents Decoction with Persica and Carthamus	*táo hóng sì wù tāng*
Great Guffaw Powder	*shī xiào sǎn*
Carapax Amydae Decocted Pills	*biē-jiǎ jiān wán*
Generalized-Pain-Relieving Stasis-Expelling Decoction	*shēn tòng zhú yū tāng*
Leaden Obturation Tested Formula	*zhuó bì yàn fāng*

Origin-Restorative Blood-Quickening Decoction is effective for impact traumas. Four Agents Decoction with Persica and Carthamus is effectively used to treat menstrual disorders by quickening the blood. Great Guffaw Powder quickens the blood and relieves pain. Carapax Amydae Decocted Pills are effective in dispersing masses. Generalized-Pain-Relieving Stasis-Expelling Decoction and Leaden Obturation Tested Formula treat obturation patterns characterized by enduring pain penetrating the connecting channels.

Acumoxatherapy

In traumatology, bleeding local points and cupping, or warming the affected area with moxa is combined with needling local points to move qi and blood and disperse stagnation. Distal points, such as those previously mentioned under "Warming the channels and dissipating cold," are also commonly employed.

Menstrual disorders resulting from blood stasis are treated with local points such as CV-4‡, CV-2‡, and M-CA-18‡ *(zi-gong)*, combined with such points as SP-6‡, SP-8‡, and LV-3 to move stasis and regulate the blood. ST-30 is often used to harmonize the qi of the penetrating vessel and course obstruction and stagnation of construction-blood.

SP-8 and SP-10 may be combined with SP-1‡ and LV-1‡ in hemorrhagic diseases with signs of blood stasis.

Softening

Indications

Treatment by the method of softening would be indicated for scrofulous swellings, phlegm nodules, and strumae (including lymphadenhypertrophy and thyrocele), urinary calculi and colelithiasis, and abdominal concretions, including hepatomegaly, splenomegaly, and masses.

Agents used

Agents Treating Scrofula, Phlegm Nodules, and Struma	
Herba Sargassii	*hǎi zǎo*
Thallus Algae	*kūn bù*
Spica Prunellae	*xià kū cǎo*
Bulbus Fritillariae	*bèi mǔ*
Concha Ostreae	*mǔ lì*
Bulbus Shan Tz'u Ku	*shān cí gū*
Tuber Colocasiae	*yù nǎi*
Tuber Dioscoreae Bulbiferae	*huáng yào zǐ*

These are commonly used for scrofulous swellings, phlegm nodules, and strumae, and are often combined with blood-quickening stasis transformers and heat-clearing detoxicants. The following agents disperse calculii:

Agents Treating Calculus	
Herba Chin Ch'ien Ts'ao	*jīn qián cǎo*
Endothelium Gigeriae Galli	*jī nèi jīn*
Sal Petrae	*xiāo shí*

To treat urinary calculi, these agents are frequently combined with water disinhibiting antistrangurics; to treat biliary tract calculi, they may be combined with liver-coursing qi rectifiers, and in some cases with draining precipitants such as Rhizoma Rhei *(dà huáng)*, Fructus Citri Immaturus *(zhǐ shí)*, and Mirabilitum *(máng xiāo)*.

For agents that disperse concretions, see above, "Transforming stasis."

Representative formulae

Softening Formulae	
Sargassium Jade Teapot Decoction	hǎi-zǎo yù hú tāng
Scrofula-Dispersing Pills	nèi xiāo luǒ lì wán
Biliary Calculus Decoction	dān dào pái shí tāng
Pyrrosia Powder	shí-wěi sǎn

Sargassium Jade Teapot Decoction is used for dispersing strumae. Scrofula-Dispersing Pills disperse scrofulous swellings. Biliary Calculus Decoction expels gallstones. Pyrrosia Powder disperses urinary tract calculi. All these are specific-use formulae.

Acumoxatherapy

Strong stimulation of local points is favored to disperse nodules. SP-6‡ and M-BW-16‡ *(pi-gen)* may be included.

Transformation of phlegm

Phlegm is transformed in different ways depending on its location. Phlegm in the lung is treated by the method of transforming phlegm and suppressing cough. Phlegm confounding the cardiac portals is treated by the method of transforming phlegm and opening the portals. Phlegm scurrying through the channels, characterized by wry mouth and eyes, stiff tongue, and impeded speech, is treated by the method of dispelling wind and transforming phlegm. Phlegm lodging in the stomach, characterized by symptoms such as vomiting and nausea, is treated by the method of harmonizing the stomach and transforming phlegm. Phlegm binding in masses, such as phlegm nodules, scrofulous swellings, and strumae, is treated by the method of softening hardness and transforming phlegm. For details about phlegm confounding the cardiac portals, see forward to the section, "Portal opening," and for phlegm nodules, scrofulous swellings, and strumae, see above subsection, "Softening hardness."

Transforming phlegm and suppressing cough

Indications

Cough and phlegm expectoration.

Agents used

Warm phlegm transformers that treat cold phlegm and damp phlegm include:

Warm Phlegm Transformers	
Semen Sinapis Albae	*bái jiè zǐ*
Rhizoma Arisaematis	*nán xīng*
Rhizoma Pinelliae	*bàn xià*
Fructus Perillae Crispae	*sū zǐ*
Pericarpium Citri Reticulatae	*chén pí*
Rhizoma Zingiberis Exsiccatum	*gān jiāng*
Fructus Gleditsiae	*zào jiá*

Cool phlegm transformers that are used to treat heat phlegm and dryness phlegm include:

Cold Phlegm Transformers	
Herba Rorippae	*hān cài*
Semen T'ing Li Tzu	*tíng lì zǐ*
Bulbus Fritillariae	*bèi mǔ*
Fructus Trichosanthis	*guā lóu*
Fructus Arctii	*niú bàng zǐ*
Semen Benincasae	*dōng guā rén*
Radix Adenophorae	*shā shēn*

The following are milder in nature and may be used in most cases:

Balanced Phlegm Transformers	
Radix Platycodi	*jié gěng*
Semen Pruni Armeniacae	*xìng rén*
Radix Peucedani	*qián hú*
Radix Asteris	*zǐ wǎn*
Flos Tussilagi Farfarae	*kuǎn dōng huā*

Representative formulae

Phlegm-Transforming Formulae	
Minor Cyan Dragon Decoction	*xiǎo qīng lóng tāng*
Stomach-Calming Powder	*píng wèi sǎn*
Lonicera and Phragmites Combination	*yín wěi hé jì*
Dryness-Clearing Lung-Restorative Decoction	*qīng zào jiù fèi tāng*
Phlegm-Cough Powder	*zhǐ sòu sǎn*

Minor Cyan Dragon Decoction treats cold phlegm. Stomach-Calming Powder is effective for damp phlegm. Lonicera and Phragmites Combination may be used for heat phlegm. Dryness-Clearing Lung-Restorative Decoction treats dryness phlegm. Phlegm-Cough Powder is a general phlegm-transforming antitussive remedy.

Acumoxatherapy

Treatment of expectoration accords with the location of the pathogen. Exterior patterns with cough and phlegm are treated with points such as BL-12, BL-13, and LI-4, LU-9, and LU-7 to resolve the exterior, dispel wind, and diffuse lung qi. Points such as SP-5, CV-12, and SP-9 are added to transform damp.

Cough is diagnosed as being either due to yin vacuity or yang vacuity. Yin vacuity cough is treated by using points that nourish yin and supplement lung and kidney qi, such as BL-13, BL-23, and KI-3. LV-2 may be included to course liver fire, and LU-5 may be added to clear upper-burner heat. Yang vacuity cough is treated by applying supplementing stimulus to points such as BL-13‡, BL-20‡, and ST-36‡, and moxibustion at CV-4 and CV-12, to warm the yang of the lung, spleen, and kidney. ST-40 is a particularly effective point for transforming phlegm and downbearing turbidity.

Dispelling wind and transforming phlegm

Indications

Wry mouth and eyes, stiff tongue and impeded speech, and child fright wind.

Agents used

The main agents used are:

Wind Dispellants and Phlegm Transformers	
Rhizoma Aconiti Coreani	*bái fù zǐ*
Bombyx Batryticatus	*jiāng cán*
Concretio Siliceae Bambusae	*tiān zhú huáng*
Pulvis Arisaemae cum Felle Bovis	*dǎn nán xīng*

These are often combined with wind extinguishers:

Wind-Extinguishing Agents	
Buthus	*quán xiē*
Scolopendra	*wú gōng*

Formulae may also include heat clearers and portal openers.

Representative formula

Anti-Contracture Powder *(qiān zhèng sǎn)*.

Acumoxatherapy

Treatment is directed towards resolving the exterior, transforming phlegm, and clearing any heat present. Exterior resolution can be achieved through stimulus at LI-4 and TB-5, while a classical phlegm transforming point is ST-40. Heat can be cleared through GV-20, M-HN-3 *(yin-tang)*, M-UE-1 *(shi-xuan)*, GV-14, TB-5, and LI-11. Other points are added according to the symptoms. For example, for paralysis of the tongue, M-HN-22 *(wai-jin-jin, yu-ye)* can be added.

Harmonizing the stomach and transforming phlegm

Indications

Cough with copious phlegm, oppression in the chest, nausea and vomiting, dizziness, and palpitations.

Agents used

Basic agents are phlegm transformers such as:

Phlegm Transformers	
Rhizoma Pinelliae	*bàn xià*
Pericarpium Citri Reticulatae	*chén pí*
Sclerotium Poriae	*fú líng*

Damp turbidity harassing the upper body, characterized by dizziness and headache, is treated with Rhizoma Atractylodis Macrocephalae *(bái zhú)* and Rhizoma Gastrodiae *(tiān má)*. When manifesting as insomnia and palpitations, Fructus Citri Immaturus *(zhǐ shí)* and Caulis Bambusae in Taenis *(zhú rú)* are often added.

Representative formula

Double Vintage Decoction *(èr chén tāng)*.

Acumoxatherapy

Points such as CV-12 are used to harmonize the stomach and transform damp. Supplementation at BL-20 and CV-13 can move earth to transform damp, and strong stimulus at SP-9 will disinhibit urine and move water. PC-6 opens the chest and diaphragm and relieves nausea. If there is dizziness or headache, local points such as M-HN-9 *(tai-yang)*, M-HN-3 *(yin-tang)*, GB-20, and GV-20 may be used in combination with distal points such as LV-2 and ST-41. Where phlegm-heat harassing the upper body gives rise to dizziness, strong stimulation at points such as GV-24, ST-40, SI-7, and BL-48 is called for. ST-40 is often a useful point in the treatment of phlegm and damp patterns.

Transformation of damp

Transforming damp is the method of dispelling the damp pathogen with dry, bitter agents, aromatics, or bland percolators.

Indications

The most common patterns include persistent fever, generalized sensation of heaviness, fatigued or heavy limbs, bag-over-the-head sensation, musculocutaneous water swelling, slimy tongue fur, and soggy pulse. Damp in the spleen, stomach, liver, or gallbladder is characterized by such symptoms as dyspeptic anorexia, oppression in the chest, abdominal distention, thin stool, nausea, vomiting, and jaundice. Damp in the lower burner may be characterized by oliguria, yellow or dark-colored urine, urinary frequency, painful urination, and foul-smelling diarrhea with burning sensation. Eczema (damp papules) and swollen joints with a sensation of extreme heaviness are also signs of the damp pathogen.

Agents used

Damp transformers fall into three categories: warm, bitter damp dryers, aromatic damp transformers, and bland percolating damp disinhibitors. Warm, bitter damp dryers include:

Warm, Bitter Damp Dryers	
Rhizoma Atractylodis	*cāng zhú*
Rhizoma Pinelliae	*bàn xià*
Cortex Magnoliae	*hòu pò*
Pericarpium Citri Reticulatae	*chén pí*

Aromatic damp transformers include:

Aromatic Damp Transformers	
Herba Agastaches	*huò xiāng*
Herba Eupatorii	*pèi lán*
Fructus Amomi	*shā rén*
Fructus Amomi Cardamomi	*kòu rén*

Bland percolating damp disinhibitors include:

Bland Percolating Damp Disinhibitors	
Sclerotium Poriae	fú líng
Sclerotium Polypori Umbellati	zhū líng
Talcum	huá shí
Medulla Tetrapanacis	tōng cǎo
Semen Coicis	yì yǐ rén

Warm, bitter damp dryers have a strong damp-transforming effect and are used to dispel exuberant pathogens. Aromatic damp transformers have a lesser damp-transforming effect, but promote qi-aspect perfusion as well as fortify the spleen and harmonize the stomach. Bland percolating damp disinhibitors cause the damp pathogen to be expelled through the urine, so that they can be used for any type of damp pattern. Hence it is said, "Without diuresis, damp disorders cannot be cured." If damp is located in the lower burner, the need for bland percolating damp disinhibitors is all the greater. For further elaboration on this subject see ahead to the subsection, "Disinhibition of water."

The location of the disorder within the triple burner is given special consideration when selecting appropriate medication. It is important to determine whether the emergence of the damp pattern is attributable to non-diffusion of lung qi in the upper burner, impaired splenic movement in the middle burner, or to an impairment of the transformative action of bladder qi in the lower burner, so that agents capable of promoting the transformative action of qi in the relevant burner may be selected. The following promote lung qi perfusion in the upper burner:

Upper-Burner Qi Perfusion Agents	
Semen Pruni Armeniacae	xìng rén
Folium Nelumbinis	hé yè
Herba Agastaches	huò xiāng
Herba Menthae	bò hé
Herba Eupatorii	pèi lán

The following agents promote movement and transformation:

Middle-Burner Movement and Transformation Agents	
Rhizoma Atractylodis Macrocephalae	bái zhú
Semen Dolichoris	biǎn dòu
Fructus Amomi Cardamomi	kòu rén
Fructus Citri	zhǐ ké
Fructus Amomi	shā rén
Cortex Magnoliae	hòu pò

Bland percolating damp disinhibitors combined with yang-freeing water disinhibitors promote perfusion in the qi aspect of the lower burner.

Lower-Burner Qi Perfusion Agents	
Ramulus Cinnamomi	guì zhī
Cortex Cinnamomi	ròu guì

The possibility of complex patterns also calls for consideration. Damp-heat patterns are treated with agents that clear heat and dry damp, such as:

Heat Clearers and Damp Driers	
Rhizoma Coptidis	huáng lián
Radix Scutellariae	huáng qín
Fructus Gardeniae	zhī zǐ
Cortex Phellodendri	huáng bó
Rhizoma Rhei	dà huáng
Herba Artemisiae Capillaris	yīn chén
Radix Sophorae Flavescentis	kǔ shēn
Cortex Fraxini	qín pí

Cold-damp may be treated with warm, bitter damp dryers combined with drugs that warm and move the kidney and spleen, such as:

Warming Splenorenal Movers	
Rhizoma Zingiberis Exsiccatum	gān jiāng
Radix Aconiti Fu Tzu	fù zǐ
Semen Alpiniae Katsumadai	cǎo dòu kòu

Formulae for treating wind-damp contain agents that dispel wind and dissipate damp, such as:

Wind Dispellants and Damp Dissipators	
Radix Ledebouriellae	fáng fēng
Radix Fang Chi	fáng jǐ
Rhizoma et Radix Notopterygii	qiāng huó
Radix Angelicae	bái zhǐ

Representative formulae

Damp-Transforming Formulae	
Stomach-Calming Powder	píng wèi sǎn
Agastache, Magnolia, Pinellia and Poria Decoction	huò pò xià líng tāng
Poria Five Powder	wǔ líng sǎn
Three Kernel Decoction	sān rén tāng

Stomach-Calming Powder is a formula that dries damp with warm, bitter agents. Agastache, Magnolia, Pinellia and Poria Decoction transforms damp with aromatics. Poria Five Powder frees yang and disinhibits water. Three Kernel Decoction transforms damp by promoting triple-burner qi perfusion.

Acumoxatherapy

Damp is often treated by disinhibiting urine, using points such as SP-9, BL-53, BL-28, and CV-9. Another treatment method is to strengthen the organs that are involved in water transformation and movement, primarily the triple burner, kidney, spleen, and lung. The large intestine and bladder are considered less important.

The back-associated points of the above organs are useful, depending on the location of the damp pathogen, and its particular symptoms. Other points, such as KI-3, CV-2, ST-36, ST-28, LU-9, SP-6, CV-6, CV-12, ST-40, TB-10, and CV-11 all are used to dispel water damp, transform damp, or transform phlegm damp in the channels.

In cases of splenic vacuity vaginal discharge, for example, ST-36 and BL-20 are used to fortify the spleen, move damp, and transform turbidity. In the instance of damp-heat prolapse of the rectum, SP-9 is used to transform damp-heat. To treat enduring yin water-swelling, BL-23‡ and BL-20‡ can be combined with ST-36‡ to fortify spleen earth and thus promote transformation of water qi. In acute yang water-swelling, the emphasis is on points that disinhibit urine such as SP-9 and ST-28, points that promote lung qi diffusion such as LU-7, and points that support the bladder and dispel damp such as BL-28 and KI-7.

Disinhibiting water with bland percolators

This is one of two basic forms of water disinhibition, the other being clearing heat and freeing strangury.

Indications

Water-damp collection, oliguria, and water swelling are patterns that call for treatment using the method of disinhibiting water with bland percolators.

Agents used

Bland Percolating Water Disinhibitors	
Sclerotium Polypori Umbellati	zhū líng
Talcum	huá shí
Sclerotium Poriae	fú líng
Pericarpium Benincasae	dōng guā pí
Medulla Tetrapanacis	tōng cǎo
Semen Coicis	yì yǐ rén
Stylus Zeae	yù mǐ xū
Pericarpium Lagenariae	hú lú piáo

These are the most commonly used agents. Most of these drugs are mild in sapor and balanced in nature, so that they are termed bland percolators. They may be combined with Ramulus Cinnamomi *(guì zhī)*, which frees yang and transforms (stagnant) qi, Rhizoma Atractylodis Macrocephalae *(bái zhú)*, which fortifies the spleen and transforms damp, and with Gelatinum Corii Asini *(lǘ pí jiāo)* and Talcum *(huá shí)*, which nourish yin, clear heat, and disinhibit water.

Representative formula

Poria Four Powder *(sì líng sǎn)*.

Acumoxatherapy

Points and methods used for disinhibiting water are the same as those for transforming damp. See previous section.

Clearing heat and freeing strangury

This is the other of the two basic forms of dishibition of water.

Indications

Painful, burning sensation in the urethra, urgency and frequency, and dark-colored urine, are indications for treatment by the method of clearing heat and freeing strangury.

Agents used

Heat-Clearing and Strangury-Freeing Agents	
Caulis Mu T'ung	mù tōng
Semen/Herba Plantaginis	chē qián zǐ/cǎo
Herba Polygoni Avicularis	biǎn xù
Folium Pyrrosiae	shí wěi
Herba Dianthi	qū mài
Talcum	huá shí

Principles and Methods of Treatment

These provide the basis of treatment. They may be combined with heat clearers such as:

Heat Clearers	
Herba Andrographis	*chuān xīn lián*
Herba et Radix Taraxaci	*pú gōng yīng*
Herba Commelinae	*yā zhí cǎo*
Herba Houttuyniae	*yú xīng cǎo*
Herba Pteridis	*fèng wěi cǎo*
Flos Lonicerae	*yín huā*
Cortex Phellodendri	*huáng bó*

Patterns involving hematuria are treated with formulae that additionally contain agents such as:

Antihematurics	
Herba Euphorbiae Humifusae	*dì jǐn cǎo*
Herba Cephalanoploris	*xiǎo jì cǎo*
Nodus Rhizomatis Nelumbinis	*ǒu jié*

Representative formula

Eight Corrections Powder *(bā zhèng sǎn)*.

Acumoxatherapy

Heat in the lower burner is treated by supplementation at KI-3 and BL-23, to enrich the kidney and thereby clear internal heat. CV-4 and BL-27, respectively the front-alarm and back-associated points of the small intestine, can drain heat from the small intestine and are especially appropriate in cases of fire spreading from the heart to the small intestine. Here, BL-15, the back-associated point of the heart, would also be added. If there is damp heat, SP-6 and SP-9 may be added.

Remarks concerning the use of water disinhibition

Short micturition with scant urine or urinary block from impairment of the transformative action of qi cannot be treated with water disinhibitors alone and require the addition of yang warmers, since kidney yang vacuity is the underlying cause. When short micturition with scant urine is attributable to insufficiency of fluids, water disinhibitors are contraindicated.

Portal opening

The method of opening the portals employs pungent, aromatic, penetrating agents, which open the portals and free the joints (principally the jaw). It is applied in the treatment of sudden clouding inversion (syncope) in diseases such as fright wind, epilepsy, windstrike, or angina pectoris, or stupor of the spirit-disposition caused by inner-body block occurring in exogenous heat disease. Its principal effect is to resuscitate, and eliminate distention and oppression in the chest and abdomen caused by foul turbidity. Aromatic portal-openers penetrate the heart and free the portals, repel foulness, and open blocks. This method, which in most cases represents emergency symptomatic treatment (treatment of the branches), takes three major forms: clearing the heart and opening the portals, sweeping phlegm and opening the portals, and repelling foulness and opening the portals. In most cases, prescribed medication comes in the form of prepared formulae.

Clearing the heart and opening the portals

Indications

Exogenous heat disease patterns such as heat entering the pericardium, characterized by high fever and clouding of the spirit, or tetanic inversion or convulsive spasm, call for treatment using the method of clearing the heart and opening the portals. Other patterns include coma from cerebrovascular trauma, accompanied by heat signs.

Representative formulae

Heart-Clearing and Portal-Opening Formulae	
Peaceful Palace Bovine Bezoar Pills	*ān gōng niú-huáng wán*
Purple Snow Elixir	*zǐ xuě dān*
Divine Rhinoceros Elixir	*shēn xī dān*
Crown Jewel Elixir	*zhì bǎo dān*

These formulae may be combined with blood coolers, heat clearers, and detoxicants where necessary. Cerebrovascular trauma is treated with Crown Jewel Elixir combined with liver-calming wind extinguishers.

Acumoxatherapy

Such exogenous heat diseases as heat entering the pericardium are treated with points that open the portals, such as PC-9. GV-26 can clear interior heat and spirit-disposition. HT-7 and PC-6 can be added to quiet the spirit and clear the pericardium.

In cases of cerebrovascular trauma, M-UE-1 *(shi-xuan)* (bleed), GV-20, and KI-1 are commonly used.

Sweeping phlegm and opening the portals

Indications

Treatment using the method of sweeping phlegm and opening the portals is indicated in patterns of paroxysms of angina pectoris with sudden clouding inversion; exogenous heat disease patterns with phlegm turbidity clouding the upper body, characterized by coma, the sound of phlegm gurgling in the throat, and thick, slimy tongue fur; cerebrovascular trauma with sudden fainting, obtundation of the essence-spirit or coma, copious phlegm, and thick slimy tongue fur; and phlegm clouding the cardiac portals, characterized by torpor of the essence-spirit, incoherent speech (as distinct from manic agitation), and thick, slimy tongue fur.

Representative formulae

Phlegm-Sweeping and Portal-Opening Formulae	
Liquid Styrax Pills	sū hé xiāng wán
Crown Jewel Elixir	zhì bǎo dān

Liquid Styrax Pills are the medication of choice; Crown Jewel Elixir may be used if necessary. The following may be added as needed:

Additional Agents	
Bulbus Fritillariae Cirrhosae	chuān bèi mǔ
Concretio Siliceae Bambusae	tiān zhú huáng
Rhizoma Acori Graminei	chāng pú
Tuber Curcumae	yù jīn
Succus Bambusae	zhú lì
Radix Polygalae	yuǎn zhì
Rhizoma Arisaematis	nán xīng

Acumoxatherapy

Paroxysms of angina pectoris are treated with points such as PC-6, CV-14, HT-1, and GV-26. HT-8, PC-6, GV-20, BL-15, and BL-39 are all commonly used to sweep phlegm and open the cardiac portals. ST-40 is a major point for treating any phlegm condition.

Repelling foulness and opening the portals

Indications

Contraction of foul turbidity qi in hot weather, precipitating sudden oppression and distention in the chest and abdomen, ungratified urge to vomit and evacuate, and in serious cases, sudden loss of consciousness, copious phlegm and saliva causing congestion, and trismus, call for treatment using the method of repelling foulness and opening the portals.

Representative formulae

Foulness-Repelling and Portal-Opening Formulae	
Jade Axis Elixir	yù shū dān
Troop Deployment Powder	xíng jūn sǎn
Liquid Styrax Pills	sū hé xiāng wán

Acumoxatherapy

PC-6 is a major point for opening the chest and relieving nausea. GV-14, LI-11, and LV-3 are added to clear wind and heat from the yang channels, and ST-36 is included to supplement qi.

Remarks concerning the use of portal opening

Portal opening may be used only for block patterns caused by strong pathogens, and is contraindicated for patterns characterized by gaping mouth, limp hands, weak breathing, and clouding of the spirit, which should be first treated by supplementing qi to check vacuity desertion. It should also be noted that portal opening is only a means of restoring normal consciousness and does not treat the root. Portal openers are abortifacient and therefore contraindicated in pregnancy.

Securing Astriction

The aim of securing astriction is to check desertion, i.e., to stem loss of qi, blood, and fluids. It is used in the treatment of both spontaneous sweating and night sweating, persistent cough, enduring diarrhea efflux desertion, seminal emission, seminal efflux, heavy micturition, enuresis, bleeding, metrorrhagia, and persistent vaginal discharge. All these diseases are, at root, vacuity disorders, so that securing astringents are usually combined with supplementers.

Constraining perspiration

Indications

Spontaneous or night sweating calls for treatment using the method of constraining perspiration.

Principles and Methods of Treatment

Agents used

Spontaneous sweating is usually attributable to qi vacuity, and is therefore primarily treated by boosting qi and securing the exterior, so that Radix Astragali *(huáng qí)* is the ideal agent. Night sweating is usually a consequence of yin vacuity, and is therefore treated by enriching yin and constraining perspiration, using such agents as Radix Paeoniae Albae *(bái sháo)*, Testa Glycines *(lǜ dòu yī)*, and Semen Tritici *(huái xiǎo mài)*. Treatment of both spontaneous and night sweating may include agents such as Fructus Schisandrae *(wǔ wèi zǐ)*, Radix et Rhizoma Oryzae Glutinosae *(nuò dào gēn)*, Os Draconis tempered *(duàn lóng gǔ)*, and Concha Ostreae tempered *(duàn mǔ lì)*.

Representative formula

Oystershell Powder *(mǔ lì sǎn)*.

Securing astriction is only one method of checking spontaneous and night sweating. By harmonizing construction and defense, Cinnamon-Twig Decoction *(guì-zhī tāng)* can also check perspiration. Jade Wind-Barrier Powder *(yù píng fēng sǎn)* can check sweating by boosting qi and securing the exterior. Night sweating may also be treated by the yin-nourishing and fire-draining effect of Yellow Sextet plus Angelica Decoction *(dāng-guī liù huáng tāng)*.

Acumoxatherapy

LI-4 and KI-7 are commonly used to constrain perspiration. Because spontaneous and night sweating are both usually due to vacuity, points should be included to supply the particular vacuity.

Constraining the lung

Indications

Persistent cough with little or no phlegm, resulting from lung vacuity, calls for treatment using the method of constraining the lung.

Agents used

Formulae containing lung-constraining antitussives such as:

Lung-Constraining Antitussives	
Fructus Schisandrae	*wǔ wèi zǐ*
Fructus Terminaliae Chebulae	*hē zǐ*
Pericarpium Papaveris	*yīng sù ké*

These are used with general antitussives:

General Antitussives	
Radix Stemonae	bǎi bù
Radix Asteris	zǐ wǎn
Fructus Aristolochiae	mǎ dōu líng
Folium Eriobotryae	pí pa yè
Flos Tussilagi Farfarae	kuǎn dōng huā

In clinical practice, phlegm dispellants are found to enhance the antitussive action of lung constrainers. Although exclusive use of lung constrainers brings some measure of relief from coughing, it fails to facilitate phlegm ejection and leaves a feeling of oppression in the chest. Lung constrainers are usually contraindicated when an exogenous pathogen is lodged in the lung.

Representative formula

Nine Immortals Powder *(jiǔ xiān sǎn)*.

Acumoxatherapy

LU-7 and LU-9 are major points for diffusing lung qi, transforming phlegm, and suppressing cough. CV-22 is another effective point, but is used less frequently because it is located near the great vessels and must be needled carefully. For further information, refer to the earlier section, "Transforming phlegm and suppressing cough."

Intestinal astriction

Indications

Enduring diarrhea and fecal incontinence culminating in efflux desertion and prolapse of the rectum are symptoms that call for treatment using the method of intestinal astriction.

Agents used

Warming splenorenal supplementers such as the following may be used:

Warming Splenorenal Supplementers	
Radix Codonopsis Pilosulae	dǎng shēn
Rhizoma Atractylodis Macrocephalae	bái zhú
Radix Aconiti Fu Tzu	fù zǐ
Ramulus Cinnamomi	guì zhī
Rhizoma Zingiberis Exsiccatum	gān jiāng

To these should be added securing astringent agents to astringe the bowels and secure against desertion, such as:

Principles and Methods of Treatment

Securing Astringents	
Fructus Psoraleae	*bǔ gǔ zhǐ*
Semen Myristicae	*ròu dòu kòu*
Fructus Schisandrae	*wǔ wèi zǐ*
Pericarpium Papaveris	*yīng sù ké*
Halloysitum Rubrum	*chì shí zhī*
Limonitum	*yǔ yú liáng*
Radix Dioscoreae	*shān yào*
Semen Euryalis	*qiàn shí*
Semen Nelumbinis	*lián zǐ ròu*

Representative formula

True Man Viscera-Nourishing Decoction *(zhēn rén yǎng zàng tāng)*.

Acumoxatherapy

Treatment is directed toward warming and supplementing the spleen and kidney, using points such as GV-4‡, CV-4‡, BL-23‡, BL-20‡, and ST-36‡. For enduring diarrhea, the front-alarm and back-associated points of the large intestine, ST-25 and BL-25 respectively, may be used. GV-20 is used to uplift yang qi, particularly when there is prolapse of the rectum. SP-9 and SP-4 are used when damp restricts the qi-moving function of the spleen.

Securing essence

Indications

Seminal emission and seminal efflux due to vacuity are indications that may be treated using the method of securing essence.

Agents used

Essence-securing agents include:

Essence Securers	
Os Draconis	*lóng gǔ*
Concha Ostreae	*mǔ lì*
Fructus Rosae Laevigatae	*jīn yīng zǐ*
Semen Euryalis	*qiàn shí*
Stamen Nelumbinis	*lián xū*

These are frequently combined with kidney supplementers, such as:

Kidney Supplementers	
Semen Cuscutae	tù sī zǐ
Semen Astragali Complanati	tóng jí lí
Mesocarpium Corni	yú ròu

Representative formula

Golden Lock Essence-Securing Pills (jīn suǒ gù jīng wán).

Acumoxatherapy

The kidney is strengthened and essence secured by supplementation through points such as BL-23, KI-12, SP-6, BL-30, and KI-3. Moxibustion is used at CV-4 and CV-6 to strengthen the conception vessel and the original qi. ST-30, which secures the portals of essence, is often added.

Urine reduction

Indications

Enuresis and frequent long micturition with copious clear urine call for treatment using the method of urine reduction.

Agents used

The drugs used in the urine-reducing method are largely the same as those used for securing essence. The following are more commonly used to reduce urine and check enuresis:

Urine Reducers	
Oötheca Mantidis	sāng piāo xiāo
Radix Dioscoreae	shān yào
Bombyx Batryticatus	jiāng cán

Representative formulae

Urine-Reducing Formulae	
Oötheca Mantidis Powder	sāng-piāo-xiāo sǎn
Stream-Reducing Pills	suō quán wán

Oötheca Mantidis Powder also has the added action of promoting cardiorenal interaction, and is mostly used for infantile enuresis. Stream-Reducing Pills, which warm and supplement kidney qi, are used to treat vacuity polyuria in old age.

Principles and Methods of Treatment

Acumoxatherapy

Treatment focuses on strengthening the bladder and kidney with points such as BL-23, BL-28, and CV-3. SP-6, a point of intersection of the three yin channels of the foot, is used to supplement original qi and boost the kidney. Moxibustion at LV-1 is added to enhance the curative effect. If there is urination while dreaming, HT-7 is included to quiet the spirit.

Hemorrhage arrest

Indications

Any form of hemorrhage calls for treatment using the method of hemorrhage arrest.

Agents used

Hemorrhage is treated with different agents depending on the cause. Agents that clear heat and cool the blood are used to treat hemorrhage occuring in heat patterns. Ones that transform stasis and arrest hemorrhage are selected when bleeding is caused by blood stasis. Qi-boosting and spleen-fortifying agents contain the blood in vacuity patterns. Formulae usually contain relatively strong antihemorrhagics. Qi downbearers and agents that calm, clear, and nourish the liver are used in some cases.

In choosing antihemorrhagics, consideration should be given first to the need for warm or cool agents. Cool agents, which account for the majority, include:

Cool Antihemorrhagics	
Herba Ecliptae	*hàn lián cǎo*
Cacumen Biotae	*cè bó yè*
Rhizoma Imperatae	*máo gēn*
Fibra Stipulae Trachycarpi	*zōng lǘ pí*
Folium Nelumbinis	*hé yè*
Herba Cephalanoploris	*xiǎo jì cǎo*
Flos Sophorae Immatura	*huái huā*
Radix Rumicis	*tǔ dà huáng*

Warm antihemorrhagics include:

Warm Antihemorrhagics	
Folium Artemisiae Argyi	*ài yè*
Herba Agrimoniae	*xiān hè cǎo*

Warm Antihemorrhagics (continued)	
Radix Pseudoginseng	sān qī
Rhizoma Zingiberis carbonisatum	páo jiāng tàn
Terra Flava Usta	zào xīn tǔ

Drug selection also depends on the location of the bleeding. Agents frequently used for vaginal bleeding are:

Antihemorrhagics for Vaginal Bleeding	
Folium Artemisiae Argyi	ài yè
Os in Cornu Bovis	niú jiǎo sāi

The following agents are often used for hematuria:

Antihemorrhagics for Hematuria	
Pollen Typhae	pú huáng
Herba Cirsii Japonici	dà jì
Herba Cephalanoploris	xiǎo jì cǎo

The following drugs treat hematemesis and expectoration of blood:

Antihemorrhagics for Blood Vomiting and Expectoration of Blood	
Rhizoma Bletillae	bái jí
Rhizoma Imperatae	máo gēn

The following are mostly used for hemafecia:

Antihemorrhagics for Hemafecia	
Radix Sanguisorbae	dì yú
Flos Sophorae Immatura	huái huā
Terra Flava Usta	zào xīn tǔ

However, most antihemorrhagics are interchangeable. The following all have a pronounced securing astringent effect:

Securing Astringent Antihemorrhagics	
Cacumen Biotae	cè bó yè
Fibra Stipulae Trachycarpi	zōng lǘ pí
Folium Nelumbinis	hé yè
Rhizoma Bletillae	bái jí
Terra Flava Usta	zào xīn tǔ

Carbonization is frequently used to increase the astringent and hemostatic effect of other drugs.

Representative formula

Ten Cinders Pills *(shí huī wán)*.

Acumoxatherapy

The spleen is fortified through such points as SP-6, SP-4, and SP-9. SP-10 is frequently used to cool the blood and arrest hemorrhage. Moxibustion at LV-1 and SP-1 has a special antihemorrhagic effect.

This is an example of treating the branches first, in an acute situation. Once the crisis is past, the root must be determined and treated accordingly. Trauma, blood heat, and splenic vacuity are among the possible causes.

Securing the menses

Indications

One way that menorrhagia and persistent metrorrhagia may be treated is to use the method of securing the menses. However, this represents symptomatic treatment, and is mostly used for heavy bleeding only.

Agents used

General antihemorrhagics:

Antihemorrhagics	
Gelatinum Corii Asini	*lǘ pí jiāo*
Radix Rehmanniae Cruda	*shēng dì*
Herba Agrimoniae	*xiān hè cǎo*

In addition, securing astringents may be used:

Securing Astringents	
Os in Cornu Bovis	*niú jiǎo sāi*
Limonitum	*yǔ yú liáng*
Halloysitum Rubrum	*chì shí zhī*
Fluoritum	*zǐ shí yīng*

Representative formula

Awakening Spirit Elixir *(zhèn líng dān)*.

Acumoxatherapy

Menorrhagia and persistent metrorrhagia are generally treated according to their presenting symptoms. For example, if there are heat signs, strong stimulation of SP-10 and LV-1 is appropriate. If the spleen is unable to contain the blood, points such as BL-20‡, SP-6‡, and SP-1‡ can be used. SP-8, GV-20‡, LV-3, GV-4‡, and CV-6 may also be added, according to the symptoms. The *Great Compendium of Acumoxatherapy* mentions M-CA-18 *(zi-gong)* and LI-2 as points effective for this type of condition.

Checking vaginal discharge

Indications

Persistent, clear, thin white flow without foul smell, leading to physical weakness, calls for treatment using the method of checking vaginal discharge.

Agents used

Qi and kidney supplementers are combined with securing astringents such as:

Securing Astringents	
Os Sepiae tempered	duàn zéi gǔ
Concha Ostreae tempered	duàn mǔ lì
Semen Euryalis	qiàn shí
Semen Gingko	bái guǒ
Cera Chinensis Aurea	huáng là

Representative formula

Leukorrhea Tablets *(zhǐ dài piàn)*.

Acumoxatherapy

Vaginal discharge is caused by spleen or kidney vacuity and is treated accordingly. Points such as CV-6‡, GB-26‡, and SP-6‡ are used, with the addition of BL-20‡ and ST-36‡ in cases of spleen vacuity, and KI-2‡ and BL-23‡ in cases of kidney vacuity. An alternative treatment is moxibustion at GV-4, CV-8, and CV-2.

Remarks concerning the use of securing astriction

Normally, securing astringents are not used at the onset of disease. In repletion patterns characterized by a strong pathogen, such as exuberant phlegm-turbidity in the inner body, they should be used with caution.

Settling and Absorption

Settling and absorption uses minerals and animal shells to achieve the aim of heavy settling, subduing yang, extinguishing wind, and promoting the absorption of qi.

Settling fright and calming the spirit

Indications

Palpitations, racing of the heart, insomnia, mania, and withdrawal are symptoms that call for treatment using the method of settling fright and calming the spirit.

Agents used

Heavy Settlers	
Magnetitum	*cí shí*
Os Draconis	*lóng gǔ*
Dens Draconis	*lóng chǐ*
Concha Ostreae	*mǔ lì*
Concha Margaritifera	*zhēn zhū mǔ*
Cinnabaris	*zhū shā*
Ferric Oxide	*shēng tiě luò*

These may be combined with heart yang freers:

Heart Yang Freers	
Ramulus Cinnamomi	*guì zhī*
Rhizoma Acori Graminei	*chāng pú*

Heart qi boosters are also used:

Heart Qi Boosters	
Radix Codonopsis Pilosulae	*dǎng shēn*
Radix Glycyrrhizae	*gān cǎo*

In addition, heart blood nourishers are employed:

Heart Blood Nourishers	
Radix Salviae Miltiorrhizae	*dān shēn*
Radix Rehmanniae Cruda	*shēng dì*
Radix Angelicae Sinensis	*dāng guī*
Gelatinum Corii Asini	*lǘ pí jiāo*

Heart spirit quietants include:

Heart Spirit Quietants	
Semen Zizyphi Jujubae	*zǎo rén*
Semen Biotae	*bó zǐ rén*

In some cases is is helpful to use agents that clear heat and transform phlegm:

Heat Clearers and Phlegm Transformers	
Rhizoma Coptidis	*huáng lián*
Caulis Bambusae in Taenis	*zhú rú*

Representative formula

Magnetite and Cinnabar Pills *(cí zhū wán)*.

Acumoxatherapy

HT-7, PC-6, and BL-15 are fundamental points used to settle fright and quiet the spirit. Other points are added according to the specific condition.

If the underlying cause is breakdown of cardiorenal interaction, BL-23, KI-3, BL-15, and PC-8 may be used. If there is heart yin-blood vacuity, BL-20, BL-17, and SP-6 are appropriate. Hepatocystic heat is treated with strong stimulation at LV-3, LV-2, BL-18, and BL-19.

Insomnia from splenogastric disharmony may be treated with CV-12, ST-25, ST-40, and BL-20 as primary points to reestablish gastrosplenic harmony, adding HT-7 and PC-6 secondarily to quiet the spirit.

Subduing yang and extinguishing wind

Indications

Subduing yang and extinguishing wind is a treatment method useful for symptom patterns including the following: rising hyperactivity of liver yang and liver wind stirring within (endogenous liver wind) characterized by headache, dizziness, agitation, twitching muscles, and trembling hands; high fever, clouding of the spirit, tetanic inversion, and convulsive spasm of the limbs occurring when extreme heat engenders wind in exogenous heat diseases; and heat in the palms of the hands and soles of the feet, trembling limbs, or tetanic inversion occurring when yin vacuity stirs wind in final-stage exogenous heat diseases.

Agents used

Yang-subduing wind extinguishers such as the following are often used:

Yang-Subduing and Wind-Extinguishing Agents	
Concha Ostreae	mǔ lì
Concha Margaritifera	zhēn zhū mǔ
Dens Draconis	lóng chǐ
Magnetitum	cí shí

These are often combined with liver clearers such as:

Liver Clearers	
Ramulus et Uncus Uncariae	gōu téng
Flos Chrysanthemi	jú huā
Folium Mori	sāng yè
Spica Prunellae	xià kū cǎo
Cortex Radicis Mu Tan	mǔ dān pí
Fructus Gardeniae	zhī zǐ

Yang-subduing wind extinguishers are also combined with yin enrichers such as:

Yin Enrichers	
Radix Rehmanniae Cruda	shēng dì
Radix Scrophulariae	xuán shēn
Tuber Ophiopogonis	mài dōng
Fructus Ligustri Lucidi	nǔ zhēn zǐ
Plastrum Testudinis	guī bǎn
Gelatinum Corii Asini	lǘ pí jiāo

If necessary, wind-extinguishing tetany settlers may also be employed:

Wind-Extinguishing and Tetany-Settling Agents	
Buthus	quán xiē
Bombyx Batryticatus	jiāng cán
Lumbricus	dì lóng
Cornu Antelopis	líng yáng jiǎo

Representative formulae

Yang-Subduing and Wind-Extinguishing Formulae	
Gastrodia and Uncaria Cool Decoction	tiān-má gōu-téng yǐn
Triple-Armored Pulse-Restorative Decoction	sān jiǎ fù mài tāng

Gastrodia and Uncaria Cool Decoction is used to treat liver yang transforming into wind, whereas Triple-Armored Pulse-Restorative Decoction treats yin vacuity stirring wind.

Acumoxatherapy

Ascendant hyperactivity of liver yang and liver wind stirring within are treated with LV-2 and BL-18 to drain the liver, KI-3 and BL-23 to enrich water and thereby moisten wood, and GB-20 and GV-20 to disperse wind and yang in the head. KI-1 is often warmed with indirect moxibustion to downbear liver yang. If phlegm-damp is present, points such as SP-9 and PC-6 are included.

Yin vacuity spasm requires the use of points such as GV-8 to drain governing vessel qi, GV-14 and BL-60 to course and drain tai yang channel qi, and BL-23, BL-17, SP-10, and KI-3 to supplement yin-blood.

Initial-stage heat diseases are treated with points that clear heat. BL-23 and KI-3 may be included to enrich yin. Points on the liver channel are usually used to treat spasms. LI-4 is also a useful general point.

Securing the kidney to promote qi absorption

Indications

Failure of renal governance of qi absorption, characterized by short, rapid breathing, dyspnea at the slightest exertion, vacuity sweating, and frigid limbs, are patterns that call for treatment using the method of securing the kidney to promote qi absorption. Such patterns are associated with a drained or dark cyan complexion or upbearing fire-flush. The pulse is deep and fine.

Agents used

Kidney supplementers may be used, including:

Principles and Methods of Treatment

Kidney Supplementers	
Radix Aconiti Fu Tzu	*fù zǐ*
Cortex Cinnamomi	*ròu guì*
Radix Rehmanniae Conquita	*shóu dì*
Mesocarpium Corni	*yú ròu*
Semen Juglandis	*hú táo ròu*
Gecko	*gé jiè*

These may be combined with heavy settlers such as:

Heavy Settlers	
Magnetitum	*cí shí*
Fluoritum	*zǐ shí yīng*
Stalactitum	*zhōng rǔ shí*
Galenitum	*qīng qiān*

The heavy settlers are added to promote qi absorption.

Representative formula

Black Tin Elixir *(hēi-xí dān)*.

Acumoxatherapy

Kidney vacuity diseases with the above symptoms are treated using mild stimulation at points such as BL-23, CV-4, GV-4, CV-6, BL-38, and ST-36 to supplement the kidney and the original qi. Moxibustion is used if there are cold symptoms, KI-3 is included if there is yin vacuity, and KI-7 is added to enrich the kidney, moisten dryness, and check sweating.

Principles and Methods of Treatment

Summary

The above eleven methods of treatment are the most commonly used in clinical practice. Generally speaking, cold patterns are treated by warming, heat patterns by clearage, vacuity patterns by supplementation, and repletion patterns mostly by precipitation. However, diseases are rarely so simply classified, and treatment accordingly requires an appropriate blend of methods.

For instance, diaphoresis combined with clearage or precipitation is known as "dual resolution of interior and exterior," in which formulae such as Ledebouriella Wondrous Panacea Powder *(fáng-fēng tōng shèng sǎn)* are used. Dual cooling of qi and blood involves clearing both qi and blood heat with formulae such as Scourge-Clearing Detoxifying Cool Decoction *(qīng wēn bài dú yǐn)* which treats dual blaze of qi and blood in exogenous heat diseases. Warming and clearage may also be combined, using such formulae as Yellow Earth Decoction *(huáng tǔ tāng)* which, containing both Radix Aconiti Fu Tzu *(fù zǐ)* and Radix Scutellariae *(huáng qín)*, treats hemafecia. Two Immortals Decoction *(èr xiān tāng)* which contains Rhizoma Curculiginis *(xiān máo)* and Herba Epimedii *(xiān líng pí)* as well as Rhizoma Anemarrhenae *(zhī mǔ)* and Cortex Phellodendri *(huáng bó)*, relieves hypertension. Carriage-Halting Pills *(zhù chē wán)* with Rhizoma Coptidis *(huáng lián)* and Rhizoma Zingiberis blast-fried *(páo jiāng)* cures persistent dysentery. Offensive treatment (mainly precipitation) and supplementation may sometimes be applied simultaneously as in the case with cirrhosis of the liver, which can be treated by blood-breaking and stasis-transforming agents together with qi-supplementing and yin-nourishing agents.

Notes

[1] "Outthrust" denotes the movement or bringing out of pathogens to or through the exterior, and the eruption of papules and macules, which in some diseases, accompanies this process. "Effusion" denotes gentle outward movement such as sweat through the striations. The concept of sweating, both natural and induced, is expressed in Chinese as "effusing sweat." In the phrase, "pungent, dissipating outthrust and effusion," the terms "pungent" and "dissipating" describe drug properties, while "effusion" and "outthrust" describe their action of promoting perspiration and expelling the pathogen.

[2] To induce evacuation, the *Gateway to Medicine* recommends the "penetrating heaven coldness method" described in O'Connor and Bensky, *Acupuncture, A Comprehensive Text*, p. 525.

[3] KI-14 is a point of intersection with the penetrating vessel irregular channel, and thus has a strong effect on the abdomen. Because the penetrating vessel passes through the uterus, this point is also used to treat menstrual problems.

Appendices

Appendix One

Introduction

This section is divided into two related glossaries. The first, **Glossary of Terms,** is presented in alphabetical order and contains extended explanations of the Chinese medical terms used in this text. Included for each entry are the transliteration of the term and a reference number, for example, "**abduction**: dǎo (432)." The reference number, in this case "432," indicates that the Chinese character from which this term is derived may be found by locating the same number in the **Stroke-Order Glossary.** Thus, students of Chinese who are as yet not comfortable with stroke-order searches may find the characters easily.

A **Stroke-Order Glossary** has been included for the benefit of translators, teachers or students who wish to reference the Chinese medical terminology. This glossary is presented in Chinese dictionary order and contains the Chinese characters, the transliteration, and the English term or phrase used to translate the Chinese medical concept. Each entry also includes the sequential reference number previously described. Please note that a few terms (such as those that describe tongue or pulse qualities) do not have a separate English glossary entry and are not followed by a reference number. These terms usually qualify another term. Where there are lists of terms that qualify a major entry, these are noted by the use of a tilde (˜) in advance of the transliteration. Thus, " ˜ pàng dà" (enlarged) qualifies the major entry "shé" (tongue body).

Glossary of Terms

abduction: dǎo (432)

The removal of pathogens after they have been dispersed. See **dispersion**.

abscess: yōng (484)

A pyogenic inflammatory lesion of the skin and subcutaneous tissue. Abscesses result when channel blockage gives rise to congealing and stagnation of qi and blood. Channel blockage can occur when damp-heat and fire toxin resulting from excessive consumption of rich foods become depressed in the inner body, or when toxin is contracted through unclean wounds. Abscesses start with swelling and redness. Then pus begins to form, the skin becomes redder, resulting in a head that produces a rippling sensation under pressure. The healing process begins after the head bursts. There are internal and external abscesses.

accumulation: jī (439)

Collection or amassment, especially of waste in the digestive tract; also refers to stable, unyielding abdominal masses, in contradistinction to **gathering** which denotes unstable, yielding masses. See also **flow stoppage** and **concretions and gatherings**.

acid regurgitation: tūn suān (125)

The flowing back of sour fluid into the mouth, which is swallowed before there is time to eject it. This represents a symptom similar to, but more severe than **acid upflow** (q.v.).

acid upflow: fǎn suān (168)

The upflow of acid from the stomach into the mouth; similar to, yet milder than **acid regurgitation**.

affect: qíng (268)

[*qíng*, fact, reason, emotion, affection] Mental state, particularly as a reaction to the environment. The seven affects are: joy, anger, anxiety, preoccupation, sorrow, fear, and fright. Five of these correspond to the "five dispositions" (see **disposition**). The associations of the word *qíng* emphasize reality and factuality, while disposition *(zhì)* emphasizes will and subjectivity. The rendering of the names of the five affects in English is inconsistent. For instance, preoccupation *(sī)*, the affect of the spleen, is rendered by some writers as "worry." By others, the same English word is used to denote anxiety *(yōu)*, the affect associated with the lung. These other renderings of the terms are not necessarily without foundation, but, when reading, care is needed to avoid confusion.

affect damage: nèi shāng qī qíng (52)

Damage to yin, yang, qi, and blood, etc., by excesses of the seven affects.

agitation: fán zào (366)

A subjective feeling of restlessness *(fán)* outwardly expressed by pronounced abnormal movement *(zào)*.

amassment: xù (416)

Accumulate, collect. See **blood amassment**.

animal odor: sāo wèi (456)

The odors characteristically associated with sheep and foxes.

ascites: fù shuǐ (384)

Accumulation of water in the abdomen. See **water**.

aspect: fēn

Physiologic activity viewed from a particular functional context. Thermic disease theory observes bodily function from four distinct viewpoints: the defense aspect, the qi aspect, the construction aspect, and the blood aspect. Each of these may be considered as separate but interrelated functional entities. Each of these four functional aspects can be affected by the heat pathogen, presenting its own characteristic signs and symptoms. Because pathogen penetration is usually sequential, other translators have chosen to render this term as "level," although the Chinese word only means a "part" or "division," implying no notion of depth.

assail: qīn xí (176)

Intrude, as of pathogens into the exterior of the body. See **exuberance and debilitation**.

assail: xí (481)

Attack or invade; especially of pathogens entering the body through the exterior.

atony: wěi (379)

Weakness and limpness. **Atony** patterns are characterized by limpness and weakness in the legs. In severe cases, the condition may also affect the hands, and additional signs such as numbness of the flesh and dry, lusterless skin may be observed. Atony patterns may occur after high fever or childbirth. Pathomechanisms include: scorching of the blood vessels by pathogenic heat, such as may occur in lung heat parching the lobes; sinew damage by yang ming damp-heat, causing permanent relaxation of the muscles; or insufficiency of essence-blood due to hepatorenal depletion, whereby the sinews are deprived of nourishment.

attack: gōng (139)

Treatment of patterns characterized by repletion of pathogenic qi and vacuity of correct qi, using superlative agents.

audio-olfactive examination: wén zhěn (410)

[*wén,* listen, smell; *zhěn,* examine] Examining the body by listening and smelling.

bad odor, malodorous: chòu (248)

A general term for unpleasant or offensive smells. See **fishy odor, animal odor, putrid odor,** and **foul odor**.

bag-over-the-head sensation: tóu zhòng rú guǒ (443)

Heavy-headedness characterized by a feeling of encumbrance, as though the head was covered with a bag.

balloon-head scourge: dà tóu wēn (22)

A disease resulting from invasion of the spleen and stomach channels by seasonal wind-thermia toxin; characterized by swelling and redness of the head, and sometimes by painful swelling of the throat; in severe cases, additional symptoms include deafness, trismus, clouding of the spirit, and delirious raving.

banking-up earth: péi tǔ (261)

Supplementing the stomach and spleen.

bind: jié (330)

[*jié,* to knot, freeze, congeal, form, bear fruit] 1) To become tight, hard, or stiff. 2) To cohere or make cohere. 3) To constipate. **Bind** principally refers to the concentration of pathogens in a specific location, giving rise to hardness. When phlegm and qi bind, phlegm nodules form. When heat binds in the intestines, the stool becomes dry and solid, and difficult to evacuate. In the term "binding depression of qi dynamic," it refers to the restricted movement of substances caused by a reduced activity of qi. See **flow stoppage**.

binding depression of liver qi: gān qì yù jié (146)

The liver governs free-coursing and upbearing effusion, which may readily be affected by anger, annoyance, and general emotional constraint, giving rise to liver depression. The main general signs are distention and fullness or scurrying pain in the lateral costal region, usually emotion-related. Globus hystericus may occur when liver qi ascends counterflow. Ventral pain, vomiting of sour fluid, and poor appetite are observed when liver qi invades the stomach, affecting gastric harmony and downbearing. Binding depression of liver qi may cause qi stagnation and blood stasis. In such cases, there is stabbing pain in the lateral costal region, with the possibility of formation of concretions and gatherings. Finally, menstrual disorders, neurosis, hepatocystic diseases, hepatosplenomegalia, and indigestion are often related to binding depression of liver qi.

bitter fullness in the chest and lateral costal region:
xōng xié kǔ mǎn (245)

Fullness and oppression the the chest and lateral costal region associated with disruption of qi dynamic in the foot shao yang gallbladder channel and with gallbladder fire.

blast-fry: pāo (187)

To stir-fry (medicinal agents) in an iron wok over a fierce fire allowing them to give off smoke. Rhizoma Zingiberis Exsiccatum *(gān jiāng)*, Radix Aconiti Fu Tzu *(fù zǐ)*, and Radix Aconiti Negri *(tiān xióng)* may be prepared in this way to reduce their harshness.

blaze: fán (438)

Describes heat in the exuberant heat stage of thermic diseases. See **heat**.

block: bì (291)

Closure (of pathways through the exterior); used to describe symptoms, such as in the term "menstrual block" (amenorrhea), "fecal block" (constipation); also denotes "pathogen block" (or "inner-body block"), whose various different forms are referred to as **block patterns**. These may occur when, as a result of drastic debilitation of correct qi, a pathogen falls into the inner body, where it becomes trapped and severely disrupts organ function. The chief signs are: stupor of the spirit-disposition or coma, clenched jaws and hands, and exuberant phlegm-drool. The pulse is either urgent and wiry, or surging and rapid. See **flow stoppage**.

block clouding inversion: nèi bì hūn jué (50)

Clouding inversion (syncope) due to inner-body block.

block patterns: bì zhèng (292)

See **block**.

blood amassment: xù xùe (417)

A form of inner-body stasis heat occurring in exogenous heat diseases when pathogenic heat interiorizes and contends with the blood. Signs include lower abdominal pain and distention, together with chills and fever. The symptoms may be moderate in the daytime, but at night the patient may suffer from mania, delirium, and confused speech; he may be aggressive in speech and behavior. Blood amassment is also used loosely to denote any substantial or insubstantial forms of inner- or outer-body static blood.

blood quickening: huó xuè (192)

Stimulating blood flow.

blood strangury: xuè lín (116)

Strangury with hematuria. See **strangury**.

blood tympany: xuè gǔ (117)

Severe abdominal distention due to blood amassment, attended by such signs as black stool, dark-colored urine, and caput medusae.

body: xíng tǐ (120)

Xíng denotes the corporeal body, while *tǐ* denotes the constitutional body. The combined term accordingly refers to the physical body and constitution.

body inch: cùn (23)

A proportional unit of measurement used to determine the location of acupoints on the body, roughly equivalent to the length of the medial phalange of the middle finger.

boil: jiān áo (369)

The action of heat on blood, particularly when phlegm arises as a result. See **heat**.

boosting: yì (230)

Supplementation (especially of qi, organs, etc.), to ensure their normal, vigorous activity. See **supplementation**.

bowel: fǔ (336)

Any of the organs of the exterior (stomach, small and large intestine, gallbladder, bladder and triple burner). NB: only the latterly addition of the "flesh" radical to this Chinese ideogram distinguished it from the ideogram meaning "dwelling place."

breaking: pò (235)

See **dispersion**.

brew: yùn (476)

To gather, ferment (usually in a concealed or inconspicuous way). Brew describes certain forms of inner-body (and especially lung) heat. See **heat**.

bruxism: yǎo yá (178)

Involuntary grinding of the teeth, especially in sleep.

calculous strangury: shí lín (102)

Strangury with urinary calculous. See **strangury**.

calming the liver and extinguishing wind: píng gān xí fēng (94)

A method of treating liver wind due to ascendant hyperactivity of liver yang.

cardiac portals: xīn qiào (71)

The clear portals in relation to the heart and spirit.

cardialgia: xīn tòng (68)

Pain in the pit of the stomach or the region of the heart. **Cardiodynia** refers specifically to pain in the heart itself.

cardiodynia: zhēn xīn tòng (234)

Pain in the heart. Cf. **cardialgia**.

carphologia: xún yī mō chuáng (308.1)

Involuntary picking at bedclothes.

center: zhōng (38)

The spleen and stomach; the middle burner.

changes in urine and micturition:
pái niào yǔ niào yè bìng biàn

The normal, healthy individual voids from four to six times a day, mostly during the daytime. Western medicine establishes that the adult voids between 700 to 2000 ml. per day. A daily volume in excess of 2500 ml. is termed "polyuria"' and less than 500 ml. is termed "oliguria." "Anuria" refers to a daily volume of less than 100 ml. Polyuria, and in particular "nocturia," indicate vacuous kidney yang failing to secure and contain the urine. Long micturition with clear urine is a vacuity cold sign. Frequent micturition with clear urine, or even incontinence, indicates qi vacuity. Heavy micturition (frequent copious voidings) is a sign of diabetic disease when accompanied by thirst, high fluid intake, and weight loss. Anuria and short micturition with scant urine are explained pathomechanically as fulminant desertion of the fluids, causing exhaustion of the source of urine; debilitation of kidney yang, leading to insufficiency of the transformative action of qi, and hence reduced urine production; or vesicular qi block, whereby urine is retained in the bladder.

Short micturition with scant urine is normal in hot weather if fluids lost in sweating are not replaced by adequate fluid intake. Short micturition with scant, yellow, or dark-colored urine indicates heat. Frequency (frequent urination), urgency, and painful urination are seen in qi vacuity, repletion heat, and damp-heat patterns. For example, frequent, short micturition with scant urine occurring in pregnancy indicates fetal pressure and is attributable to qi vacuity; frequent micturition with scant, dark-colored or turbid urine, associated with acute pain, indicates damp-heat in the lower burner, or specifically in the bladder.

Frequency and urgency with painful and difficult urination together with blood or calculi in the urine are signs of strangury. Sudden urinary block, or reduction of urine flow to a mere dribble, together with foul-smelling urine, pain in the bladder, and fever indicate repletion. Dribbling incontinence refers to a constant dribble of urine and inability to achieve a full stream. It is commonly due to center qi vacuity. Enuresis is attributable to insecurity of vacuous kidney qi. A gradual reduction of the amount of urine, leading to oliguria, and in severe cases, anuria, indicates vacuity. Such patterns are also characterized by cold in the lumbar region and limbs. Hematuria can be caused by a wide variety of factors, including damp-heat in the lower burner, yin vacuity fire effulgence, tumors, or calculi. Other signs must be correlated for accurate diagnosis.

channel passage: chuán jīng (347)

The movement of pathogens from one channel to another.

child fright inversion: xiǎo ér jīng jué (25)

See **fright inversion**.

child fright wind: xiǎo ér jīng fēng (24)

See **fright wind**.

chong products: chóng lèi (469)

Drugs derived from reptiles, arthropods, and shellfish.

clamoring stomach: cáo zá (391)

A sensation of discomfort in the venter or cardiac region described as being of neither hunger nor pain. It is akin to the discomfort that may normally be felt after drinking tea without milk on an empty stomach or eating fruits such as apples.

clear: qīng (280)

1) *Adj:* Pure and insubstantial (e.g., clear yang qi), in opposition to turbid, which means impure and substantial. 2) *vb:* To eliminate pathogens.

clearage: qīng (281)

A method of eliminating pathogens, especially heat.

clear-food diarrhea: xià lì qīng gǔ (9)

Diarrhea characterized by watery, light brown stool containing partially digested food.

cloud: méng (413)

To cover, cloud, obscure; describes the effect of phlegm and phlegm turbidity, such as in the term "phlegm clouding the pericardium," a pattern characterized by oppression in the chest, confusion, and in serious cases, coma. See **exuberance and debilitation.**

clouding: hūn (164)

Describes severe lack of clarity (of vision or consciousness).

clove lesions: dīng chuāng (147)

Small, hard, deep-rooted, pyogenic lesions. The name is derived from the fact that they are shaped like nails or cloves.

cold: hán

The quality of cold; the quality that produces a cooling effect. Cf. **frigid.**

cold enveloping fire: hán bāo huǒ (307)

A pattern of outer-body cold due to contraction of wind-cold with accumulated heat in the inner body. The outer-body cold is seen as "enveloping" the depressed inner-body heat.

cold form: xíng hán (119)

Outwardly manifest signs of cold, e.g., aversion to cold, desire for warm beverages, curled, recumbent posture, frigid limbs, etc.

cold shan: hán shàn (308)

1) Accumulation in the abdomen of the cold pathogen from repeated wind-cold contractions due to vacuity cold in the spleen and stomach, or to postpartum blood vacuity. It is characterized by cold in the umbilical region, cold sweating, and counterflow cold in the limbs. The pulse is deep and tight. In severe cases, there is generalized cold in the body and numbness in the limbs. Occurring in blood vacuity patients, the abdominal

pain stretches up the lateral costal region and is accompanied by cramp in the lower abdomen.

2) A pain pattern due to cold pathogen invading the jue yin channel. The signs are painful, cold, hard swelling of the scrotum, with pain in the testicles, impotence, desire for warmth and aversion to cold, and cold form and frigid limbs.

collapse: wáng (17)

Critical exhaustion (of yin, yang, blood, or fluids). See also **desertion**.

collect: tíng (257)

Accumulation, as of water, in specific locations; e.g., water collecting around the stomach. See **flow stoppage**.

column rheum: zhī yǐn (72)

Water in the infracardiac region (diaphragm and lungs), giving rise to symptoms such as cough, copious phlegm, rapid breathing, inability to lie flat, and facial edema.

concretions and gatherings: zhēng jiǎ jī jù (475)

The collective term for concretions *(zhēng)*, conglomerations *(jiǎ)*, accumulations *(jī)*, and gatherings *(jù)*, all four of which refer to abdominal masses associated with pain and distention. Concretions and accumulations are masses of definite form and fixed location, associated with pain of fixed location. They stem from disease in the viscera and at blood level. Conglomerations and gatherings are masses of indefinite form, which gather and dissipate at irregular intervals and which are attended by pain of unfixed location. They are attributed to disease in the bowels and at qi level. Accumulations and gatherings chiefly occur in the middle burner. Concretions and conglomerations chiefly occur in the lower burner, and in many cases are the result of gynecologic disorders. In general, concretions and gatherings arise when emotional depression or intemperate eating causes damage to the liver and spleen. The resultant organ disharmony leads to obstruction and stagnation of qi which in turn causes static blood to collect gradually in the inner body. Invariably the root cause is insufficiency of correct qi.

confound: mí (250)

To render stuporous, to cloud severely; occurs in the term "phlegm confounding the cardiac portals," characterized, amongst other symptoms, by stupor or coma. See **exuberance and debilitation**.

congealing: níng (430)

Viscid, becoming or making viscid, describes the viscid nature of pathogens such as damp, and their inhibitive effect on normal flow of blood and qi. When applied to the blood, this term denotes thickening but not necessarily coagulation.

congestion: yōng (431)

The clogging effect of pathogens, especially those affecting the lung. See **flow stoppage.**

connect: luò (331)

To link; of channels, to link up with the exterior organ corresponding to the governing viscus, e.g., the hand tai yin lung channel connects with the large intestine.

constitutional body: tǐ (489)

The human body in its constitutional aspect, as opposed to the formal body, which denotes the purely physical manifestation of human life.

constraining: lián (446)

Astriction, especially of the lung, as in the terms "constraining the lung and suppressing cough," and "constraining perspiration."

construction: yìng (451)

An abbreviation for construction qi, which is an essential qi formed from the essence of digestate and which flows in the vessels. Construction is considered to be an aspect of the blood.

contain: shè (478)

To hold in; used specifically to denote, in physiology, qi's action of keeping the blood flowing within the vessels, and in therapy, the promotion of this and analogous functions.

contention: xiāng bó (194)

Struggle, especially of two pathogens simultaneously present in the body, such as contention of wind and damp. See **exuberance and debilitation.**

contraction: gǎn (353)

Being affected (by exogenous pathogens), e.g., wind-cold contraction, a disease caused by exogenous wind-cold.

contracture: lüān suō (483)

Permanent contraction of a muscle; a term used in Western medicine.

contracture and tautness: shōu yǐn (109)

Permanent contraction or hypertension of the muscles, generally associated with kidney yang vacuity.

conversion: zhuǎn huà (470)

In yin-yang theory, change from yin or yang to its complement; in eight-parameter pattern identification, displacement of symptoms of one parameter by those of its opposite.

convulsive spasm: chōu chù (160)

Violent involuntary contraction or series of contractions of muscles.

correct: zhèng (95)

Normal or rendering normal. "Correct complexion" refers to the normal complexion of the healthy individual. "Correct qi" denotes the forces that maintain the normal functioning of the human body and seek to re-establish normal function when pathogenic qi is present. "The correct" refers specifically to correct qi, where qi is understood in its broader sense of meaning activity, or substance in its active aspect.

correct qi: zhèng qì (95.1)

See **correct**.

cosmic qi: dà qì (20)

The qi of the environment, air.

cough (and expectoration): ké sòu (179)

Classically, *ké* is explained as being with sound but without matter, while *sòu* is with matter but without sound. The combined term is often used loosely in the sense of cough with or without expectoration.

counterflow: nì (252)

Flow counter to the normal direction. See also **inversion**.

counterflow frigidity of the limbs: sì zhī nì lěng (88)

See **inversion frigidity of the limbs**.

coursing: shū (317)

Promotion of free flow, such as hepatic free-coursing; also denotes elimination of pathogens, especially wind, or the liberation of parts of the body from them. Coursing is closely associated with the liver and wind, the pathogen by which it ails. This concept is often rendered as "dredging" by other writers.

cramp: zhuǎn jīn, chōu jīn (471)

Painful contraction and contortion of muscles; due to insufficiency of qi and blood, fatigue, or exposure to damp or cold; usually affects only the calves, but in severe cases, the abdomen too.

crimson: jiàng (333)

A deep shade of red.

cumbersome: kùn (127)

The heaviness and fatigue felt in the limbs, particularly when the spleen fails to transform water-damp.

cutaneous cornification: jī fū jiǎ cuò (114)

Roughness and peeling of the skin associated with emaciation due to major illness or malnutrition.

cyan: qīng (175)

Green-blue, greenish blue. Often translated as either "green" or "blue," **cyan** is the most accurate rendering of the original Chinese, and is closest to the actual physical appearance it describes (hence: cyanosis, cyanotic complexion).

dai-yang: dài yáng (461)

[*dài*, to wear on the head; to look upwards] A disease pattern characterized by tidal flushing of the cheeks and attributable to upfloating of vacuous yang. Like **repelled yang,** it is a critical condition of cold falsely presenting as heat. *Dài yáng* is attributable to true cold in the lower body with false heat in the upper body. The tidal flushing is characterized by pale red patches, giving the cheeks the appearance of having been dabbed with rouge. The patches often constantly change location. Other symptoms include counterflow frigidity of the lower limbs and long micturition with clear urine. False heat signs include nosebleed and bleeding gums, and painful swollen throat. The pulse is large and floating, but feeble and vacuous. In serious cases, it is faint and fine, verging on expiry.

damage: shāng (349)

Injury of any kind, e.g., damage to liquid.

damp forming with cold: shī cóng hán huà (447)

The development of cold-damp in patients suffering from impaired fluid transformation due to devitalization of splenic yang. In such cases the damp pathogen may be completely endogenous (i.e., due to vacuity), or of exogenous origin. Exogenous and endogenous damp are mutually conducive. Splenic transformation failure represents an intrinsic factor facilitating the invasion of exogenous damp, while failure to eliminate exogenous damp may damage the spleen, thereby giving rise to endogenous damp.

damp forming with heat: shī cóng rè huà (448)

The development of damp-heat in patients suffering from intense stomach heat due to excessive consumption of sweet or fatty foods. Exogenous damp or damp-heat may or may not be involved.

damp phlegm: shī tán (449)

Phlegm-rheum developing through accumulation of endogenous damp which arises when the spleen's capacity to move and transform water-damp is impaired. Symptoms include copious, thin, white phlegm, thoracic oppression or nausea, cough and dyspnea, and an enlarged tongue with a glossy or slimy fur.

damp turbidity: shī zhuó (450)

Dampness, especially where it is heavy or viscid in nature and obstructs clear, light, yang qi.

daybreak diarrhea: chén xiè (273)

Also known as **fifth-watch diarrhea** and effectively synonymous with **kidney diarrhea**; occurs in the early morning and is heralded by borborygmi. The main cause is vacuous kidney yang and insufficiency of the vital-gate fire, causing a reduction in the supply of warmth and nourishment to spleen and stomach. See also **diarrhea**.

debilitation: shuāi (249)

In yin-yang theory, debilitation describes (usually severe) weakness of yang; also used in physiology to describe weakness of qi and other yang aspects of the organism. See **exuberance and debilitation.**

decoct: jiān (368)

To boil (medicinal agents) in water in order to extract their active properties.

deep-lying: fú (103)

Describes pathogens at a deep level of the inner body; latent.

defense: wèi (427)

An abbreviation for **defense qi,** which is formed from kidney yang qi, continually replenished by the essence of digestate, and dependent on pulmonary perfusion. Defense is thus rooted in the lower burner, nourished in the middle burner, and effused by the upper burner. It is a form of yang qi which is described as being "fierce and bold in nature" and "fast moving." It is not confined to the channels and vessels, and pervades the whole of the body including the bowels and viscera, and the muscular exterior and striations. It warms the organs, moistens the skin and nourishes the striations, and controls the opening and closing of the pores. It defends the muscular exterior against attack by exogenous pathogens and hence represents the body's first line of defense. Other texts refer to **defense** as "wei" or "protective" qi.

defense-construction disharmony: yíng wèi bù hé (452)

Exterior patterns characterized by spontaneous sweating and occurring in one of two forms: a) strong defense and weak construction, where yang qi is depressed in the muscular exterior and forces sweat out of the pores, giving rise to perspiration whenever fever occurs; and b) weak defense and strong construction, characterized by spontaneous sweating without fever, whereby sweat flows forth unconstrained by defense qi.

deficit: piān shuāi (255)

In yin-yang theory, relative weakening (of either yin or yang). Deficit of yin is often referred to as vacuity, while that of yang is often termed debilitation.

deflagration: fén (314)

Describes heat in the exuberant heat stage of thermic diseases. See **heat**.

depletion: kuī (458)

Severe loss; used primarily in the context of the kidney, e.g., "kidney depletion," which refers to insufficiency of kidney essence. See **exuberance and debilitation**.

depression: yù (493)

Reduction of normal activity characterized by unvented stagnation. In physiology, depression refers either to "binding depression" of qi dynamic or to flow stoppage due to congestion. The term also describes inhibition of normal emotional activity, expressing itself in the form of melancholy, oppression, frustration, and irascibility. Though often associated with psychosomatic disorders, this term bears broader connotations in Chinese Medicine than it has in Western psychology. See also the **six depressions, depression patterns**, and **flow stoppage**.

depression patterns: yù zhèng (494)

1) Generally denotes patterns caused by depression of normal physiological activity. See also **six depressions** and **depression**. 2) Specifically denotes patterns of disruption of the essence-spirit and organ dysfunction.

depurative downbearing: sù jiàng (346)

A function of the lung comprising two aspects: a) ensuring regular flow through the waterways (i.e., ensuring the passage of fluids down to the kidney); and b) sending qi absorbed from the air down to the kidney.

desertion: tuō (285)

Patterns characterized by critical depletion of yin, yang, qi, or blood, mainly characterized by pearly sweat, inversion frigidity of the limbs, gaping mouth and closed eyes, limp, open hands and enuresis, and a fine pulse verging on expiry. Desertion associated with loss of fluids such as through diarrhea, spermatorrhea, metrorrhagia, or urinary incontinence is known as **efflux desertion** (see also **efflux**). In the case of diarrhea or metrorrhagia, efflux desertion is sometimes associated with prolapse of the rectum or the womb. Desertion of rapid onset and development is known as fulminant desertion. Desertion due to gradual debilitation of original qi through enduring illness is known as vacuity desertion. The related term **collapse** is applied to specific aspects of the body such as yin, yang, and the blood, and stresses the cause rather than the result. Hence, "yang collapse vacuity desertion" denotes a desertion pattern attributed to exhaustion of yang qi. Desertion frequently corresponds to "shock" in Western medicine. See **exuberance and debilitation**.

desiccated: kū (185)

Dried out, dehydrated. See **exuberance and debilitation**.

detoxification: jiě dú (388)

Resolution of toxin.

detriment: sǔn (354)

Loss and damage (to blood, fluids, etc.). See **exuberance and debilitation**.

devitalization: bú zhèn (34)

Deprivation of vigor or force. See **exuberance and debilitation**.

diabetic disease: xiāo kě (222)

[*xiāo*, disperse; *kě*, thirst] 1) Generally denotes diseases characterized by thirst, increased fluid intake, and polyuria, and categorized as upper-burner, middle-burner, and lower-burner diabetic diseases depending on the operant pathomechanism; Western medical correspondences include diabetes insipidus and hypoadrenocorticism. 2) Specifically denotes a disease characterized by increased intake of both fluids and solids, emaciation, polyuria, and glycosuria and broadly corresponding to diabetes mellitus in Western medicine. Pathomechanisms include: a) accumulated heat in the middle burner occurring in patients fond of alcohol or sweet, fatty foods; b) fire formation following depression of physiologic activity due to dispositional excess; c) wearing of kidney essence due to excessive sexual activity, causing frenetic vacuity fire. All three pathomechanisms involve the mutual exacerbation of yin vacuity and dryness heat scorching kidney yin essence and the fluids of the lung and stomach. Yin vacuity is primarily associated with the kidney, and according to the principle that detriment to yin affects yang, kidney yang vacuity is also invariably observed in enduring cases.

diarrhea: xiè xiè (166)

Diarrhea is a global term denoting deviation from established bowel rhythm, characterized by increased frequency and fluidity of the stool. The Chinese term is made up of two characters, the first meaning "flowing away like water," and the second meaning "constant flow." Other sources explain the first character as meaning intermittent diarrhea, and the second character as "pouring down of watery stool." In compound terms such as kidney diarrhea *(shèn xiè),* the notion of diarrhea is often represented by the first character alone.

Diarrhea is classified in three distinct ways: a) according to cause or pathomechanism, e.g., summerheat diarrhea, ingesta damage diarrhea, cold diarrhea, heat diarrhea, and vacuity diarrhea; b) according to the associated morbid organ, e.g., splenic diarrhea, gastric diarrhea, small intestine diarrhea, large intestine diarrhea, and kidney diarrhea; c) according to signs, e.g., daybreak diarrhea, enduring diarrhea, efflux diarrhea, outpour diarrhea, swill diarrhea, clear-food diarrhea, clear-water diarrhea, and duck-stool diarrhea.

These categories are not necessarily mutually exclusive. Ingesta damage diarrhea, for example, is the result of damage to the digestive system by ingested food, as opposed to pre-existing dysfunction. It may therefore include certain forms of gastric, large intestine, and small intestine diarrhea, but excludes large intestine diarrhea due to lung qi vacuity (these two organs standing in exterior-interior relationship). Association between causes and form of diarrhea is variable. For example, kidney diarrhea always presents with the same basic symptoms, so that the term is synonymous with daybreak diarrhea. By contrast, thin-stool diarrhea may form part of either heat or cold patterns.

diminished qi: shǎo qì (65)

Feeble speech, together with weak, short, rapid, distressed breathing; mainly attributable to visceral qi vacuity, especially of center and pulmorenal qi.

direct strike: zhí zhòng (151)

Direct penetration of exogenous pathogens to the yin channels, without first affecting the yang channels as is normally the case.

discharge: xiè

Relase or leakage; spontaneous or induced outward or downward movement.

disharmony: bù hé (32)

Functional imbalance between organ or body levels (construction, defense, qi and blood).

disinhibition: lì (121)

Promoting fluency, movement, or activity. Promoting the free elimination (of urine, damp, etc.). See also **inhibition**.

disinhibition of urine: lì niào (122)

Diuresis.

dispel: qū (236)

To eliminate (pathogens from the body).

dispersion: xiāo (fǎ) (221)

A general method of eliminating pathogens, especially substantial ones such as phlegm and static blood. **Breaking** and **disintegration** refer to stronger forms of the same.

disposition: zhì (137)

The five dispositions (with five-phase correspondences) are joy (fire), anger (wood), anxiety (metal), preoccupation (earth), and fear (water). These are the same in name as the seven affects: joy, anger, anxiety, preoccupation, sorrow, fear, and fright. However, **disposition** refers to a deeper level of emotional activity than **affect** (q.v.). The compound term *qíng-zhì* (lit. "affect-disposition"), which embraces both concepts, is rendered as "emotion." The term *zhì*, whose ideographic meaning is fixity or direction of the heart, conveys the notion of will and determination, in which sense it is most commonly used outside medicine. Hence the broader meaning of the term is the power of will and the deeper emotions to which it is subject. This meaning is to be found in the compound term **spirit-disposition**, which refers to consciousness, will, and the state of the emotions.

dispositional excess: wǔ zhì guò jí (43)

A potentially pathogenic excess of one or more of the five dispositions. See **disposition**.

disquieting: bù ān (29)

Unrest, jeopardy; refers, for example, to restlessness, palpitations, etc., due to yin vacuity.

dissipation: sàn (310)

1) The pervasive spreading of qi. 2) gentle elimination (of pathogens).

distention: zhàng (334)

The state of being stretched out or inflated; implies both objective swelling and subjective sensation of **fullness**.

distress: pò (197)

Occurs in pattern descriptions such as "heat distressing the large intestine," where damp-heat damages the stomach and large intestine, affecting conveyance of waste. The term **distress** refers to the chief symptoms, which are abdominal pain, severe diarrhea with yellow, malodorous stool, and a burning sensation in the anus.

dolorous obturation: tòng bì (318)

Cold obturation characterized by severe pain.

dormant papules: yǐn zhěn (480)

Remittent outthrust of faint papules in changing locations.

dorsal styloid pulse: fǎn guān mài (64)

A congenital anomaly in which the radial pulse is located on the posterior face of the medial styloid process.

downbearing: jiàng (199)

The downward movement of qi (including waste products through the digestive tract), and the promotion of such movement in therapy. Cf. **upbearing**.

downpour: xià zhù (10)

Downward movement (of damp-heat). For example, "downpour of damp heat" denotes a variety of lower burner damp-heat patterns, such as damp-heat dysentery, damp-heat diarrhea, unctuous strangury, urinary block, genital itch, and vaginal discharge.

downpour diarrhea: zhù xià (169)

Diarrhea characterized by stool flowing out like water.

downward fall: xià xiàn (12)

Downward movement, as of insufficient center qi; frequently abbreviated to **fall**, as in the term **qi fall**.

drainage: xiè (463)

[*xiè*, to flow or allow to flow along, down, or away] Elimination (of heat or fire).

drained white: huǎng bái

Bloodless white. See also **pale white** and **somber white**.

dream emission: mèng yí

Seminal emission associated with dreaming.

dribbling incontinence: xiǎo biàn lín lì (bu jin) (26)

A constant dribble of urine and inability to achieve a full stream. See **changes in urine and micturition**.

dribbling metrorrhagia: lòu xià (401)

Scant non-menstrual bleeding. See **metrorrhagia**.

drool: xián (223)

That part of the saliva which is the humor of the spleen. In the term **phlegm-drool** it refers to expectorated fluids thinner than those normally described as phlegm.

dry miliaria: kū péi (186)

Miliaria whose vesicles are white in color and contain no fluid; an unfavorable sign.

duck stool: yā táng (445)

Greenish stool bearing the the appearance of duck droppings; generally forms part of a cold-damp pattern due to splenic damp and cold in the large intestine and including other signs such as clear urine and a deep, slow pulse.

dwelling place: fǔ (159)

Occurs in the phrase "the vessels are the dwelling place of the blood." It should be noted that this term in ancient Chinese was undifferentiated from the term rendered in the present text as **bowel**.

dysentery: lì (323)

Diarrhea with either pus and mucus or blood in the stool, accompanied by abdominal pain and tenesmus; usually occurs in summer.

dyspeptic anorexia: nà dāi (241)

[*nà*, receive; *dāi*, dull, torpid] Impairment of the stomach's governance of ingestion, characterized by indigestion and loss of appetite.

dyspnea: chuǎn (306)

Labored breathing characterized by rapidity and distress frequently associated with wheezing; sometimes rendered in other texts as "asthma."

edema: fú (219)

See **water**.

edematous swelling: fú zhǒng (220)

See **water**.

efflux: huá (362)

Denotes uncontrollable loss (of urine, and especially stool or semen). The term occurs in the phrases "incontinent seminal efflux," "efflux desertion" (see **desertion**), and "efflux diarrhea" (see **diarrhea**). See also **exuberance and debilitation**.

efflux desertion: huá tuō (364)

See **desertion**.

efflux diarrhea: huá xiè (363)

Diarrhea with loss of voluntary continence. See also **efflux**.

effulgent: wàng (163)

Exuberance of heat or fire. See **heat**.

effusion: fā (326)

Natural or induced gentle outward movement, as of sweat through the striations.

ejection: tù (fǎ) (105)

The spontaneous expulsion of matter from the digestive tract through the mouth; induced expulsion of matter from the digestive tract, throat, or lungs through the mouth.

elixir: dān (37)

Originally, any formula containing sublimed minerals; by extension, a formula containing superlative or harsh agents used in small quantities.

emolliating the liver: róu gān (188)

The method of treating liver yin vacuity (or insufficiency of liver blood) characterized by loss of visual acuity, dry eyes, night blindness, periodic mental dizziness and tinnitus, and pale nails, or poor sleep, excessive dreaming, dry mouth with lack of fluid, and a fine, weak pulse. Since the liver is the unyielding viscus and relies on the blood for nourishment, liver yin vacuity is treated with blood-nourishing agents.

emotion: qíng zhì (269)

Affects and dispositions collectively.

emotional constraint: qíng zhì bù shū

Impairment of normal emotional activity, making the individual ill at ease, frustrated, irascible, etc.

encumbrance: kùn (126)

Describes the effect of damp on the spleen. Translated by other writers as "distress." See **exuberance and debilitation.**

endogenous: nèi (48)

Arising in the inner body, especially of diseases due to excesses of the seven affects (endogenous damage) and pathogens simulating their exogenous counterparts (e.g., endogenous wind, endogenous damp). See Chapter 5.

enduring: jiǔ (14)

Chronic or persistent; indicates duration, not degree, of acuteness.

enduring diarrhea: jiǔ xiè (15)

Chronic or persistent diarrhea. See **enduring.**

enduring diarrhea efflux desertion: jiǔ xiè huá tuō (16)

Desertion due to fluid loss through persistent diarrhea.

engender: shēng (97)

To produce or give rise to. See **supplementation.**

enrichment: zī (361)

A method of supplementation applied specifically to yin.

entry: rù (1)

One of the four movements.

enuresis: yí niào (441)

Urinary incontinence; especially, the involuntary discharge of urine during sleep at night. See **changes in urine and micturition.**

environmental excesses: yín qì (279)

Refers to excesses of the six qi (wind, cold, summerheat, damp, dryness, and fire).

esophageal constriction: yē gè (418)

[*Ye*, esophagus; *gè*, diaphragm] Constriction of the upper esophagus characterized by a sensation of blockage when swallowing, and/or blockage at the diaphragm preventing the downflow of digestate. Upper esophageal constriction may occur alone, although it usually portends the development of the dual condition. Causes include damage to the spleen by excessive preoccupation, excessive consumption of tobacco and alcohol, qi stagnation and heat depression, hard foodstuffs, and phlegm-rheum and blood stasis.

essence-spirit: jīng shén (406)

The spirit *(shén)* and its deeper physical foundation *(jīng)*. The closest equivalent of *jīng shén* in English is "mental energy" or "vitality," although it is often rendered as "mind," because it is now used as such by the Chinese in modern psychology. However, both Chinese medicine and popular usage still retain the original meaning of the term. For example, the term *jīng shén bú zhèn* (devitalization of essence-spirit) is commonly used to denote lack of mental energy or vitality. The mind, with respect to its emotional or thought content, is traditionally expressed in Chinese as *xīn* (heart) or *nǎo hǎi* (lit. brain sea).

essential qi: jīng qì (407)

A general term denoting all essential elements of the body; usually refers to acquired essence and the essence stored by the viscera which is derived from it. The connection with the reproductive essence of the kidney is very strong. Only when the essential qi of the organs is abundant can the body fulfill its reproductive function.

exhaustion: jié (405)

Severe depletion, as of blood, fluids, or essence.

exogenous: wài (90)

Originating outside (the body); describes different forms of qi present in the human environment in respect to their influence on the human organism, and the diseases they cause.

exogenous heat diseases: wài gǎn rè bìng (91)

Diseases of exogenous origin usually (but not always) characterized by fever and stage-by-stage development (initial stage, exuberant fever stage, and recovery stage). See **heat**.

expectoration: luò (178), sòu (390)

See **cough** and **expectoration**.

expiry: jué (332)

Complete exhaustion, disappearance, death. See **exuberance and debilitation**.

expulsion: zhú (288)

Forceful elimination, as of water.

exterior: biǎo (173)

The outer part of the body as opposed to the interior; includes the **muscular exterior**, i.e., the skin and exterior muscles of the head, limbs and trunk, and also the **bowels**, which are the organs of the exterior through which nutrients are absorbed and waste is expelled.

extinguishing wind: xí fēng (402)

Method of eliminating endogenous wind.

exuberance: shèng (327)

A strengthening of yin and yang in excess of their normal flux, i.e., marked "prevalence" (q.v.). Exuberance also denotes the strength of pathogens.

exuberance and debilitation: shèng shūai

Exuberance denotes strength or profusion; debilitation denotes weakness and scarcity. Both describe strength or weakness of organs or physiologic elements (qi, blood, fluid, essence), but in the main, exuberance qualifies pathogens.

Exuberant pathogens, physiologic elements, and yin-yang aspects of the organs are often described in terms of the way in which they affect the parts of the organism. **Invasion** and **assailment** both describe the intrusion of an exuberant pathogen into the body; **invasion** also describes intrusion of the liver qi into the stomach. **Fettering** denotes the inhibitive effect of an exogenous pathogen on the lung or exterior. **Interiorization** and **inward fall** both describe movement of pathogens into the interior (innerbody), the former being associated with cold damage theory and the latter with thermic disease theory. **Encumbrance** refers to the inhibitive effect of damp (or damp-heat) on the splenic function of moving water-damp (often manifesting as heavy, cumbersome limbs). **Congealing** is an attribute of damp, but often describes the damping effect of cold on the movement of blood or qi. **Clouding** and **confounding** both denote the effect of phlegm on the cardiac portals resulting in essence-spirit derangement or coma. **Harassment** describes the effect of heat or phlegm giving rise to dizziness or essence-spirit derangement. **Flood** denotes water accumulations due to kidney yang vacuity. **Shooting and intimidation** describe the effect of water flood on the lung and heart respectively. **Upsurge** describes the upward movement of depressed liver qi, one form of qi inversion. **Bind** suggests intensification or concentration when applied to qi, emotions or pathogens, and also describes the substantial hardening produced as a result (e.g., phlegm nodules). **Contention** describes the mutually inhibitive effect as of phlegm and qi which results in the binding of the two to produce scrofulous swellings, phlegm nodules, etc. **Mutual exacerbation** frequently describes the interaction of wind and fire. **Stirring** describes the development of wind, either as a result of blood vacuity or of upflaming liver fire (repletion); it also describes the effect of exuberant heat on the blood, giving rise to frenetic blood. Terms describing the effect of heat may be found under **heat**. See also **transformation**.

Terms related to debilitation describe degree and nature of weakness. **Debilitation** itself is a general word, but is often applied to serious conditions. **Devitalization** usually describes a weakened state of the essence-spirit, i.e., lack of mental or general vigor; in the context of splenic yang, it describes a relatively serious weakness. **Insecurity** denotes failure to retain sweat, stool, or essence, or resist invading pathogens. **Downward fall** is the downward movement of vacuous qi manifesting in the form of prolapse, etc. Both insecurity and downward fall are results of debilitation. **Detriment** describes the reductive effect of damaging influences. **Retrenchment** is sudden or hard detriment to body elements. **Wearing** denotes gradual detriment. **Taxation** is severe, usually gradual detriment to the organs, often in diseases Western medicine would describe as consumptive. **Depletion** and **exhaustion** describe severe, usually gradual reduction, the former usually being applied to kidney essence, and the latter to the blood, fluids, or essence. **Collapse** denotes critical insufficiency of yin, yang, blood, or fluids. **Desertion** is similar to collapse, but suggests the resultant loss to the body; it is also particularly associated with loss of physiologic elements, and hence is often used in conjunction with the term **efflux**, referring to loss of liquids or blood. **Floating** sometimes describes extreme yang vacuity characterized by vacuity heat signs in the upper body or outer body, but may also describe exterior repletion heat in initial-stage exogenous heat diseases. **Expiry** refers to critical weakness, usually of organ functions, which portends death.

fen: fēn, candareen (54)

One hundredth of a *liang*, or 0.375 grams.

fetal qi: tāi qì (196)

The fetus seen in its capacity to affect the organism.

fetter: shù (141)

Describes the inhibitive effect of pathogens, especially on the exterior of the body or the lung. See **exuberance and debilitation**.

fever in the five hearts: wǔ xīn fán rè (42)

Palpable heat in palms of hand or soles of feet, and feverishness in chest.

feverishness: fán rè (367)

Restlessness *(fán)* accompanied by fever *(rè)*, or agitation with a subjective feeling of heat and oppression.

fifth-watch diarrhea: wǔ gēng (jīng) xiè (44)

See **daybreak diarrhea**.

fire: huǒ (79)

In physiology, fire represents a mutation of yang qi. As such it may be explained as a vital force, e.g., imperial fire, ministerial fire, and lesser fire. In pathology, fire denotes one of the six environmental excesses, which, like summerheat, is a form of heat in the eight-parameter sense. It may also denote a pathologic transformation of yang qi, seen in what Western medicine would describe as functional hyperactivity. Under given circumstances, all pathogens and endogenous damage by the seven affects (or excesses of the five dispositions) may lead to fire formation. See **heat**.

fishy odor: xīng wèi

The odor characteristic of fish or blood.

five forms of taxation damage: wǔ láo suǒ shāng (45)

Disorders of qi, blood, sinews, and bones caused by irregularities of work and leisure. The *Inner Canon* states: "Prolonged vision damages the blood; prolonged lying damages qi; prolonged sitting damages the flesh; prolonged standing damages the bones; and prolonged walking damages the sinews. These are the five forms of taxation damage."

five hearts: wǔ xīn (41)

The soles of the feet, the palms of the hand, and the center of the chest.

floating: fú (218)

Location in, or tendency to move towards, the upper or outer body. Examples include: "floating heat," which denotes either exterior heat occurring in the initial stages of exogenous heat diseases or a form of cold falsely presenting as heat where there is exuberant cold in the inner body and vacuous yang qi floats to the outer body; "floating pulse," which denotes a pulse pronounced at the superficial level, but relatively weak at the deep level.

flood: fàn (167)

Describes the behavior of excess fluid in the body, as in the term "renal vacuity water flood," which denotes water swelling caused by kidney vacuity. See **exuberance and debilitation.**

flow restoration: tōng (289)

Ensuring the normal access of qi to where it is needed. This may (or may not) involve removing obstruction (**unstopping,** q.v.).

flow stoppage: bù tōng

Cessation of movement of body elements (qi, blood, fluids) and their derivates phlegm and rheum, due either to intrinsic vacuity or to extrinsic obstruction. For example, qi may stop because it is vacuous, or may be stopped by static blood.

Terms denoting specific forms of flow stoppage highlight the degree and nature of the stoppage. **Inhibition** is the mildest form of flow stoppage, and is applied mainly to the movement of fluids (particularly urine) and the blood; it also describes motor impairment. **Stagnation** describes the impaired movement of qi and of the digestate (turbid qi). **Stasis** most commonly denotes impairment or complete cessation of blood flow due to heat, cold, qi stagnation, or trauma; it sometimes describes cessation of movement resulting from exuberant heat. **Depression** describes reduced or frustrated activity of physiologic elements, particularly qi, as well as pathogens (such as inner-body heat), and the emotions (in which context the word has wider connotations than mere low spirits). **Bind** describes the intensity of depression (particularly in the context of the emotions and liver qi), the concentration of pathogens and the hardening that results from either of these (e.g., phlegm nodules; hard, bound stool). **Accumulation** denotes the buildup of waste in the digestive tract. **Gathering** denotes the coming together in one place of pathogens. Both gathering and accumulation also denote certain forms of abdominal masses. **Collection** usually denotes buildup of water in specific locations, particularly in the region of the stomach. **Congestion** denotes clogging by exuberant pathogens, especially in the lung. **Block** denotes failure of body elements to issue through the exterior (e.g., fecal block, menstrual block, inner-body heat block); it is the opposite of insecurity, insofar as the latter denotes failure to retain physiologic substances. **Obstruction** denotes the inhibitive effect of a substantial pathogen on pathways (e.g., the striations) or organs (e.g., the lung or spleen). **Obturation** denotes blockage or disruption of channel flow, usually giving rise to symptoms such as numbness or pain.

flowery vision: mù huā (101)

A general term embracing various kinds of visual disturbances such as blurring, distortion, floaters, etc.

Glossary of Terms

fluids: jīn yè (191)

The generic name of all fluids of the human body, comprising **liquid** *(jīn)*, the thinner fluids, and **humor** *(yè)*, the thick, turbid ones.

flushing: dàng dí (440)

Forceful elimination (of pathogens).

foot-qi disease: jiǎo qì (382)

A disease characterized by numbness of the legs, water swelling, and heart disease; found, by synthesized research, to be due to vitamin B1 deficiency. Serious cases are marked by abstraction of spirit-disposition, and deranged speech. Different forms include damp foot-qi disease, cold-damp foot-qi disease, and phlegm-damp foot-qi disease. Foot-qi disease corresponds in Western medicine largely to beriberi, which is attributed to vitamin B1 deficiency.

form: xíng

Shape and substantial quality; the formal body, in contrast to the **constitutional body,** q.v..

formal body: xíng (118)

The physical body, as the outward manifestation of the individual, in contradistinction to the constitutional body, the physiologic makeup of the individual.

formation: hùa (56)

See **transformation**.

fortification: jiàn (258)

Supplementation (of spleen, stomach, or center). See **fortifying the spleen** and **supplementation.**

fostering: yù (172)

Supplementation (especially of yin). See **supplementation.**

foul odor: huì chòu (464)

The smell of filth, as distinct from fishy, animal, or putrid smells.

foul turbidity: huì zhuó (465)

A term used to describe damp turbidity, certain forms of qi such as mountain forest miasma, and excreta or body smells. The term "foul," used in the sense of filthy or dirty, describes color, odor, and particularly when

479

coupled with the word **turbidity,** the obstructive effect of pathogens on clear, light yang qi. See also **damp turbidity** and **foul odor.**

free downflow: tōng jiàng (290)

The natural downflow (of the digestate from the stomach through the intestines).

freeing: tōng

See flow restoration.

frenetic blood heat: xuè rè wàng xíng (115)

Frenetic movement of the blood due to blood heat. See **frenetic movement.**

frenetic movement: wàng xíng (107)

Denotes a pathologic movement or activity of the blood manifesting in the form of hemorrhage or maculopapular eruptions; when due to blood heat, as is usually the case, it is also referred to as frenetic blood heat.

fright inversion: jīng jué (488)

1) Syncope occurring when strong emotional stimulus disrupts the flow of qi and blood. 2) The signs associated with **fright wind.**

fright wind: jīng fēng (487)

A childhood disease characterized by fright inversion, convulsive spasm, and obtundation of the spirit-disposition; attributable to manifold causes including high fever, neurologic disorders, nutritional disturbances, and drug or food poisoning.

frigid: lěng

Pronounced or overt cold. See **cold.**

frog rattle: hóu zhōng yǒu shuǐ jī shēng (305)

A continuous high-pitched rale produced by phlegm blocking the respiratory tracts. It occurs in diseases classified in in Western medicine as asthma and asthmatic bronchitis. So named by the virtue of the similarity to the sound of frogs crying in chorus.

fullness: mǎn (400)

A subjective sensation of expansion and pressure, which may or may not be associated with objectively perceptible distention.

fulminant: bào (420)

Developing suddenly and severely.

fulminant downpour: bào zhù (421)

Acute abdominal pain, with sudden bouts of diarrhea characterized by a forceful stream of watery stool or explosive evacuation.

fume: xūn (467)

Describes the behavior of heat and its effect on organs.

gan: gān (226)

1) Indented mucosal ulceration, often accompanied by putrefaction of the flesh and mild suppuration, e.g., **periodontal gān** which refers to ulceration of the gums. 2) *Gān* accumulation.

gan accumulation: gān jī (227)

A pediatric disease caused by splenogastric vacuity. Signs include yellow complexion, emaciation, dry hair, abdominal distention with visible superficial veins, and loss of essence-spirit vitality. It corresponds to child malnutrition as well as some parasitic and debilitating diseases in Western medicine.

gangrenous lesion: jū (228)

A deep, inflammatory, pyogenic lesion of the flesh identified by its concave surface.

gastric reflux: fǎn wèi (63)

A pattern characterized by distention and fullness after eating, the vomiting in the evening of food ingested in the morning, or the vomiting in the morning of food ingested the previous evening; undigested food in the vomitus, spiritual fatigue, and lack of bodily strength. The tongue is pale in color, and the pulse is fine and without force. The principal cause is splenogastric vacuity cold, but may also occur when congealing damp-heat stagnation leads to impairment of gastric harmony and downbearing.

gathering: jù (409)

Collection, accumulation. Specifically refers to unstable, yielding abdominal masses in contradistinction to **accumulation,** which denotes stable, unyielding masses. See also **concretions and gatherings** and **flow stoppage.**

glomus: pǐ (324)

The sensation of a lump, generally of limited size, in the abdominothoracic cavity. When palpable, it is referred to as **lump glomus.**

govern: zhǔ (82)

To control or be closely associated with. Early texts commonly use political government as a source of metaphors to express physiologic activity and relationships. For example, the *Inner Canon* states: "The stomach and spleen hold the office of the granaries; they manage the five sapors {food}." Thus, "the stomach governs ingestion of food" and "the spleen governs movement and transformation of the essence of digestate."

governance: zhǔ (83)

The governing by the organs of functions or parts of the body. For example, "hepatic governance of free-coursing" (or simply "hepatic free-coursing") refers to the liver's control over qi and blood flow throughout the body. See **govern**.

governor: zhǔ (84)

The (organ) that governs.

great heat: dà rè (21)

Great fever; one of the "four greatnesses" associated with yang ming channel patterns.

great restlessness and thirst: dà fán kě (20.1)

One of the "four greatnesses" associated with yang ming channel patterns.

grossness: yǒng zhǒng (455)

Severe obesity.

hacking: kà (303)

Short, often frequent, coughing.

hacking blood: kà xuè (304)

Expectoration of blood in short coughs.

harass: rǎo (462)

Trouble, worry, torment (as by phlegm and phlegm fire). For example, "phlegm fire harassing the heart," a pattern characterized by disturbances of spirit-disposition, deranged speech, and in severe cases, manic agitation with wild physical movements, and often corresponding to what Western medicine describes as schizophrenia. See **exuberance and debilitation**.

hardness: jiān (262)

Any hard swelling or mass, treated by the method of softening.

harmonization: hé (fǎ) (154)

A method of treatment that involves coursing and disinhibiting qi, and harmonizing the functions of the organs; mainly used in the treatment of shao yang midstage exogenous disease patterns; also used to treat hepatosplenic disharmony, hepatogastric disharmony, and malarial disease. This method should not be used in cases where an exogenous pathogen is still located in the exterior and has not yet entered the shao yang, nor where it has already interiorized, giving rise to yang ming exuberant heat symptoms. Misuse may induce interiorization or prolong the condition.

heart: xīn (66)

The term *xīn* refers not only to the heart proper, but in describing symptoms also refers to the region of the heart, i.e., the upper venter (the upper part of the stomach and lower section of the esophagus).

heat: rè (424)

In eight-parameter pattern identification, **heat** denotes the nature of diseases, in contradistinction to **cold**. In this sense it embraces the concepts of **fire** and **summerheat**. The latter two are both exogenous pathogens which, being of the nature of heat, are commonly referred to as such. "Endogenous fire" denotes a pathologic mutation of yang qi manifesting in forms of what in Western medicine would be described as hyperactivity. Endogenous fire may occur as a result of endogenous damage (emotional disturbance), or as a result of transformation of any exogenous pathogen. For this reason, the term **heat** is sometimes used in describing interior patterns in which there is no exogenous fire. This distinction is reflected in methods of treatment, where "heat clearage" is used both as a global term including fire drainage, blood cooling, detoxification, etc., and in contradistinction to "fire drainage." In its broadest sense, **heat** denotes any manifestation of disease characterized by a rise in temperature, such as fever, localized palable heat, and subjective sensations of heat. Fever, for example, may attend cold as well as heat patterns (in the eight-parameter sense). This is especially common in the case of exogenous wind-cold diseases. It should be pointed out that the word *rè* in Chinese is rendered in this text both as "heat" and as "fever," but that the term **heat** is meant to include fever in some contexts.

A number of terms describe the degree of heat (or fire) and its effect on the individual. Exuberance is a general term applied to a strong heat (or any other pathogen). **Intensity** means pronounced exuberance. **Blaze** and **deflagration** both describe intense heat, and are used in terms denoting specific four-aspect patterns. **Vigorous** describes the fever associated with exuberant heat. **Brewing** describes inner-body heat, especially when combined with damp, and like deep-lying, suggests that outward heat signs are not pronounced. **Upflaming** describes the way in which (repletion) fire produces upper-body heat signs, and is especially associated with heart or liver fire. **Fuming, steaming,** and **sweltering** also describe the way in which heat rises or affects organs, the latter two being particularly associated with damp-heat. **Burning** describes the effect of heat on organs, while **scorching** describes its effects on organs or on blood and the fluids. **Boil** describes the effect of heat on the blood, especially when phlegm is produced as a result. **Stirring,** more commonly used to describe wind, describes the way in which heat gives rise to frenetic movement of the blood. **Bind,** when applied to heat, most commonly describes the way in which it produces hardening of the stool (gastrointestinal heat-bind). **Effulgence** is a term similar to exuberance, describing either vacuity or repletion heat. **Floating** describes the way in which extreme yang vacuity produces upper-body or outer-body heat signs, or exterior repletion heat in initial-stage exogenous heat diseases. Note that most of these terms describe repletion heat. Terms describing vacuity patterns usually point to the nature of the insufficiency that gives rise to the heat. These, and terms that describe exuberance or pathogens other than heat, are listed under **exuberance and debilitation.**

heat formation: huà rè (58)

Development of fire in exogenous diseases. The term is particularly common in the thermic disease theory where it describes the passage to the exuberant fever stage as the pathogen enters qi level. Signs include aversion to heat, thirst, and dry lips, restlessness, red tongue with yellow fur, and a fast pulse. Constipation or darkening of the urine may also occur.

heat-block tetanic inversion: rè bì jìng jué (425)

Tetanic inversion (spasm and syncope) due to heat block.

heavy micturition: duō niào (106)

Frequent, copious voidings of urine. See **changes in urine and micturition**.

heavy settlers: zhòng zhèn yào (198)

Mineral or shell products used, for example, to quiet the spirit in patterns characterized by palpitation and manic agitation.

hematuria: niào xuè (132.1); sōu xuè (360)

Blood in the urine. See **changes in urine and micturition**.

home: shǔ (477)

Of channels, to meet the organs to which they belong, e.g., the foot tai yin lung channel homes to the lung.

humor: yè (276)

The thicker fluid of the human body.

hyperactivity: kàng (46)

In yin-yang theory, pronounced prevalence (strengthening) of yang; equivalent to the term **exuberance**, which is applied to both yin and yang.

hypertonicity: jū (jū jí, jū lüán) (161)

Inhibited bending and stretching of the limbs; usually caused by a wind pathogen.

incontinent seminal efflux: jīng húa bú jìn (162)

Severe seminal efflux.

increasing humor: zēng yè (419)

Method of treating insufficiency of fluids.

infracardiac region: xīn xià (67)

The area below the heart, the venter. See also **heart**.

ingesta damage diarrhea: shí xiè (201)

Diarrhea due to ingesta damage, i.e., food poisoning, excessive consumption of alcohol or fatty and spicy foods, or ingestion of food that is too hot or too cold in temperature, or by voracious eating. It includes some forms of gastric, large intestinal, and small intestinal diarrhea. The dividing line between ingesta damage diarrhea and splenic diarrhea is sometimes hazy in the case of diarrhea caused by fatty foods. If due to excesses in respect to general dietary norms, it is classed as ingesta damage diarrhea; if due to organic dysfunction, e.g., vacuity or damp, it is classed as splenic diarrhea. See also **diarrhea**.

inhibition: bú lì (30)

Disfluency (of liquids or damp) or difficulty (of physical movement, urination, and speech). Methods of treating such conditions are often described as **disinhibition**. See **flow stoppage**.

inner body: nèi (47)

The inner part of the body; synonymous with interior, but used especially in the context of deep-lying and endogenous disease. Used widely in thermic disease in preference to **interior**.

inner-body block: nèi bì (49)

See **block**.

insecurity: bú gù (33)

Failure to secure or be secured; vulnerability (to invasion by pathogens or loss of essential elements). For example, "insecurity of defense qi" denotes weakness of defense qi and a consequent loosening of the striations, laying the body open to invasion by exogenous pathogens. Under such circumstances, contraction of exogenous pathogens gives rise to spontaneous sweating and aversion to wind. "Insecurity of kidney qi" refers to impairment of the kidney's function of storing essence, and is characterized by seminal emission, seminal efflux, and premature ejaculation, or urinary frequency, enuresis, and incontinence. "Intestinal insecurity" denotes a loosening of the bowels, and is therefore characterized by diarrhea.

insufficiency: bù zú (31)

Lack (of substance) or incompleteness (of function); opposite of **superabundance**. Cf. **vacuity and repletion**.

intense heat: chì (437)

Heat more intense than **exuberant heat**.

interior: lǐ (386)

The inner part of the body as opposed to the exterior; refers to the deeper levels of the organism, i.e., the five viscera by which the rest of the body is largely governed. In six-channel pattern identification of cold damage theory, **interior** refers to yang ming and the yin channels, while shao yang is considered the point of midstage penetration. In thermic disease theory, the term "inner body" is of equivalent meaning.

interiorization: rù lǐ (2)

Movement (of pathogens) into the interior; used particularly in cold damage theory, and similar in meaning to the term **inward fall** used more prevalently in thermic disease theory. See **exuberance and debilitation**.

intestinal vacuity efflux desertion: cháng xū huá tuō (383)

Efflux desertion due to intestinal vacuity.

intimidate: líng (202)

Describes the harmful effects of water qi, as in the expression "water qi intimidating the heart," a pattern in which water qi developing as a result of splenorenal yang vacuity collects above the diaphragm impeding heart yang. It is characterized by palpitations and distressed, rapid breathing.

invasion: fàn (96)

Intrusion; describes pathogens entering the body, and liver qi entering the stomach.

inversion: jué (302)

Severe disruption of qi dynamic chiefly associated with **clouding inversion** (i.e., syncope) and **inversion frigidity of the limbs** (severe cold in the limbs associated with desertion patterns), in which adequate supplies of qi and blood fail to reach the head and extremities. "Inversion patterns" are those characterized by these symptoms. For example, "cold inversion" refers to a pattern characterized by clouding inversion and inversion frigidity of the limbs, attributable to yang qi vacuity. "Blood inversion" refers to patterns caused by blood disease (repletion or vacuity) and characterized by the two symptoms of inversion. The notion of inversion is closely associated with that of **counterflow. Inversion frigidity of the limbs** and **counterflow frigidity of the limbs** are identical in meaning. However, counterflow is otherwise associated with disruption of the qi dynamic of organs such as the liver, stomach, and lung. Both the ideograms for *jué* and *nì* (q.v.) carry connotations of adversity and of going against the grain; *jué* carries connotations of disruption, breaking off, and finality. It should also be pointed out that the ideogram *jué* is that occurring in the term *jue yin channel*, interestingly rendered by Porkert as *yin flectens* (bending yin).

inversion frigidity of the limbs: sì zhī jué lěng (87)

Severe cold in the limbs associated with desertion, etc. Synonym: **counterflow frigidity of the limbs.** See **inversion.**

invigorating yang: zhuàng yáng (129)

Strengthening the yang qi of the body with warming and supplementing agents. It usually refers to strengthening the yang qi of the heart and kidney, and especially the latter. See **supplementation.**

inward fall: nèi xiàn (51)

Passage (of pathogens) into the inner body, due to vacuity of the correct.

iron-band sensation: tóu tòng rú chè (444)

Headache characterized by pressure or tension, as though the head was squeezed by a tight iron band.

issue: chū (86)

One of the four movements.

jerking sinews and twitching muscles: jīn tì ròu rùn (329)

Spasmatic jerking of the muscles not necessarily causing articular movement; due to blood or fluid insufficiency, cold-damp, or in some cases yang vacuity.

kidney diarrhea: shèn xiè (335)

Diarrhea due to kidney yang vacuity. See **daybreak diarrhea**.

kidney vacuity water flood: shèn xū shuǐ fàn

Failure of the kidney to govern water, giving rise to edematous swelling (particularly from the lumbar region downwards).

leaden: zhuó (385)

[*zhuó*, contact, press down] Incapable, or rendering incapable, of performing normal physical movements; heavy.

lesion: chuāng (yáng) (426)

Any interruption of normal tissue structure.

liang: *liǎng*, tael (150.1)

A unit of weight equal to 31.25 gr. and divided into 10 *qian* and 100 *fen*.

linger: liú liàn (225)

To rest and resist elimination; said of pathogens and fever.

liquid: jīn (190)

The thinner fluids of the human body.

lodge: liú (224)

To rest and remain fixed; said of pathogens.

long micturition with clear urine : xiǎo biàn qīng cháng (28)

Long, usually copious voidings of clear urine. See **changes in urine and micturition**.

lower body: xià (6)

The lower part of the body (yin) as opposed to the upper body (yang). It sometimes specifically refers to the lower burner.

lower body distress: xià pò (11)

Evacuative difficulty and abdominal distress, associated with fever.

lump glomus: pǐ kuài (325)

See **glomus**.

maculopapular eruptions: bān zhěn (312)

Macules are unraised discolorations of the skin. Papules are raised, papular eruptions. Both are especially associated with exogenous heat diseases.

malarial disease: nüè jí (403)

A recurrent disease characterized by shivering, vigorous fever, and sweating; classically attributed to contraction of summerheat during the hot season, contact with mountain forest miasma, or contraction of cold-damp. In Western medicine, it is explained as being caused by any of various protozoans (genus *Plasmodium*) transmitted to man by the bite of an infected mosquito, especially the anopheles, prevalent in conditions that Chinese medicine regards as being the direct cause.

malign: è (309)

Noxious, severe, difficult to cure. Not to be confused with the term "malignant" as used in Western medicine.

mania: kuáng (144)

An essence-spirit disorder chiefly caused by affect-related binding depression, disposition-related fire formation, or phlegm clouding the cardiac portals. Signs include reduced recumbency and hunger, frenzy and presumption, angry bellowing, destructive and aggressive behavior, tendency to spring walls and climb roofs, increased physical strength. The tongue is red with a yellow fur, and the pulse is wiry, large, slippery and rapid.

mania and withdrawal: diān kuáng (490)

Mania and withdrawal are both forms of derangement of the essence-spirit. Mania denotes states of excitement characterized by noisy, unruly, and even aggressive behavior, and offensive speech, constant singing and laughter, irascibility, and inability to remain tidily dressed. This is a yang-pattern overexteriorization of the heart spirit due to hyperactivity of yang qi. Withdrawal refers to mental depression, indifference, deranged speech, taciturnity, and obliviousness of hunger or satiety. It is a vacuity pattern caused by binding of depressed qi and phlegm or cardiosplenic vacuity.

manic agitation: kuáng zào (145)

Agitation with signs of mania.

massotherapy: tuī ná (271)

Therapeutic massage.

mental dizziness: yūn (355)

A subjective whirling sensation, such as is experienced when travelling by ship. Cf. **visual dizziness**.

metrorrhagia: bēng lòu (265)

Non-menstrual uterine bleeding. *Bēng* means profuse metrorrhagia. *Lòu* means scant, or dribbling, metrorrhagia.

miliaria: péi (371)

Small white vesicles appearing on the neck and sometimes the arms of patients suffering from damp thermia.

miliaria alba: bái péi (98)

See **miliaria**.

miliaria crystallina: jīng péi (313)

Crystallina characterized by plump, glossy, damp vesicles; also known as sudamina. See **miliaria alba**.

ministerial fire: xiàng huǒ (193)

The fire of the kidney, i.e., kidney yang. This is generally explained as being synonymous with the vital gate fire. The fire of the liver, gallbladder, and triple burner are also referred to as the ministerial fire when seen as being derived from the ministerial fire.

mix-fry: zhì (152)

To stir-fry (medicinal agents) with an additive. For example, Radix Glycyrrhizae *(gān cǎo)* mix-fried is prepared by stir-frying with honey, together with a small quantity of water to ensure an even spread.

moving the spleen: yùn pí

Method of treating splenic damp encumbrance characterized by distention, inability to taste food, nausea, bland taste and sticky sensation in the mouth, clouded head, fatigued body, diarrhea, or abdominal distention, edematous swelling of the extremities, scant urine, a white, slimy tongue fur, and a soggy pulse. This method uses agents such as Rhizoma Atractylodis *(cāng zhú)*, Cortex Magnoliae *(hòu pò)*, Pericarpium Citri Tangerinae *(chén pí)*, Herba Agastaches *(huò xiāng)*, Herba Eupatorii *(pèi lán)*, Fructus Amomi Cardamomi *(kòu rén)*, and Sclerotium Poriae *(fú líng)*. Cf. **splenic fortification**.

muscle and skin: jī fū (113)

The muscle and the skin retaining it, seen in their capacity to reflect the body's nutritional reserves.

muscular exterior: jī biǎo (112)

The exterior of the body seen essentially as being comprised of the muscles of the face, neck, back, abdomen, and limbs; the outward-facing exterior of the body, as opposed to the organs of the exterior (i.e., principally the digestive tract).

muscular tetany: jìng (319)

Severe tetanic spasm, chiefly manifesting in the form of stiffness and tension in the neck, trismus, convulsive spasm of the limbs, and opisthotonos. Occurring in repletion patterns, it is chiefly attributable to loss of supply of nourishment and moisture to the sinews and stirring of vacuity wind in the inner body, developing as a result of excessive sweating, loss of blood, vacuous constitution, qi vacuity and shortage of blood, and insufficiency of the fluids. Muscular tetany may occur as a symptom of a variety of different diseases, and should not be associated with tetanus (i.e., lockjaw) alone.

mutation: biàn huà

A combined term denoting transmutation *(biàn)* and transformation *(huà)*, i.e., all gradual and major change.

nocturia: yè jiān duō niào (156)

Excessive urination at night. See **changes in urine and micturition**.

nourish: yǎng (428)

To supply nutritive elements; to supplement (yin aspects of the body). See **supplementation**.

numbness: má mù (296)

Loss of normal sensation in the skin and flesh. *Má* denotes **tingling** (q.v.), while *mù*, literally meaning "wood," denotes absence of sensation. See also **palsy**.

obstruction: zǔ (174)

Blockage by pathogens (such as damp or phlegm) of the airways, striations, spleen, etc., causing disruption of normal functions.

obturation: bì (372)

Pain and numbness, specifically that characteristic of obturation patterns (cf. **palsy**). Also, blockage or disruption of channel flow (q.v. **stoppage**).

obturation patterns: bì zhèng (373)

Conditions attributable to pathogenic qi causing blockage in the limbs and trunk or in the organ channels. Obturation patterns are generally the result of a combination of wind, cold, and damp pathogens invading the exterior channels and joints, giving rise to articular or muscular pain, severe swelling, and leaden heaviness.

ocular rubor: mù chì (100)

Any reddening of the eyes, including bloodshot eyes and the reddening that occurs in conjunctivitis. It has manifold causes.

offensive treatment: gōng (140)

See **attack**.

oliguria: niào shǎo (131)

Scant urine. See **changes in urine and micturition**.

oral gan: kǒu gān (18)

Ulceration of the oral mucosa occurring in the course of, or subsequent to, *gan* accumulation diarrhea in children, and attributable to *gan* heat passing to the heart channel.

outer body: wài (89)

The outer part of the body, the exterior.

outthrust: tòu (287)

The spontaneous or induced forcing of pathogens to and through the exterior of the body, including those which provoke maculopapular outthrust on so doing.

overflow incontinence: lóng bì ér shī jìn (454)

Incontinence associated with urinary block occurring when intravesicular pressure exceeds outlet resistance.

overpassage: yuè chuán jīng (342)

Denotes, in six-channel pattern identification, the missing of a channel in the normal sequence of passage, e.g., when tai yang disease passes directly to shao yang without first affecting yang ming.

painful urination: niào tòng (135)

Also known as dysuria. See **changes in urine and micturition**.

pale white: dàn bái (278)

Colorless white. "Pale" denotes the absence of color, whereas "white" is regarded as a distinct color often bearing five-phase associations. Cf. **somber white** and **drained white**.

palpable heat: zhuó rè (143)

Heat that can be felt through palpation.

palpitation: xīn jì (69)

Rapid or throbbing pulsation of the heart; usually occurs in paroxysms associated with emotional states or overexertion. See also **racing of the heart.**

palsy: má bì (297)

Loss of normal muscle sensation associated with tingling or pain, as well as loss of muscle power. *Má* denotes **tingling** (q.v.), while *bì* denotes pain and numbness. See also **obturation.**

papules: bān (311)

See **maculopapular eruptions**.

paralysis: tān huàn (492)

Loss of muscle power and sensation.

parching: jiāo (315)

Describes the burning and drying effect of heat, as in the expression "lung heat parching the lobes."

paste: gāo (411)

Any pharmaceutical preparation made by reducing the extract of medicinal substances to the desired consistency or by blending triturated agents with a binding agent such as honey, cottonseed oil, or peanut oil.

pathogen: xié (150)

Any harmful influence opposing the correct.

pathogenic qi: xié qì

Pathogen. See **qì**.

pathomechanism: bìng jī (229)

The process by which a disease arises and develops.

pattern: zhèng (473)

A meaningful symptom or group of symptoms; e.g., a "heat pattern" is a symptom or set of symptoms indicating the presence of heat.

percolation: shèn (399)

Disinhibition, especially of damp and water.

perduring ailment: sù jí (263)

Any disease that persists over many months or years.

perfusion: xuān tōng (182)

Pervasive spreading (of qi), and the promotion of such action through therapy. Non-perfusion is treated by promoting perfusion. See **supplementation.**

periodontal gan: yá gān (81)

Swelling, reddening, and ulceration of the gums, usually caused by wind-heat.

periodontal xuan: yá xuān (80)

A disease of the gums characterized initially by swelling, bleeding, and suppuration, and in advanced stages by ulceration and atrophy, leaving the roots of the teeth exposed. Generally caused by stomach-channel heat accumulation and insufficiency of kidney qi.

perished complexion: yāo sè

[*yāo*, to die young] A dry complexion, showing no sign of vital qi (vitality), an unfavorable sign.

perverted appetite: shì shí yì wù (351)

Craving for strange foods.

phlegm-drool: tán xián (369.1)

Thin, white, usually copious expectorate. "Phlegm" refers to thick expectorate while "drool" refers to thin expectorate.

phlegm-rheum: tán yǐn (370)

Generally denotes any water-rheum disease, i.e., those involving accumulation of fluid in the trunk or limbs; occurs when the lung, spleen, and kidney fail to move fluids; specifically denotes water-rheum in the chest and lateral costal region, the venter, and intestines.

pills: wán (13)

Finely triturated substances mixed with a binding agent such as honey, water, flour paste, or medicinal extract and pressed into spherical form.

-plegia: bú suì (36)

A combining form denoting paralysis, e.g., **hemiplegia.**

plum-blossom needle: méi huā zhēn (274)

An instrument traditionally made by binding 5 to 7 sewing needles to a bamboo stick, and used to provide a therapeutic stimulus when lightly tapped on the skin.

plum-stone globus: méi hé qì (275)

Dryness and a sensation of a foreign body present in the throat which can be neither swallowed or ejected. The intensity of the signs fluctuates. The main cause is binding depression of liver qi.

polyuria: niào duō (132)

Copious urine. See **changes in urine and micturition**.

portal: qiào (466)

Any one of the organ openings, i.e., points of contact with the environment. The clear portals are the eyes, ears, nose, and mouth, while the turbid portals refers to the genitals and anus. These are collectively referred to as the "nine portals."

precipitation: xià (fǎ) (7)

[xia, to cause to descend] A method of treatment used to eliminate pathogens through the bowels (and urinary system). Compound terms such as "draining precipitation" and "flow-restorative precipitation" place different emphasis on pathogen elimination and promotion of bowel movement. **Precipitation** is often rendered in other literature as "purgation."

premature ejaculation: zǎo xiè (110)

Inability to prevent ejaculation of semen at the beginning of copulation, or prior to it.

prevalence: shèng (299)

A strengthening of yin or yang in excess of their natural flux.

prickles: máng cì (148)

The papillae of the tongue when pathologically enlarged.

principal, support, assistant, and conductor (drug roles): zhǔ fǔ zuǒ yǐn (85)

See **sovereign, minister, assistant, and courier** (drug roles).

profuse metrorrhagia: bēng zhōng (264)

Profuse non-menstrual uterine bleeding.

profuse perspiration: dà hàn (19)

One of the "four greatnesses" associated with yang ming channel patterns.

profuse spermatorrhea: jīng yè dà xiè (408)

Continuous seminal efflux; the most severe form of **seminal loss**.

putrid odor: fǔ chòu (410.1)

The odor characteristic of putrefaction.

qi: qì (208)

[Pronounced *chee,* and spelt *ch'i* according to Wade-Giles] No satisfactory definition of *qì* is to be found in any Chinese text. While classical texts take its existence for granted, modern literature from mainland China explains it as being a "substance." Since no such substance has ever been isolated, this definition can be presumed to have been prompted by a desire for scientific credibility and conformity to dialectic materialism. The word *qi* appears in such terms as: the "six qi" (environmental influences); "correct qi," "original qi," "ancestral qi," and other forms of physiologic qi; "damp qi," "pestilential qi," "water qi," and other damaging influences of endogenous or exogenous origin; "turbid qi" (q.v.); and the "four qi" (the four natures of drugs). *Qi* denotes a vast variety of phenomena. It includes not only different forms of physiologic qi inherent in the organism (the meaning most commonly associated with the term in the West) but also to other phenomena within and outside the body. Strictly, qi is explained as forces in configuration or as potential or actual activity. A given configuration may or may not possess substantial continuity. Thus damp qi may be viewed as damp in its active aspect or as qi indissociable from the material phenomenon of damp, while ancestral qi possesses no continuity other than that of its function. Chinese medicine is founded on a holistic approach which focuses on general dynamics within the body as directly perceived by the human observer. The analytical quest for the primary nature of substances and their interaction, characteristic of Western medicine, is alien to Chinese medicine. Qi, ultimately, can be defined as neither matter nor energy; it is their dynamic seen in substantive (but not necessarily substantial) form.

The different forms of physiologic qi (e.g., original qi, essential qi, true qi, organ qi, etc.) are often explained in Chinese texts merely in terms of each other. However, if we accept the hypothesis that qi is substance/activity, certain correspondences with Western medicine become apparent. **Cosmic qi,** in terms of the body's needs, represents oxygen, while **grain qi** (food qi) represents ingested nutrients (fluid, protein, vitamins, fats, minerals). Regular supplies of cosmic qi and grain qi are needed to keep the body alive. **Essential qi** (essence) roughly corresponds to the "genetic information" needed to transform cosmic and grain qi into human cells. Here, the parallels are clearest in Western and Chinese medical explanation of reproduction and development. In Chinese medicine, the aging process is explained in terms of the debilitation of essence.

Though this process is not fully understood by Western medicine, the fact that the danger of giving birth to children with congenital defects increases with age indicates a possible further connection between essential qi and genetics.

If these correspondences are correct, **original qi,** as a combination of the three above forms of qi, represents normal bodily function based on adequate supplies of nutrients and the "genetic information" required for their normal processing. **Correct qi** is original qi in its aspect of protecting the body against disease.

Defense qi is the body's resistance to extraneous influences; it is one aspect of correct qi. Since it is said to "warm the bowels and viscera" and "control the opening and closing of the striations," it protects the body by regulating body temperature, a factor Western medicine would accept as helping to prevent contraction of viruses. Furthermore, because it "flows outside the vessels," it may also correspond to the resistance to bacteria and other foreign bodies that is offered not only by the blood but also by tissue cells. Defense qi therefore differs from what Western medicine refers to as the "body's defenses" in that it is narrower in scope and cannot be analyzed into contributing functions. While Western medicine provides exhaustive detail about the body's defensive reactions to viruses, bacteria, and transplanted organs, Chinese medicine employs a simple concept that is useful in providing effective treatment.

qi absorption: nà qì (242)

Normal respiration is dependent on the health of the lung, and as well on the kidney absorption of the qi it draws in from the air. If the kidney fails to absorb qi, then qi drawn in by the lung accumulates in the chest, giving rise to pulmonary distention, dyspnea and fullness, and congestion. The dyspnea is characterized by short, rapid, distressed breathing, and exacerbated by physical movement. Other signs include frigidity of the limbs, aversion to wind and cold, and edematous swelling of the face. The tongue is pale and the pulse is deficient. Failure of renal governance of qi absorption (frequently referred to as "qi absorption failure") is seen in patients suffering from kidney qi vacuity and is treated by the method of promoting qi absorption.

qi ascent: shàng qì (5)

Dyspnea due to counterflow ascent of qi; corresponds roughly to expiratory dyspnea in Western medicine.

qi dynamic: qì jī (217)

The activity, particularly the flow, of qi. See **qi.**

qi inversion: qì jué (213)

Sudden loss of consciousness and inversion frigidity of the limbs due to qi vacuity or derangement of qi dynamic. Two pathomechanisms are known: a) disruption of qi dynamic due to excessive emotional stimulus, whereby congestion of qi in the chest and heart gives rise to clouding the clear portals, i.e., loss of consciousness; b) insufficient food or excessive fatigue in patients regularly suffering from original qi vacuity, causing downward fall of qi and impaired upbearing of clear yang, manifesting in sudden loss of consciousness and inversion frigidity of the limbs, perspiration, and a faint pulse. The first is a repletion pattern while the latter is a vacuity pattern.

qi pain: qì tòng (215)

Pain due to qi stagnation.

qi shortage: qì shǎo (210)

Shortage of breath, i.e., shallow, rapid breathing.

qi strangury: qì lín (212)

Strangury associated with distention of the abdomen and scrotum; frequently attributable to bladder qi stagnation. See **strangury patterns**.

qi swelling: qì zhǒng (216)

See **water**.

qi temerity: qì què (211)

Qi vacuity, especially as manifest in the form of shortage of breath, and fearfulness or lack of courage.

qi thoroughfare: qì jiē (214)

The region between the base of the lower abdomen and the buttocks, i.e., the inguinal region.

qian: *qián,* mace (442.1)

A unit of weight equal to the tenth part of a *liang;* 3.75 grams.

quelling the liver: fá gān (104)

Controlling excessive exuberance of liver qi.

quieting the spirit: ān shén (108)

A method of treating disquieting of spirit-disposition, using supplementing agents, sometimes combined with heavy settlers.

racing of the heart: zhēng chōng (158)

Violent throbbing of the heart felt not only in the chest but even as far down as the umbilical region; attributable to heart blood or heart yin vacuity. Racing of the heart similar to, but more severe than palpitation. It generally forms part of a vacuity pattern, and is continuous in nature. By contrast, palpitation may be attributable either to vacuity or to repletion, and is paroxysmal. Palpitation is generally due to nervous or functional disorders, while racing of the heart is organic. In ancient texts, palpitation and racing of the heart were sometimes used interchangeably.

rectifying qi: lǐ qì (282)

A method of treating qi stagnation, counterflow, and vacuity with qi-moving and depression-resolving agents, qi-downbearing, center-regulating agents, or center-supplementing and qi-boosting agents. This is rendered in other texts as regulating the qi.

rectifying the blood: lǐ xuè (283)

Denotes methods of treating blood-level diseases; includes blood supplementation, blood cooling, blood warming, dispelling stasis and quickening the blood, and arresting hemorrhage.

regular presence: sù yǒu

Permanent or persistent suffering from, or disposition to (a particular condition or disease).

repelled yang: gé yáng (207)

An abbreviation of "exuberant yin repelling yang," a pattern in which exuberant inner-body cold forces yang qi to the outer body; signs are those of true inner-body cold and false outer-body heat.

repelling foulness: bì huì (389)

Eliminating foul turbidity.

reinforcing yang: zhù yáng (123)

A method of supplementing yang qi.

repletion: shí (396)

See **vacuity and repletion**.

repletion swelling: shí zhǒng (397)

See **water**.

repressing the liver: yì gān (138)

See **quelling the liver**.

resolution: jiě (387)

A general term denoting the termination of patterns, the elimination of pathogens, and the freeing of parts of the body from pathogens.

restlessness: xīn fán (70)

[*xīn,* heart; *fán,* troubled] Inability to rest or be at ease; cf. **agitation**.

retching: ǒu (392)

See vomiting.

retching of blood: ǒu xuè (394)

The bringing up of blood from the stomach in cases of gastric hemorrhage. Digestate may be seen in the vomitus, but its relative absence explains the use of the term *ǒu* (retching), as opposed to *tù* (ejection). See **vomiting**.

retrenchment: duó (395)

Severe or sudden depletion (of blood, fluid, or essence), as in the phrase, "retrenchment of the blood diminishes sweating and retrenchment of sweat diminishes the blood;" also, elimination of pathogens. See **exuberance and debilitation.**

rigid: jiàng zhí (267)

Severe stiffness, such as of the neck or back.

sabulous strangury: shā lín (195)

Strangury with fine calculi in the urine. See **strangury**.

sapor: wèi (153)

That quality in a substance which produces taste or flavor. The five sapors are pungent, sweet, sour, bitter, and salty, and act on the lung (metal), spleen (earth), liver (wood), heart (fire), and kidney (water) respectively, hence their importance in determining the action of drugs. "Bland" denotes the relative absence of sapor, but is of significance in regard to drug action in that it is associated with **percolation**. In the classics, the "five sapors" is an expression that often refers to food.

scorch: zhuó (142)

Describes the potent damaging effect of pathogenic heat on the blood and fluids. See **heat.**

sea of grain and water: shuǐ gǔ zhī hǎi (74)

The stomach.

securing: gù (155)

Preventing or arresting the loss of blood, qi, fluids, or essence, and invasion of pathogens, as through the exterior. Examples: "securing essence," a method of treatment used to arrest seminal loss (also called "astringing essence"); "securing against metrorrhagia," which refers to checking metrorrhagia; "securing the exterior," which treats insecurity of exterior qi, characterized by spontaneous or night sweating. See also **insecurity**.

seminal efflux: huà jīng (365)

Seminal loss occurring in the daytime.

seminal emission: yí jīng (442)

Seminal loss, especially during sleep and unassociated with dreaming.

seminal loss: shī jīng (93)

The generic term for all involuntary loss of semen, embracing dream emission, incontinent seminal efflux, profuse spermatorrhea, seminal efflux, and seminal emission. It may also refer specifically to seminal emission.

settle: zhèn (472)

Describes methods of calming the heart with heavy settlers.

settling pathogens: kè xié (181)

Exogenous pathogens assailing and settling in the body.

shaking: diào (270)

From the *Inner Canon*: "Wind patterns with shaking and visual dizziness are associated with the liver." Shaking denotes shaking of the head, tremor, and tremulous or shaking movement of the limbs.

shan: shàn (170)

Shan classically referred to various forms of abdominal pain and protrusion of organs or tissues through the abdominal wall, i.e., hernia. "Shan qi" is often used to denote the same, owing to the association with qi pain (hence "shan qi pain"), and has been adopted as the Western medical equivalent of hernia.

shan qi: shàn qì (171)

See **shan**.

shift: chuán biàn (348)

Passage and transmutation (q.v.), i.e., all regular and irregular developments in cold-damage diseases. Shift includes the normal passage of disease through the channels, such as tai yang passage to yang ming or shao yang, and major or irregular changes such as of yang patterns into yin patterns or cold-heat complexes.

shooting: shè (205)

Occurs in the expression "water-cold shooting (into) the lung," a pattern that occurs after contraction of the cold pathogen in patients regularly suffering from phlegm-rheum or water swelling. In such cases, the cold pathogen stirs the water-rheum and both pathogens rise counterflow into the lung, causing non-pervasion of lung qi characterized by cough, dyspnea, and copious, thin white phlegm and drool.

short micturition with scant urine: xiǎo biàn duǎn shǎo (27)

Oliguria characterized by short voidings. See **changes in urine and micturition**.

sinew-vascular: jīn mài

Of or relating to the sinews and vessels.

sinews: jīn (328)

In their physical aspect, the sinews correspond to the tendons and fasciae of Western medicine. In their functional aspect, they represent muscular power, as distinct from flesh, which denotes that which gives the body shape and reflects the state of the body's nutritional reserves. The sinews are governed by the liver, so that their power is much dependent on the strength of the essential qi of the liver.

six depressions: liù yù (53)

Qi, blood, damp, fire, phlegm, and digestate depression. The concept of "free flow" is of key significance particularly in the qi-blood, channel, and triple burner theories. **Flow stoppage** is thus a major focus of attention in pathology. **Depression** describes flow stoppage associated with congestion or impairment of flow associated with binding depression. The six depressions, which are the six most typical forms, are readily identifiable: "qi depression," by pain in the chest and lateral costal region, and a deep, rough pulse; "damp depression," by general heaviness and pain, or pain in the joints, usually associated with damp weather, and a deep, fine pulse; "fire" (or "heat") depression, by visual distortion, oppression, and restlessness, dark-colored urine, and a deep, fast pulse; "phlegm depression," by dyspnea associated with physical exertion, and a deep, slippery pulse; "blood depression," by loss of power in the lower limbs, hemafecia, and a deep, scallion-stalk pulse; and "digestate depression," which denotes perduring digestate, by eructation of sour gas, abdominal distention, and no thought of food and drink. Of these six, qi depression is the most important, as it underlies all the others; when qi depression is eliminated, the other forms naturally disappear. See also **depression**.

softening (of hardness): ruǎn jiān (286)

Denotes methods used to treat hard swellings and masses.

somber white: cāng bái (415)

[*cāng,* blue, black; *bái,* white] A white complexion with a hint of dull blue, often seen, for example, in desertion patterns. Cf. **drained white** and **pale white.**

somnolence: shì shuì (352)

Drowsiness and excessive sleep.

soot black: lí hēi (200.2)

Describes dull, extremely dark complexions.

sovereign, minister, assistant and courier (drug roles): jūn chén zuǒ shǐ (124)

The term "drug roles" denotes the function of drugs in relation to those of drugs in a medicinal formula. The four roles are sovereign, minister, assistant, and courier. The sovereign, consisting of one or more agents, represents the main action of the formula and therefore addresses the principal pattern. Sovereign agents are also known as principal agents. The minister supports the action of the sovereign, while the assistant addresses secondary patterns or reduces the toxicity or harshness of the sovereign. The courier, sometimes known as the conductor, makes other agents act on the desired part of the body or harmonizes the other drugs.

spasm: jìng lüán (322)

Western medical term now widely used in Chinese medicine.

spillage rheum: yì yǐn (359)

Water in the limbs, characterized by heavy, painful, swollen limbs.

spirit: shén (237)

The principle of consciousness and of healthy physical and mental functioning; e.g., "the spirited patient thrives, while the spiritless patient is doomed." See also **essence-spirit, disposition,** and **affect.**

spirit light: shén míng (238)

Spirit, especially as seen in the light of the eyes.

Glossary of Terms

spirit-affect: shén qíng (239)

The spirit and the outwardly manifest emotions.

spirit-disposition: shén zhì (240)

The spirit, will, and emotions; roughly equivalent to consciousness.

spittle: tuò (260)

That part of the saliva which is the humor of the spleen.

splenic diarrhea: pí xiè (337)

Diarrhea due to splenic vacuity.

splenic fortification: jiàn pí

Method of treating impaired splenic movement and transformation characterized by a withered yellow facial complexion, lack of strength in the limbs, reduced appetite, stomachache relieved by pressure or eating, thin stool, a pale tongue with white fur and a soggy, weak pulse. Splenic fortification makes use of agents such as Radix Codonopsis Pilosulae *(dǎng shēn)*, Rhizoma Atractylodis Macrocephalae *(bái zhú)*, Sclerotium Poriae *(fú líng)*, Radix Dioscoreae *(shān yào)*, and Semen Coicis *(yì yǐ ren)*. Cf. **moving the spleen**.

stabilizing wind: dìng fēng (157)

In the final stages of thermic heat diseases, damage to yin by exuberant heat invariably gives rise to the stirring of vacuity wind in the upper body. Stabilizing wind, the method used to treat such patterns, is similar to enriching yin and extinguishing wind.

stagnant-looking: zhì

Dull, blotchy, as of complexions occurring in stagnation patterns.

stagnation: zhì (398)

Sluggishness of movement, particularly of qi and the digestate. See **flow-stoppage**.

stasis: yū (375)

Sluggishness or cessation of movement (of the blood).

stasis clots: yū kuài (377)

Clotting of menstrual discharge indicating the presence of static blood.

stasis macules: yū bān (376)

Sluggishness or cessation of movement (of the blood).

stasis speckles: yū diǎn (378)

Cyan-purple speckles on the tongue indicating the presence of static blood.

steam: zhēng (414)

Describes the behavior of damp-heat and its effect on organs. See **heat**.

steaming bone tidal fever: gǔ zhēng cháo rè (254)

Yin vacuity tidal fever, whereby heat qi thrusts out from the interior. This type of fever is invariably associated with night sweating.

steaming bones: gǔ zhēng (253)

Heat that arises in the inner body and is difficult to eliminate. Characterized by spontaneous sweating, heat in the cheeks, the palms of the hands, and soles of the feet, and an intermittent subjective feeling of fever unsubstantiated by any abnormally high body temperature; sometimes associated with emotional factors; usually attributed to yin vacuity.

stirring: dòng (259)

Provocation or development (of wind); agitation (of blood).

stoppage: bù tōng (35)

See **flow stoppage**.

strangury patterns: lín zhèng (277)

Patterns characterized by urinary frequency, urgency, and difficulty in voiding, as well as dribbling incontinence; includes calculous strangury (which also includes sabulous strangury), qi strangury, blood strangury, unctuous strangury, and taxation strangury, known collectively as the "five stranguries."

striations: còu lǐ (380)

The interstices of the flesh. The terms corresponds, among other things, to the sweat ducts in Western medicine.

strike: zhòng (39)

Affliction, usually sudden or severe, e.g., wind-strike.

subduing yang: qián yáng (422)

A method of treating such patterns as ascendant hyperactivity of liver yang due to yin vacuity; may be used where symptoms include headache and dizziness, tinnitus and deafness, and numbness or tremor of the limbs.

505

summerheat diarrhea: shǔ xiè (356)

Diarrhea occurring in a summerheat pattern. Contraction of summerheat heat may give rise to diarrhea characterized by watery or thick, slimy stool, accompanied by such signs as restlessness and thirst, dark-colored urine, spontaneous sweating, dirty-looking complexion and soggy, fast pulse. Conventionally, the term also refers to diarrhea caused by heatstroke, excessive consumption of fluid, raw foods, or cold foods in summer.

superabundance: yǒu yú (111)

Excess (of qi, blood, or fluids), cf. **vacuity and repletion**.

superlative: jùn (206)

Highly potent, as of drug action and methods of treatment; applied most commonly to draining and supplementing.

supplementation: bǔ (fǎ) (341)

The general method of treating vacuity patterns, in accordance with the principle of supplying insufficiency. Specific terms highlight the way in which aspects and elements are supplemented.

Supplementation of yin is often referred to as **nourishing, fostering,** or **enriching yin**, the last of these referring in particular to supplementation of kidney yin. **Strengthening yin** is a method of supplementing yin essence in patterns characterized by lumbar pain, seminal emission, copious urine, etc. **Emolliating** the liver is a method used to treat insufficiency of liver blood. **Engendering** liquid denotes supplementation of the fluids.

Supplementation of yang is often referred to as **reinforcing** yang. **Yang salvage,** or **yang restoration,** is the method used to treat yang collapse; a commonly used formula is Aconite Center-Rectifying Decoction *(fu-zi li zhong tang)*. Since yang vacuity is characterized by pronounced cold signs, the method of **warming** is used. **Freeing yang** and **perfusing yang** refer to the method of eliminating yang qi flow stoppage. Supplementation of qi, usually referred to as **qi boosting,** uses agents that are less hot. **Fortification** is usually applied to the spleen or center. Fortifying the center and boosting qi is a method of treatment whereby qi is boosted by enhancing the assimilative function of the spleen. **Moving the spleen** refers to supplementation of the spleen to improve movement and transformation of water-damp. **Upraising center qi** is the method of fortifying the center to treat prolapse conditions. **Quieting the spirit** is a method of treating disquiet of the spirit-disposition, using supplementing agents, sometimes combined with heavy settlers.

surface skin and body hair: pí máo (99)

The aspect of the body's exterior integument governed by the lung; closely associated with defense qi, which repels invading pathogens.

surfeit: piān shèng (256)

In yin-yang theory, relative strengthening (of either yin or yang). Same as **prevalence**.

suspended rheum: xuán yǐn (474)

Water in the chest and lateral costal region causing local pain and cough with copious phlegm.

sweeping: huò (459)

Forceful elimination of pathogens, such as phlegm.

swelling: zhǒng (381)

See **water**.

swelter: xūn zhēng (468)

Describes the behavior of damp-heat and its effect on organs.

swill diarrhea: sūn xiè (345)

Diarrhea characterized by clean-looking stool containing some undigested food; often occurs shortly after eating.

taxation: láo (300)

1) Severe, usually gradual detriment to the viscera, e.g., the five taxations (cardiac, hepatic, splenic, pulmonary, and renal taxation); 2) taxation fatigue, denoting fatigue due to overexertion. Cf. **five forms of taxation damage**.

taxation strangury: láo lín (301)

Strangury associated with taxation fatigue.

temper: duàn (316)

To treat (medicinal agents) by heating them to red heat in a fire or in a heat-resistant pot, in order to make them brittle or to alter their properties.

tetanic disease: jìng bìng (320)

See **muscular tetany**.

tetanic inversion: jìng jué (321)

Muscular tetany accompanied by syncope.

thin-stool diarrhea: táng xiè (357)

Mild diarrhea characterized by thin stool.

thoracic water: xiōng shuǐ (244)

See **water**.

through-flux diarrhea: dòng xiè (189)

Diarrhea due to indigestion. Refers specifically to: a) a form of cold diarrhea characterized by evacuation shortly after eating, or b) soft stool diarrhea *(rú xiè)*.

tidal fever: cháo rè (423)

Fever, sometimes only felt subjectively, occurring at regular intervals, usually in the afternoon or evening; may form part of both vacuity and repletion patterns.

tingling: má (295)

The sensation, typified by "pins and needles," which attends incomplete, or follows complete numbness; traditionally described as being neither pain nor itching, and as like insects running through the flesh.

toxin: dú (165)

1) A factor of disease, e.g., toxic qi. 2) Denotes inflammatory conditions characterized by redness, swelling and pain, or serous discharge.

transformation: huà (55)

Transformation denotes change of a gentle or gradual nature, in relative contrast to "transmutation," which denotes sudden or major qualitative change. Transformation implies progressive (productive) and regressive (destructive) change, and in the former case is frequently rendered as "formation." Hence, "fire formation" refers to the natural transformation of pathogens or yang qi into fire (progressive change), while "transformation of phlegm" refers to a method of treatment to eliminate phlegm (i.e., regressive change).

transformation into fire: huà huǒ (57)

See **fire formation**.

transformation into heat: huà rè (59)

See **heat formation**.

transformative action of qi: qì huà (209)

The function of qi as manifest in splenogastric upbearing and downbearing, the distribution of qi and blood by the lung and heart, the opening and closing action of the kidney (i.e., bladder function), and the control of the movement of water and fluids by the lung, spleen, and kidney. The transformative action of qi is also seen in the power of sight, locomotive ability, etc. See **qi**.

transmutation: biàn (485)

Major, sudden, or untoward change. See **transformation**.

transmuted pattern: biàn zhèng (486)

Conversion of repletion into vacuity or a simple condition into a complex one owing to inappropriate treatment (incorrect use of diaphoresis, ejection, or precipitation, or use of supplementation in the treatment of repletion patterns) or insufficiency of correct qi. For example, excessive use of diaphoretics in the treatment of tai yang cold damage patterns can cause detriment to heart yang and give rise to palpitations and racing of the heart, and oppression in the chest. Another example is that of the measles, where if papule outthrust is not complete, the papule toxin falls inward giving rise to a dyspnea counterflow pattern. In both cases, the resulting condition is known as a transmuted pattern.

true: zhēn (232)

Pertaining to that upon which the health of the whole organism rests, in particular the kidney. For example, "true yin" and "true yang" refer to kidney yin and yang.

true origin: zhēn yuán (233)

Original qi in its relationship to the kidney.

true qi: zhēn qì (234.1)

One form of qi within the body. The *Inner Canon* states, "True qi is the product of that which is received from Heaven combined with grain qi, and which makes the body full." "Heaven" is explained as meaning congenital source qi.

turbid: zhuó (435)

Murky, unclean, in opposition to "clear." "Turbid" is commonly used to describe alimentary waste as opposed to the nutritive elements extracted from the digestate, but may also be used to describe the blood as opposed to qi. In describing pathogens, it is closely associated with phlegm, the heaviest and most intractable of pathogens. "Turbid" is closely associated with yin, while "clear" is associated with yang. The combined terms "turbid yin" and "clear yang" are generally used to describe different elements of the body and matter present in it. See also **damp turbidity**.

tympany: gǔ (457)

Severe abdominal swelling with a withered yellow coloration of the skin, and prominent vessels. Causes include: damage to the liver and spleen when emotional depression gives rise to disruption of qi dynamic; damage to stomach and spleen due to intemperate eating and alcohol consumption; damage to liver and spleen when qi and blood flow is disrupted in parasite accumulation patterns and other infectious diseases. Tympany is the result of stagnation and accumulation of qi, blood, and water turbidity in the abdomen, due to interrelated pathologies of the liver, spleen, and kidney.

unclean: gòu

In the tongue examination, unclean describes a dirty-looking tongue fur.

unstopping: tōng

See **flow restoration**.

unctuous strangury: gāo lín (412)

Strangury associated with milky urine. See **strangury patterns**.

unsurfaced fever: shēn rè bú (wài) yáng (149)

Generalized fever in which heat is felt only by prolonged palpation; mostly due to binding of damp and heat, where the damp is blocked on the outside. Since the heat lies deep within the damp it cannot easily be felt on the surface of the body.

upbearing: shēng (60)

The normal upward movement of qi, and the promotion of such movement in therapy; also describes the tendency of drugs to act on the upper body.

upbearing fire flush: miàn hóng shēng huó (200)

A flushed complexion due to fire in the organs.

upflame: shàng yán (4)

To flame upwards. In five phase theory, "fire is the flaming upwards." Accordingly, patterns such as upflaming of liver fire are characterized by severe headache, red complexion, ocular rubor, and dry mouth. See **heat**.

uplifting: shēng jǔ (62)

See **upraising**.

Glossary of Terms

upper body: shàng (3)

The upper part of the body (yang) as opposed to the lower body (yin); sometimes specifically denotes the upper burner.

upper ventral vexation: ào nóng (433)

A symptom described as a burning sensation in the infracardiac region associated with nervous tension. The condition is often relieved by vomiting.

upraising: shēng tí (61)

Upbearing and raising; promoting normal upbearing of spleen qi and lifting prolapsed organs. "Upbearing eliminates downbearing," e.g., center qi fall can be treated with Center-Supplementing Qi-Boosting Decoction *(bǔ zhōng yì qì tāng)*, and downward fall of thoracic qi can be treated with Fall-Upbearing Decoction *(shēng xián tāng)*.

upstirring: shēng dòng

Upbearing and stirring. These are the attributes of liver yang. When liver yin-blood (or hepatorenal yin humor) is depleted, upstirring of liver yang is unchecked. The resulting pattern is called ascendant hyperactivity of liver yang.

upward-fixed eyes: dài yǎn (460)

A condition in which both eyes are fixed in an upturned direction. This condition is principally associated with *dai-yang* expiry patterns. Also seen in child fright inversion.

urinary block: niào bì, lóng bì (134)

Urine retention, urodialysis. See **changes in urine and micturition** and **block**.

urinary frequency: niào pín (136)

Increased frequency of urination usually in short voidings; often referred to simply as "frequency." See **changes in urine and micturition**.

urinary incontinence: shī sōu (92)

Involuntary loss of urine; generally denotes a pronounced condition of diurnal incontinence, as opposed to **enuresis**, which refers to loss of urine during sleep.

urinary urgency: niào jí (133)

Increased frequency or urination; often referred to simply as urgency.

vacuity and repletion: xū shí

Vacuity: weakness or emptiness; repletion: strength or fullness. Vacuity is used in yin-yang theory to denote weakness of one or another complement, and when applied to yang is synonymous with debilitation. In eight-parameter pattern identification, vacuity and repletion describe the weakness of correct qi and strength of pathogenic qi. Cf. **insufficiency** and **superabundance.**

vacuity desertion: xū tuō (340)

See **desertion**.

vacuity edema: xū fú (339)

See **water**.

vaginal discharge: dài xià (266)

Distinction is made between white, black, cyan, red, yellow, and multicolored vaginal discharge, white and red being the most common.

venter: guǎn (284)

The stomach cavity and adjoining sections of the duodenum and esophagus; divided into upper, middle, and lower venters. As used in Chinese medicine, this term carries a meaning different to that of its usage in Western medicine.

vessel: mài (mò) (247)

The pathways of the blood or of qi.

vigorous fever: zhuàng rè (130)

High fever occurring in repletion patterns and characteristic of qi-level heat in thermic diseases.

vigorous fire: zhuàng huǒ (128)

Pathological fire standing in opposition to the lesser fire, which is the healthy fire of physiologic activity; it can wear correct qi and affect physiologic functions.

visceral malaise: zàng zào (482)

A paroxysmal essence-spirit disorder most prevalent in women; heralded by essence-spirit melancholy and depression, illusions, emotionalism, and increased or diminished sensitivity. Attacks are characterized by restlessness and feelings of oppression, rashness and impatience, sighing for no apparent reason, and sadness with an urge to weep. In serious cases there may be convulsive spasms which, unlike those occurring in epilepsy, are accompanied by pallor or complete loss of consciousness. Cardiohepatic blood vacuity and emotional depression constitute the prime causes.

visceral manifestation theory: zàng xiàng xúe shūo

The body of theories concerning normal and abnormal functions of the viscera (in the broad sense of the word) as they appear to the observer; the Chinese medical equivalent of physiology and pathology.

viscus: zàng (479)

[Plural: viscera] Any of the organs of the interior (lung, kidney, liver, heart, and spleen). NB: The Chinese ideogram was only latterly distinguished from that meaning to store *(cáng)* by the addition of the flesh radical.

visual distortion: mào (404)

Deranged, flowery vision.

visual dizziness: xuàn (231)

Clouded, flowery vision; often associated with mental dizziness.

vomiting: ǒu tù (393)

The Chinese term is composed of two characters, *ǒu*, meaning retching (sound without matter, and *tù*, meaning ejection (matter without sound). However, the combined term, as the English **vomiting**, tends to exclude retching. While retching denotes a relative absence of expelled matter, "dry retching" *(gǎn ǒu)* denotes its complete absence.

water: shuǐ (73)

Any form of fluid, in particular ingested fluids (such as in the expression **sea of grain and water**), waste fluids or urine (as in "waterways"), and pathologic accumulation of water (as in **water swelling**). In five-phase theory, the kidney corresponds to water. Hence in many texts, **water** refers to the kidney and its corresponding exterior organ, the bladder. Pathologically, water (or more commonly, **water qi**) refers to fluid accumulations attributable to morbidity of the lung, spleen, or kidney. In such contexts, distinction is made between "yin water" and "yang water." Yin water patterns are ones of vacuity or patterns that develop slowly and are difficult to treat. Yang water patterns are ones of repletion or patterns that develop rapidly and can be eliminated swiftly. "Abdominothoracic water" includes ascites (abdominal water) and thoracic water, as well as water collecting around the stomach. These patterns are characterized by distention and fullness, although such signs may also be due to other causes. Swelling other than abdominothoracic water is referred to as "edematous swelling." Distinction is made between repletion and vacuity swelling. Repletion swelling, which is one form of yang water, is characterized by resilience of the flesh on application of pressure. Vacuity swelling, a form of yin water, is resilient only when light pressure is applied. After releasing greater pressure, the flesh is slow to assume its original contours. "Qi swelling" refers to accumulation of water in the superficial layers of skin, attributable to obstruction or constraint of striations (impaired sweat secretion) in exogenous diseases. It is marked by visibility of fluid movement under strong lamplight. Water swelling, in the broader sense, is synonymous with edematous swelling as a generic term, yet often specifically denotes swelling of the eyes due to cardiorenal vacuity. The Chinese term rendered as "water swelling" is used in Western medicine as the equivalent of edema, and hence is often rendered as such by translators of Chinese medical texts. "Deficiency edema" refers to qi swelling or vacuity swelling. Generally speaking, repletion swelling is characterized by a predominance of blood over water, while vacuity swelling is characterized by a greater proportion of water. Qi swelling is characterized by the presence only of water. All water patterns described above are interrelated. Under given circumstances, one form of water accumulation may give rise to another. For instance, ascites in severe cases may develop into generalized edematous swelling.

water qi: shuǐ qì (75)

Pathologic excesses of water in the body and diseases provoked by them. The main cause is impairment of movement and transformation of water due to splenorenal yang vacuity. See **water**.

water swelling: shuǐ zhǒng (76)

See **water**.

water-damp: shuǐ shī (78)

A collective term for water and damp commonly used in the context of the spleen, especially regarding its function of governing the movement and transformation of fluids and its intolerance of damp.

water-rheum: shuǐ yǐn (77)

Fluid exuded by diseased organs. Thin, clear fluid is known as "water" while thin, sticky fluid is known as "rheum." These differ in name and form, but are in essence the same; hence the compound term.

wearing: hào (243)

Describes gradual loss of, or damage (to the blood, fluids, etc.) associated with enduring illness. See **exuberance and debilitation**.

wheezing: xiāo (203)

See **dyspnea**.

wheezing dyspnea: xiāo chuǎn (204)

See **dyspnea**.

wind numbness: má fēng (298)

Leprosy.

wind-strike: zhòng fēng (40)

1) Disease characterized by sudden loss of consciousness, hemaplegia, or wry mouth, and impeded speech; occurs under the following circumstances: a) when depletion of yin essence or sudden anger causes hyperactivity of liver yang which stirs liver wind; b) when, owing to a predilection for rich, fatty foods, phlegm heat congests in the inner body and transforms into wind; c) when vacuity of qi and blood give rise to vacuity wind; d) when a patient suffering from inner-body vacuity suddenly contracts exogenous wind. Distinction is made between "connecting-channel strike," "major channel strike," "bowel strike," and "visceral strike" (in ascending order of severity). Correspondences in Western medicine include cerebral hemorrhage, cerebral embolism, and cerebral thrombosis, as well as a number of diseases of the brain and cranial nerves. Patterns including initial-stage fever invariably correspond to cerebrovascular disease. 2) Exogenous wind contraction, characterized by fever, headache, moderate floating pulse (*Treatise on Cold Damage*).

withdrawal: diān (491)

See **mania and withdrawal**.

withered yellow: wěi huáng

A pale brownish yellow; the color of withered leaves. A withered yellow complexion is a dry, brownish yellow complexion.

yang vacuity water flood: yáng xū shuǐ fàn (344)

Water accumulation due to yang vacuity. See **water**.

yang water: yáng shuǐ (343)

See **water**.

yin vacuity fire effulgence: yīn xū huǒ wàng (294)

Effulgence of fire due to yin vacuity.

yin humor: yīn yè

Humor (the thicker fluids of the body); all nutritious fluids of the body.

yin water: yīn shuǐ (293)

See **water**.

Stroke-Order Glossary of Chinese Medical Terms

二筆　　　　Two Strokes

入	rù	entry (1)
入裡	rù lǐ	interiorization (2)

三筆　　　　Three Strokes

上	shàng	upper body; ascent, rise (3)
上炎	shàng yán	upflame (4)
上氣	shàng qì	qi ascent (5)
下	xià	lower body; precipitation (6)
下利清谷	xià lì qīng gǔ	clear-food diarrhea (9)
下注	xià zhù	downpour (10)
下迫	xià pò	lower body distress (11)
下陷	xià xiàn	downward fall (12)
丸	wán	pills (13)
久	jiǔ	enduring (14)
久泄	jiǔ xiè	enduring diarrhea (15)
久泄滑脫	jiǔ xiè huá tuō	enduring diarrhea efflux desertion (16)
亡	wáng	collapse (17)
亡陰	wáng yīn	yin collapse
亡陽	wáng yáng	yang collapse
口疳	kǒu gān	oral *gan* (18)
口腐	kǒu fǔ	cottage cheese fur
口糜	kǒu mí	oral putrefaction
大汗	dà hàn	profuse perspiration (19)
大風	dà fēng	great wind (leprosy)
大氣	dà qì	cosmic qi (20)
大煩渴	dà fán kě	great restlessness and thirst (20.1)
大熱	dà rè	great heat (21)
大頭瘟	dà tóu wēn	balloon-head scourge (22)
寸	cùn	body inch (23)
小兒驚風	xiǎo ér jīng fēng	child fright wind (24)
小兒驚厥	xiǎo ér jīng jué	child fright inversion (25)
小便淋漓不禁	xiǎo biàn lín lì (bú jìn)	dribbling incontinence (26)

小便短少	xiǎo biàn duǎn shǎo	short micturition with scant urine (27)
小便清長	xiǎo biàn qīng cháng	long micturition with clear urine (28)

四筆 Four Strokes

不安	bù ān	disquieted, disquieting (29)
不利	bú lì	inhibited, inhibition (30)
不足	bù zú	insufficient, insufficiency (31)
不和	bù hé	disharmony (32)
不固	bú gù	insecurity (33)
不振	bú zhèn	devitalized, devitalization (34)
不秘	bú mì	untight, unsound
不通	bù tōng	stoppage, flow stoppage (35)
不遂	bú suì	-plegia (36)
不寧	bù níng	disquieting
丹	dān	elixir (37)
中	zhōng	center (38)
中	zhòng	strike (39)
中氣下陷	zhōng qì xià xiàn	center qi fall
中風	zhòng fēng	wind-strike (40)
五心	wǔ xīn	five hearts (41)
五心煩熱	wǔ xīn fán rè	fever in the five hearts (42)
五志過極	wǔ zhì guò jí	dispositional excess (43)
五更泄	wǔ gēng (jīng) xiè	fifth-watch diarrhea (44)
五勞所傷	wǔ láo suǒ shāng	five forms of taxation damage (45)
亢盛	kàng shèng	hyperactivity (46)
內	nèi	endogenous; inner body (47)
內閉	nèi bì	inner-body block (49)
內閉昏厥	nèi bì hūn jué	block clouding inversion (50)
內陷	nèi xiàn	inward fall (51)
內傷七情	nèi shāng qī qíng	affect damage (52)
六鬱	liù yù	six depressions (53)
分	fēn	*fen;* candareen (54)
化	huà	formation; transformation (55)
化火	huà huǒ	transformation into fire (57)
化熱	huà rè	heat formation; transformation into heat (58)
升	shēng	upbearing (60)
升動	shēng dòng	upstirring
升提	shēng tí	upraising (61)

升舉	shēng jǔ	uplifting (62)
升舉無力	shēng jǔ wú lì	diminution of uplift
反胃	fǎn wèi	gastric reflux (63)
反關脈	fǎn guān mài	dorsal styloid pulse (64)
太陰病	tài yīn bìng	tai yin disease
太陽病	tài yáng bìng	tai yang disease
少氣	shǎo qì	diminished qi (65)
少陰病	shào yīn bìng	shao yin disease
少陽病	shào yáng bìng	shao yang disease
心	xīn	heart (66)
心下	xīn xià	infracardiac region (67)
心火上炎	xīn huǒ shàng yán	upflaming of heart fire
心包證	xīn bāo zhèng	pericardiac pattern
心血虛	xīn xuè xū	heart blood vacuity
心肝火旺	xīn gān huǒ wàng	cardiohepatic fire effulgence
心肺氣虛	xīn fèi qì xū	cardiopulmonary qi vacuity
心氣虛	xīn qì xū	heart qi vacuity
心痛	xīn tòng	cardialgia (68)
心悸	xīn jì	palpitations (69)
心陰虛	xīn yīn xū	heart yin vacuity
心腎不交	xīn shèn bù jiāo	breakdown of cardiorenal interaction
心腎陰虛	xīn shèn yīn xū	cardiorenal yin vacuity
心腎陽虛	xīn shèn yáng xū	cardiorenal yang vacuity
心脾血虛	xīn pí xuè xū	cardiosplenic blood vacuity
心陽虛	xīn yáng xū	heart yang vacuity
心煩	xīn fán	restlessness (70)
心痺	xīn bì	cardiac obturation
心竅	xīn qiào	cardiac portals (71)
支飲	zhī yǐn	column rheum (72)
止	zhǐ	arrest, stop, suppress, relieve
水	shuǐ	water (73)
水谷之海	shuǐ gǔ zhī hǎi	sea of grain and water (74)
水氣	shuǐ qì	water qi (75)
水液	shuǐ yè	fluid
水腫	shuǐ zhǒng	water swelling (76)
水飲	shuǐ yǐn	water-rheum (77)
水濕	shuǐ shī	water-damp (78)
火	huǒ	fire (79)
牙宣	yá xuān	periodontal *xuan* (80)
牙疳	yá gān	periodontal *gan* (81)

Five Strokes 五筆

主	zhǔ	govern, governance, governor (82)
主輔佐引	zhǔ fǔ zuǒ yǐn	principal, support, assistant, and conducting agents
出	chū	issue (86)
四肢厥冷	sì zhī jué lěng	inversion frigidity of the limbs (87)
四肢逆冷	sì zhī nì lěng	counterflow frigidity of the limbs (88)
外	wài	outer body; exogenous (89)
外感風邪	wài gǎn fēng xié	exogenous wind contraction
外感寒邪	wài gǎn hán xié	exogenous cold contraction
外感熱病	wài gǎn rè bìng	exogenous heat disease (91)
失	shī	impairment, failure, breakdown
失溲	shī sōu	urinary incontinence (92)
失精	shī jīng	seminal loss (93)
平肝熄風	píng gān xí fēng	calming the liver and extinguishing wind (94)
本經自發	běn jīng zì fā	originate in channel
正	zhèng	correct (95)
正氣	zhèng qì	correct qi (95.1)
犯	fàn	invasion; invade (96)
生	shēng	engender (97)
用藥	yòng yào	drug use
白㾦	bái péi	miliaria alba (98)
皮毛	pí máo	surface skin and body hair (99)
目赤	mù chì	ocular rubor (100)
目花	mù huā	flowery vision (101)
石淋	shí lín	calculous strangury (102)

Six Strokes 六筆

伏	fú	deep-lying (103)
伐肝	fā gān	quelling the liver (104)
合病	hé bìng	combination disease
吐	tù	eject; vomit; spit (105)
吐血	tù xuè	hematemesis
多尿	duō niào	heavy micturition (106)
妄行	wàng xíng	frenetic movement (107)
安	ān	quieting (108)
收引	shōu yǐn	contracture and hypertonicity (109)

Stroke-Order Glossary

早泄	zǎo xiè	premature ejaculation (110)
有餘	yǒu yú	superabundance (111)
汗	hàn	sweat, perspiration, diaphoresis
肌表	jī biǎo	muscular exterior (112)
肌膚	jī fū	skin and muscle (113)
肌膚甲錯	jī fū jiǎ cuò	cutaneous cornification (114)
血分證	xuè fēn zhèng	blood-aspect pattern
血淋	xuè lín	blood strangury (116)
血虛	xuè xū	blood vacuity
血虛生風	xuè xū shēng fēng	blood vacuity engendering wind
血瘀	xuè yū	blood stasis
血熱	xuè rè	blood heat
血燥	xuè zào	blood dryness
血燥生風	xuè zào shēng fēng	blood dryness engendering wind
血臌(蠱)	xuè gǔ	blood tympany (117)
血熱妄行	xuè rè wàng xíng	frenetic blood heat (115)
舌(質)	shé (zhí)	tongue (body)
胖大	~pàng dà	enlarged
瘦癟	~shòu biě	shrunken
有點刺	~yǒu diǎn cì	having speckles and prickles
裂	~liè	fissured
光滑	~guāng huá	mirror tongue
鏡面舌	~jìng miàn shé	mirror tongue
強	~jiàng	stiff
痿	~wěi	limp
顫動	~zhàn (chàn) dòng	trembling
歪斜	~wāi xié	wry
卷縮	~juǎn suō	curling, contraction
弄舌	~nòng shé	worrying
吐舌	~tù shé	protracted
淡	~dàn	pale
紅	~hóng	red
絳	~jiàng	crimson
紫	~zǐ	purple
青紫	~qīng zǐ	cyan-purple
舌苔	shé tāi	tongue fur
潤	~rùn	moist
滑	~huá	glossy
燥	~zào	dry

糙	~ cāo	rough
厚	~ hòu	thick
薄	~ bó (báo)	thin
化	~ huà	transforming
淨	~ jìng	clean
膩	~ nì	slimy
垢	~ gòu	unclean
濁	~ zhuó	turbid
捎	~ kěn	generalized slimy
剝	~ bō	peeling
白	~ bái	white
腐	~ fǔ	cottage cheese
黃	~ huáng	yellow
老黃	~ lǎo huáng	old yellow
焦黃	~ jiāo huáng	burnt yellow
黃白相間	~ huáng bái xiāng jiān	mixed yellow and white
黑	~ hēi	black
灰白相兼	~ huī bái xiāng jiān	mixed gray and white
行	xíng	move

七筆 Seven Strokes

形	xíng	form; formal body (118)
形寒	xíng hán	cold form (119)
形體	xíng tǐ	body (120)
利	lì	disinhibition (121)
利水	lì shuǐ	disinhibition of water
利尿	lì niào	disinhibition of urine (122)
助陽	zhù yáng	reinforcing yang (123)
君臣佐使	jūn chén zuǒ shǐ	sovereign, minister, assistant and courier (124)
吞酸	tūn suān	acid regurgitation (125)
困	kùn	encumbrance, cumbersome (126)
壯火	zhuàng huǒ	invigorating fire (128)
壯陽	zhuàng yáng	invigorating yang (129)
壯熱	zhuàng rè	vigorous fever (130)
尿少	niào shǎo	oliguria, scant urine (131)
尿多	niào duō	polyuria, copious urine (132)
尿血	niào xuè	hematuria (360)
尿急	niào jí	urinary urgency (133)

Stroke-Order Glossary

尿閉	niào bì	urinary block (134)
尿痛	niào tòng	painful urination (135)
尿頻	niào pín	urinary frequency (136)
志	zhì	disposition (137)
抑肝	yì gān	repressing the liver (138)
攻	gōng	attack; offensive treatment (139)
束	shù	fetter (141)
束表	shù biǎo	fettering of the exterior
灼	zhuó	scorch (142)
灼熱	zhuó rè	palpable heat (143)
狂	kuáng	mania (144)
狂躁	kuáng zào	manic agitation (145)
肝火上炎	gān huǒ shàng yán	upflaming of liver fire
肝血虛	gān xuè xū	liver blood vacuity
肝胆濕熱	gān dǎn shī rè	hepatocystic damp-heat
肝風內動	gān fēng nèi dòng	stirring of endogenous liver wind
肝氣犯胃	gān qì fàn wèi	invasion of the stomach by liver qi
肝氣鬱結	gān qì yù jié	binding depression of liver qi (146)
肝脾不和	gān pí bù hé	hepatosplenic disharmony
肝陽上亢	gān yáng shàng kàng	ascendant hyperactivity of liver yang
疔瘡	dīng chuāng	clove lesion (147)
芒刺	máng cì	prickles (148)
身熱不(外)揚	shēn rè bù (wài) yáng	unsurfaced fever (149)
邪	xié	pathogen (150)

八筆 Eight Strokes

兩	liǎng	*liang;* tael (150.1)
兩感	liǎng gǎn	dual affection
直中	zhí zhòng	direct strike (151)
炙	zhì	mix-fry (152)
味	wèi	sapor (153)
和	hé	harmonization, harmony (154)
固	gù	securing, security, secure (155)
夜間多尿	yè jiān duō niào	nocturia (156)
定風	dìng fēng	stabilizing wind (157)
怔忡	zhēng chōng	racing of the heart (158)
府	fǔ	dwelling place (159)

Stroke-Order Glossary

抽搐	chōu chù	convulsive spasm (160)
抽筋	chōu jīn	cramp
拘(拘急,拘攣)	jū (jū jí, jū lüán)	hypertonicity (161)
旺	wàng	effulgent, effulgence (163)
昏	hūn	clouding (164)
毒	dú	toxin, toxic (165)
泄瀉	xiè xiè	diarrhea (166)
泛	fàn	flooding (167)
泛酸	fàn suān	acid upflow (168)
注下	zhù xià	outpour diarrhea (169)
疝	shàn	*shan* (170)
疝氣	shàn qì	*shan qi* (171)
育	yù	fostering (172)
臥	wò	recumbency
舍	shè	abide, abode
表	biǎo	exterior (173)
阻	zǔ	obstruction (174)

九筆 Nine Strokes

削	xuè (xiāo)	disintegrate
青	qīng	cyan (175)
侵襲	qīn xí	assail, invade (176)
咬牙	yǎo yá	bruxism (178)
咯	luò	expectoration (390)
咳	ké	cough (179)
咳嗽	ké sòu	cough (and expectoration)
咽	yān	pharynx
客邪	kè xié	settling pathogens (181)
宣	xuān	diffusion; perfusion
宣通	xuān tōng	perfusion; (182) promoting perfusion
宣散	xuān sàn	diffusion; (183) promoting diffusion
急	jí	acute (disease); distress (lower body); rapid (breathing); tension (muscles); urgent (micturition)
枯	kū	desiccated (185)
枯瘠	kū péi	dry miliaria (186)
柔肝	róu gān	emolliating the liver (188)

Stroke-Order Glossary

洞泄	dòng xiè	through-flux diarrhea (189)
津	jīn	liquid (190)
津液	jīn yè	fluids (191)
活血	huó xuè	blood quickening (192)
炮	pāo	blast-fry
相火	xiāng huǒ	ministerial fire (193)
相爭	xiāng zhēng	struggle
相搏	xiāng bó	contention (194)
相煽	xiāng shān	mutual exacerbation
砂淋	shā lín	sabulous strangury (195)
肺失肅降	fèi shī sù jiàng	impaired depurative downbearing of lung qi
肺胃熱盛	fèi wèi rè shèng	exuberant pulmogastric heat
肺氣不宣	fèi qì bù xuān	non-diffusion of lung qi
肺氣虛	fèi qì xū	lung qi vacuity
肺陰虛	fèi yīn xū	lung yin vacuity
胃火	wèi huǒ	stomach fire
胃失和降	wèi shī hé jiàng	breakdown of gastric harmony and downbearing
胃氣上逆	wèi qì shàng nì	counterflow ascent of stomach qi
胃氣虛寒	wèi qì xū hán	gastric qi vacuity cold
胃陰不足	wèi yīn bù zú	insufficiency of stomach yin
胃熱	wèi rè	stomach heat
胃熱乘心	wèi rè chéng xīn	stomach heat overwhelming the heart
胎氣	tāi qì	fetal qi (196)
迫	pò	distress (197)
重鎮藥	zhòng zhèn yào	heavy settler (198)
降	jiàng	downbearing (199)
面色	miàn sè	complexion
白	~bái	white
黃白	~huáng bái	drained white
淡白	~dàn bái	pale white
無華	~wú huá	lusterless
蒼白	~cāng bái	somber white
青	~qīng	cyan
青紫	~qīng zǐ	cyan-purple
晦暗	~huì àn	dark
灰	~huī	gray
紅	~hóng	red
潮紅	~cháo hóng	tidal flushing

兩顴潮紅	˜liǎng quán cháo hóng	tidal flushing of the cheeks
紅如塗油彩	˜hóng rú tú yóu cǎi	unusually rosy
面紅升火	˜miàn hóng shēng huǒ	upbearing fire flush
黃	˜huáng	yellow
陰黃	˜yīn huáng	yin yellow
陽黃	˜yáng huáng	yang yellow
淡黃	˜dàn huáng	pale yellow
萎黃	˜wēi huáng	withered yellow
黑	˜hēi	black
黎黑	˜lí hēi	soot black
紫黑	˜zǐ hēi	purple-black
風火赤眼	fēng huǒ chì yǎn	wind-fire ocular rubor
風火齒痛	fēng huǒ chǐ tòng	wind-fire toothache
風邪入經絡	fēng xié rù jīng luò	entry of wind pathogen into the channels
風溫	fēng wēn	wind thermia
風寒	fēng hán	wind-cold
風痰	fēng tán	wind phlegm
風熱	fēng rè	wind-heat
食泄	shí xiè	ingesta damage diarrhea (201)
食滯	shí zhì	digestate stagnation
食積	shí jī	digestate accumulation

十筆 Ten Strokes

凌	líng	intimidate (202)
哮	xiào	wheezing (203)
哮喘	xiào chuǎn	wheezing and dyspnea (204)
射	shè	shoot (205)
竣	jùn	superlative (206)
格陽	gé yáng	repelled yang (207)
氣	qì	qi (208)
氣不攝血	qì bú shè xuè	blood management failure
氣分大熱	qì fēn dà rè	great heat in the qi aspect
氣分初熱	qì fēn chū rè	first-stage qi-aspect heat
氣分證	qì fēn zhèng	qi-aspect pattern
氣化	qì huà	transformative action of qi (209)
氣少	qì shǎo	qi shortage (210)

氣血同病	qì xuè tóng bìng	dual disease patterns of qi and blood
氣血俱虛	qì xuè jù xū	dual vacuity of qi and blood
氣怯	qì què	qi temerity (211)
氣促	qì cù	distressed, rapid breathing
氣急	qì jí	rapid breathing
氣淋	qì lín	qi strangury (212)
氣粗	qì cū	rough breathing
氣厥	qì jué	qi inversion (213)
氣街	qì jiē	qi thoroughfare (214)
氣痛	qì tòng	qi pain (215)
氣腫	qì zhǒng	qi swelling (216)
氣滯	qì zhì	qi stagnation
氣滯血瘀	qì zhì xuè yū	qi stagnation and blood stasis
氣機	qì jī	qi dynamic (217)
氣隨血脫	qì suí xuè tuō	sequential desertion of blood and qi
浮	fú	edema; floating (218)
浮腫	fú zhǒng	edematous swelling (220)
消	xiāo	dispersion (221)
消渴	xiāo kě	diabetic disease; thirsting dispersion (222)
涎	xián	drool (223)
留	liú	lodge (224)
留戀	liú liàn	linger (225)
疳	gān	*gan* (226)
疳積	gān jī	*gan* accumulation (227)
疽	jū	gangrenous lesion; ju (228)
病機	bìng jī	pathomechanism (229)
益	yì	boosting (230)
眩	xuàn	visual dizziness (231)
眞	zhēn	true (232)
眞元	zhēn yuán	true origin (233)
眞心痛	zhēn xīn tòng	cardiodynia (234)
眞氣	zhēn qì	true qi
破	pò	breaking (235)
破血	pò xuè	blood breaking
祛	qū	dispel (236)
神	shén	spirit, spiritual (237)
神明	shén míng	spirit light (238)
神情	shén qíng	spirit-affect (239)

神志	shén zhì	spirit-disposition (240)
納呆	nà dāi	dyspeptic anorexia (241)
納氣	nà qì	qi absorption, promoting qi absorption (242)
耗	hào	wearing (243)
胸水	xiōng shuǐ	thoracic water (244)
胸脅苦滿	xiōng xié kǔ mǎn	bitter fullness in the chest and lateral costal region (245)
胸腹水	xiōng fù shuǐ	abdominothoracic water (246)
脈	mài	vessel (247)
脈象	mài xiàng	pulse (reading)
浮	~fú	floating
沉	~chén	deep
遲	~chí	slow
數	~shuò	rapid
虛	~xū	vacuous
實	~shí	replete
滑	~huá	slippery
澀	~sè	rough (choppy)
強	~qiáng	strong
濡	~rú	soggy
洪	~hóng	surging
微	~wéi	faint
欲絕	~yù jué	verging on expiry
細	~xì	fine
弱	~ruò	weak
大	~dà	large
散	~sàn	scattered, dissipated
緊	~jǐn	tight
芤	~kòu	scallion-stalk
革	~gé	drumskin
牢	~láo	confined
疾	~jí	racing
動	~dòng	stirred
伏	~fú	hidden
緩	~huǎn	moderate
促	~cù	skipping (rapid, interrupted)
結	~jié	bound (slow, interrupted)
代	~dài	regularly interrupted
長	~cháng	long
短	~duǎn	short

臭	chòu	bad odor, malodorous (248)
衰	shuāi	debilitation (249)
迷	mí	confound (250)
追	zhuī	expulsion (251)
逆	nì	counterflow (252)
逆傳	nì chuán	irregular passage
逆傳心包	nì chuán xīn bāo	anticipated passage to the pericardium
骨蒸	gǔ zhēng	steaming bones (253)
骨蒸潮熱	gǔ zhēng cháo rè	steaming bone tidal fever (254)

十一筆 Eleven Strokes

乾嘔	gān ǒu	dry retching
偏衰	piān shuāi	deficit, debilitation (255)
偏勝	piān shèng	surfeit, prevalence (256)
停	tíng	collect (257)
健	jiàn	fortification (258)
健脾	jiàn pí	splenic fortification
動	dòng	stirring (259)
唾	tuò	spittle (260)
唾血	tuò xuè	spitting of blood
培土	péi tǔ	banking up earth (261)
堅	jiān	hardness (262)
宿疾	sù jí	perduring ailment, previous disease (263)
崩中	bēng zhōng	profuse metrorrhagia (264)
崩漏	bēng lòu	metrorrhagia (265)
帶下	dài xià	vaginal discharge (266)
強	qiáng	strong, strengthening
強直	jiàng zhí	rigid (267)
情	qíng	affect (268)
情志	qíng zhì	emotion (269)
掉	diào	shaking (270)
推拿	tuī ná	massotherapy (271)
晨泄	chén xiè	daybreak diarrhea (273)
梅花針	méi huā zhēn	plum-blossom needle (274)
梅核氣	méi hé qì	plum-stone globus (275)
涸	hé	aridity
液	yè (yì)	humor (276)
涵	hán	moisten
淋證	lín zhèng	strangury pattern (277)

淡	dàn	pale; bland (278)
淫氣	yín qì	environmental excesses (279)
清	qīng	clear; clearage (280)
理氣	lǐ qì	rectifying qi (282)
理血	lǐ xuè	rectifying the blood (283)
脘	wǎn (guǎn)	venter (284)
脫	tuō	desertion (285)
軟堅	ruǎn jiān	softening (hardness) (286)
透	tòu	outthrust (287)
逐	zhú	expulsion (288)
通	tōng	restoring flow, freeing, unstopping (289)
通降	tōng jiàng	free downflow (290)
閉	bì	block (291)
閉證	bì zhèng	block pattern (292)
陰水	yīn shuǐ	yin water (293)
陰液	yīn yè	yin humor
陰虛火旺	yīn xū huǒ wàng	yin vacuity fire effulgence (294)
陷	xiàn	fall
麻	má	tingling (295)
麻木	má mù	numbness (296)
麻痺	má bì	palsy (297)
麻風	má fēng	wind numbness (298)
勝	shèng	prevalence, overcoming (299)

十二筆 Twelve Strokes

勞	láo	taxation (300)
勞淋	láo lín	taxation strangury (301)
厥	jué	inversion (302)
厥陰病	jué yīn bìng	jue yin disease
喀	kà	hacking (303)
喀血	kà xuè	hacking blood (304)
喉	hóu	larynx
喉中有水雞聲	hóu zhōng yǒu shuǐ jī shēng	frog rattle (305)
喘	chuǎn	dyspnea (306)
寒包火	hán bāo huǒ	cold enveloping fire (307)
寒疝	hán shàn	cold *shan* (308)
寒痛	hán tòng	cold pain
寒痰	hán tán	cold phlegm
寒痹	hán bì	cold obturation

Stroke-Order Glossary

寒戰	hán zhàn	shivering
寒泄	hán xiè	cold diarrhea
循衣摸床	xún yī mō chuáng	carphologia (308.1)
惡	è	malign (309)
惡	wù	aversion; ail
散	sǎn	powder
散	sàn	dissipation (310)
斑	bān	papules (311)
斑疹	bān zhěn	maculopapular eruptions (312)
晶㾦	jīng péi	miliaria crystallina (313)
焚	fén	deflagrate (314)
焦	jiāo	parch, parched; burnt; burner (315)
煅	duàn	temper (316)
疏	shū	coursing (317)
痛痹	tòng bì	dolorous obturation (318)
痙	jìng	muscular tetany (319)
痙病	jìng bìng	tetanic disease (320)
痙厥	jìng jué	tetanic inversion (321)
痙攣	jìng lüán	spasm (322)
痢	lì	dysentery (323)
痞	pǐ	glomus (324)
痞塊	pǐ kuài	lump glomus (325)
發	fā	effusion (326)
發汗	fā hàn	sweat, perspiration, diaphoresis
盛	shèng	exuberance (327)
筋	jīn	sinews (328)
筋惕肉瞤	jīn tì ròu rùn	jerking sinews and twitching muscles (329)
結	jié	bind (330)
絡	luò	connect (331)
絡脈	luò mài	connecting channel
絕	jué	expiry (332)
絳	jiàng	crimson (333)
脹	zhàng	distention (334)
腎不納氣	shèn bú nà qì	qi absorption failure
腎泄	shèn xiè	kidney diarrhea (335)
腎氣不固	shèn qì bú gù	insecurity of kidney qi
腎陰虛	shèn yīn xū	kidney yin vacuity
腎虛水泛	shèn xū shuǐ fàn	kidney vacuity water flood
腎陽虛	shèn yáng xū	kidney yang vacuity

Stroke-Order Glossary

腎精不足	shèn jīng bù zú	insufficiency of kidney essence
腑	fǔ	bowel (336)
脾不統血	pí bù tǒng xuè	blood management failure
脾失健運	pí shī jiàn yùn	splenic transformation failure
脾泄	pí xiè	splenic diarrhea (337)
脾氣虛弱	pí qì xū ruò	splenic qi vacuity
脾虛夾實	pí xū jiā shí	splenic vacuity with ingesta damage complication
脾腎陽虛	pí shèn yáng xū	splenorenal yang vacuity
脾陽不振	pí yáng bú zhèn	devitalization of splenic yang
虛	xū	vacuity
虛浮	xū fú	vacuity edema (339)
虛脫	xū tuō	vacuity desertion (340)
虛熱	xū rè	vacuity heat
補	bǔ	supplementation (341)
越傳經	yuè chuán jīng	overpassage (342)
陽水	yáng shuǐ	yang water (343)
陽明病	yáng míng bìng	yang ming disease
陽氣虛脫	yáng qì xū tuō	yang qi vacuity desertion
陽虛水泛	yáng xū shuǐ fàn	yang vacuity water flood (344)
飧泄	sūn xiè	swill diarrhea (345)

十三筆   Thirteen Strokes

肅降	sù jiàng	depurative downbearing (346)
傳經	chuán jīng	channel passage (347)
傳變	chuán biàn	shift (348)
傷	shāng	damage (349)
傷食	shāng shí	ingesta damage
傷津	shāng jīn	damage to liquid
傷陰	shāng yīn	damage to yin
飲	yǐn	cool decoction (350)
嗜食異物	shì shí yì wù	perverted appetite (351)
嗜睡	shì shuì	somnolence (352)
感	gǎn	contraction (353)
感受燥邪	gǎn shòu zào xié	contraction of exogenous dryness
損	sǔn	detriment; reduction (354)
暈	yūn	mental dizziness (355)
暑泄	shǔ xiè	summerheat diarrhea (356)
暑熱	shǔ rè	summerheat-heat
暑濕	shǔ shī	summerheat-damp

Stroke-Order Glossary

溫	wēn	warm, warming; thermia
溫熱	wēn rè	thermic heat
溏泄	táng xiè	thin-stool diarrhea (357)
溢	yì	spillage (358)
溢飲	yì yǐn	spillage rheum (359)
溲血	sōu xuè	hematuria (360)
滋	zī	enrich, enrichment (361)
滑	huá	efflux (stool, semen); glossy (tongue); slippery (pulse) (362)
滑泄	huá xiè	efflux diarrhea (363)
滑脫	huá tuō	efflux desertion (364)
滑精	huá jīng	seminal efflux (365)
煩躁	fán zào	agitation (366)
煩熱	fán rè	feverishness (367)
煎	jiān	decoct (368)
煎熬	jiān áo	boil (369)
痰	tán	phlegm
痰涎	tán xián	phlegm-drool (369.1)
痰迷心竅	tán mí xīn qiào	phlegm confounding the cardiac portals
痰留肢體	tán liú zhī tǐ	phlegm lodging in the limbs
痰留胸脅	tán liú xiōng xié	phlegm lodging in the chest and lateral costal region
痰留經絡	tán liú jīng luò	phlegm lodging in the channels
痰飲	tán yǐn	phlegm-rheum (370)
痰濁上擾	tán zhuó shàng rǎo	upper-body harassment by phlegm turbidity
痰濁蒙蔽心包	tán zhuó méng bì xīn bāo	clouding of the pericardium by phlegm turbidity
痦	péi	miliaria (371)
痹	bì	obturation (372)
痹證	bì zhèng	obturation patterns (373)
瘀	yū	stasis (374)
瘀斑	yū bān	stasis macules (376)
瘀塊	yū kuài	stasis clots (377)
瘀點	yū diǎn	stasis speckles (378)
痿	wěi	atony (379)
經	jīng	major channel; channel; menses
腠理	còu lǐ	striations (380)
腫	zhǒng	swelling (381)

腳氣	jiǎo qì	foot qi disease (382)
腸胃積滯	cháng wèi jī zhì	gastrointestinal accumulation
腸液虧耗	cháng yè kuī hào	intestinal humor depletion
腸虛滑脫	cháng xū huá tuō	intestinal vacuity (383) efflux desertion
腹水	fù shuǐ	ascites (384)
著	zhuó	leaden (385)
著痹	zhuó bì	leaden obturation
裡	lǐ	interior (386)
解	jiě	resolution (387)
解毒	jiě dú	detoxification (388)
辟穢	bì huì	repelling foulness (389)
電針	diàn zhēn	electroacupuncture

十四筆 Fourteen Strokes

嗽	sòu	expectoration (390)
嘈雜	cáo zá	clamoring stomach (391)
嘔	ǒu	retching (392)
嘔吐	ǒu tù	vomiting (393)
嘔血	ǒu xuè	retching of blood (394)
奪	duó	retrenchment (395)
寧	níng	quiet, quieting
實	shí	repletion (396)
實熱	shí rè	repletion heat
實腫	shí zhǒng	repletion swelling (397)
滯	zhì	stagnation (398)
滲	shèn	percolation (399)
滿	mǎn	fullness (400)
漏下	lòu xià	dribbling (or scant) (401) metrorrhagia
熄風	xí fēng	extinguishing wind (402)
瘧疾	nüè jí	malarial disease (403)
瞀	mào	visual distortion (404)
竭	jié	exhaustion (405)
精	jīng	essence; semen
精神	jīng shén	essence-spirit (406)
精氣	jīng qì	essential qi (407)
精液大泄	jīng yè dà xiè	profuse spermatorrhea (408)
聚	jù	gathering (409)
聞診	wén zhěn	audio-olfactive examination (410)
腐	fǔ	putrefaction, putrid

腐臭	fǔ chòu	putrid odor, putrid smelling (410.1)
膈	gé	diaphragm
膏	gāo	paste (411)
膏淋	gāo lín	turbid strangury (412)
蒙	méng	cloud (413)
蒸	zhēng	steam (414)
蓄	xù	amassment (416)
蓄血	xù xuè	blood amassment (417)

十五筆 Fifteen Strokes

噎膈	yē gé	esophageal constriction (418)
墜	zhuì	sagging
增液	zēng yè	increasing humor (419)
暴	bào	fulminant (420)
暴注	bào zhù	fulminant downpour (421)
潔腑	jié fǔ	cleansing the bladder
潛陽	qián yáng	subduing yang (422)
潤	rùn	moistening
潮熱	cháo rè	tidal fever (423)
熱	rè	heat (424)
熱入心包	rè rù xīn bāo	heat entering the pericardium
熱結腸胃	rè jié cháng wèi	gastrointestinal heat bind
熱閉痙厥	rè bì jìng jué	heat-block tetanic inversion (425)
熱痰	rè tán	heat phlegm
瘟	wēn	scourge
瘡瘍	chuāng yáng	lesion (426)
緩	huǎn	non-acute; moderate
蝦蟆瘟	há má wēn	toad-head scourge
衛	wèi	defense (427)
衛氣	wèi qì	defense qi
衛分證	wèi fēn zhèng	defense pattern
衛表	wèi biǎo	defensive exterior
養	yǎng	nourish (428)

十六筆 Sixteen Strokes

戰汗	zhàn hàn	shiver sweating
凝	níng	congealing (430)
噦逆	yuē nì	hiccup
壅	yǒng	congestion (431)

導	dǎo	abduction (432)
懊憹	ào nóng	upper ventral vexation (433)
澤	zé	moisturize (434)
濁	zhuó	turbid, turbidity (435)
熾	chì	intense heat (437)
燔	fán	blaze (438)
積	jī	accumulation (439)
膩	nì	rich, fatty (foods); sickly (taste in mouth); slimy (tongue fur)
蕩滌	dàng dí	flushing (440)
辨證	biàn zhèng	pattern identification
遺尿	yí niào	enuresis (441)
遺精	yí jīng	seminal emission (442)
醒	xǐng	rouse; resuscitate
錢	qián	*qian*; mace (442.1)
頭重如裹	tóu zhòng rú guǒ	bag-over-the-head sensation (443)
頭痛如掣	tóu tòng rú chè	iron-band sensation (444)
鴨溏	yā táng	duck stool (445)

十七筆 Seventeen Strokes

斂	liàn	constraining (446)
澀（濇）	sè	astringe; astringent (drugs); rough (pulse)
濡	rú	moisten
濕注下焦	shī zhù xià jiāo	downpour of damp into the lower burner
濕阻	shī zǔ	damp obstruction
濕阻中焦	shī zǔ zhōng jiāo	middle burner damp obstruction
濕從寒化	shī cóng hán huà	damp forming with cold (447)
濕從熱化	shī cóng rè huà	damp forming with heat (448)
濕溫	shī wēn	damp thermia
濕痰	shī tán	damp phlegm (449)
濕熱	shī rè	damp-heat
濕熱下注大腸	shī rè xià zhù dà cháng	downpour of damp-heat into large intestine
濕熱下注膀胱	shī rè xià zhù páng guāng	downpour of damp-heat the bladder
濕熱阻滯脾胃	shī rè zǔ zhì pí wèi	splenogastric damp-heat obstruction

濕熱留戀三焦	shī rè liú liàn sān jiāo	damp-heat lingering in the triple burner
濕熱留戀氣分	shī rè liú liàn qì fēn	damp-heat lodged in the qi aspect
濕熱蘊結肝胆	shī rè yùn jié gān dǎn	brewing hepatocystic damp-heat
濕蒙上焦	shī méng shàng jiāo	damp clouding the upper burner
濕濁	shī zhuó	damp turbidity (450)
營	yíng	construction (451)
營分證	yíng fēn zhèng	construction-aspect pattern
營衛不和	yíng wèi bù hé	defense-construction (452) disharmony
燥邪犯肺	zào xié fàn fèi	invasion of the lung by a dryness pathogen
燥痰	zào tán	dryness phlegm
癃閉	lóng bì	urinary block (453)
癃閉而失禁	lóng bì ér shī jīn	overflow incontinence (454)
癰腫	yǒng zhǒng	massiveness (455)
臊味	sāo wèi	animal odor (456)
臌（蠱）	gǔ	tympany (457)
虧	kuī	depletion (458)
豁	huò	sweeping (459)

Eighteen Strokes
十八筆

戴眼	dài yǎn	upward-fixed eyes (460)
戴陽	dài yáng	*dai-yang* (461)
擾	rǎo	harass (462)
瀉	xiè	draining (463)
癖	pǐ	elusive swelling
癘風	lì fēng	pestilential wind (leprosy)
癘氣	lì qì	pestilential qi
穢臭	huì chòu	foul odor (464)
穢濁	huì zhuó	foul turbidity (465)
竅	qiào	portal (466)
薰	xūn	fume (467)
薰蒸	xūn zhēng	swelter (468)
藏	cáng	store, storage
蟲類	chóng lèi	*chong* products (469)
轉化	zhuǎn huà	conversion (470)
轉胞	zhuǎn bāo	fetal pressure

轉筋	zhuǎn jīn	cramp (471)
轉變	zhuǎn biàn	transmutation
鎮	zhèn	settling (472)
鎮納	zhèn nà	settling and promoting qi absorption

十九筆 Nineteen Strokes

證	zhèng	pattern; sign (473)

二十筆 Twenty Strokes

懸飲	xuán yǐn	suspended rheum (474)
癥瘕積聚	zhēng jiǎ jī jù	concretions and gatherings (concretions, conglomerations, accumulations, and gatherings) (475)
蘊	yùn	brew (476)

二十一筆 Twenty-one Strokes

屬	shǔ	homing (477)
攝	shè	containment (478)

二十二筆 Twenty-two Strokes

臟	zàng	viscus (pl. viscera) (479)
臟腑學說	zàng xiàng xué shuō	visceral manifestation theory (479.1)
臟躁	zàng zào	visceral malaise
癮疹	yǐn zhěn	dormant papules (480)
襲	xí	assail (481)

二十三筆 Twenty-three Strokes

攣縮	lüán suō	contracture (483)
癰	yōng	abscess (484)
變	biàn	transmutation (485)
變證	biàn zhèng	transmuted pattern (486)
驚風	jīng fēng	fright wind (487)
驚厥	jīng jué	fright inversion (488)
體	tǐ	constitutional body (489)

Twenty-four strokes

二十四筆

癲	diān	withdrawal (490)
癲狂	diān kuáng	mania and withdrawal (491)
癱瘓	tān huàn	paralysis (492)

Twenty-nine Strokes

二十九筆

鬱	yù	depression (493)
鬱痰	yù tán	depressed phlegm (494)

Introduction

There are six related indexes in this section. These are:

Latin-Chinese Index of Chinese Drugs
Chinese-Latin Index of Chinese Drugs
English-Chinese Index of Chinese Medicinal Formulae
Chinese-English Index of Chinese Medicinal Formulae
Acumoxatherapy Index
Chinese Medical Concept Index

Each of these indexes contains page references to the text.

Foreword to the Drug Indexes

Most of the drug names in these listings are composed of the Latin name of the substance or plant, together with the part used. Chinese classifications do not always correspond to botanical classification: one entry in a Chinese pharmacopeia may be seen as various different plants according to botanical classification. Likewise, one botanical entity may appear under different headings in the pharmacopeia. These difficulties are further aggravated by the fact that botanical sources disagree on certain classifications, and that inconsistencies are to be found even in Chinese pharmacological sources. Thus, renderings have been chosen that properly highlight the distinctions in the Chinese pharmacopeia. *These do not necessarily reflect their exact botanical classification.* Wade-Giles transcriptions of the Chinese names are used where no single botanical term can adequately render the Chinese, or where unity of association would be jeopardized.

While effort has been made to ensure consistency with other listings currently used, some new distinctions have been made. For example, place names denoting the origin of drugs, often omitted in other listings, have been added. One plant may vary in properties or quality depending on its origin. In this context, it should be noted that, for example, the words *australis* (southern) and *septentrionalis* (northern), refer to southern China or locations south of China, and northern China, or locations north of China, respectively.

Following is a list of commonly used Latin terms with their English equivalents.

arillus ....aril	*carapax* ....carapace (dorsal shell)
ater ....black	
aureus ....golden, yellow	*carbonisatus* ......carbonized
australis ....southern	*caulis*...............stem
bulbus..............bulb	*concretio* ....concretion
cacumen..........cacumen	*corium* ....skin, hide

Introduction to the Indexes

cormus	corm	*orientalis*	eastern
cortex	bark	*os*	bone
crassus	thick	*pasta*	cake
cuticula	skin	*pedicellus*	pedicel (small stalk)
dens	tooth		
derma	skin	*pedunculus*	peduncle (flower stalk)
dulcis	sweet		
embryon	embryo	*pericarpium*	pericarp
exocarpium	exocarp; epicarp (outermost layer of pericarp)	*periostracum*	snake slough
		pinguis	oily, greasy
		plastrum	plastron (ventral shell)
exsiccatus	dried (out)		
extractum	extract	*preparatio*	preparation
fibra	fiber	*preparatus*	prepared
flavus	yellow, light brown	*pulvis*	powder
flos	flower	*radix*	root
folium	leaf	*ramulus*	twig
fossilia	fossil	*ramus*	branch
fructificatio	fructification	*recens*	fresh (not dried)
fructus	fruit	*receptaculum*	receptacle
gluten	glue	*rhizoma*	rhizome
gummi	gum	*sclerotium*	sclerotium
herba	herb	*secretio*	secretion
hiemalis	winter	*sectus*	cut, sliced
hominis	human	*semen*	seed
insulsus	unsalted, bland	*spina*	thorn, prickle
iecur	liver	*squama*	scale, scaly armor
in taenis	shavings	*stylus*	style; botanical term denoting filiform extension of ovary
lapis	stone		
lignum	wood		
medulla	pith		
mesocarpium	mesocarp; middle layer of pericarp	*testa*	testa; outer, usually hard, integument of a seed
niger	black	*vivus*	fresh

Foreword to the Medical Concepts Index

For some entries the glossary page reference is included (e.g. "pn-543"), as is the reference number for the Chinese characters (e.g. "gl-161"). Entries are contextual, that is, as stated in the text or as used in technical conversation. Thus "fine, weak pulse" is located in the "fine" division, not as "pulse; fine, weak."

Latin — Chinese Index
of
Chinese Drugs

Agkistrodon — fù shé: 272
Arillus Euphoriae Longanae — lóng yǎn: 194, 207, 412
Bombyx Batryticatus — jiāng cán: 240, 274, 312-313, 425, 439, 446
Bulbus Allii Macrostemi — xiè bái: 210
Bulbus Fritillariae — bèi mǔ: 422, 424
Bulbus Fritillariae Cirrhosae — chuān bèi mǔ: 213, 215, 217, 300, 311, 434
Bulbus Fritillariae Thunbergii — xiàng bèi mǔ: 212, 267
Bulbus Lilii — bǎi hé: 207, 217, 414
Bulbus Shan Tz'u Ku — shān cí gū: 422
Buthus — quán xiē: 240, 270, 274, 312-313, 409, 425, 446
Cacumen Biotae — cè bó yè: 440-441
Carapax Amydae — biē jiǎ: 172, 238, 240-241, 244, 388, 413
Catharsius — qiāng láng: 421
Caulis Bambusae in Taenis — zhú fú 229, 403, 426, 445
Caulis Mu T'ung — mù tōng: 208, 296, 431
Caulis Perillae — sū gěng: 234
Caulis Piperis Kadsurae — hǎi fēng téng: 270
Caulis Polygoni Multiflori — yè jiāo téng: 207
Caulis Sargentodoxae — hóng téng: 383
Cera Chinensis Aurea — huáng là: 443
Cinnabaris — zhū shā: 205, 207, 444
Concha Arcae — wǎ léng zǐ: 225
Concha Haliotidis — shí jué míng: 238
Concha Margaritifera — zhēn zhū mǔ: 238, 444, 446
Concha Ostreae — mǔ lì: 176, 205, 238, 240, 249, 287, 407, 422, 438, 444, 446
Concha Ostreae tempered — duàn mǔ lì: 436, 443
Concretio Siliceae Bambusae — tiān zhú huáng: 425, 434
Cornu Antelopis — líng yáng jiǎo: 238, 240, 355, 446
Cornu Cervi — lù jiǎo: 172, 248, 376, 415
Cornu Rhinoceri — xī jiǎo: 385
Cortex Cinnamomi — ròu guì: 167, 172, 211, 221, 246, 276-278, 280, 287, 394, 406-407, 415, 429, 448
Cortex Eucommiae — dù zhòng: 248
Cortex Fraxini — qín pí: 295, 429

Cortex Magnoliae — hòu pò: 285, 290, 293, 297, 309, 338, 386-387, 392, 427-428

Cortex Perillae — bái sū pí: 387

Cortex Phellodendri — huáng bó: 169, 217, 283, 294-295, 382, 386, 429, 432, 449

Cortex Radicis Lycii — dì gǔ pí: 169, 283, 388

Cortex Radicis Mori — sāng bái pí: 213, 311

Cortex Radicis Mu Tan — mǔ dān pí: 197, 209, 236, 283, 382, 385, 392-393, 402, 420, 446

Dens Draconis — lóng chǐ: 238, 444, 446

Egg Yolk — jī zǐ huáng: 302

Embryon Nelumbinis — lián zǐ xīn: 208

Endothelium Gigeriae Galli — jī nèi jīn: 305, 418, 422

Epicarpium Citri Tangerinae — jú hóng: 297

Eupolyphaga — dì biē chóng: 196, 398, 421

Excrementum Trogopteri — wǔ líng zhī: 420

Exocarpium Citrulli Vulgaris — xī guā cuì yī: 284

Exocarpium Pyri — lí pí: 214, 300

Ferric Oxide — shēng tiě luò: 444

Fibra Stipulae Trachycarpi — zōng lǘ pí: 440-441

Flos Carthami — hóng huā: 196, 210, 242, 398, 402, 420

Flos Caryophylli — dīng xiāng: 276

Flos Chrysanthemi — jú huā: 236, 272, 446

Flos Daphnes Genkwa — yuán huā: 395

Flos Inulae — xuán fù huā: 229

Flos Lonicerae — yín huā: 268, 282, 311, 353, 379, 382, 385, 392, 419, 432

Flos Sophorae Immatura — huái huā: 440-441

Flos Tussilagi Farfarae — kuǎn dōng huā: 214-215, 424, 437

Fluoritum — zǐ shí yīng: 442, 448

Folium Artemisiae Argyi — ài yè: 440-441

Folium Bambusae — zhú yè: 208

Folium Bambusae Vivum — xiān zhú yè: 284

Folium Clerodendri Trichotoni — chòu wú tóng: 270

Folium Eriobotryae — pí pa yè: 213, 215, 437

Folium Mori — sāng yè: 163, 209, 213, 236, 268, 272, 300, 379, 446

Folium Nelumbinis — hé yè: 428, 440-441

Folium Perillae — sū yè: 162, 267, 377-378, 381

Folium Pyrrosiae — shí wěi: 296, 431

Folium Ta Ch'ing Yeh — dà qīng yè: 268, 282, 382, 385, 392

Fructus Akebiae — bā yuè zhā: 234
Fructus Alpiniae Oxyphyllae — yì zhì rén: 246
Fructus Amomi — shā rén: 220, 307, 373, 417, 427-428
Fructus Amomi Cardamomi — kòu rén: 292, 297, 386, 427-428
Fructus Arctii — niú bàng zǐ: 163, 212, 268, 286, 300, 379, 393, 424
Fructus Aristolochiae — mǎ dōu líng: 213, 215, 437
Fructus Citri — zhǐ ké: 191, 230, 234, 373, 417, 428
Fructus Citri Immaturus — zhǐ shí: 294, 305, 307, 392, 401, 419, 422, 426
Fructus Crataegi — shān zhā: 210, 305, 418
Fructus Crataegi Carbonisatus — shān zhā tàn: 419
Fructus Cubebae — bì chéng: 276
Fructus Evodiae — wú zhū yú: 167, 224, 229, 276, 278, 280, 403
Fructus Foeniculi — xiǎo huí xiāng: 278
Fructus Forsythiae — lián qiào: 208, 268, 282, 286, 353, 379, 382
Fructus Gardeniae — zhī zǐ: 209, 226, 236, 282, 286, 292-294, 296, 353, 379, 382-384, 393, 402, 429, 446
Fructus Gleditsiae — zào jiá: 424
Fructus Hordei Germinatus — mài yá: 305, 307, 418
Fructus Ligustri Lucidi — nǚ zhēn zǐ: 238, 241, 245, 413, 446
Fructus Liquidambaris — lù lù tōng: 234
Fructus Lycii — qǐ zǐ: 194, 235, 238, 241, 248, 303-304, 376, 412, 416
Fructus Meliae Toosendan — chuān liàn zǐ: 192, 225, 234, 402
Fructus Mori — sāng shēn zǐ: 194, 241, 304, 413
Fructus Oryzae Sativae Germinatus — gǔ yá: 307, 418-419
Fructus Perillae Crispae — sū zǐ: 214, 310, 424
Fructus Psoraleae — bǔ gǔ zhī: 246, 438
Fructus Rosae Laevigatae — jīn yīng zǐ: 249, 438
Fructus Schisandrae — wǔ wèi zǐ: 216, 287, 408, 436, 438
Fructus Terminaliae Chebulae — hē zǐ: 230, 436
Fructus Tribuli — jí lí: 238
Fructus Trichosanthis — guā lóu: 210, 311, 396, 424
Fructus Xanthii — cāng ěr zǐ: 272
Fructus Zanthoxyli Szechuanensis — chuān jiāo: 276, 406
Fructus Zizyphi Jujubae — dà zǎo: 224, 401
Galenitum — qīng qiān: 448
Gecko — gé jiè: 448
Gelatinum Corii Asini — lǘ pí jiāo: 177, 119, 193, 199, 217, 223, 240-241, 302, 412-413, 416-417, 431, 442, 444, 446

Gummi Olibanum — rǔ xiāng: 420
Gypsum — shí gāo: 39, 168, 226, 284, 383-384
Haematitum — dài zhě shí: 229, 237
Halloysitum Rubrum — chì shí zhī: 230, 438, 442
Herba Agastaches — huò xiāng: 285, 290, 292-293, 297, 351, 386, 427-428
Herba Agrimoniae — xiān hè cǎo: 440, 442
Herba Allii Fistulosi — cōng bái: 286, 378, 381
Herba Aloes — lú huì: 394
Herba Andrographis — chuān xīn lián: 282, 432
Herba Artemisiae Apiaceae — qīng hāo: 169, 283, 285, 292, 384, 388, 401
Herba Artemisiae Capillaris — yīn chén: 294, 429
Herba Asari — xì xīn: 275, 280, 310, 317, 409
Herba Cephalanoploris — xiǎo jì cǎo: 196-197, 296, 432, 440-441
Herba Chin Ch'ien Ts'ao — jīn qián cǎo: 296, 422
Herba Cirsii Japonici — dà jì: 441
Herba Cistanches — cōng róng: 231, 248, 304, 396, 415
Herba Commelinae — yā zhí cǎo: 432
Herba Cynomorii — suǒ yáng: 248, 417
Herba Dendrobii — shí hú: 172, 227, 283-284, 413, 417
Herba Dendrobii Viva — xiān shí hú: 301, 384
Herba Dianthi — qū mài: 296, 431
Herba Ecliptae — hàn lián cǎo: 193, 241, 245, 413, 417, 440
Herba Elsholtziae — xiāng rú: 285
Herba Ephedrae — má huáng: 162, 212, 267, 275, 280, 310, 317, 338, 378, 380
Herba Epimedii — xiān líng pí: 246, 415, 417, 449
Herba Eupatorii — pèi lán: 285, 290, 292, 297, 386, 427-428
Herba Euphorbiae Humifusae — dì jǐn cǎo: 432
Herba Gentianae Macrophyllae — qín jiāo: 270, 388
Herba Houttuyniae — yú xīng cǎo: 311, 432
Herba Lemnae — fú píng: 272
Herba Leonuri — yì mǔ cǎo: 196, 420
Herba Lophatheri — dàn zhú yè: 386
Herba Lycopi — zé lán: 196, 420
Herba Menthae — bò hé: 163, 268, 272, 286, 379, 381, 428
Herba Perillae Crispae — zǐ sū: 403
Herba Polygoni Avicularis — biǎn xù: 296, 431
Herba Polygoni Hydropiperis — là liǎo: 277
Herba Portulacae — mǎ chǐ xiàn: 295, 383
Herba Pteridis — fèng wěi cǎo: 432

Herba Rorippae — hān cài: 424
Herba Sargassii — hǎi zǎo: 316, 422
Herba Schizonepetae — jīng jiè: 162, 267, 271, 377, 380
Herba Sedi Sarmentosi — chuí pén cǎo: 294
Herba Siegesbeckiae — xī xiān cǎo: 270
Herba et Radix Taraxaci — pú gōng yīng: 268, 311, 379, 382, 392, 432
Hirudo — shuǐ zhì: 421
Lapis Chloriti — méng shí: 315, 397
Lignum Aquilariae — chén xiāng: 192, 237
Lignum Dalbergiae Odoriferae — jiàng xiāng: 210
Limonitum — yǔ yú liáng: 230, 438, 442
Lumbricus — dì lóng: 240, 270, 274, 446
Magnetitum — cí shí: 205, 207, 287, 444, 446, 448
Massa Fermentata — liù qū: 305, 418
Massa Fermentata Ustulata — jiāo liù qū: 419
Medulla Junci — dēng xīn: 208
Medulla Tetrapanacis — tōng cǎo: 290, 298, 386, 428, 431
Mesocarpium Corni — yú ròu: 241, 245, 248, 416-417, 439, 448
Mirabilitum — máng xiāo: 40, 196, 282, 316, 391, 398-399, 401, 422
Myrrha — mò yào: 420
Nodus Rhizomatis Nelumbinis — ǒu jié: 432
Oötheca Mantidis — sāng piāo xiāo: 249, 439
Os Draconis — lóng gǔ: 176, 205, 249, 287, 407, 438, 444
Os Draconis tempered — duàn lóng gǔ: 436
Os Sepiae — wū zéi gǔ: 225
Os Sepiae tempered — duàn zéi gǔ: 443
Os in Cornu Bovis — niú jiǎo sāi: 441-442
Pericarpium Alpiniae — kòu ké: 287
Pericarpium Benincasae — dōng guā pí: 431
Pericarpium Citri Reticulatae Viride — qīng pí: 192, 234, 402
Pericarpium Citri Reticulatae — chén pí: 191, 214, 220, 225, 229-230, 307, 309, 313, 373, 404, 417, 424, 426-427
Pericarpium Lagenariae — hú lú piáo: 431
Pericarpium Papaveris — yīng sù ké: 230, 436, 438
Pericarpium Punicae Granati — shí liú pí: 230
Pericarpium Trichosanthis — guā lóu pí: 300
Periostracum Cicadae — chán yī: 270, 272, 286
Placenta Hominis — zǐ hé jū: 248, 416-417

Plastrum Testudinis — guī bǎn: 172, 217, 238, 240-241, 244, 248, 302, 413, 416, 446
Pollen Typhae — pú huáng: 196-197, 296, 420, 441
Poria cum Radice Pini — fú shén: 205, 207
Pulvis Arisaemae cum Felle Bovis — dǎn nán xīng: 315, 425
Pulvis Seminis Crotonis — bā dòu shuāng: 394, 397
Radix Achyranthis — tǔ niú xī: 393
Radix Achyranthis Bidentatae — niú xī: 242
Radix Aconiti Fu Tzu — fù zǐ: 167, 172, 176, 205, 211, 221, 223, 246, 275, 277, 280, 287, 317, 343, 372, 394, 406-408, 415-416, 429, 437, 448-449
Radix Aconiti Wu T'ou — wū tóu: 275
Radix Aconiti Wu T'ou Szechuanensis — chuān wū: 409
Radix Adenophorae — shā shēn: 214, 217, 227, 284, 300, 413, 417, 424
Radix Adenophorae Viva — xiān shā shēn: 301, 384
Radix Angelicae — bái zhǐ: 39, 429
Radix Angelicae Sinensis — dāng guī: 172, 193, 196, 199, 207, 210, 235, 241, 303-304, 399, 402, 409, 412, 417, 444
Radix Angelicae Sinensis Pinguis — yóu dāng guī: 396
Radix Asteris — zǐ wǎn: 214, 424, 437
Radix Astragali — huáng qí: 171, 190, 199, 205, 216, 223, 280, 409, 411, 416, 436
Radix Bupleuri — chái hú: 192, 222, 234, 287, 294, 401-402, 404
Radix Caraganae Sinicae — jīn què gēn: 270
Radix Clematidis — wēi líng xiān: 270
Radix Codonopsis Pilosulae — dǎng shēn: 167, 171, 190, 199, 205, 211, 216, 220, 223, 280, 307, 407, 409, 411, 437, 444
Radix Cynanchi Atrati — bái wéi: 169, 388
Radix Dioscoreae — shān yào: 219, 249, 307, 438-439
Radix Dipsaci — xù duàn: 242
Radix Euphorbiae — dà jǐ: 317, 395
Radix Euphorbiae Kan Sui — gān suì: 317, 395
Radix Fagopyri Vulgaris — yě qiáo: 383
Radix Fang Chi — fáng jǐ: 429
Radix Gentianae — lóng dǎn cǎo: 209, 236, 294, 386, 394
Radix Ginseng — rén shēn: 167, 176, 205, 287, 340, 344, 372, 401, 407, 416
Radix Glycyrrhizae — gān cǎo: 167, 171, 190, 199, 211, 216, 220, 223-224, 280, 284, 287, 401, 407, 411, 444
Radix Glycyrrhizae mix-fried — zhì gān cǎo: 205, 406
Radix Glycyrrhizae Recens — shēng gān cǎo: 208

Radix Isatidis — bǎn lán gēn: 268, 282, 294, 379, 382, 385
Radix Ledebouriellae — fáng fēng: 39, 162, 267, 270-271, 377, 380, 429
Radix Linderae — wū yào: 234, 278
Radix Lithospermi — zǐ cǎo: 385, 392
Radix Morindae — bā jǐ ròu: 248
Radix Paeoniae — sháo yào: 177, 402
Radix Paeoniae Albae — bái sháo: 193, 224, 235, 238, 240-241, 303-304, 338, 378, 404, 409, 436
Radix Paeoniae Rubrae — chì sháo: 196-197, 236, 382, 385, 420
Radix Peucedani — qián hú: 267, 424
Radix Platycodi — jié gěng: 212, 267, 287, 297, 424
Radix Polygalae — yuǎn zhì: 207, 223, 315, 434
Radix Polygoni Multiflori — shǒu wū: 193, 241, 245, 303-304, 412, 417
Radix Polygoni Multiflori Viva — xiān shǒu wū: 231, 396
Radix Pseudoginseng — sān qī: 196, 420, 441
Radix Puerariae — gé gēn: 39, 287, 338, 379, 381, 384
Radix Pulsatillae — bái tóu wēng: 295, 383
Radix Rehmanniae — dì huáng: 177, 240-241, 244, 304
Radix Rehmanniae Conquita — shóu dì: 172, 193, 199, 207, 248, 303, 376, 392, 408, 416-417, 448
Radix Rehmanniae Cruda — shēng dì: 172, 207, 217, 223, 226-227, 235-236, 238, 283, 303, 381, 412-413, 417, 442, 444, 446
Radix Rehmanniae Viva — xiān shēng dì: 197, 231, 301, 385
Radix Rubiae — qiàn cǎo: 196, 402
Radix Rumicis — tǔ dà huáng: 440
Radix Salviae Miltiorrhizae — dān shēn: 194, 196, 205, 207, 210, 303, 402, 420, 444
Radix Sanguisorbae — dì yú: 197, 295, 441
Radix Saussureae — mù xiāng: 191, 225, 230, 373
Radix Scrophulariae — xuán shēn: 172, 217, 226, 231, 244, 283, 302, 385, 393, 396, 413-414, 417, 446
Radix Scutellariae — huáng qín: 168, 213, 217, 226, 236, 282, 285, 292-295, 311, 353, 355, 379, 382, 386-387, 392, 401, 405, 419, 429, 449
Radix Sophorae Flavescentis — kǔ shēn: 387, 429
Radix Stellariae Dichotomae — yín chái hú: 169, 388
Radix Stemonae — bǎi bù: 213, 437
Radix Trichosanthis — tiān huā fěn: 227, 300-301, 384
Radix Tu Huo — dú huó: 270, 409
Radix et Caulis Chi Hsüeh T'eng — jī xuè téng: 194, 242, 320
Radix et Rhizoma Oryzae Glutinosae — nuò dào gēn: 436

Ramulus Cinnamomi — guì zhī: 162, 205, 210, 224, 267, 275, 280, 299, 310, 317, 338, 378, 408-409, 416, 429, 431, 437, 444
Ramulus Mori — sāng zhī: 270
Ramulus et Folium Tamaricis — xī hé liǔ: 286, 379
Ramulus et Uncus Uncariae — gōu téng: 238, 240, 274, 313, 355, 446
Ramus Loranthi — sāng jì shēng: 242
Rhizoma Aconiti Coreani — bái fù zǐ: 270, 312, 425
Rhizoma Acori Graminei — chāng pú: 210, 315, 357, 434, 444
Rhizoma Alismatis — zé xiè: 296, 298, 408
Rhizoma Alpiniae Officinari — liáng jiāng: 167, 224, 276, 406
Rhizoma Anemarrhenae — zhī mǔ: 39, 168-169, 217, 226, 282-284, 383-384, 449
Rhizoma Arisaematis — nán xīng: 312, 424, 434
Rhizoma Atractylodis — cāng zhú: 285, 290, 293, 297, 309, 351, 386, 427
Rhizoma Atractylodis Macrocephalae — bái zhú: 167, 190, 219, 277, 280, 290, 299, 307, 313, 404, 406, 417, 426, 428, 431, 437
Rhizoma Bletillae — bái jí: 441
Rhizoma Cimicifugae — shēng má: 39, 222, 287
Rhizoma Coptidis — huáng lián: 119, 168, 208, 226, 229, 282, 284-285, 293, 295, 355, 382, 386-387, 392, 403, 405, 429, 445, 449
Rhizoma Corydalis — yán hú suǒ: 225, 234, 402, 420
Rhizoma Curculiginis — xiān máo: 246, 415, 417, 449
Rhizoma Curcumae Zedoariae — é zhú: 196, 398, 421
Rhizoma Cyperi — xiāng fù: 191, 225, 234, 402
Rhizoma Dioscoreae Pi Hsieh — bì xiè: 296
Rhizoma Gastrodiae — tiān má: 238, 240, 313, 426
Rhizoma Imperatae Vivum — xiān máo gēn: 197
Rhizoma Imperatae — máo gēn: 300, 440-441
Rhizoma Ligustici Wallichii Szechuanensis — chuān xiōng: 420
Rhizoma Phragmitis — lú gēn: 39, 226, 300, 384
Rhizoma Phragmitis Vivum — xiān lú gēn: 301, 311
Rhizoma Pinelliae — bàn xià: 214, 229, 285, 290, 292-293, 309-310, 312-313, 315, 386-387, 401, 403, 405, 424, 426-427
Rhizoma Polygonati Odorati — yù zhú: 217, 227, 381, 413
Rhizoma Polygoni Cuspidati — hǔ zhàng: 294
Rhizoma Rhei — dà huáng: 40, 168, 196, 226, 282, 294, 391-395, 398-399, 401, 420, 422, 429
Rhizoma Smilacis Glabrae — tǔ fú líng: 387
Rhizoma Sparganii — sān léng: 196, 398, 421

Rhizoma Zingiberis blast-fried — pāo jiāng: 221, 223, 276-277, 406, 449

Rhizoma Zingiberis Carbonisatum — pāo jiāng tàn: 441

Rhizoma Zingiberis Exsiccatum — gān jiāng: 167, 280, 310, 317, 345, 394, 405-408, 424, 429, 437

Rhizoma Zingiberis Recens — shēng jiāng: 167, 211, 224, 229, 280, 377, 382, 401, 403

Rhizoma et Radix Notopterygii — qiāng huó: 162, 267, 270-271, 287, 377, 380, 429

Saccharum Granorum — yí táng: 224

Sal Petrae — xiāo shí: 422

Sclerotium Polypori Umbellati — zhū líng: 296, 428, 431

Sclerotium Poriae — fú líng: 190, 285, 290, 298-299, 307, 309, 313, 315-316, 351, 386, 404, 406, 408, 426, 428, 431

Scolopendra — wú gōng: 270, 274, 425

Semen Alpiniae Katsumadai — cǎo dòu kòu: 429

Semen Arecae — bīn láng: 192, 305, 419

Semen Astragali Complanati — tóng jí lí: 249, 439

Semen Benincasae — dōng guā rén: 311, 424

Semen Biotae — bó zǐ rén: 207, 231, 414, 445

Semen Cannabis — má rén: 231, 396

Semen Cassiae — jué míng zǐ: 394

Semen Celosiae — qīng xiāng zǐ: 236

Semen Citri — jú hé: 234, 278, 287

Semen Coicis — yì yǐ rén: 290, 292, 428, 431

Semen Cuscutae — tù sī zǐ: 248, 376, 439

Semen Dolichoris — biǎn dòu: 219, 290, 307, 428

Semen Euryalis — qiàn shí: 249, 438, 443

Semen Gingko — bái guǒ: 443

Semen Glycenes Germinatum — dà dòu juǎn: 351

Semen Hydnocarpi — dà fēng zǐ: 272

Semen Juglandis — hú táo ròu: 448

Semen Myristicae — ròu dòu kòu: 230, 438

Semen Nelumbinis — lián zǐ ròu: 438

Semen Persicae — táo rén: 196, 210, 231, 398, 420

Semen Pharbitidis — qiān niú zǐ: 317, 395

Semen Plantaginis — chē qián zǐ: 290, 298, 408

Semen Pruni Armeniacae — xìng rén: 214, 267, 292, 297, 338, 396, 424, 428

Semen Raphani — lái fú zǐ: 305, 419

Semen Sesame Atrum — hēi zhī má: 303
Semen Sinapis Albae — bái jiè zǐ: 214, 310, 316-317, 424
Semen Sojae Praeparatum — dòu shǐ: 163, 268, 286, 379, 381, 384
Semen T'ing Li Tzu — tíng lì zǐ: 311, 317, 397, 424
Semen Trichosanthis — guā lóu rén: 231
Semen Trigonellae — hú lú bā: 246, 278, 417
Semen Tritici — huái xiǎo mài: 207, 436
Semen Zizyphi Jujubae — zǎo rén: 194, 205, 207, 223, 445
Semen/Herba Plantaginis — chē qián zǐ/cǎo: 296, 431
Spica Prunellae — xià kū cǎo: 236, 316, 394, 422, 446
Squama Manitis — shān jiǎ: 196, 398
Stalactitum — zhōng rǔ shí: 448
Stamen Nelumbinis — lián xū: 249, 438
Stylus Zeae — yù mǐ xū: 431
Styrax Liquidis — hé xiāng: 210
Succus Bambusae — zhú lì: 311-312, 315, 434
Succus Zingiberis — jiāng zhī: 312, 315, 399
Sulfur Praeparatum — zhì liú huáng: 396
Tabanus — méng chóng: 421
Talcum — huá shí: 290, 296, 298, 351, 386, 428, 431
Terra Flava Usta — zào xīn tǔ: 223, 441
Testa Glycines — lǜ dòu yī: 436
Thallus Algae — kūn bù: 316, 422
Tuber Asparagi — tiān dōng: 217, 238, 244, 413
Tuber Colocasiae — yù nǎi: 422
Tuber Curcumae — yù jīn: 192, 210, 234, 294, 315, 357, 402, 434
Tuber Dioscoreae Bulbiferae — huáng yào zǐ: 422
Tuber Ophiopogonis — mài dōng: 172, 207, 214, 217, 226-227, 231, 238, 283-284, 381, 413-414, 417, 446
Zaocys — wū shāo shé: 270

Chinese — Latin Index
of
Chinese Drugs

ài yè — Folium Artemisiae Argyi: 440-441
bā dòu shuāng — Pulvis Seminis Crotonis: 394, 397
bā jǐ ròu — Radix Morindae: 248
bā yuè zhā — Fructus Akebiae: 234
bǎi bù — Radix Stemonae: 213, 437
bái fù zǐ — Rhizoma Aconiti Coreani: 270, 312, 425
bái guǒ — Semen Gingko: 443
bǎi hé — Bulbus Lilii: 207, 217, 414
bái jí — Rhizoma Bletillae: 441
bái jiè zǐ — Semen Sinapis Albae: 214, 310, 316-317, 424
bái sháo — Radix Paeoniae Albae: 193, 224, 235, 238, 240-241, 303-304, 338, 378, 404, 409, 436
bái sū pí — Cortex Perillae: 387
bái tóu wēng — Radix Pulsatillae: 295, 383
bái wéi — Radix Cynanchi Atrati: 169, 388
bái zhǐ — Radix Angelicae: 39, 429
bái zhú — Rhizoma Atractylodis Macrocephalae: 167, 190, 219, 277, 280, 290, 299, 307, 313, 404, 406, 417, 426, 428, 431, 437
bǎn lán gēn — Radix Isatidis: 268, 282, 294, 379, 382, 385
bàn xià — Rhizoma Pinelliae: 214, 229, 285, 290, 292-293, 309-310, 312-313, 315, 386-387, 401, 403, 405, 424, 426-427
bèi mǔ — Bulbus Fritillariae: 422, 424
bì chéng — Fructus Cubebae: 276
bì xiè — Rhizoma Dioscoreae Pi Hsieh: 296
biǎn dòu — Semen Dolichoris: 219, 290, 307, 428
biǎn xù — Herba Polygoni Avicularis: 296, 431
biē jiǎ — Carapax Amydae: 172, 238, 240-241, 244, 388, 413
bīn láng — Semen Arecae: 192, 305, 419
bò hé — Herba Menthae: 163, 268, 272, 286, 379, 381, 428
bó zǐ rén — Semen Biotae: 207, 231, 414, 445
bǔ gǔ zhǐ — Fructus Psoraleae: 246, 438
cāng ěr zǐ — Fructus Xanthii: 272
cāng zhú — Rhizoma Atractylodis: 285, 290, 293, 297, 309, 351, 386, 427
cǎo dòu kòu — Semen Alpiniae Katsumadai: 429
cè bó yè — Cacumen Biotae: 440-441
chái hú — Radix Bupleuri: 192, 222, 234, 287, 294, 401-402, 404

chán yī — Periostracum Cicadae: 270, 272, 286
chāng pú — Rhizoma Acori Graminei: 210, 315, 357, 434, 444
chē qián zǐ — Semen Plantaginis: 290, 298, 408
chē qián zǐ/cǎo — Semen/Herba Plantaginis: 296, 431
chén pí — Pericarpium Citri Reticulatae: 191, 214, 220, 225, 229-230, 307, 309, 313, 373, 404, 417, 424, 426-427
chén xiāng — Lignum Aquilariae: 192, 237
chì sháo — Radix Paeoniae Rubrae: 196-197, 236, 382, 385, 420
chì shí zhǐ — Halloysitum Rubrum: 230, 438, 442
chòu wú tóng — Folium Clerodendri Trichotoni: 270
chuān bèi mǔ — Bulbus Fritillariae Cirrhosae: 213, 215, 217, 300, 311, 434
chuān jiāo — Fructus Zanthoxyli Szechuanensis: 276, 406
chuān liàn zǐ — Fructus Meliae Toosendan: 192, 225, 234, 402
chuān wū — Radix Aconiti Wu T'ou Szechuanensis: 409
chuān xīn lián — Herba Andrographis: 282, 432
chuān xiōng — Rhizoma Ligustici Wallichii Szechuanensis: 420
chuí pén cǎo — Herba Sedi Sarmentosi: 294
cí shí — Magnetitum: 205, 207, 287, 444, 446, 448
cōng bái — Herba Allii Fistulosi: 286, 378, 381
cōng róng — Herba Cistanches: 231, 248, 304, 396, 415
dà dòu juǎn — Semen Glycenes Germinatum: 351
dà fēng zǐ — Semen Hydnocarpi: 272
dà huáng — Rhizoma Rhei: 40, 168, 196, 226, 282, 294, 391-395, 398-399, 401, 420, 422, 429
dà jì — Herba Cirsii Japonici: 441
dà jǐ — Radix Euphorbiae: 317, 395
dà qīng yè — Folium Ta Ch'ing Yeh: 268, 282, 382, 385, 392
dà zǎo — Fructus Zizyphi Jujubae: 224, 401
dài zhě shí — Haematitum: 229, 237
dǎn nán xīng — Pulvis Arisaemae cum Felle Bovis: 315, 425
dān shēn — Radix Salviae Miltiorrhizae: 194, 196, 205, 207, 210, 303, 399, 402, 420, 444
dàn zhú yè — Herba Lophatheri: 386
dāng guī — Radix Angelicae Sinensis: 172, 193, 196, 199, 207, 210, 235, 241, 303-304, 399, 402, 409, 412, 417, 444
dǎng shēn — Radix Codonopsis Pilosulae: 167, 171, 190, 199, 205, 211, 216, 220, 223, 280, 307, 407, 409, 411, 437, 444
dēng xīn — Medulla Junci: 208
dì biē chóng — Eupolyphaga: 196, 398, 421
dì gǔ pí — Cortex Radicis Lycii: 169, 283, 388

dì huáng — Radix Rehmanniae: 177, 240-241, 244, 304
dì jǐn cǎo — Herba Euphorbiae Humifusae: 432
dì lóng — Lumbricus: 240, 270, 274, 446
dì yú — Radix Sanguisorbae: 197, 295, 441
dīng xiāng — Flos Caryophylli: 276
dōng guā pí — Pericarpium Benincasae: 431
dōng guā rén — Semen Benincasae: 311, 424
dòu shì — Semen Sojae Praeparatum: 163, 268, 286, 379, 381, 384
dú huó — Radix Tu Huo: 270, 409
dù zhòng — Cortex Eucommiae: 248
duàn lóng gǔ — Os Draconis tempered: 436
duàn mǔ lì — Concha Ostreae tempered: 436, 443
duàn zéi gǔ — Os Sepiae tempered: 443
é zhú — Rhizoma Curcumae Zedoariae: 196, 398, 421
fáng fēng — Radix Ledebouriellae: 39, 162, 267, 270-271, 377, 380, 429
fáng jǐ — Radix Fang Chi: 429
fèng wěi cǎo — Herba Pteridis: 432
fú líng — Sclerotium Poriae: 190, 285, 290, 298-299, 307, 309, 313, 315-316, 351, 386, 404, 406, 408, 426, 428, 431
fú píng — Herba Lemnae: 272
fù shé — Agkistrodon: 272
fú shén — Poria cum Radice Pini: 205, 207
fù zǐ — Radix Aconiti Fu Tzu: 167, 172, 176, 205, 211, 221, 223, 246, 275, 277, 280, 287, 317, 343, 372, 394, 406-408, 415-416, 429, 437, 448-449
gān cǎo — Radix Glycyrrhizae: 167, 171, 190, 199, 211, 216, 220, 223-224, 280, 284, 287, 401, 407, 411, 444
gé gēn — Radix Puerariae: 39, 287, 338, 379, 381, 384
gān jiāng — Rhizoma Zingiberis Exsiccatum: 167, 280, 310, 317, 345, 394, 405-408, 424, 429, 437
gān suì — Radix Euphorbiae Kan Sui: 317, 395
gé jiè — Gecko: 448
gōu téng — Ramulus et Uncus Uncariae: 238, 240, 274, 313, 355, 446
gǔ yá — Fructus Oryzae Sativae Germinatus: 307, 418-419
guā lóu — Fructus Trichosanthis: 210, 311, 396, 424
guā lóu pí — Pericarpium Trichosanthis: 300
guā lóu rén — Semen Trichosanthis: 231
guī bǎn — Plastrum Testudinis: 172, 217, 238, 240-241, 244, 248, 302, 413, 416, 446

guì zhī — Ramulus Cinnamomi: 162, 205, 210, 224, 267, 275, 280, 299, 310, 317, 338, 378, 408-409, 416, 429, 431, 437, 444
hǎi fēng téng — Caulis Piperis Kadsurae: 270
hǎi zǎo — Herba Sargassii: 316, 422
hān cài — Herba Rorippae: 424
hàn lián cǎo — Herba Ecliptae: 193, 241, 245, 413, 417, 440
hē zǐ — Fructus Terminaliae Chebulae: 230, 436
hé xiāng — Styrax Liquidis: 210
hé yè — Folium Nelumbinis: 428, 440-441
hēi zhī má — Semen Sesame Atrum: 303
hóng huā — Flos Carthami: 196, 210, 242, 398, 402, 420
hóng téng — Caulis Sargentodoxae: 383
hòu pò — Cortex Magnoliae: 285, 290, 293, 297, 309, 338, 386-387, 392, 427-428
hú lú bā — Semen Trigonellae: 246, 278, 417
hú lú piáo — Pericarpium Lagenariae: 431
hú táo ròu — Semen Juglandis: 448
hǔ zhàng — Rhizoma Polygoni Cuspidati: 294
huá shí — Talcum: 290, 296, 298, 351, 386, 428, 431
huái huā — Flos Sophorae Immatura: 440-441
huái xiǎo mài — Semen Tritici: 207, 436
huáng bó — Cortex Phellodendri: 169, 217, 283, 294-295, 382, 386, 429, 432, 449
huáng là — Cera Chinensis Aurea: 443
huáng lián — Rhizoma Coptidis: 119, 168, 208, 226, 229, 282, 284-285, 293, 295, 355, 382, 386-387, 392, 403, 405, 429, 445, 449
huáng qí — Radix Astragali: 171, 190, 199, 205, 216, 223, 280, 409, 411, 416, 436
huáng qín — Radix Scutellariae: 168, 213, 217, 226, 236, 282, 285, 292-295, 311, 353, 355, 379, 382, 386-387, 392, 401, 405, 419, 429, 449
huáng yào zǐ — Tuber Dioscoreae Bulbiferae: 422
huò xiāng — Herba Agastaches: 285, 290, 292-293, 297, 351, 386, 427-428
jí lí — Fructus Tribuli: 238
jī nèi jīn — Endothelium Gigeriae Galli: 305, 418, 422
ji què gēn — Radix Caraganae Sinicae: 270
jī xuè téng — Radix et Caulis Chi Hsüeh T'eng: 194, 242, 320
jī zǐ huáng — Egg Yolk: 302

jiāng cán — Bombyx Batryticatus: 240, 274, 312-313, 425, 439, 446
jiāng zhī — Succus Zingiberis: 312, 315, 399
jiàng xiāng — Lignum Dalbergiae Odoriferae: 210
jiāo liù qū — Massa Fermentata Ustulata: 419
jié gěng — Radix Platycodi: 212, 267, 287, 297, 424
jīn qián cǎo — Herba Chin Ch'ien Ts'ao: 296, 422
jīn yīng zǐ — Fructus Rosae Laevigatae: 249, 438
jīng jiè — Herba Schizonepetae: 162, 267, 271, 377, 380
jú hé — Semen Citri: 234, 278, 287
jú hóng — Epicarpium Citri Tangerinae: 297
jú huā — Flos Chrysanthemi: 236, 272, 446
jué míng zǐ — Semen Cassiae: 394
kòu ké — Pericarpium Alpiniae: 287
kòu rén — Fructus Amomi Cardamomi: 292, 297, 386, 427-428
kǔ shēn — Radix Sophorae Flavescentis: 387, 429
kuǎn dōng huā — Flos Tussilagi Farfarae: 214-215, 424, 437
kūn bù — Thallus Algae: 316, 422
là liǎo — Herba Polygoni Hydropiperis: 277
lái fú zǐ — Semen Raphani: 305, 419
lí pí — Exocarpium Pyri: 214, 300
lián qiào — Fructus Forsythiae: 208, 268, 282, 286, 353, 379, 382
lián xū — Stamen Nelumbinis: 249, 438
lián zǐ ròu — Semen Nelumbinis: 438
lián zǐ xīn — Embryon Nelumbinis: 208
liáng jiāng — Rhizoma Alpiniae Officinari: 167, 224, 276, 406
líng yáng jiǎo — Cornu Antelopis: 238, 240, 355, 446
liù qū — Massa Fermentata: 305, 418
lóng chǐ — Dens Draconis: 238, 444, 446
lóng dǎn cǎo — Radix Gentianae: 209, 236, 294, 386, 394
lóng gǔ — Os Draconis: 176, 205, 249, 287, 407, 438, 444
lóng yǎn — Arillus Euphoriae Longanae: 194, 207, 412
lǜ dòu yī — Testa Glycines: 436
lú gēn — Rhizoma Phragmitis: 39, 226, 300, 384
lú huì — Herba Aloes: 394
lù jiǎo — Cornu Cervi: 172, 248, 376, 415
lù lù tōng — Fructus Liquidambaris: 234
lǘ pí jiāo — Gelatinum Corii Asini: 177, 119, 193, 199, 217, 223, 240-241, 302, 412-413, 416-417, 431, 442, 444, 446
mǎ chǐ xiàn — Herba Portulacae: 295, 383

mǎ dōu líng — Fructus Aristolochiae: 213, 215, 437
má huáng — Herba Ephedrae: 162, 212, 267, 275, 280, 310, 317, 338, 378, 380
má rén — Semen Cannabis: 231, 396
mài dōng — Tuber Ophiopogonis: 172, 207, 214, 217, 226-227, 231, 238, 283-284, 381, 413-414, 417, 446
mài yá — Fructus Hordei Germinatus: 305, 307, 418
máng xiāo — Mirabilitum: 40, 196, 282, 316, 391, 398-399, 401, 422
máo gēn — Rhizoma Imperatae: 300, 440-441
méng chóng — Tabanus: 421
méng shí — Lapis Chloriti: 315, 397
mò yào — Myrrha: 420
mǔ dān pí — Cortex Radicis Mu Tan: 197, 209, 236, 283, 382, 385, 392-393, 402, 420, 446
mǔ lì — Concha Ostreae: 176, 205, 238, 240, 249, 287, 407, 422, 438, 444, 446
mù tōng — Caulis Mu T'ung: 208, 296, 431
mù xiāng — Radix Saussureae: 191, 225, 230, 373
nán xīng — Rhizoma Arisaematis: 312, 424, 434
niú bàng zǐ — Fructus Arctii: 163, 212, 268, 286, 300, 379, 393, 424
niú jiǎo sāi — Os in Cornu Bovis: 441-442
niú xī — Radix Achyranthis Bidentatae: 242
nǚ zhēn zǐ — Fructus Ligustri Lucidi: 238, 241, 245, 413, 446
nuò dào gēn — Radix et Rhizoma Oryzae Glutinosae: 436
ǒu jié — Nodus Rhizomatis Nelumbinis: 432
pāo jiāng — Rhizoma Zingiberis blast-fried: 221, 223, 276-277, 406, 449
pāo jiāng tàn — Rhizoma Zingiberis Carbonisatum: 441
pèi lán — Herba Eupatorii: 285, 290, 292, 297, 386, 427-428
pí pa yè — Folium Eriobotryae: 213, 215, 437
pú gōng yīng — Herba et Radix Taraxaci: 268, 311, 379, 382, 392, 432
pú huáng — Pollen Typhae: 196-197, 296, 420, 441
qǐ zǐ — Fructus Lycii: 194, 235, 238, 241, 248, 303-304, 376, 412, 416
qiān niú zǐ — Semen Pharbitidis: 317, 395
qiāng huó — Rhizoma et Radix Notopterygii: 162, 267, 270-271, 287, 377, 380, 429
qiāng láng — Catharsius: 421
qiàn cǎo — Radix Rubiae: 196, 402
qiàn shí — Semen Euryalis: 249, 438, 443
qián hú — Radix Peucedani: 267, 424
qín jiāo — Herba Gentianae Macrophyllae: 270, 388

qín pí — Cortex Fraxini: 295, 429
qīng hāo — Herba Artemisiae Apiaceae: 169, 283, 285, 292, 384, 388, 401
qīng pí — Pericarpium Citri Reticulatae Viride: 192, 234, 402
qīng qiān — Galenitum: 448
qīng xiāng zǐ — Semen Celosiae: 236
qū mài — Herba Dianthi: 296, 431
quán xiē — Buthus: 240, 270, 274, 312-313, 409, 425, 446
rén shēn — Radix Ginseng: 167, 176, 205, 287, 340, 344, 372, 401, 407, 416
ròu dòu kòu — Semen Myristicae: 230, 438
ròu guì — Cortex Cinnamomi: 167, 172, 211, 221, 246, 276-278, 280, 287, 394, 406-407, 415, 429, 448
rǔ xiāng — Gummi Olibanum: 420
sān léng — Rhizoma Sparganii: 196, 398, 421
sān qī — Radix Pseudoginseng: 196, 420, 441
sāng bái pí — Cortex Radicis Mori: 213, 311
sāng jì shēng — Ramus Loranthi: 242
sāng piāo xiāo — Oötheca Mantidis: 249, 439
sāng shēn zǐ — Fructus Mori: 194, 241, 304, 413
sāng yè — Folium Mori: 163, 209, 213, 236, 268, 272, 300, 379, 446
sāng zhī — Ramulus Mori: 270
shā rén — Fructus Amomi: 220, 307, 373, 417, 427-428
shā shēn — Radix Adenophorae: 214, 217, 227, 284, 300, 413, 417, 424
shān cí gū — Bulbus Shan Tz'u Ku: 422
shān jiǎ — Squama Manitis: 196, 398
sháo yào — Radix Paeoniae: 177, 402
shān yào — Radix Dioscoreae: 219, 249, 307, 438-439
shān zhā — Fructus Crataegi: 210, 305, 418
shān zhā tàn — Fructus Crataegi Carbonisatus: 419
shēng dì — Radix Rehmanniae Cruda: 172, 207, 217, 223, 226-227, 235-236, 238, 283, 303, 381, 412-413, 417, 442, 444, 446
shēng gān cǎo — Radix Glycyrrhizae Recens: 208
shēng jiāng — Rhizoma Zingiberis Recens: 167, 211, 224, 229, 280, 377, 382, 401, 403
shēng má — Rhizoma Cimicifugae: 39, 222, 287
shēng tiě luò — Ferric Oxide: 444
shí gāo — Gypsum: 39, 168, 226, 284, 383-384
shí hú — Herba Dendrobii: 172, 227, 283-284, 413, 417
shí jué míng — Concha Haliotidis: 238

shí liú pí — Pericarpium Punicae Granati: 230
shí wěi — Folium Pyrrosiae: 296, 431
shóu dì — Radix Rehmanniae Conquita: 172, 193, 199, 207, 248, 303, 376, 392, 408, 416-417, 448
shǒu wū — Radix Polygoni Multiflori: 193, 241, 245, 303-304, 412, 417
sū gěng — Caulis Perillae: 234
sū yè — Folium Perillae: 162, 267, 377-378, 381
sū zǐ — Fructus Perillae Crispae: 214, 310, 424
shuǐ zhì — Hirudo: 421
suǒ yáng — Herba Cynomorii: 248, 417
táo rén — Semen Persicae: 196, 210, 231, 398, 420
tiān dōng — Tuber Asparagi: 217, 238, 244, 413
tiān huā fěn — Radix Trichosanthis: 227, 300-301, 384
tiān má — Rhizoma Gastrodiae: 238, 240, 313, 426
tiān zhú huáng — Concretio Siliceae Bambusae: 425, 434
tíng lì zǐ — Semen T'ing Li Tzu: 311, 317, 397, 424
tōng cǎo — Medulla Tetrapanacis: 290, 298, 386, 428, 431
tóng jí lí — Semen Astragali Complanati: 249, 439
tǔ dà huáng — Radix Rumicis: 440
tǔ fú líng — Rhizoma Smilacis Glabrae: 387
tǔ niú xī — Radix Achyranthis: 393
tù sī zǐ — Semen Cuscutae: 248, 376, 439
wǎ léng zǐ — Concha Arcae: 225
wēi líng xiān — Radix Clematidis: 270
wú gōng — Scolopendra: 270, 274, 425
wū shāo shé — Zaocys: 270
wǔ líng zhī — Excrementum Trogopteri: 420
wū tóu — Radix Aconiti Wu T'ou: 275
wū yào — Radix Linderae: 234, 278
wū zéi gǔ — Os Sepiae: 225
wú zhū yú — Fructus Evodiae: 167, 224, 229, 276, 278, 280, 403
wǔ wèi zǐ — Fructus Schisandrae: 216, 287, 408, 436, 438
xī guā cuì yī — Exocarpium Citrulli Vulgaris: 284
xī hé liǔ — Ramulus et Folium Tamaricis: 286, 379
xī jiǎo — Cornu Rhinoceri: 385
xī xiān cǎo — Herba Siegesbeckiae: 270
xì xīn — Herba Asari: 275, 280, 310, 317, 409
xià kū cǎo — Spica Prunellae: 236, 316, 394, 422, 446
xiān hè cǎo — Herba Agrimoniae: 440, 442

xiān líng pí — Herba Epimedii: 246, 415, 417, 449
xiān lú gēn — Rhizoma Phragmitis Vivum: 301, 311
xiān máo — Rhizoma Curculiginis: 246, 415, 417, 449
xiān máo gēn — Rhizoma Imperatae Vivum: 197
xiān shā shēn — Radix Adenophorae Viva: 301, 384
xiān shēng dì — Radix Rehmanniae Viva: 197, 231, 301, 385
xiān shí hú — Herba Dendrobii Viva: 301, 384
xiān shǒu wū — Radix Polygoni Multiflori Viva: 231, 396
xiān zhú yè — Folium Bambusae Vivum: 284
xiàng bèi mǔ — Bulbus Fritillariae Thunbergii: 212, 267
xiāng fù — Rhizoma Cyperi: 191, 225, 234, 402
xiāng rú — Herba Elsholtziae: 285
xiǎo huí xiāng — Fructus Foeniculi: 278
xiǎo jì cǎo — Herba Cephalanoploris: 196-197, 296, 432, 440-441
xiāo shí — Sal Petrae: 422
xiè bái — Bulbus Allii Macrostemi: 210
xìng rén — Semen Pruni Armeniacae: 214, 267, 292, 297, 338, 396,
    424, 428
xù duàn — Radix Dipsaci: 242
xuán fù huā — Flos Inulae: 229
xuán shēn — Radix Scrophulariae: 172, 217, 226, 231, 244, 283, 302,
    385, 393, 396, 413-414, 417, 446
yā zhí cǎo — Herba Commelinae: 432
yán hú suǒ — Rhizoma Corydalis: 225, 234, 402, 420
yè jiāo téng — Caulis Polygoni Multiflori: 207
yě qiáo — Radix Fagopyri Vulgaris: 383
yì mǔ cǎo — Herba Leonuri: 196, 420
yí táng — Saccharum Granorum: 224
yì yǐ rén — Semen Coicis: 290, 292, 428, 431
yì zhì rén — Fructus Alpiniae Oxyphyllae: 246
yín chái hú — Radix Stellariae Dichotomae: 169, 388
yīn chén — Herba Artemisiae Capillaris: 294, 429
yín huā — Flos Lonicerae: 268, 282, 311, 353, 379, 382, 385,
    392, 419, 432
yīng sù ké — Pericarpium Papaveris: 230, 436, 438
yóu dāng guī — Radix Angelicae Sinensis Pinguis: 396
yù jīn — Tuber Curcumae: 192, 210, 234, 294, 315, 357, 402, 434
yù mǐ xū — Stylus Zeae: 431
yù nǎi — Tuber Colocasiae: 422
yù zhú — Rhizoma Polygonati Odorati: 217, 227, 381, 413

yú ròu — Mesocarpium Corni: 241, 245, 248, 416-417, 439, 448
yú xīng cǎo — Herba Houttuyniae: 311, 432
yǔ yú liáng — Limonitum: 230, 438, 442
yuán huā — Flos Daphnes Genkwa: 395
yuǎn zhì — Radix Polygalae: 207, 223, 315, 434
zào jiá — Fructus Gleditsiae: 424
zào xīn tǔ — Terra Flava Usta: 223, 441
zǎo rén — Semen Zizyphi Jujubae: 194, 205, 207, 223, 445
zé lán — Herba Lycopi: 196, 420
zé xiè — Rhizoma Alismatis: 296, 298, 408
zhēn zhū mǔ — Concha Margaritifera: 238, 444, 446
zhì gān cǎo — Radix Glycyrrhizae mix-fried: 205, 406
zhǐ ké — Fructus Citri: 191, 230, 234, 373, 417, 428
zhì liú huáng — Sulfur Praeparatum: 396
zhī mǔ — Rhizoma Anemarrhenae: 39, 168-169, 217, 226, 282-284, 383-384, 449
zhī zǐ — Fructus Gardeniae: 209, 226, 236, 282, 286, 292-294, 296, 353, 379, 382-384, 393, 402, 429, 446
zhǐ shí — Fructus Citri Immaturus: 294, 305, 307, 392, 401, 419, 422, 426
zhōng rǔ shí — Stalactitum: 448
zhū líng — Sclerotium Polypori Umbellati: 296, 428, 431
zhū shā — Cinnabaris: 205, 207, 444
zhù lì — Succus Bambusae: 315
zǐ cǎo — Radix Lithospermi: 385, 392
zǐ hé jū — Placenta Hominis: 248, 416-417
zǐ sū — Herba Perillae Crispae: 403
zǐ shí yīng — Fluoritum: 442, 448
zǐ wǎn — Radix Asteris: 214, 424, 437
zhú lì — Succus Bambusae: 311-312, 315, 434
zhú rú — Caulis Bambusae in Taenis: 229, 403, 426, 445
zhú yè — Folium Bambusae: 208
zōng lǘ pí — Fibra Stipulae Trachycarpi: 440-441

English — Chinese Index
of
Chinese Medical Formulae

Aconite Center-Rectifying Decoction — fù-zǐ lǐ zhōng tāng: 343

Aconite Center-Rectifying Pills — fù-zǐ lǐ zhōng wán: 221, 254

Aconite and Cinnamon Eight Pills — fù guì bā wèi wán: 172, 246, 262, 415

Agastache, Magnolia, Pinellia, and Poria Decoction —
    huò pò xià líng tāng: 325, 365

Alpinia and Cyperus Pills — liáng fù wán: 167, 276, 320

Anemarrhena, Phellodendron, and Rehmannia Pills — zhī bó dì-huáng wán:
    245, 414, 416

Angelica Blood-Supplementing Decoction — dāng-guī bǔ xuè tāng: 199

Angelica Splenic Decoction — guī pí tāng: 194, 199, 207, 223,
    251, 255, 412

Angelica, Gentiana, and Aloe Pills — dāng-guī lóng huì wán: 394

Antelope Horn Decoction — líng-yáng-jiǎo tāng: 240, 260

Anti-Contracture Powder — qiān zhèng sǎn: 271, 426, 319

Anti-Obturation Decoction — juān bì tāng: 271, 319

Artemisia Apiacea and Scutellaria Gallbladder-Clearing Decoction —
    hāo qín qīng dǎn tāng: 323, 367

Astragalus Center-Fortifying Decoction — huáng qí jiàn zhōng tāng: 225

Atractylodes Seven Powder — qī wèi bái-zhú sǎn: 220

Awakening Spirit Elixir — zhèn líng dān: 442

Biliary Calculus Decoction — dǎn dào pái shí tāng: 423

Black Free Wanderer Powder — hēi xiāo yáo sǎn: 242, 260

Black Paste Formula — hēi gāo fāng: 355

Black Tin Elixir — hēi-xí dān: 247, 262, 448

Boats and Carts Pills — zhōu chē wán: 395

Bone-Clearing Powder — qīng gǔ sǎn: 388

Bupleurum Liver-Coursing Decoction — chái-hú shū gān tāng: 192, 234, 257

Bupleurum and Cinnamon Decoction — chái-hú guì-zhī tāng: 342, 362

Cannabis Pills — má-zǐ-rén wán: 231, 397

Carapax Amydae Decocted Pills — biē-jiǎ jiān wán: 421

Carriage-Halting Pills — zhù chē wán: 449

Celestial Emperor Heart-Supplementing Elixir — tiān wáng bǔ xīn dān:
    194, 207, 251, 261

Center-Rectifying Pills — lǐ zhōng wán: 167, 221, 254, 277, 321, 343, 363, 407
Center-Supplementing Qi-Boosting Decoction — bǔ zhōng yì qì tāng: 199, 222, 254, 411
Cephalanoplos Cool Decoction — xiǎo-jì yǐn zǐ: 198
Cervix Ginseng Powder — shēn lù sǎn: 389
Chlorite Phlegm-Expelling Pills — méng-shí gǔn tán wán: 397
Cinnamon Eight Pills — guì-zhī bā wèi wán: 376
Cinnamon-Twig and Ginseng Decoction — guì-zhī rén-shēn tāng: 375
Cinnamon-Twig Decoction — guì-zhī tāng: 163, 338, 361, 378, 436
Clear and Quiet Pills — qīng níng wán: 237
Clove and Persimmon Decoction — dīng-xiāng shì-dì tāng: 229, 256
Construction-Clearing Decoction — qīng yíng tāng: 355, 368, 385
Coptis Detoxifying Decoction — huáng-lián jiě dú tāng: 198, 282, 322, 353, 367, 385
Coptis Detoxifying Powder — huáng-lián jiě dú sǎn: 383
Coptis Gallbladder-Warming Decoction — huáng-lián wēn dǎn tāng: 313, 331
Coptis and Ass-Hide Glue Decoction — huáng-lián ē-jiāo tāng: 209, 252, 344, 362
Coptis and Evodia Pills — zuǒ jīn wán: 256-257, 229, 234
Coptis and Magnolia Cool Decoction — lián pò yǐn: 293, 325, 353, 367, 387
Counterflow Cold Decoction — sì nì tāng: 344-345, 363, 408
Counterflow Cold Powder — sì nì sǎn: 192
Counterfow Cold Decoction with Ginseng — sì nì jiā rén-shēn tāng: 167
Crown Jewel Elixir — zhì bǎo dān: 315, 331, 433-434
Dead-On Pills — dǐ-dāng wán: 398
Defiant Three Decoction — sān ào tāng: 212, 253
Diaphragm-Cooling Powder — liáng gé sǎn: 226, 394
Divine Rhinoceros Elixir — shēn xī dān: 355, 357, 369, 433
Double Supreme Pills — èr zhì wán: 245, 261
Double Vintage Decoction — èr chén tāng: 309, 426
Double-Armored Pulse-Restorative Decoction — èr jiǎ fù mài tāng: 356
Drool-Controlling Elixir — kòng xián dān: 317, 332, 395
Dryness-Clearing Lung-Restorative Decoction — qīng zào jiù fèi tāng: 214, 217, 303, 327, 424
Dryness-Moistening Construction-Nourishing Decoction — zī zào yǎng yíng tāng: 303, 323, 323
Eight Corrections Powder — bā zhèng sǎn: 296, 326, 432
Eight Jewel Decoction — bā zhēn tāng: 199, 412

Elsholtzia Cool Decoction — xiāng-rú yǐn: 285
Ephedra Decoction — má-huáng tāng: 162, 267, 319-320, 338, 361, 375, 378
Ephedra, Apricot, Gypsum and Liquorice Decoction —
    má xìng shí gān tāng: 366
Evodia Decoction — wú-zhū-yú tāng: 229, 256, 407
Fang Chi and Astragalus Decoction — fáng-jǐ huáng-qí tāng: 221
Fit-Settling Pills — dìng xián wán: 312, 331
Five Cortices Cool Decoction — wǔ pí yǐn: 221
Five Kernel Pills — wǔ rén wán: 231
Five-Tigers-Chasing-The-Wind Decoction — wǔ hǔ zhuī fēng sǎn: 271, 319
Five Torrents Cool Decoction — wǔ mó yǐn zǐ: 192
Fluids Decoction — jīn yè tāng: 302
Four Agents Decoction — sì wù tāng: 172, 194, 242, 260, 412
Four Divinity Pills — sì shén wán: 246, 262
Four Nobles Decoction — sì jūn zǐ tāng: 172, 190, 220, 254, 373, 411
Four-Seven Decoction — sì qī tāng: 234, 258, 403
Free Wanderer Powder — xiāo yáo sǎn: 234, 258, 402, 404
Gallbladder-Warming Decoction — wēn dǎn tāng: 229
Gardenia and Fermented Soybean Decoction — zhī-zǐ shǐ tāng: 353, 366, 384
Gastrodia and Uncaria Cool Decoction — tiān-má gōu-téng yǐn: 238, 259, 447
Generalized-Pain-Relieving Stasis-Expelling Decoction —
    shēn tòng zhú yū tāng: 421
Gentian Liver-Draining Decoction — lóng dǎn xiè gān tāng: 236, 259, 296, 387
Ginseng, Aconite, Dragon Bone and Oystershell Decoction —
    shēn fù lóng mǔ tāng: 250
Ginseng Solo Decoction — dú shēn tāng: 200, 205, 411
Ginseng and Aconite Decoction — shēn fù tāng: 167, 177, 205, 247, 250, 262
Ginseng and Gecko Powder — shēn jiè sǎn: 206, 247, 262
Ginseng and Perilla Leaf Cool Decoction — shēn sū yǐn: 380
Ginseng, Poria and Atractylodes Powder — shēn líng bái-zhú sǎn: 220, 307
Golden Lock Essence-Securing Pills — jīn suǒ gù jīng wán: 249, 263, 439
Great Guffaw Powder — shī xiào sǎn: 421
Great Quieting Pills — dà ān wán: 307, 419
Great Wind-Stabilizing Pills — dà dìng fēng zhū: 239-240, 260
Great Yin Supplementation Pills — dà bǔ yīn wán: 283, 332, 414, 416
Greatly Fortifying Placenta Pills — hé-jū dà zào wán: 248

Gynecological Decoction — shēng huà tāng: 398
Harmony-Preserving Pills — bǎo hé wán: 229, 305, 329, 419
Heart-Draining Decoction — xiè xīn tāng: 168, 209, 252, 282, 322, 353, 367, 393
Heart-Nourishing Decoction — yǎng xīn tāng: 205, 250
Heart-Supplementing Pills — bǔ xīn wán: 245
Heat-Abducting Powder — dǎo chì sǎn: 209, 252
Honeyed Liquorice Decoction — zhì gān cǎo tāng: 205, 250
Humor-Increasing Decoction — zēng yè tāng: 327, 399, 414
Humor-Increasing Purgative Decoction —
  zēng yè chéng qì tāng: 375, 399
Immature Citrus Stagnation-Abducting Pills — zhǐ-shí dào zhì wán: 306, 329, 419
Inula and Hematite Decoction — xuán fù dài-zhě tāng: 229, 256
Jade Axis Elixir — yù shū dān: 229, 256, 358, 364, 435
Jade Lady Decoction — yù nǚ jiān: 226, 255, 376
Jade Wind-Barrier Powder — yù píng fēng sǎn: 216, 436
Kidney Pills — zuǒ guī wán: 242, 263, 248, 376, 403, 416
Leaden Obturation Tested Formula — zhuó bì yàn fāng: 421
Ledebouriella Wondrous Panacea Powder — fáng-fēng tōng shèng sǎn: 449
Leukorrhea Tablets — zhǐ dài piàn: 443
Life-Saver Kidney Qi Pills — jì shēng shèn qì wán: 206, 247, 263, 408
Lily Bulb Metal-Securing Decoction — bǎi-hé gù jīn tāng: 217, 245, 253, 261
Liquid Styrax Pills — sū hé xiāng wán: 210, 252, 315, 358, 369, 434-435
Liver-Supplementing Decoction — bǔ gān tāng: 242, 262
Liver-Warming Decoction — nuǎn gān jiān: 278
Lonicera and Forsythia Powder — yín qiào sǎn: 163, 212, 268, 350, 380
Lonicera and Phragmites Combination — yín wěi hé jì: 212, 311, 365, 424
Lung-Draining Powder — xiè bái sǎn: 214, 253
Lung-Supplementing Decoction — bǔ fèi tāng: 216, 253
Lycium, Chrysanthemum, and Rehmannia Pills —
  qǐ jú dì-huáng wán: 238, 242, 245, 259-261
Magnetite and Cinnabar Pills — cí zhū wán: 445
Major Bupleurum Decoction — dà chái-hú tāng: 294, 342, 359, 362, 401
Major Cyan Dragon Decoction — dà qīng lóng tāng: 338
Major Purgative Decoction — dà chéng qì tāng: 340, 359, 361, 367, 369, 374-375, 392
Melia Toosendan Powder — jīn-líng-zǐ sǎn: 198
Minor Bupleurum Decoction — xiǎo chái-hú tāng: 165, 342, 362, 401
Minor Center-Fortifying Decoction — xiǎo jiàn zhōng tāng: 224

Minor Chest-Bind Decoction — xiǎo xiàn xiōng tāng: 353
Minor Cyan Dragon Decoction — xiǎo qīng lóng tāng: 212, 310, 317, 338, 385, 424
Minor Pinellia Decoction with Poria — xiǎo bàn-xià jiā fú-líng tāng: 229, 256
Minor Purgative Decoction — xiǎo chéng qì tāng: 306, 340, 392
Mulberry and Apricot Kernel Decoction — sāng xìng tāng: 214, 300
Mulberry and Chrysanthemum Cool Decoction — sāng jú yǐn: 163, 268, 350, 364, 380
Mume Pills — wū-méi wán: 346, 359, 364
Mysterious Trinity Pills — sān miào wán: 296
Nectar Paste — qióng yù gāo: 415
Nine Immortals Powder — jiǔ xiān sǎn: 437
Nine Pains Pills — jiǔ tòng wán: 398
Ophiopogon Decoction — mài-mén-dōng tāng: 227, 255
Oötheca Mantidis Powder — sāng-piāo-xiāo sǎn: 249, 263, 439
Origin-Restorative Blood-Quickening Decoction — fù yuán huó xuè tāng: 421
Oystershell Powder — mǔ lì sǎn: 436
Pain and Diarrhea Formula — tòng xiè yào fāng: 234, 257, 404
Pathfinder Poria Pills — zhǐ mí fú-líng wán: 316
Peaceful Palace Bovine Bezoar Pills — ān gōng niú-huáng wán: 355, 357, 369, 433
Peach Blossom Decoction — táo huā tāng: 230
Peach Pit Purgative Decoction — táo-rén chéng qì tāng: 196, 398
Pedicellus Cucumeris Powder — guā-dì sǎn: 389
Perilla Fruit Qi-Downbearing Decoction — sū-zǐ jiàng qì tāng: 214, 253
Phlegm-Cough Powder — zhǐ sòu sǎn: 214, 424
Pinellia Heart-Draining Decoction — xiè xīn tāng: 405
Pinellia and Sulfur Pills — bàn liú wán: 397
Pinellia, Atractylodes, and Gastrodia Decoction — bàn-xià bái-zhú tiān-má tāng: 313
Placenta Solo Powder — dān wèi hé-jū fěn: 248
Polygonatum Odoratum Decoction — wěi ruǐ tāng: 381
Poria, Cinnamon, Atractylodes, and Liquorice Decoction — líng guì zhú gān tāng: 222
Poria Five Powder — wǔ líng sǎn: 430
Poria Four Powder — sì líng sǎn: 221, 431
Portal-Opening Blood-Quickening Decoction — tōng qiào huó xuè tāng: 210, 252
Prunella Paste — xià-kū-cǎo gāo: 316
Pulsatilla Decoction — bái-tóu-wēng tāng: 295

Pulse-Engendering Powder — shēng mài sǎn: 176, 218, 288, 415
Pulse-Restorative Decoction — fù mài tāng: 302, 356, 368
Purple Snow Elixir — zǐ xuě dān: 284, 355, 357, 369, 433
Pyrrosia Powder — shí-wěi sǎn: 296, 423
Realgar Detoxifying Pills — xióng-huáng jiě dú wán: 390
Rehmannia Six Pills — liù wèi dì-huáng wán: 172, 245, 261, 376, 414
Rhinoceros Horn and Rehmannia Decoction —
    xī-jiǎo dì-huáng tāng: 198, 356, 368, 385
Rhizoma Rhei and Eupolyphaga Pills — dà-huáng zhè-chóng wán: 196
Rhizoma Rhei and Mu Tan Decoction — dà-huáng mǔ-dān tāng: 393
Sanguine Mansion Stasis-Expelling Decoction — xuè fǔ zhú yū tāng: 196
Sargassium Jade Teapot Decoction — hǎi-zǎo yù hú tāng: 234, 258, 423
Saussurea and Areca Pills — mù-xiāng bīn-láng wán: 306
Schizonepeta and Ledebouriella Detoxifying Powder —
    jīng fáng bài dú sǎn: 162, 267, 378
Scourge-Clearing Detoxifying Cool Decoction —
    qīng wēn bài dú yǐn: 385, 449
Scrofula-Dispersing Pills — nèi xiāo luǒ lì wán: 316, 423
Six-to-One Powder — liù yī sǎn: 284-285, 292
Spleen-Reinforcing Cool Decoction — shí pí yǐn: 221
Spleen-Warming Decoction — wēn pí tāng: 395
Stomach-Calming Powder — píng wèi sǎn: 309, 424, 430
Stomach-Clearing Powder — qīng wèi sǎn: 226, 255
Stomach-Nourishing Decoction — yǎng wèi tāng: 227, 255, 414
Stomach-Regulating Purgative Decoction — tiáo wèi chéng qì tāng:
    226, 340, 392, 399
Stream-Reducing Pills — suō quán wán: 249, 263, 439
Sweet Dew Toxin-Dispersing Elixir — gān lù xiāo dú dān: 292, 353, 367, 387
T'ien T'ai Lindera Powder — tiān-tái-wū-yào sǎn: 278, 321
T.B. Tested Formula — fèi láo yàn fāng: 214
Tea-Blended Ligusticum Powder — chuān-xiōng chá tiáo sǎn: 267
Ten Cinders Pills — shí huī wán: 442
Ten Jujubes Pills — shí zǎo wán: 395
Thin Drool Powder — xī xián sǎn: 390
Three Kernel Decoction — sān rén tāng: 292, 353, 367, 387, 430
Three Seed Filial Devotion Decoction — sān zǐ yǎng qīn tāng: 214
Toilette Pills — gēng yī wán: 237, 394

Trichosanthes, Allium, and Pinellia Decoction —
    guā-lóu xiè-bái bàn-xià tāng: 210, 252
Triple-Armored Pulse-Restorative Decoction —
    sān jiǎ fù mài tāng: 302, 356, 447
Troop Deployment Powder — xíng jūn sǎn: 435
True Man Viscera-Nourishing Decoction — zhēn rén yǎng zàng tāng:
    230, 438
True Warrior Decoction — zhēn wǔ tāng: 206, 221, 247, 263, 345, 376, 408
Two Immortals Decoction — èr xiān tāng: 416, 449
Two-A Decoction — qīng-hāo biē-jiǎ tāng: 169, 283, 388
Universal Salvation Detoxifying Cool Decoction — pǔ jì xiāo dú yǐn: 269
Vital Gate Pills — yòu guī wán: 247-248, 376, 415-416
Wheat and Jujube Decoction — gān-mài dà-zǎo tāng: 207
White Tiger Decoction — bái hǔ tāng: 168, 284, 302, 340, 353, 361,
    366, 375, 384-385
Winning Streak Powder — dà shùn sǎn: 407
Wu T'ou Aconite Decoction — wū-tóu tāng: 275, 409
Yellow Dragon Decoction — huáng lóng tāng: 375
Yellow Earth Decoction — huáng tǔ tāng: 223, 255, 449
Yellow Sextet plus Angelica Decoction — dāng-guī liù huáng tāng: 436

Chinese — English Index of Chinese Medical Formulae

ān gōng niú-huáng wán — Peaceful Palace Bovine Bezoar Pills: 355, 357, 369, 433

bā zhēn tāng — Eight Jewel Decoction: 199, 412

bā zhèng sǎn — Eight Corrections Powder: 296, 326, 432

bái hǔ tāng — White Tiger Decoction: 168, 284, 302, 340, 353, 361, 366, 375, 384-385

bái-tóu-wēng tāng — Pulsatilla Decoction: 295

bǎi-hé gù jīn tāng — Lily Bulb Metal-Securing Decoction: 217, 245, 253, 261

bàn liú wán — Pinellia and Sulfur Pills: 397

bàn-xià bái-zhú tiān-má tāng — Pinellia, Atractylodes, and Gastrodia Decoction: 313

bǎo hé wán — Harmony-Preserving Pills: 229, 305, 329, 419

biē-jiǎ jiān wán — Carapax Amydae Decocted Pills: 421

bǔ fèi tāng — Lung-Supplementing Decoction: 216, 253

bǔ gān tāng — Liver-Supplementing Decoction: 242, 260

bǔ xīn wán — Heart-Supplementing Pills: 245

bǔ zhōng yì qì tāng — Center-Supplementing Qi-Boosting Decoction: 199, 222, 254, 411

cí zhū wán — Magnetite and Cinnabar Pills: 445

chái-hú guì-zhī tāng — Bupleurum and Cinnamon Decoction: 342, 362

chái-hú shū gān tāng — Bupleurum Liver-Coursing Decoction: 192, 234, 257

chuān-xiōng chá tiáo sǎn — Tea-Blended Ligusticum Powder: 267

dà ān wán — Great Quieting Pills: 307, 419

dà bǔ yīn wán — Great Yin Supplementation Pills: 283, 332, 414, 416

dà chái-hú tāng — Major Bupleurum Decoction: 294, 342, 359, 362, 401

dà chéng qì tāng — Major Purgative Decoction: 340, 359, 361, 367, 369, 374-375, 392

dà dìng fēng zhū — Great Wind-Stabilizing Pills: 239-240, 260

dà-huáng mǔ-dān tāng — Rhizoma Rhei and Mu Tan Decoction: 393

dà-huáng zhè-chóng wán — Rhizoma Rhei and Eupolyphaga Pills: 196

dà qīng lóng tāng — Major Cyan Dragon Decoction: 338

dà shùn sǎn — Winning Streak Powder: 407

dān dào pái shí tāng — Biliary Calculus Decoction: 423

dān wèi hé-jū fěn — Placenta Solo Powder: 248

dāng-guī bǔ xuè tāng — Angelica Blood-Supplementing Decoction: 199

dāng-guī lóng huì wán — Angelica, Gentiana, and Aloe Pills: 394

dāng-guī liù huáng tāng — Yellow Sextet plus Angelica Decoction: 436
dǎo chì sǎn — Heat-Abducting Powder: 209, 252
dīng-xiāng shì-dì tāng — Clove and Persimmon Decoction: 229, 256
dìng xián wán — Fit-Settling Pills: 312, 331
dǐ-dāng wán — Dead-On Pills: 398
dú shēn tāng — Ginseng Solo Decoction: 200, 205, 411
èr chén tāng — Double Vintage Decoction: 309, 426
èr jiǎ fù mài tāng — Double-Armored Pulse-Restorative Decoction: 356
èr xiān tāng — Two Immortals Decoction: 416, 449
èr zhì wán — Double Supreme Pills: 245, 261
fáng-fēng tōng shèng sǎn — Ledebouriella Wondrous Panacea Powder: 449
fáng-jǐ huáng-qí tāng — Fang Chi and Astragalus Decoction: 221
fèi láo yàn fāng — T.B. Tested Formula: 214
fù mài tāng — Pulse-Restorative Decoction: 302, 356
fù yuán huó xuè tāng — Origin-Restorative Blood-Quickening Decoction: 421
fù-zǐ lǐ zhōng tāng — Aconite Center-Rectifying Decoction: 254, 343
gān lù xiāo dú dān — Sweet Dew Toxin-Dispersing Elixir: 292, 353, 367, 387
gān-mài dà-zǎo tāng — Wheat and Jujube Decoction: 207
gēng yī wán — Toilette Pills: 237, 394
guā-dì sǎn — Pedicellus Cucumeris Powder: 389
guā-lóu xiè-bái bàn-xià tāng — Trichosanthes, Allium, and Pinellia Decoction: 210, 252
guī pí tāng — Angelica Splenic Decoction: 194, 199, 207, 223, 251, 255, 412
fù guì bā wèi wán — Aconite and Cinnamon Eight Pills: 172, 246, 262, 415
guì-zhī bā wèi wán — Cinnamon Eight Pills: 376
guì-zhī rén-shēn tāng — Cinnamon-Twig and Ginseng Decoction: 375
guì-zhī tāng — Cinnamon-Twig Decoction: 163, 338, 361, 378, 436
hǎi-zǎo yù hú tāng — Sargassium Jade Teapot Decoction: 234, 258, 423
hāo qín qīng dǎn tāng — Artemisia Apiacea and Scutellaria Gallbladder-Clearing Decoction: 323, 367
hé-jū dà zào wán — Greatly Fortifying Placenta Pills: 248
hēi gāo fāng — Black Paste Formula: 355
hēi-xí dān — Black Tin Elixir: 247, 262, 448
hēi xiāo yáo sǎn — Black Free Wanderer Powder: 242, 260
huáng-lián ē-jiāo tāng — Coptis and Ass-Hide Glue Decoction: 209, 252, 344, 363
huáng-lián jiě dú sǎn — Coptis Detoxifying Powder: 383
huáng-lián jiě dú tāng — Coptis Detoxifying Decoction: 198, 282, 322, 353, 367, 385
huáng-lián wēn dǎn tāng — Coptis Gallbladder-Warming Decoction: 313, 331

huáng lóng tāng — Yellow Dragon Decoction: 375
huáng qí jiàn zhōng tāng — Astragalus Center-Fortifying Decoction: 225
huáng tǔ tāng — Yellow Earth Decoction: 223, 255, 449
huò pò xià líng tāng — Agastache, Magnolia, Pinellia and Poria Decoction: 325, 365
jì shēng shèn qì wán — Life-Saver Kidney Qi Pills: 206, 247, 263, 408
jīn suǒ gù jīng wán — Golden Lock Essence-Securing Pills: 249, 263, 439
jīn-líng-zǐ sǎn — Melia Toosendan Powder: 198
jīn yè tāng — Fluids Decoction: 302
jīng fáng bài dú sǎn — Schizonepeta and Ledebouriella Detoxifying Powder: 162, 267, 378
jiǔ tòng wán — Nine Pains Pills: 398
jiǔ xiān sǎn — Nine Immortals Powder: 437
juān bì tāng — Anti-Obturation Decoction: 271, 319
kòng xián dān — Drool-Controlling Elixir: 317, 332, 395
lǐ zhōng wán — Center-Rectifying Pills: 167, 221, 254, 277, 321, 343, 362, 407
lián pò yǐn — Coptis and Magnolia Cool Decoction: 293, 325, 353, 367, 387
liáng fù wán — Alpinia and Cyperus Pills: 167, 276, 320
liáng gé sǎn — Diaphragm-Cooling Powder: 226, 394
líng guì zhú gān tāng — Poria, Cinnamon, Atractylodes, and Liquorice Decoction: 222
líng-yáng-jiǎo tāng — Antelope Horn Decoction: 240, 260
liù wèi dì-huáng wán — Rehmannia Six Pills: 172, 245, 261, 376, 414
liù yī sǎn — Six-to-One Powder: 284-285, 292
lóng dǎn xié gān tāng — Gentian Liver-Draining Decoction: 236, 259, 296, 387
má-huáng tāng — Ephedra Decoction: 162, 267, 319-320, 338, 361, 375, 378
má xìng shí gān tāng — Ephedra, Apricot, Gypsum, and Liquorice Decoction: 366
má-zǐ-rén wán — Cannabis Pills: 231, 397
mài-mén-dōng tāng — Ophiopogon Decoction: 227, 255
méng-shí gǔn tán wán — Chlorite Phlegm-Expelling Pills: 397
mǔ lì sǎn — Oystershell Powder: 436
mù-xiāng bīn-láng wán — Saussurea and Areca Pills: 306
nèi xiāo luǒ lì wán — Scrofula-Dispersing Pills: 316, 423
nuǎn gān jiān — Liver-Warming Decoction: 278
píng wèi sǎn — Stomach-Calming Powder: 309, 424, 430
pǔ jì xiāo dú yǐn — Universal Salvation Detoxifying Cool Decoction: 269
qǐ jú dì-huáng wán — Lycium, Chrysanthemum, and Rehmannia Pills: 238, 242, 245, 259-261

qī wèi bái-zhú sǎn — Atractylodes Seven Powder: 220
qiān zhèng sǎn — Anti-Contracture Powder: 271, 426, 319
qīng gǔ sǎn — Bone-Clearing Powder: 388
qīng-hāo biē-jiǎ tāng — Two-A Decoction: 169, 283, 388
qīng níng wán — Clear and Quiet Pills: 237
qīng wēn bài dú yǐn — Scourge-Clearing Detoxifying Cool Decoction: 385, 449
qīng wèi sǎn — Stomach-Clearing Powder: 226, 255
qīng yíng tāng — Construction-Clearing Decoction: 355, 368, 385
qīng zào jiù fèi tāng — Dryness-Clearing Lung-Restorative Decoction: 214, 217, 303, 327, 424
qióng yù gāo — Nectar Paste: 415
sān ào tāng — Defiant Three Decoction: 212, 253
sān jiǎ fù mài tāng — Triple-Armored Pulse-Restorative Decoction: 302, 356, 368, 447
sān miào wán — Mysterious Trinity Pills: 296
sān rén tāng — Three Kernel Decoction: 292, 353, 367, 387, 430
sān zǐ yǎng qīn tāng — Three Seed Filial Devotion Decoction: 214
sāng jú yǐn — Mulberry and Chrysanthemum Cool Decoction: 163, 268, 350, 364, 380
sāng-piāo-xiāo sǎn — Oötheca Mantidis Powder: 249, 263, 439
sāng xìng tāng — Mulberry and Apricot Kernel Decoction: 214, 300
sì jūn zǐ tāng — Four Nobles Decoction: 172, 190, 220, 254, 373, 411
sì líng sǎn — Poria Four Powder: 221, 431
sì qī tāng — Four-Seven Decoction: 234, 258, 403
sì nì jiā rén-shēn tāng — Counterfow Cold Decoction with Ginseng: 167
sì nì sǎn — Counterflow Cold Powder: 192
sì nì tāng — Counterflow Cold Decoction: 344-345, 363, 408
sì shén wán — Four Divinity Pills: 246, 262
sì wù tāng — Four Agents Decoction: 172, 194, 242, 260, 412
shēn fù lóng mǔ tāng — Ginseng, Aconite, Dragon Bone, and Oystershell Decoction: 250
shēn fù tāng — Ginseng and Aconite Decoction: 167, 177, 205, 247, 250, 262
shēn jiè sǎn — Ginseng and Gecko Powder: 206, 247, 262
shēn líng bái-zhú sǎn — Ginseng, Poria, and Atractylodes Powder: 220, 307
shēn lù sǎn — Cervix Ginseng Powder: 389
shēn sū yǐn — Ginseng and Perilla Leaf Cool Decoction: 380
shēn tòng zhú yū tāng — Generalized-Pain-Relieving Stasis-Expelling Decoction: 421

shēn xī dān — Divine Rhinoceros Elixir: 355, 357, 369, 433
shēng huà tāng — Gynecological Decoction: 398
shēng mài sǎn — Pulse-Engendering Powder: 176, 218, 288, 415
shí huī wán — Ten Cinders Pills: 442
shí pí yǐn — Spleen-Reinforcing Cool Decoction: 221
shí zǎo wán — Ten Jujubes Pills: 395
shí-wěi sǎn — Pyrrosia Powder: 296, 423
shī xiào sǎn — Great Guffaw Powder: 421
sū hé xiāng wán — Liquid Styrax Pills: 210, 252, 315, 358, 369, 434-435
sū-zǐ jiàng qì tāng — Perilla Fruit Qi-Downbearing Decoction: 214, 253
suō quán wán — Stream-Reducing Pills: 249, 263, 439
táo huā tāng — Peach Blossom Decoction: 230
táo-rén chéng qì tāng — Peach Pit Purgative Decoction: 196, 398
tiān wáng bǔ xīn dān — Celestial Emperor Heart-Supplementing
    Elixir: 194, 207, 251, 261
tiān-má gōu-téng yǐn — Gastrodia and Uncaria Cool Decoction: 238,
    259, 447
tiān-tái-wū-yào sǎn — T'ien T'ai Lindera Powder: 278, 321
tiáo wèi chéng qì tāng — Stomach-Regulating Purgative Decoction:
    226, 340, 392, 399
tōng qiào huó xuè tāng — Portal-Opening Blood-Quickening Decoction:
    210, 252
tòng xiè yào fāng — Pain and Diarrhea Formula: 234, 257, 404
wěi ruǐ tāng — Polygonatum Odoratum Decoction: 381
wēn dǎn tāng — Gallbladder-Warming Decoction: 229
wēn pí tāng — Spleen-Warming Decoction: 395
wǔ hǔ zhuī fēng sǎn — Five-Tigers-Chasing-The-Wind Decoction:
    271, 319
wǔ líng sǎn — Poria Five Powder: 430
wū-méi wán — Mume Pills: 346, 359, 364
wǔ mó yǐn zǐ — Five Torrents Cool Decoction: 192
wū-tóu tāng — Wu T'ou Aconite Decoction: 275, 409
wǔ pí yǐn — Five Cortices Cool Decoction: 221
wǔ rén wán — Five Kernel Pills: 231
wú-zhū-yú tāng — Evodia Decoction: 229, 256, 407
xī-jiǎo dì-huáng tāng — Rhinoceros Horn and Rehmannia Decoction:
    198, 356, 368, 385
xī xián sǎn — Thin Drool Powder: 390
xiāng-rú yǐn — Elsholtzia Cool Decoction: 285
xià-kū-cǎo gāo — Prunella Paste: 316

xiǎo bàn-xià jiā fú-líng tāng — Minor Pinellia Decoction with Poria: 229, 256
xiǎo chái-hú tāng — Minor Bupleurum Decoction: 165, 342, 363, 401
xiǎo chéng qì tāng — Minor Purgative Decoction: 306, 340, 392
xiǎo-jì yǐn zǐ — Cephalanoplos Cool Decoction: 198
xiǎo jiàn zhōng tāng — Minor Center-Fortifying Decoction: 224
xiǎo qīng lóng tāng — Minor Cyan Dragon Decoction: 212, 310, 317, 338, 385, 424
xiǎo xiàn xiōng tāng — Minor Chest-Bind Decoction: 353
xiāo yáo sǎn — Free Wanderer Powder: 234, 258, 402, 404
xiè bái sǎn — Lung-Draining Powder: 214, 253
xiè xīn tāng — Heart-Draining Decoction: 168, 209, 252, 282, 322, 353, 367, 393
xiè xīn tāng — Pinellia Heart-Draining Decoction: 405
xióng-huáng jiě dú wán — Realgar Detoxifying Pills: 390
xíng jūn sǎn — Troop Deployment Powder: 435
xuán fù dài-zhě tāng — Inula and Hematite Decoction: 229, 256
xuè fǔ zhú yū tāng — Sanguine Mansion Stasis-Expelling Decoction: 196
yǎng wèi tāng — Stomach-Nourishing Decoction: 227, 255, 414
yǎng xīn tāng — Heart-Nourishing Decoction: 205, 250
yīn-chén-hāo tāng — Artemisia Capillaris Decoction: 294, 326, 387
yín qiào sǎn — Lonicera and Forsythia Powder: 163, 212, 268, 350, 365, 380
yín wěi hé jì — Lonicera and Phragmites Combination: 212, 311, 424
yòu guī wán — Vital Gate Pills: 247-248, 376, 415-416
yù nǚ jiān — Jade Lady Decoction: 226, 255, 376
yù píng fēng sǎn — Jade Wind-Barrier Powder: 216, 436
yù shū dān — Jade Axis Elixir: 229, 256, 358, 369, 435
zēng yè chéng qì tāng — Humor-Increasing Purgative Decoction: 375, 399
zēng yè tāng — Humor-Increasing Decoction: 327, 399, 414
zhèn líng dān — Awakening Spirit Elixir: 442
zhēn rén yǎng zàng tāng — True Man Viscera-Nourishing Decoction: 230, 438
zhēn wǔ tāng — True Warrior Decoction: 206, 221, 247, 263, 345, 376, 408
zhì bǎo dān — Crown Jewel Elixir: 315, 331, 433-434

zhī bó dì-huáng wán — Anemarrhena, Phellodendron, and Rehmannia Pills: 245, 414, 416

zhǐ dài piàn — Leukorrhea Tablets: 443

zhì gān cǎo tāng — Honeyed Liquorice Decoction: 205, 250

zhǐ mí fú-líng wán — Pathfinder Poria Pills: 316

zhǐ-shí dào zhì wán — Immature Citrus Stagnation-Abducting Pills: 306, 329, 419

zhǐ sòu sǎn — Phlegm-Cough Powder: 214, 424

zhī-zǐ shì tāng — Gardenia and Fermented Soybean Decoction: 353, 366, 384

zhōu chē wán — Boats and Carts Pills: 395

zhù chē wán — Carriage-Halting Pills: 449

zī zào yǎng yíng tāng — Dryness-Moistening Construction-Nourishing Decoction: 303, 323, 323

zǐ xuě dān — Purple Snow Elixir: 284, 355, 357, 369, 433

zhuó bì yàn fāng — Leaden Obturation Tested Formula: 421

zuǒ guī wán — Kidney Pills: 242, 248, 263, 376, 403, 416

zuǒ jīn wán — Coptis and Evodia Pills: 229, 234, 256-257

Acumoxatherapy Index

Bladder

BL-1: 45, 47-48, 269
BL-2: 172, 269
BL-7: 267
BL-10: 241, 268
BL-11: 47, 340
BL-12: 163, 213, 216, 253, 267, 272, 280, 310, 338, 378, 425
BL-13: 163, 212-213, 215-216, 218, 253, 268, 272, 301, 309-311, 327, 330, 351, 365, 378, 425
BL-15: 206, 208-209, 247, 250, 262, 312, 397, 432, 434, 445
BL-17: 199, 208, 232, 237, 242, 255, 340-341, 356, 385, 412, 445, 447
BL-18: 151, 194, 198, 232, 239-240, 242, 260, 294, 303, 326, 347, 364, 404, 412, 445, 447
BL-19: 151, 387, 445
BL-20: 168, 191, 194, 198-199, 208, 220, 222-223, 225, 229, 231-232, 235, 242-243, 247, 254-255, 257, 262, 277, 280, 291, 293, 303, 305, 307, 309-310, 321, 325, 328-330, 345, 404, 407, 419, 425-426, 430, 438, 443, 445
BL-21: 225, 227, 229, 235, 255, 257, 314, 325
BL-22: 229, 345
BL-23: 172, 206, 216, 221-223, 231, 240, 242, 245, 247-249, 261-263, 271, 276-277, 280, 396, 409, 411, 415, 425, 430, 432, 438-440, 443, 445, 447-448
BL-24: 411
BL-25: 230, 232, 247, 277, 295, 305, 320, 326, 329, 340, 345, 347, 388, 392, 395, 397-398, 400, 405, 419, 438
BL-27: 209, 388, 432
BL-28: 296, 345, 409, 430, 440
BL-29: 345, 347
BL-30: 249, 296, 347, 439
BL-31: 52
BL-32: 235, 296
BL-34: 52
BL-36: 47, 434
BL-38: 172, 177, 206, 309-310, 408, 411, 448
BL-43: 294, 387
BL-46: 228
BL-47: 245, 261
BL-48: 427
BL-49: 276
BL-53: 51, 292, 294, 345, 354, 387, 430
BL-54: 169, 198, 269, 272, 284-285, 295-297, 303, 319, 323, 326, 328, 339, 356, 368, 383, 385, 388, 393
BL-57: 339-341, 343, 361, 410
BL-58: 314, 331
BL-60: 197, 271, 276, 339, 410, 447
BL-62: 57, 276, 312, 339, 345

BL-63: 57
BL-65: 276
BL-67: 49, 339-340, 354, 366-367, 409

Conception Vessel

CV-1: 54-55
CV-2: 53, 223, 249, 291, 422, 430, 443
CV-3: 46, 49, 53, 235, 242, 278, 296, 326, 341, 345, 354, 409, 440
CV-4: 46, 49, 53, 168, 172, 177, 191, 194, 199, 206, 216, 221, 223, 225, 229, 247-248, 254-255, 258, 262-263, 277-278, 280, 296, 321, 345, 347, 381, 399, 411-412, 415, 422, 425, 432, 438-439, 448
CV-6: 168, 172, 194, 198-199, 206, 221, 229, 231, 243, 248, 254, 256, 258, 263, 277, 296, 321, 343, 345, 347, 363, 381, 411, 415, 430, 439, 443, 448
CV-8: 231, 277, 339-340, 345, 347, 363, 381, 395, 443
CV-9: 221-222, 247, 263, 347, 396, 430
CV-10: 277, 364, 398-399, 404, 419
CV-11: 294, 387, 397, 430
CV-12: 45, 47, 177, 215, 220, 225, 228-230, 235, 248, 255-257, 277, 280, 291-293, 295, 305, 307, 309-312, 314, 321, 325, 329-331, 339-340, 345, 347, 351, 354-355, 364, 390, 395, 403, 405, 407, 411, 415, 425-426, 430, 445
CV-13: 45, 47, 211, 227, 255-256, 294, 317, 339, 341-342, 362, 426
CV-14: 209, 211, 347, 397, 434
CV-15: 211
CV-17: 51, 211-212, 229, 235, 252-253, 262, 309-311, 317, 332
CV-21: 229, 305, 329, 419
CV-22: 57, 215, 235, 253, 258, 262, 330, 339, 390, 437
CV-23: 57, 235, 339
CV-24: 45, 269

Gallbladder

GB-1: 47, 237, 269
GB-3: 45, 51
GB-6: 45, 51
GB-7: 48
GB-8: 48
GB-10: 48
GB-11: 48
GB-12: 48
GB-13: 58
GB-14: 51, 58
GB-15: 48, 58, 163, 269, 314, 342

GB-16: 58
GB-17: 58
GB-18: 58
GB-19: 58
GB-20: 57-58, 163, 194, 213, 239-240, 260, 267, 269, 271, 276, 280, 291, 312, 314, 319-320, 338, 342-343, 361, 378, 381, 397, 426, 447
GB-21: 50, 58, 141, 241
GB-24: 46
GB-26: 56, 296, 443
GB-27: 56
GB-28: 56
GB-29: 276
GB-30: 48, 52, 276, 319
GB-31: 272, 276
GB-34: 192, 194, 235, 242, 257, 276, 282, 285, 294, 317, 322-323, 326, 332, 339-340, 342, 362, 384, 387, 393, 400-401, 404, 410
GB-35: 276
GB-38: 297
GB-39: 58, 241, 271, 388
GB-40: 235, 257, 276, 294, 326, 403
GB-41: 52, 235, 237, 342, 347, 362
GB-42: 269
GB-44: 52

Governing Vessel

GV-1: 49, 54, 231, 345
GV-4: 168, 172, 177, 206, 221-223, 231, 247-250, 254, 262-263, 277, 280, 345, 363, 408, 415, 438, 443, 448
GV-5: 345
GV-6: 345
GV-8: 447
GV-12: 338, 393, 411
GV-13: 48
GV-14: 44-45, 47-48, 50-51, 54, 163, 169, 172, 177, 213, 241, 250, 260, 268-269, 282, 284, 301, 312, 314, 319, 322-323, 339, 341-342, 355, 368, 378, 384, 393, 414, 426, 435, 447
GV-15: 58, 378, 397
GV-16: 54, 57-58, 88, 267, 271, 312, 319, 338, 361
GV-17: 48
GV-20: 48, 54, 172, 177, 200, 222-223, 231, 237, 239-240, 242, 249, 254, 260, 268-269, 277, 284-285, 312, 314-315, 358, 369, 383, 394, 408, 411, 415, 426, 434, 438, 443, 447
GV-24: 45, 48, 314, 331, 427
GV-25: 194, 208
GV-26: 177, 197, 200, 271, 284-285, 312, 315, 319, 331, 358, 369, 396-397, 433-434

Heart

HT-1: 211, 434
HT-3: 276
HT-5: 169, 209, 248, 252, 312, 315, 322, 366-368
HT-6: 209, 228, 252, 255, 282, 339, 354-355
HT-7: 194, 197, 206, 208-209, 223, 242, 247-248, 251, 261-262, 283-284, 312, 315, 322, 339, 345, 355, 358, 369, 397, 403, 414, 433, 440, 445
HT-8: 209, 211, 252, 434

Kidney

KI-1: 177, 200, 240, 312, 315, 331, 408, 434, 447
KI-2: 49, 276, 443
KI-3: 169, 172, 177, 208-209, 215, 218, 228, 239-240, 242, 245, 247-249, 251-252, 259-261, 263, 283, 302, 322, 327-328, 345, 356, 363, 381, 389, 394, 411-412, 414, 425, 430, 432, 439, 445, 447-448
KI-4: 315
KI-6: 56, 215, 218, 232, 245, 253, 261, 278, 312, 321, 339, 345, 397
KI-7: 163, 177, 215, 218, 221, 245, 253, 261, 267, 296, 302, 326-328, 339, 378, 396, 411, 430, 436, 448
KI-9: 57
KI-10 245
KI-11: 55
KI-12: 439
KI-14: 398, 450

Large Intestine

LI-1: 39, 347
LI-2: 269, 414, 443
LI-3: 276, 345
LI-4: 39, 141, 163, 169, 172, 177, 191-192, 200, 220, 226, 232, 235, 237, 239, 249, 257-258, 267, 269, 271-272, 276-277, 280, 284, 291-293, 295, 301, 309-310, 316, 319-320, 322-323, 325, 332, 338-339, 342-343, 345, 347, 351, 355, 361-362, 364-365, 368, 378, 381, 389, 392-394, 397, 399-400, 405, 408, 410-411, 425-426, 436, 447
LI-5: 275
LI-6: 169
LI-9: 326
LI-10: 235, 269, 272, 276, 282, 319, 327
LI-11: 192, 197-198, 232, 235, 240, 258, 269, 272, 276, 282, 284-285, 291-293, 295, 301-302, 305, 315, 319, 322-323, 327, 339-340, 342, 347, 351, 355-356, 361, 368, 378, 383-385, 388, 397, 426, 435
LI-15: 276, 312, 319, 340, 361
LI-17: 235
LI-20: 268

Lung

LU-1: 46, 212, 253
LU-5: 163, 213, 215, 268, 276, 282, 301, 311, 322, 330, 378, 384, 388, 425
LU-6: 301, 340
LU-7: 163, 212, 245, 253, 267, 269, 272, 280, 309-311, 319-320, 345, 396, 425, 430, 437
LU-8: 339
LU-9: 163, 206, 215-216, 218, 253, 261, 267, 301, 309-311, 330, 339, 345, 388, 425, 430, 437
LU-10: 163, 215, 218, 253, 272, 283, 301-302, 311, 322, 327-328, 345, 351, 365, 378, 385, 394, 414
LU-11: 163, 311, 365

Liver

LV-1: 52, 198, 200, 223, 255, 278, 321, 406, 422, 440, 442-443
LV-2: 192, 197, 229, 235, 237, 240, 245, 257, 259, 278, 283, 296-297, 394, 403, 425, 427, 447
LV-3: 169, 172, 192, 194, 197-198, 225, 235, 237, 239, 257, 259-261, 283, 294, 312, 314-315, 319, 322, 326, 328, 331, 347, 356, 368, 387, 389, 399, 403, 422, 435, 443, 445
LV-4: 268
LV-5: 242, 319, 404
LV-8: 194, 235, 239, 242, 294, 303, 328, 356, 368, 388, 399, 414
LV-13: 52, 229, 235, 294, 332
LV-14: 46, 57, 151, 192, 235, 239, 321, 347, 364, 403

Miscellaneous

M-BW-16 423
M-BW-29 312
M-CA-18 242, 399, 422, 443
M-HN-22 426
M-HN-3 267, 426
M-HN-9 237, 240, 242, 245, 267, 269, 314, 394, 426
M-LE-13 151
M-LE-5 208
M-LE-8 276
M-UE-1 211, 284, 393, 426, 434
M-UE-22 276
N-HN-54 208

Pericardium

PC-1: 52
PC-3: 250, 272
PC-5: 197, 296, 312, 339-342, 345, 347, 356, 362, 368
PC-6: 194, 206, 208-209, 211, 225-226, 229, 235, 240, 242, 247, 250-252, 256-257, 262, 272, 284, 286, 291-294, 305, 310-312, 314-315, 317, 325, 329-331, 339, 341-343, 345, 347, 351, 354-355, 358, 365, 369, 388-390, 394, 397, 401, 403, 405, 414, 419, 426, 433-435, 445, 447
PC-7: 172, 197, 209, 242, 252, 261, 275, 284, 302, 311, 315, 327-328, 330-331, 340, 354, 358, 366-369, 394, 414
PC-8: 209, 272, 282-283, 315, 331, 358, 369, 397, 445
PC-9: 433

Small Intestine

SI-1: 47
SI-3: 163, 241, 268-269, 271, 276, 284, 315, 339, 351, 355, 365, 368, 378, 383, 397, 410
SI-4: 275, 340
SI-5: 235, 275, 347
SI-7: 314, 331, 427
SI-9: 48, 276
SI-10: 58
SI-12: 44, 50-51
SI-17: 51
SI-18: 51
SI-19: 51, 237, 260, 314

Spleen

SP-1: 45, 197-198, 200, 223, 255, 406, 422, 442
SP-2: 307
SP-4: 194, 211, 229, 235, 252, 256-258, 276-277, 293, 295, 305, 314, 321, 325, 329, 340-343, 354, 395-396, 403-404, 407, 419, 438, 442
SP-5: 276, 310, 425
SP-6: 49, 52, 141, 163, 168-169, 172, 191, 194, 198-199, 208, 220, 222-223, 231-232, 235, 239, 242, 247, 249, 251, 254-255, 257, 259-260, 262, 268, 278, 285, 291, 293-296, 303, 305, 307, 309-310, 312, 315, 320-321, 325, 328-329, 341, 343, 354, 356, 362, 368, 378, 381, 396, 398-399, 403-404, 407, 409, 411-412, 422-423, 430, 432, 439-440, 442-443, 445
SP-8: 194, 197, 235, 317, 399, 422, 443
SP-9: 221-222, 247, 249, 252, 263, 269, 272, 276, 285, 291-292, 294, 296-297, 309-311, 317, 323, 325, 332, 341, 347, 351, 354-355, 388, 396, 409, 412, 425-426, 430, 432, 438, 442, 447
SP-10: 172, 194, 199-200, 235, 237, 242, 260, 272-273, 284, 296-297, 303, 328, 368, 385, 412, 422, 443, 447
SP-12: 53, 57

SP-13: 53, 57
SP-15: 57, 232, 388, 397
SP-16: 57, 258

Stomach

ST-4: 44, 347
ST-5: 45, 52
ST-6: 39, 45, 258, 269
ST-7: 39, 51
ST-8: 51, 58, 338-339, 361
ST-9: 45, 56
ST-12: 44-45, 47, 50-52, 56
ST-13: 44
ST-21: 225, 228
ST-22: 277
ST-24: 397
ST-25: 169, 220, 226, 228, 230, 232, 247, 255, 277, 295, 301, 305, 320, 326, 329, 340, 343, 345, 347, 354, 362, 388, 392, 397-400, 404-405, 407, 419, 438, 445
ST-28: 221, 278, 296, 321, 430
ST-29: 194, 278
ST-30: 45, 56, 235, 399, 422, 439
ST-31: 45
ST-32: 45
ST-33: 278, 321
ST-35: 276
ST-36: 39, 45, 151, 163, 168, 172, 177, 191-192, 199-200, 206, 216, 220, 222, 225, 228-229, 231, 235, 243, 247-249, 254-257, 259, 262, 276-277, 291, 297, 305, 307, 316, 319-321, 329, 332, 339-343, 345, 347, 354, 362-364, 366-367, 381, 389, 392, 395, 397, 399-400, 403, 405, 407-408, 411-412, 419, 425, 430, 435, 438, 443, 448
ST-37: 44, 226, 277, 305, 397-398, 405, 419
ST-38: 271
ST-39: 209, 252
ST-40: 211, 215, 227, 229, 256, 285, 309-312, 314, 317, 323, 330-332, 339-340, 388, 390, 397, 400, 425-427, 430, 434, 445
ST-41: 169, 227, 229, 255, 269, 276, 297, 399, 427
ST-42: 45, 397
ST-43: 226, 293
ST-44: 39, 226, 232, 255-256, 282-283, 296, 322, 339-340, 361, 388, 394, 397, 419
ST-45: 226, 255, 347, 383, 414

Triple Burner

TB-2: 172, 218, 253, 283, 301-302, 322, 327-328, 340, 342, 347, 355, 361, 366-368, 394, 401
TB-3: 218, 239, 245, 258-259, 261, 271, 342, 383, 410
TB-4: 271, 275
TB-5: 229, 267, 269, 317, 319, 332, 338-340, 342-343, 361, 364, 378, 401, 426
TB-6: 169, 192, 228, 232, 235, 255, 292, 305, 317, 325, 327-329, 332, 340-343, 361, 392, 397, 400-401
TB-10: 241, 272, 276, 342, 430
TB-13: 235
TB-14: 276
TB-15: 58
TB-17: 51, 314
TB-22: 51
TB-23: 51

Bibliography

Works Cited in the Text

Axioms of Medicine *Yī Mén Fǎ Lù* [醫門法律]. Yu Chang, Qing, 1658.

Bin Hu Sphygmology *Bīn Hú Mò Xué* [瀕湖脈學]. Li Shi-Zhen (sobriquet Bin Hu), Ming, 1564.

Canon of Perplexities *Nàn Jīng* [難經]. attrib. Qin Yue-Ren, Eastern Han, c. 100.

Canon of the Golden Coffer and Jade Sheath *Jīn Guì Yù Hán Jīng* [金匱玉函經]. Northern Sung (c. 960-1126), revision of a section in Zhang Ji's *Shāng Hán Zá Bìng Lùn* (Treatise on Cold Damage and Miscellaneous Diseases) [傷寒雜病論]. Eastern Han, c. 220.

Case Studies for Clinical Guidance *Lín Zhèng Zhǐ Nán Yī Àn* [臨證指南醫案]. Ye Gui (Tian Shi), Qing, 1766.

Essential Prescriptions of the Golden Coffer *Jīn Guì Yào Luè* [金匱要略]. Zhang Ji (Zhong Jing), Later Han, c. 220.

Gateway to Medicine *Yī Xué Rù Mén* [醫學入門]. Li Yan, Ming, 1575.

Great Compendium of Acumoxatherapy *Zhēn Jiǔ Dà Chéng* [鍼灸大成]. Yang Ji-Zhou, Ming, 1601.

Illustrated Supplement to the Categorized Canon *Lèi Jīng Tú Yì* [類經圖翼]. Zhang Jie-Bin (Jing Yue), Ming, 1624.

Jing Yue's Complete Compendium *Jǐng Yuè Quán Shū* [景岳全書]. Zhang Jie-Bin (Jing Yue), Ming, 1624.

Major Thermic Pestilences *Guǎng Wēn Yì Lùn* [廣溫疫論]. Dai Tian-Zhang (Bei Shan), Qing, 1722.

Origin and Outcome of Disease *Zhū Bìng Yuán Hòu Lùn* [諸病源候論]. Chao Yuan-Fang, Sui, 610.

Priceless Prescriptions *Qiān Jīn Yào Fāng* [千金要方]. Sun Si-Mo, Tang, 652.

Referenced Medical Remedies *Yī Fāng Kǎo* [醫方考]. Wu Kun, Ming, 1584.

Savior General Compendium *Shèng Jì Zǒng Lù* [聖濟總錄]. Shen Fu et al., eds., Song, 1111-1117.

Systematized Identification of Thermic Disease *Wēn Bìng Tiáo Biàn* [溫病條辨]. Wu Tang (Ju Tong), Qing, 1798.

Treatise on Cold Damage *Shāng Hán Lùn* [傷寒論]. Zhang Ji (Zhong Jing), Later Han, c. 220.

Treatise on Thermic Heat Disease *Wēn Rè Lùn* [溫熱論]. Ye Gui (Tian Shi), Qing, c. 1746.

Yellow Emperor's Inner Canon *Huáng Dì Nèi Jīng* [黃帝內經]. Authors unknown, Former Han, c. 100 B.C. Comprises **Essential Questions** *Sù Wèn* [素問] and **Spiritual Axis** *Líng Shū* [靈樞].

Translators' References

Chinese

中草藥學		啟業書局	臺北 1970
中國針灸學概要	北京中醫學院等	人民衛生出版社	北京 1980
中國醫學大辭典	謝利恆編著	商務印書館	香港 1921
中醫大辭典		啟業書局	臺北 1983
中醫內科症治		啟業書局	臺北 1982
中醫常用術語集註	王家編著	王家出版社	臺北 1984
中醫師臨床手冊	馬康慈編著	眾文圖書公司	臺北 1983
中醫診斷學講義	廣州中醫學院	上海科學技術出版社	上海 1964
中醫詞典	徐元貞等編	河南科學技術出版社	河南 1982
中醫學診斷釋義		文光圖書公司	臺北 1982
中醫學概論	南京中醫學院	人民衛生出版社	北京 1959
中藥大辭典	江蘇中醫學院	人民出版社	上海 1977
本草備要解析	張賢哲著	中國醫藥學院出版組	臺中 1979
針灸大成	(明)楊繼洲著	文光圖書公司	臺北 1982
針灸治療學	范銘著	文源書局	臺北 1982
針灸配穴		啟業書局	臺北 1983
針灸經穴學	楊維傑編著	樂羣出版公司	臺北 1979
針灸實用驗方大全	沈祖延編著	文光圖書公司	臺北 1982
針灸學	上海中醫學院	人民衛生出版社	北京 1974
康熙字典	(清)張玉等編著	啟業書局	臺北 1981
黃帝內經		聯國風出版社	臺北 1984
傷寒論新註	承澹盦著	文光圖書公司	臺北 1979
溫病學講義	南京中醫學院	上海科學技術出版社	上海 1964
新針灸臨床治療學	馬康慈編著	眾文圖書公司	臺北 1983
新編中醫學概要		人民出版社	北京 1974
道氏醫學辭典		合記圖書出版社	臺北 1979
實用中醫方劑學	游士勳等編	樂羣出版公司	臺北 1983
鄭馬潘三氏醫案		啟業書局	臺北 1981
臨床內外科針灸學	針灸研究中心主編	武陵出版社	臺北 1984
鍼灸聚英	(明)高武撰	武陵出版社	臺北 1983
醫宗金鑒	(清)吳謙等編	新文豐出版公司	臺北 1981
類經	(明)張介賓撰	莊家出版社	臺北 1984

English

Berkow, Robert, ed. *The Merck Manual,* 13th Edition. Rahway: Merck Sharp and Dohme Research Labs, 1977.

Friel, John P., ed. *Dorland's Illustrated Medical Dictionary,* 26th Edition. Philadelphia: W.B. Saunders, 1981.

Kaptchuk, Ted. *Web That Has No Weaver.* New York: Congdon and Weed, 1983.

O'Connor, J. and Dan Bensky, trans. *Acupuncture, a Comprehensive Text.* Chicago: Eastland Press, 1981.

Porkert, Manfred. *The Theoretical Foundations of Chinese Medicine.* M.I.T. East Asian Science Series, Vol. 3. Cambridge: M.I.T. Press, 1974.

Taber, Clarence W. *Taber's Cyclopedic Medical Dictionary,* 10th Edition. Philadelphia: F.A. Davis, 1965.

Williams, P and Roger Warwick, eds. *Gray's Anatomy,* 36th Edition. London: Churchill Livingstone, 1980.

Wintrobe, M.W. et al., eds. *Harrison's Principles of Internal Medicine,* 7th Edition. New York: McGraw-Hill, 1974.

References for the Introduction

Ackerknecht, Erwin H. "Psychopathology, Primitive Medicine and Primitive Culture." *Bulletin of the History of Medicine* 14 (1943): 30-67.

———. *A Short History of Psychiatry.* New York: Hafner, 1968.

Agren, Hans. "Patterns of Tradition and Modernization in Contemporary Chinese Medicine." In *Medicine in Chinese Cultures.* See Arthur Kleinman et al., 1975.

Bhardwaj, S.M. "Homoeopathy in India." *Social and Cultural Context of Medicine in India.* New Delhi: Vikas, 1981.

Baumann, Barbara. "Diversities in Conceptions of Health and Physical Illness." *Journal of Health and Human Behavior* 3 (1961): 34-46.

Beijing College of Traditional Chinese Medicine, et al. *Essentials of Chinese Acupuncture.* Beijing: Foreign Languages Press, 1980.

Blacker, Carmen. "The Catalpa Bow: A Study of Shamanic Practices in Japan." London: George Allen and Unwin, 1975.

Blendon, Robert J. "Can Chinese Health Care Be Transplanted Without China's Economic Policies?" *New England Journal of Medicine* 300, no. 26 (1979): 1453-1458.

Burkitt, D.P. "Some Diseases Characteristic of Modern Western Civilization." In *Health and the Human Condition,* edited by M. Lugen and E. Hunt. Belmont: Wadsworth, 1978.

Cassell, Eric J. "The Nature of Suffering and the Goals of Medicine." *New England Journal of Medicine* 306, no. 11 (March 18 1982): 639-645.

Caudill, William. "The Cultural and Interpersonal Context of Everyday Health and Illness in Japan and America." In *Asian Medical Systems*, edited by Charles Leslie. Berkeley: University of California Press, 1977.

Caudill, William, and Helen Weinstein. "Maternal Care and Infant Behavior in Japan and America." *Psychiatry* 32 (1969): 12-43.

Chang, Weining C. "A Cross-Cultured Study of Depressive Symptomatology." *Culture, Medicine and Psychiatry* 9 (1985): 295-317.

Chen, Meng-lei, et al. *Gu-jin Tu-shu Ji-cheng: Yi-bu Quan-lu* (Medical Part of the Collection of ancient and Modern Books, vol. 295). Beijing: People's Health Press, 1962. (This is the medical section of the imperial encyclopedia, first published in 1726 AD).

Chen, Xiu-yuan. *Yi-xue Shi-zai Yi* (Dependable and Easy Medical Studies). Fujian: Fujian Science and Technology Press, 1982. (First appeared in 1808 AD).

Cheung, F., and B. Lao. "Situational Variations of Help-Seeking Behavior Among Chinese Patients." *Comprehensive Psychiatry* 23 (1982): 252-62.

Chu, Godwin C. "The Changing Concept of Self in Contemporary China." In *Culture and Self*, edited by A. Marsella et al. New York: Tavistock, 1985.

Chin, Robert and Ai-li. *Psychological Research in Communist China: 1949-1966*. Cambridge: M.I.T. Press, 1968.

Croizier, Ralph C. *Traditional Medicine in Modern China*. Cambridge: Harvard University Press, 1968.

Davis, Winston. *Dojo: Magic and Exorcism in Modern Japan*. Palo Alto: Stanford University Press, 1980.

Eisenberg, Leon. "What Makes Persons 'Patients' and Patients 'Well'?" *American Journal of Medicine* 69 (August 1980): 227-286.

Engel, George L. "The Need for a New Medical Model: A Challenge for Biomedicine." *Science* 196, no. 4286 (April 8 1977): 129-136

———. "The Clinical Application of the Biopsychosocial Model." *American Journal of Psychiatry* 137, no. 5 (May 1980).

Englehardt, H. Tristram. "The Disease of Masturbation: Values and the Concept of Disease." *Bulletin of the History of Medicine* 48 (1974): 234-248.

Epler, D.C. "Bloodletting in Early Chinese Medicine and Its Relation to the Origin of Acupuncture." *Bulletin of the History of Medicine* 54 (1980): 337-367.

Fabrega, Horacio. *Disease and Social Behavior*. Cambridge: MIT Press, 1980.

Gernet, J. *Daily Life in China on the Eve of the Mongol Invasion.* Palo Alto: Stanford University Press, 1970.

Gilbert, Arthur N. "Doctor, Patient and Onanist Diseases in the Nineteenth Century." *Journal of the History of Medicine* 30 (1975): 217-224.

Harvey, Youngsook Kim. *Six Korean Women: The Socialization of Shamans.* St Paul: West Publishing, 1979.

Helman, Cecil E. "Psyche, Soma and Society: The Social Construction of Psychosomatic Disorders." *Culture, Medicine and Psychiatry* 9 (1985): 1-26.

Hillier, S.W., and J.A. Jewell. *Health Care and Traditional Medicine in China, 1800-1982.* London: Routledge and Keagan Paul, 1983.

Hsu, Francis L. "Suppression vs. Repression: A Limited Psychological Interpretation of Four Cultures." *Psychiatry* 12 (1949): 223-42.

———. *Religion, Science and Human Crisis.* London: Routledge and Keagan Paul, 1952.

———, 1971a. "Eros, Affect and Apo." In *Kinship and Culture.* Chicago: Aldine, 1971.

———, 1971b. "Psychosocial Homeostasis and Jen: Conceptual Tools for Advancing Psychological Anthropology." *American Anthropologist* 73 (1971): 23-44.

———. *Americans and Chinese.* Honolulu: University of Hawaii Press, 1985.

Hu, Hsien Chin. "The Chinese Concept of 'Face'." *American Anthropologist* 46 (1944): 45-63.

Huang-di Nei-jing Su-wen (Yellow Emperor's Inner Classic of Medicine). Beijing: People's Press, 1963. (First appeared c. 100 B.C.)

Huang-fu Mi. *Zhen-jiu Jia-yi Jing Jiao-shi* (Systematic Classic of Acupuncture with Annotations). Annotations by Shandong Institute of Traditional Chinese Medicine. Beijing: People's Press, 1979. (First appeared 282 A.D.)

Huard, Pierre, and Ming Wong. *Chinese Medicine.* New York: World University Library, McGraw-Hill, 1968.

Hunan Medical School. *Jing-shen Yi-xue Ji-chu* (Foundations of Psychiatry). Hunan: Hunan Science and Technology Press, 1979.

Imboden, J.B., et al., 1961b. "Convalescence from Influenza: A Study of Psychological and Clinical Determinants." *Archives of Internal Medicine* 108 (1961): 393-399.

———, 1961a. "Symptomatic Recovery from Medical Disorders: Influence of Psychological Factors." *Journal of American Medical Association* 178 (1961): 1182-84.

Inglis, Brian. *The Diseases of Civilization.* Lanton: Granada, 1981.

Jewson, N.D. "The Disappearance of the Sick Man from Medical Cosmology, 1770-1870." *Sociology* 10 (1976): 225-244.

Kendall, Laurel. "Supernatural Traffic: East Asian Shamanism." *Culture, Medicine, and Psychiatry* 5 (1981): 171-191.

Kleinman, Arthur. "Social, Cultural and Historical Themes in the Study of Medicine in Chinese Societies" and "Discussion of Papers on Chinese Cultures." In *Medicine in Chinese Cultures.* See Kleinman et al., 1975.

———. "Depression, Somatization and the 'New Cross-Cultural Psychiatry'." *Social Science and Medicine* 11 (1977): 3-10.

———, 1980a. "Indigenous and Traditional Systems of Healing." In *Health for the Whole Person,* edited by Arthur C. Hastings et al. Boulder: Westview Press, 1980.

———, 1980b. *Patients and Healers in the Context of Culture.* Berkeley: University of California Press, 1980.

———. "Neurasthenia and Depression: A Study of Somatization and Culture in China." *Culture, Medicine and Psychiatry* 6, no. 2 (1982): 117-190.

Kleinman, Arthur, et al., eds. *Medicine in Chinese Cultures.* Washington D.C.: John E. Fogarty International Center for Advanced Study in the Health Sciences, U.S. Dept. of HEW, NIH, 1975.

Lampton, David M. *The Politics of Medicine in China: The Policy Process, 1949-1977.* Folkestone: Dawson, 1977.

———. "Changing Health Policy in the Post-Mao Era." *Yale Journal of Biology and Medicine* 54 (1981): 21-26.

Lau, Bernard, et al. "How Depressive Illness Presents in Hong Kong." *Practitioner* 227 (January 1983): 112-115.

LaBarre, Weston. "Some Observations of Character Structure in the Orient." *Psychiatry* 9 (1946): 215-237.

Leigh, H., and M. F. Reiser. "Major Trends in Psychosomatic Medicine: the Psychiatrists' Evolving Role in Medicine." *Annals of Internal Medicine* 87 (1977): 233-239.

Leslie, Charles. "Medical Pluralism in World Perspective (1)." *Social Science and Medicine* 14B (1980): 191-195.

Levinson, J.M. "Traditional Medicine in the Democratic Republic of North Vietnam." *American Journal of Chinese Medicine* 2, no. 2 (1974): 159-162.

Li Shi-zhen. *Ben-cao Gang-mu* (The Great Materia Medica), vol. 4. Beijing: People's Press, 1981. (First appeared 1596 A.D.)

Ling-shu-jing Bai-hua-jie (Canon of the Spiritual Axis with Vernacular Explanation). Edited by Chen Bi-liu and Cheng Zhou-ren. Beijing: People's Hygiene Press, 1963. (First appeared c. 100 B.C.)

Liu, Xie-he. "Psychiatry in Traditional Chinese Medicine." In *British Journal of Psychiatry* 138 (1981): 429-433.

Lock, Margaret M. "Scars of Experience: The Art of Moxibustion in Japanese Medicine and Society." *Culture, Medicine and Psychiatry* 2 (1978): 151-175.

———, 1980a. *East Asian Medicine in Urban Japan.* Berkeley: University of California Press, 1980.

———, 1980b. "The Organization and Practice of East Asian Medicine in Japan: Continuity and Change." *Social Science and Medicine* 14B (1980).

Macek, Catherine. "Medical News: East Meets West to Balance Immunologic Yin and Yang." *Journal of American Medical Association* 251, no. 4 (1984): 433-441.

Malinowski, Bronislaw. *A Scientific Theory of Culture and Other Essays.* Chapel Hill: University of North Carolina Press, 1944.

Marsella, Anthony J. "Depressive Experience and Disorders Across Cultures." In *Handbook of Cross-Cultural Psychology*, vol. 6. *Culture and Psychopathology*, edited by H. Triandis and J. Draguns. Boston: Allyn and Bacon, 1980.

McCorkle, T. "Chiropractic: A Deviant Theory of Disease and Treatment in Contemporary Western Culture." *Human Organization* 20, no. 20 (1961): 20-22.

McNeill, William H. *Plaques and Peoples.* London: Penguin, 1985.

McRae, Ginger. "A Critical Overview of U.S. Acupuncture Regulation." *Journal of Health Politics, Policy and Law* 7, no. 1 (1982): 163-196.

McQueen, D. and J. Sigrist. "Social Factors in the Etiology of Chronic Disease: An Overview." *Social Science and Medicine* 14B (1980): 353-367.

Mechanic, David. "Social Psychologic Factors Affecting the Presentation of Bodily Complaints." *New England Journal of Medicine* 286, no. 21 (1972): 1131-1139.

———. "The Experience and Reporting of Common Physical Complaints." *Journal of Health and Social Behavior* 21 (1980): 146-155.

Minocha, A.A. "Medical Pluralism and Health Services in India." *Social Science and Medicine* 21, no. 4 (1985): 383-390.

Murphy, E., and G. Brown. "Life Events, Psychiatric Disturbance and Physical Illness." *British Journal of Psychiatry* 136 (1980): 326-388.

Nagi, Saad Z., et al. "A Social Epidemiology of Back Pain in a General Population." *Journal of Chronic Disease* 26 (1973): 769-779.

Nan-jing Jiao-shi (Canon of Perplexities with Annotations). Edited by Nanjing Institute of Traditional Chinese Medicine. Beijing: People's Press, 1979. (First appeared c. 200 A.D.)

Neumann, A.K., and P. Lauro. "Ethnomedicine and Biomedicine Linking." *Social Science and Medicine* 16 (1982).

Ohnuki-Tierney, Emiko. *Illness and Culture in Contemporary Japan.* Cambridge: Cambridge University Press, 1984.

Otsuka, Yasuo. "Chinese Traditional Medicine in Japan." In *Asian Medical Systems,* edited by Charles Leslie. Berkeley: University of California, 1977.

Parrish, W., and M.K. Whyte. *Village and Family in Contemporary China.* Chicago: University of Chicago Press, 1978.

Parsons, Gail Pat. "Equal Treatment for All: American Medical Remedies for Male Social Problems: 1850-1900." *Journal of the History of Medicine* 32 (1977): 55-71.

Pelletier, Kenneth R. *Holistic Medicine.* New York: Delta/Seymour Lawrence, 1979.

Palos, Stephen. *Chinese Art of Healing.* New York: Herder and Herder, 1971.

Potter, J.M. "Wind, Water, Bones and Souls: The Religious World of the Cantonese Peasant."*Journal of Oriental Studies* 8 (1970): 139-153.

Rin, Hsien. "A Study of the Aetiology of Koro in Respect to the Chinese Concept of Illness." *International Journal of Social Psychiatry* 11 (1965): 7-13.

Risse, Guenter B. "Epidemics and Medicine: the Influences of Disease on Medical Thought and Practice." *Bulletin of the History of Medicine* 53 (1979): 505-519.

Rosenthal, Marilynn M. "Political Process and the Integration of Traditional and Western Medicine in the People's Republic of China." *Social Science and Medicine* 15A (1981): 599-613.

Rubel, Arthur J. "Concepts of Disease in Mexican-American Culture." *American Anthropologist* 62 (1960): 795-814.

Sargent, Carolyn. "Between Death and Shame: Dimensions of Pain in Bariba Culture." *Social Science and Medicine* 19, no. 12 (1984): 1299-1304.

Scofield, Robert W. and Chin-wan Sun. "A Comparative Study of the Differential Effect Upon Personality of Chinese and American Child Training Practices." *Journal of Social Psychiatry* 52 (1960): 221-224.

Shepherd, M., et al. "Minor Mental Illness in London: Some Aspects of a General Practice Survey." *British Medical Journal* 2 (1964): 1359-1363.

Shweder, Richard, and Edward Bovine. "Does the Concept of the Person Vary Cross-Culturally?" In *Cultural Conceptions of Mental Health and Therapy,* edited by A. Marsella and G. White. Dordrecht: D. Piesel, 1982.

Singer, K. "Depressive Disorders from a Transcultural Perspective." *Social Science and Medicine* 9 (1975): 289-301.

Sivin N. "Why the Scientific Revolution Did Not Take Place in China - or Didn't It?" *Chinese Science* 5 (1982):45-66.

Smith, Wesley D. *The Hippocratic Tradition.* Ithaca: Cornell University Press, 1979.

Song, Kwang-Soo. *A Study on Acupuncture Treatment and Classification of 16-Sang Constitutions.* Seoul: Korea Constitution Acupuncture Association, 1979.

Song, Weizhen. "A Preliminary Study of the Character Traits of the Chinese." In *Chinese Culture and Mental Health,* edited by W.S. Tseng and D.Y.H. Wu. Orlando: Academica Press, 1985.

Spence, Jonathan. "Commentary on Historical Perspectives and Ching Medical Systems." *Medicine in Chinese Cultures.* See Kleinman et al., 1975.

Stoeckle, J.D., I.K. Zola, and G.E. Davidson. "The Quality and Significance of Psychological Distress in Medical Patients." *Journal of Chronic Disease* 17 (1964): 959-970.

Sun Si-Miao (Sun Si-Mo). *Qian-jin Yao-fang* (Thousand Ducat Prescriptions). Taipei: National Traditional Chinese Medical Research Bureau, 1965. (First appeared 652 A.D.)

———. *Qian-jin Yi-fang* (Supplemental Wings to the Thousand Ducat Prescriptions). Beijing: People's Press, 1982. (First appeared 682 A.D.)

Swartz, Leslie. "Anorexia Nervosa as a Culture-Bound Syndrome." *Social Science and Medicine* 20, no. 7 (1985): 725-730.

Tessler, R., D. Mechanic, and M. Dimond. "The Effect of Psychological Distress on Physician Utilization: A Prospective Study." *Journal of Health and Social Behavior* 17 (1976): 353-364.

Tseng, Wen-shing. "The Nature of Somatic Complaints among Psychiatric Patients: The Chinese Case." *Comprehensive Psychiatry* 16, no.3 (May/June 1975).

Tseng, Wen-shing, and Jing Hsu. "Chinese Culture, Personality Formation and Mental Illness." *Journal of Social Psychiatry* 16, no. 5 (1979): 5-14.

Unschuld, Paul U. "Medico-Cultural Conflicts in Asian Settings: An Explanatory Theory." *Social Science and Medicine* 9:303-312.

———. "Discussion on David McQueen's Paper." *Social Science and Medicine* 12 (1978): 75-77.

———. *Medicine in China: History of Ideas*. Berkeley: University of California Press, 1985.

Veith, Ilza. "The Supernatural in Far Eastern Concepts of Mental Disease." *Bulletin of the History of Medicine* 37, no.2 (March/April 1963): 139-58.

White, G. "The Role of Cultural Explanations in 'Somatization' and 'Psychologization'." *Social Sciences and Medicine* 16, no. 16 (1982): 1519-1530.

Wolff, B. Berthold and Sarah Langley. "Cultural Factors and the Response to Pain: A Review." *American Anthropologist* 70 (1964): 494-501.

Wu, Tang. *Wen-bing Tiao-bian Bai-hua-jie* (Systematized Identification on Thermic Diseases with Vernacular Explanation). Beijing: People's Health Press, 1963. (First appeared 1789 A.D.)

Yalom, Irvin D. *The Theory and Practice of Group Psychotherapy*. New York: Basic Books, 1985.

Yang, Zi-zhu. *Zhen-jiu Da-cheng* (Compendium of Acupuncture). Beijing: People's Press, 1978. (First appeared 1601 A.D.)

Yap, P.M. "Mental Disease Peculiar to Certain Cultures: A Survey of Comparative Psychiatry." *Journal of Mental Science* 97 (1951): 313-327.

Yeh, Eng-Kung. "The Chinese Mind and Human Freedom." *International Journal of Social Psychiatry* 18 (1978).

Zborowski, Mark. "Cultural Components in Response to Pain." *Journal of Social Issues* 8 (Fall 1952): 16-30.

———. *People in Pain*. San Francisco: Jossey-Bass, 1969.

Zhang Jie-Bin. *Jing-yue Quan-shu* (Complete Works of Jing-yue). Taipei: Guofeng Press, 1980. (First appeared 1624 A.D.)

Zhang Zhong-jing (Zhang Ji). *Shang-han Lun Xin-zhu* (Discussion on Cold-induced Disorders with New Commentary). Commentary by Cheng Tan-an. Hong Kong: Shaohua Cultural Service, 1955. (Main text appeared c. 220A.D.)

Zola, Irving Kenneth. "Culture and Symptoms - An Analysis of Patients' Presenting Complaints." *American Sociological Review* 31 (October 1976): 612-630.

———. *Socio-Medical Inquiries*. Philadelphia: Temple University Press, 1983.

Chinese Medical Concepts Index

abdominal distention: 46, 51, 99, 139, 174, 203, 289, 326, 325, 342, 349, 352, 367, 387, 391, 394-395, 404, 418, 427

abdominal fullness: 180, 182, 298, 339-340, 342, 361-362

abdominal glomus (lump, lump glomi): 46, 55, 173-174, 185, 191, 329, 398

abdominal pain: 43-44, 48, 53, 56-57, 76, 79, 98, 102, 114, 137-138, 165-166, 169, 179, 185, 198, 219-220, 228, 233, 254, 256-257, 276-278, 294, 320, 326, 329, 342, 394, 398, 401, 404, 406, 418

abduction *dǎo* (gl: 432, pn: 453): 229, 329, 417

abscess *yōng* (gl: 484, pn: 453): 105

absence of thirst: 164, 166-167, 176, 179, 186, 266, 324, 342-343, 394

accumulation *jī* (gl: 439, pn: 453): 29, 33-35, 80, 104, 137, 172, 189, 195, 218, 281, 307, 390-391, 394, 417-418

aching bones: 89, 99, 165, 319-320, 414

acid regurgitation *tūn suān* (gl: 125, pn: 453): 233, 418

acid upflow *fǎn suān* gl: 168, pn: 453): 138, 257

affect damage *nèi shāng qī qíng* (gl: 52, pn: 454): 95, 265, 308

agitation *fán zào* (gl: 366, pn: 454): 67, 98, 113, 168, 170, 176, 179, 185, 208, 281, 287, 314, 323, 339, 357, 391-393, 402, 445

agitated and racing pulse: 176, 360

alternating fever and chills: 52, 134, 165, 294, 341-342, 362, 400

amenorrhea: 81, 198, 260, 398

anaphylactoid purpura: 197

anemia: 115, 120, 122, 206

angina pectoris: 204, 209, 252, 433-434

animated pulse: 146, 156

anuria: 86, 136

apathetic: 112, 176

aplastic anemia: 197

appendicitis: 125, 151-152

arrhythmia: 204, 206

arteriosclerosis: 146, 148

articular pain: 58, 345, 409

ascariasis of the biliary tract: 359

ascendant hyperactivity: 5, 15, 121

ascites *fǔ shuǐ* (gl: 384, pn: 454): 149, 395; [cirrhotic]: 122

asthenia: 204, 219, 245

asthma: 122, 309; [bronchial]: 131

astringe and secure bowels: 230, 437

atony *wěi* (gl: 379, pn: 454): 46, 49, 75, 85, 87, 113

attack *gōng* (gl: 139, pn: 455): 149, 165, 173, 373-375, 390, 395

audio-olfactive examination *wén zhěn* (gl: 410, pn: 455): 111, 129, 133

aversion to cold: 43, 45, 105, 134, 161, 164-167, 178-179, 181, 183, 186, 190, 224, 246, 274, 279, 319-320, 337, 343, 349, 361, 363, 365, 371, 377, 379, 394, 405-408, 414, 416; [mild]: 178

aversion to heat: 98, 164, 179, 281, 339, 351, 361, 366-367

aversion to wind: 134, 161, 170, 265-268, 337, 361, 365

bag-over-the-head sensation *tóu zhòng rú guǒ* (gl: 443, pn: 455): 135, 427

balloon-head scourge *dà tóu wēn* (gl: 22, pn: 455): 269

banking up earth *péi tǔ* (gl: 261, pn: 455): 14-16

biliary tract diseases: 191, 233

binding depression of liver qi *gān qì yù jié* (pn455): 81, 101, 138, 140, 191-192, 232-233, 237, 257-258, 304, 402

binding phlegm-fire depression: 127, 286

bitter fullness in the chest *xiōng xié kǔ mǎn* (pn: 456): 165, 341, 362

bitter taste in the mouth: 52, 80, 138, 165, 226, 294, 326, 331, 341, 351, 366-367, 400

black complexion: 115

black tongue fur: 125, 391

bladder: 32, 41-42, 48-49, 64, 66, 71, 73-74, 76, 83-84, 86, 91-92, 96

bladder channel: 45-48, 51-52, 54, 57-63, 88

bladder fire: 38; [heat]: 341, 401

bleeding: 127-128, 197, 200, 203, 225, 255, 301, 435

bloating: 77-78, 254

block *bì* (gl: 291, pn: 456); [patterns]: 192

block clouding inversion *nèi bì hūn jué* (gl: 50, pn: 456): 169

blood: 7, 23-30, 33, 36-38, 53, 60, 65, 67, 72-75, 77, 81-83, 86, 91, 95-96, 98, 101, 134, 171, 189, 244, 344, 360, 370, 412

blood amassment *xuè xùe* (gl: 417, pn: 456): 117, 398

blood and lymphatic drainage disturbances: 119

blood and pus in the stool: 98, 294

blood and qi disharmony: 28

blood-aspect: 122, 349, 355, 358, 368

blood breaking: 196-197, 373

blood cold: 194

blood collapse: 33, 155

blood containment failure: 74, 116, 222, 219

blood cooling: 198, 356, 382, 385

blood depletion: 356

blood dissipation: 356

blood dryness: 302, 328

blood failing to nourish [eyes, liver, sinews]: 241

blood formation: 27, 28-29, 69

blood heat: 29, 192, 194, 197, 384-385

blood nourishing: 232, 274, 303, 328

Concepts Index

blood management failure: 75, 219, 222-223, 255
blood quickening *huó xuè* (gl: 192, pn: 457): 184, 196
blood retrenchment: 33
blood stasis: 29, 68, 72, 80, 98, 104, 114-115, 122, 127-128, 141, 146, 148, 194-195, 274, 419
blood storage failure: 232
blood supplementing: 194
blood transformation: 27
blood vacuity: 4, 29, 90, 114, 141, 154, 171, 192-194, 203, 206, 231, 266, 272, 302, 411
blood vessels: 24, 27
blurred vision: 53, 82, 237, 241, 244
body *xíng tǐ* (gl: 120, pn: 457): 25, 31, 40, 61, 111, 133
boosting *yì* (gl: 230, pn: 457): 14, 171, 190; [fire]: 6, 14; [qi]: 106, 222, 251, 255, 218, 380, 436
borborygmi: 44, 80, 102, 169, 404
bound pulse: 148
bowel *fǔ* (gl: 336, pn: 457): 26, 40-41, 65-66
brain: 54, 88
breast [lumps]: 102, 233, 258; [swelling]: 80, 233, 402; [distended]: 191, 198, 258; [scant milk]: 56
breathing: 25, 27, 36, 70, 73, 132
brewing hepatocystic damp-heat: 326
brittle nails: 302
bronchitis: 125, 130, 146, 213, 309
bruxism *yǎo yá* (gl: 178, pn: 458): 127
burning sensation: 225, 255, 294
burnt tongue fur: 124, 339, 368, 391
calculi: 417
calculous strangury *shí lín* (gl: 102, pn: 458): 129, 295
carcinoma: 115, 122
cardiac failure: 35, 204, 246
cardiac obturation: 148, 211, 252
cardiac pain: 204
cardiac portals *xīn qiào* (gl: 71, pn: 458): 43, 89
cardiac qi vacuity: 190
cardialgia *xīn tòng* (gl: 68, pn: 458): 47, 50, 58, 138
cardiodynia *zhēn xīn tòng* (gl: 234, pn: 458)
cardiohepatic fire effulgence: 208
cardiopulmonary qi vacuity: 128, 204, 206, 215-216
cardiorenal debilitation: 363
cardiorenal vacuity: 75
cardiorenal yang debilitation: 165, 246, 262
cardiorenal yang vacuity: 87, 128, 204, 215-216
cardiorenal yin vacuity: 15, 206, 244, 261
cardiosplenic blood vacuity: 193, 203, 206
cardiosplenic heat: 121
cardiosplenic vacuity: 69
cardiovascular diseases: 195, 420
carphologia *xún yī mō chuáng* (gl: 308.1, pn: 458): 112-113

center *zhōng* (gl: 38, pn: 458); [center-qi fall]: 77, 219, 221-222
cerebrovascular trauma with fainting: 434
channel: 24, 27, 40, 49, 52, 58, 61, 63, 79; [passage] *chuán jīng* (gl: 347, pn: 459); [qi]: 24; [theory]: 37-39
child fright wind *xiǎo ér jīng fēng* (gl: 24, pn: 459): 55, 397, 425
children: 85, 117, 121, 127-128, 140-141, 150, 247, 249, 263; [childbearing]: 89-90 102, 140
cholecystitis: 122, 219, 359
cholelithiasis: 115, 359
choppy pulse: 146
clamoring stomach *cáo zá* (gl: 391, pn: 459): 77, 137, 169, 219, 225, 288
clean tongue fur: 122-123
clear *qīng* (gl: 280, pn: 460): 34, 70, 73, 76, 78, 86, 98; [clearage]: 281, pn: 460): 96, 165, 168, 173, 197, 301-302, 340, 353, 373, 382, 385
clear-food diarrhea *xià lì qīng gǔ* (gl: 9, pn: 460): 6, 14, 68, 167, 181, 254, 340, 343-344, 374, 405
clearage of damp-heat: 386
clearing and draining damp-heat: 293
clearing and outthrusting pathogenic heat: 366
clearing blood heat: 384
clearing construction: 368
clearing dryness and restoring the lung: 303
clearing fire: 273; [heat]: 229, 282, 352, 386
clearing heat and detoxifying: 322
clearing heat and diffusing: 366
clearing heat and disinhibiting: 295, 326
clearing heat and freeing strangury: 430-431
clearing heat and resolving toxin: 311, 368, 379, 382
clearing heat and transforming: 291, 324-325, 330, 358, 387
clearing phlegm-heat: 379
clearing qi: 353, 366, 383
clearing summerheat: 284-285, 299, 323
cloud *méng* (gl: 413, pn: 460); [head]: 350; [inversion]: 50, 200, 433-434
clouding of spirit-affect: 176
clouding of spirit-disposition: 98, 204
clouding of the spirit: 45, 164, 182, 283, 301, 308, 349, 354, 368, 384, 392, 433, 435, 445
clove lesions *dīng chuāng* (gl: 147, pn: 460): 105
cold *hán* (pn: 460): 26, 29, 79, 105, 113, 134, 147, 161, 166, 268, 274-276, 355, 372; [environmental qi]: 96
cold along the thigh and knee: 46
cold and pain in the abdomen: 98, 181; [in the joints]: 274; [in the stomach and abdomen]: 405
cold blocking lung qi: 169
cold constipation: 137

cold diarrhea: 277, 279, 321
cold dissipation: 96
cold dryness: 303
cold enveloping fire *hán bāo huǒ* (gl: 307, pn: 460): 286
cold falsely presenting as heat: 170
cold form *xíng hán* (gl: 119, pn: 460): 204, 215, 220, 262, 274, 279, 309, 330
cold limbs: 181
cold obturation: 275, 279, 320
cold pain: 43, 155, 276, 279, 320
cold shan *hán shàn* (gl: 308, pn: 460): 278-279, 321
cold skin: 176, 360
cold, pungent exterior resolution: 319
cold-damp: 122, 274, 279
cold-damp obturation: 140
cold-heat complex: 169, 364, 404
cold-heat conversion: 7
cold-rheum: 211-212
cold-phlegm: 308, 317, 330, 423
coldness at the tips of the fingers: 150
colelithiasis: 422
collapse *wáng* (gl: 17, pn: 461): 176
column rheum *zhī yǐn* (gl: 72, pn: 461): 318
coma: 67, 104, 197, 314, 357, 369, 433-434
combination/complex patterns: 159-160
confined pulse: 145
conception vessel: 46, 51-53, 55, 57, 59, 61-63, 81, 84, 89-90, 102, 140, 193, 241
concretions and gatherings *zhēng jiǎ jī jù* (gl: 475, pn: 461): 80, 104, 151, 195, 417-418
congealing *níng* (gl: 430, pn: 461); [blood]: 29
congestion of lung qi: 72, 127-128, 211, 253, 265-266
conglomerations: 417-418
conjunctivitis: 269
connect *luò* (gl: 331, pn: 462); [channels]: 37, 42
constipation: 43, 48, 72, 76, 115, 120, 137, 169, 180, 186, 218, 227, 255-256, 276, 294, 305, 329, 339-341, 349, 361-362, 374, 391, 393-395, 398-399, 418
constitution: 30, 96, 112, 144, 171, 372, 375; [weak]: 26; [body] *tǐ* (gl: 489, pn: 462)
constitutional yang vacuity: 406
constraining *liǎn* (gl: 446, pn: 462): 435-436
construction *yíng* (gl: 451, pn: 462): 24, 134-135, 337-338, 355, 360, 370
construction qi: 24, 27-28, 31, 33, 104, 134, 337
construction-aspect: 122, 349, 358, 368
construction-blood: 164, 402
construction-defense disharmony: 162, 337-338
construction-defense harmonization: 178
consumption of alcohol: 102
contraction *gǎn* (gl: 353, pn: 462): 27, 71, 161
contracture and tautness *shōu yǐn* (gl: 109, pn: 462): 275; [contracture]: 98

conversion *zhuǎn huà* (gl: 470, pn: 463): 159-160, 174
convulsive spasm *chōu chù* (gl: 160, pn: 463): 82, 97, 164, 260, 266, 269, 273, 311, 319, 331, 354, 356, 368, 397, 433, 445
correct *zhèng* (gl: 95, pn: 463): 105-107, 123, 171, 174, 203, 337, 341, 373
correct qi *zhèng qì* (gl: 95.1, pn: 463): 6, 8, 25, 104-107, 111-112, 116-117, 124, 135, 142, 147, 171, 173, 335-336, 347, 373-374, 391, 395, 399
cosmic qi *dà qì* (gl: 20, pn: 463): 23
cottage cheese tongue fur: 124
cough: 27, 34-35, 43, 70, 72-73, 87, 101, 128, 131, 138, 161, 173, 203-204, 211-215, 217, 244, 265-268, 304, 308, 310, 316, 330, 338, 349-352, 365-366, 378-379, 423, 436
cough and diarrhea: 345
cough and rapid breathing: 253
cough causing pain in the chest: 308
cough with copious phlegm: 426
coughing of blood: 288
counterflow *nì* (gl: 252, pn: 463): 71, 76, 78, 132, 211, 228, 256
counterflow frigidity of the limbs *sì zhī nì lěng* (pn: 463): 49, 166-167, 345, 405, 407
counterflow qi: 204, 213; [qi cough]: 84
coursing *shū* (gl: 317, pn: 463): 26, 79-81, 83, 89-90
cracked gums: 225
crimson *jiàng* (gl: 333, pn: 464); [tongue]: 29, 34, 120-122, 164, 198, 301, 344, 354, 357, 368-369, 384, 388
crying: 128
cumbersome limbs: 99, 290
curious organs: 66
curled, recumbent: 166-167, 185, 343, 363, 407
cutaneous cornification *jī fū jiǎ cuò* (gl: 114, pn: 464): 150, 174, 195, 302
cyan *qīng* (gl: 175, pn: 464): 114; [complexion]: 114, 166-167, 169
cyan-purple complexion: 68, 183, 204, 209, 252
cyan-purple lips: 29, 72, 104, 114, 127, 204, 210, 215
cyan-purple swellings: 195
cyan-purple tongue: 29, 72, 104, 121, 175, 183
damage to fluids: 99, 281
damage to liquid: 31, 33-34, 127, 301, 327, 300, 400; [and qi]: 288
damage to yin: 5, 120-121, 123-124, 171, 142, 301, 328, 360, 368
damp arising from the center: 299
damp clouding the upper burner: 297
damp encumbrance: 147, 154, 330
damp forming with cold *shī cóng hán huà* (gl: 447, pn: 464): 298
damp forming with heat *shī cóng rè huà* (gl: 448, pn: 465): 298
damp in the liver: 427

Concepts Index

damp in the lower burner: 427
damp in the spleen: 427
damp in the stomach: 427
damp obstruction: 138, 289, 299, 325
damp obturation: 319
damp papules: 289, 427
damp pathogen: 96, 99
damp phlegm *shī tán* (gl: 449, pn: 465): 122, 308-309, 317, 330, 423, 425
damp thermia: 349-350, 352, 365
damp transformation: 96, 106, 298, 373, 428
damp turbidity *shī zhuó* (gl: 450, pn: 465): 204, 218, 426
damp-heat: 7, 116, 129, 132, 137, 174, 272, 278, 289, 291, 293-295, 299, 353-354, 386-388
damp-heat in the lower burner: 7, 129
damp-heat lodged in the qi aspect: 291, 299, 325, 358
damp-heat lodged in the triple burner: 291, 352
dark complexion: 112, 183; [cyan]: 447; [gray]: 115
dark rings around the eyes: 174
dark tongue: 276; [purple]: 195, 210; [red]: 7
dark-colored urine: 98, 100, 186, 281, 295, 367, 382-383, 427, 431
daybreak diarrhea *chén xiè* (gl: 273, pn: 465): 6, 14, 79, 87, 137, 246
deafness: 43, 51-52, 86, 139, 236, 345
debilitation *shuāi* (gl: 249, pn: 465): 103; [following illness]: 219; [organ qi]: 156; [original qi]: 103, 405; [spirit]: 344; [visceral qi]: 148; [vital gate fire]: 79
deep, fine pulse: 447
deep, full pulse: 145, 164
deep, hidden pulse: 179, 181
deep, replete pulse: 180, 343
deep, replete, forceful pulse: 361
deep, slippery and forceful pulse: 369
deep, slippery pulse: 314
deep, slippery, and rapid pulse: 352, 367
deep, slow pulse: 179, 276-277, 406
deep, tight pulse: 145
deep, weak pulse: 220, 414
deep, wiry pulse: 145, 316
deep, wiry, tight pulse: 321
deep crimson tongue: 356, 368
deep pulse: 144-145, 153, 254
deep red tongue: 120-121, 212

deep-lying *fú* (gl: 103, pn: 465); [cold]: 145; [heat]: 124
defense *wèi* (gl: 427, pn: 465): 25, 91, 134, 337, 360, 370; [against pathogens]: 25, 70
defense qi: 24, 26, 31, 71, 104, 134-135, 161-162, 337-338
defense-aspect: 349, 358, 365
defense-construction disharmony *yíng wèi bù hé* (gl: 452, pn: 466)

deficient reproductive function: 243, 247, 263
deficit *piān shuāi* (gl: 255, pn: 466): 107, 375-376
deformation of joints: 113
delayed closure of the fontanels: 85, 247, 263
delirium: 29, 45, 58, 67, 354, 357; [mania]: 69, 180, 182, 198; [speech]: 50, 185, 195, 281, 339, 361, 369
dental disorders: 85
depletion of blood and qi: 115
depletion of fluids: 34, 301
depletion of hepatorenal yin humor: 239
depletion of the blood: 193
depressed fire: 286; [heat]: 218
depression *yù* (gl: 493, pn: 466): 58, 70, 90, 281, 402
depurative downbearing *sù jiàng* (gl: 346, pn: 466): 13, 32, 70-71, 211, 213-216, 253, 308
derangement of the spirit: 130, 203
desertion *tuō* (gl: 285, pn: 467): 27, 33, 114-115
desiccated *kū* (gl: 185, pn: 467); [tongue and teeth]: 356; [intestinal humor]: 304
desire for quiet: 166-167, 185
desire for warmth: 274
desire only for sleep: 344-345
detoxification *jiě dú* (gl: 388, pn: 467): 106, 173, 197-198, 326, 382
detoxifying and draining fire: 302
devitalization of splenic yang: 164, 219-221, 254, 298, 342, 344
diabetic disease *xiāo kě* (gl: 222, pn: 467): 137, 225, 346, 364
diaphoresis: 162, 337, 377-378, 387
diarrhea *xiè xiè* (gl: 166, pn: 468): 27, 34, 43, 46, 48, 75-80, 87, 98, 102, 129, 137, 145, 164, 166, 169, 203, 218-220, 230, 245, 254, 257, 263, 274, 277, 281, 291, 305, 329, 342-343, 345-346, 349, 362-363, 372, 379, 391, 397, 404-407
diarrhea with discomfort unrelieved by evacuation: 294, 306, 342, 418
diarrhea with foul-smelling stool: 179, 292, 326, 367, 369
diet: 137; [irregularities]: 102, 191, 219, 223, 265, 304
diffusing the lung: 253, 267-268
diffusion: 13, 34-35, 70-71, 73, 91
diffusion and outthrust: 384
digestate accumulation: 102, 146, 153, 169, 228, 304, 307, 339, 417
digestion: 31, 65, 74, 76-77, 137, 218; [incomplete]: 87; [impaired]: 218-219; [indigestion]: 26, 77-78, 99, 137, 289
diminished appetite: 78, 180, 285, 291, 305, 349, 386; [diminished food intake]: 80, 293
diminished qi *shǎo qì* (gl: 65, pn: 468): 112, 283, 288
diphtheria: 127-128, 303
direct strike *zhí zhòng* (gl: 151, pn: 468): 348

direct treatment: 372
discharge *xiè* (pn: 468): 32-34, 55, 79
disharmony *bù hé* (gl: 32, pn: 469): 162
disinhibition *lì* (gl: 121, pn: 469); [of urine] *lì niào* (gl: 122, pn: 469); [of water]: 418; [of damp]: 298-299, 325, 427-428
disinhibiting water: 295, 430
disorientation of the spirit-disposition: 357
dispelling: 106, 373, 420
dispelling wind: 272, 312, 319, 331, 423, 425
dispersion *xiāo (fǎ)* (gl: 221, pn: 469): 173, 197, 258, 305, 315, 332, 391, 417-418
disposition *zhì* (gl: 137, pn: 469): 67; [excess]: 206, 281
disquieting *bù* (gl: 29, pn: 469); [of heart spirit]: 102, 206
disrupted downbearing: 341, 404
disrupted upbearing: 341, 404
disruption of fluid metabolism: 243
dissipating cold: 6, 167, 320
dissipating wind-heat: 268
dissipation of qi and blood: 155
distention *zhàng* (gl: 334, pn: 470): 27, 43, 49, 70, 77-78, 138, 221, 339
distention in the abdomen: 43, 56, 76, 78, 191, 373
distention in the chest: 53, 233, 332
distressed breathing: 70, 215
divergent channel: 37, 41, 59-62
dizziness: 7, 27, 29, 43, 47, 49, 53, 58, 68-69, 85, 87, 89, 97, 102, 113, 139, 165, 180, 184, 193, 198, 203-204, 206, 222, 237, 239, 241, 244, 246-247, 250-251, 259-262, 266, 273, 308, 312, 331, 426, 445
dolorous obturation *tòng bì* (gl: 318, pn: 470): 275
dormant papules *yǐn zhěn* (gl: 480, pn: 470): 271
dorsal styloid pulse *fǎn guān mài* (gl: 64, pn: 470): 144
downbearing *jiàng* (gl: 199, pn: 470): 6, 8, 23, 27, 33-34, 65, 73, 77-78, 83, 353
downbearing qi and transforming phlegm: 258
downpour of damp-heat: 243, 294-295, 298, 326
drainage *xiè* (gl: 463, pn: 471); [fire/heat]: 6, 72, 128, 236, 252, 282, 322
drained white *huǎng bái* (pn: 471); [complexion]: 114, 171, 181, 183, 185-186, 199, 210, 220, 246, 254, 262, 228
draining: 34, 106, 168, 173-174, 208
draining fire: 228, 256, 353, 387
dream emission *mèng yí* (pn: 471): 69, 288
dribbling incontinence *xiǎo biàn lín lì* (gl: 26, pn: 471): 86, 136, 183
drool *xián* (gl: 223, pn: 471): 127
drop in blood pressure/ body temperature: 200, 407
drumskin pulse: 147, 155
dry: 78, 105, 300, 304; [environmental qi]: 96
dry blood engendering wind: 272-273
dry cough: 213, 216, 253, 261, 300, 327
dry eyes: 57, 81-82

dry feces: 48
dry lips: 300, 310, 327-328
dry miliaria *kū péi* (gl: 186, pn: 471): 117
dry mouth: 34, 44, 49, 87, 101, 170, 208, 216, 226-227, 236, 244, 253, 255-256, 259, 268, 310, 319, 322, 327-328, 344, 349, 365, 377, 412
dry nose: 327; [and nosebleed]: 45; [dry nostrils]: 127, 288, 300
dry pharynx: 87, 165, 184, 213, 244, 341-342, 344, 400, 412; [and mouth]: 356, 363
dry skin: 33, 71, 112, 300; [and hair]: 29
dry stool: 49, 76, 236, 300, 418; [bound stool]: 34, 327-328; [hard]: 129, 231, 281, 304
dry teeth: 127
dry throat: 43, 47, 170, 300, 310; [and lips]: 261; [and mouth]: 168, 182, 282
dry tongue: 34, 101, 120-122, 124, 281, 300, 302, 310, 314, 354, 383, 391
dry tongue fur: 100, 122, 283, 327
dry, lusterless hair: 302
dry, parched-black nose: 127
dry, red tongue: 176
dry, rough skin: 195, 302; [and itching]: 272
dryness pathogen: 96, 99, 101
dryness phlegm: 308, 310, 317
drying damp: 292, 299, 325, 330, 367
dual blaze of qi: 449
dual patterns: 15, 165-166, 198
dual resolution of interior and exterior: 375, 449
dual supplementation of qi and blood: 198
dual vacuity of blood and qi: 127, 146-147, 198
dual vacuity of yin and blood: 173
dual vacuity of yin and yang: 5, 107, 147, 416
duck stool *yā táng* (gl: 445, pn: 471): 75, 129
dysentery *lì* (gl: 323, pn: 471): 129, 294, 372, 382-383, 388, 394
dyspeptic anorexia *nà dāi* (gl: 241, pn: 471): 6, 76, 78, 124, 139, 325-326, 387, 427
dyspnea *chuǎn* (gl: 306, pn: 472): 35, 43-44, 72-73, 114, 128, 131, 169, 174, 203-204, 211-213, 246, 253, 262, 288, 308, 332, 338, 352, 378
dysuria: 86
ear: 31, 86, 89, 128, 139, 237
eczema: 99, 289, 427
edema *fú* (gl: 219, pn: 472): 34, 46, 49, 51, 114, 122, 215
edematous swelling *fú zhǒng* (gl: 220, pn: 472): 46
efflux *huá* (gl: 362, pn: 472); 137, 437
effulgent *wàng* (gl: 163, pn: 472); [effusion]: 91
emaciation: 103, 112, 114, 174, 182, 184, 216, 221, 241, 244, 253-254, 282, 306, 318, 328, 388, 412
emotional disorders: 58, 232; [depression]: 148; [disturbance]: 80, 90, 191, 197, 204, 206, 219, 253; [factors]: 140, 404

Concepts Index

encumbrance *kùn* (gl: 126, pn: 473); [damp]: 174
endogenous *nèi* (gl: 48, pn: 473): 97, 160; [disease factor]: 95, 101, 107
endogenous cold: 98, 274, 372, 405
endogenous damage: 80, 101-102, 189
endogenous damp: 75, 100, 289
endogenous dryness: 101
endogenous heat: 99, 134
endogenous wind: 82, 87, 121, 273, 445
enduring *jiǔ* (gl: 14, pn: 473): 115, 130; [disease]: 26, 34, 112, 115, 153, 171, 195, 227, 301
enduring diarrhea *jiǔ xiè* (gl: 15, pn: 473): 14, 49, 86, 140, 221, 230, 285, 437
enduring diarrhea efflux desertion *jiǔ xiè huá tuō* (gl: 16, pn: 473): 27, 435; [clear-food]: 246
enriching: 14-15, 260-261, 304; [yin]: 6, 238, 251, 274, 300; [humor]: 328
enriching yin and calming: 259
enriching yin and clearing: 322, 363
enriching yin and constraining: 436
enriching yin and downbearing fire: 252
enriching yin and moistening: 253
enriching yin and nourishing: 368
enriching yin and resolving: 106, 380
enrichment *zī* (gl: 361, pn: 473): 171
enteritis: 372
entry *rù* (gl: 1, pn: 473): 8, 23, 33
enuresis *yí niào* (gl: 441, pn: 473): 49, 51, 53, 86, 136, 203, 243, 249, 263, 435, 439
environmental excesses *yín qì* (gl: 279, pn: 473): 95-96, 102, 265, 280
epilepsy: 114, 127, 311, 397, 433
epistaxis: 322, 327
erosion, oral: 15, 48, 69, 105, 124, 208, 272
eructation: 76, 78, 101, 219, 224, 228, 257, 305, 329, 403, 418
erysipelas: 382
esophageal constriction *yē gè* (gl: 418, pn: 474): 129
essence: 23, 26-28, 30-31, 36, 66, 73-76, 84, 89, 91; [congenital]: 30, 302
essence-spirit *jīng shén* (gl: 406, pn: 474): 22, 30, 65, 67-68, 79-80, 101, 103, 196, 204, 233
essence-spirit disorders: 47, 50, 55, 67, 232; [agitation;]: 357; [debilitation]: 112, 248, 360; [depression]: 90, 101, 257; [derangement]: 69, 101, 314, 331; [disturbance]: 27, 29, 69, 191, 197, 219; [excitation]: 237, 281; [fatigue]: 250; [hebetude of]: 204, 246; [obtundation]: 434; [torpor]: 181, 434
essential qi *jīng qì* (gl: 407, pn: 474): 6, 23-24, 26-27, 30-32, 66, 70, 73-74, 82, 84-87, 89-90, 139, 141, 144, 170-171, 203, 243; [expiry]: 155; [insufficiency]: 85-87
excessive dreaming: 15, 67, 69, 139, 206, 241, 244, 260-261
exhaustion *jié* (gl: 405, pn: 474): 33, 101, 199, 219, 283, 288, 301, 416

exogenous *wài* (gl: 90, pn: 474): 97, 145, 160, 231; [disease factor]: 95, 107; [pathogen]: 24, 26, 38, 71
exogenous cold: 98, 274
exogenous damp: 100, 233, 289
exogenous dryness: 101, 300
exogenous heat diseases *wài gǎn rè bìng* (gl: 91, pn: 474): 34, 42, 92, 99, 120, 130, 163-165, 189, 197, 227, 231, 301, 314, 335-337, 339, 346-348, 350-351, 360, 371, 374, 377, 382, 386, 388, 392, 396, 400, 433-434, 445
exogenous wind: 134, 273
expectoration *sòu* (gl: 390, pn: 474): 34-35, 83, 128, 161, 197, 241, 281, 308, 330
expectoration of blood: 84, 197, 236, 241, 244, 412, 441
expectoration of phlegm: 43, 104, 228, 266, 316, 330
expelling parasites: 391
expiry *jué* (gl: 332, pn: 475)
expulsion *zhú* (gl: 288, pn: 475): 338, 389, 391, 394, 398
exterior *biǎo* (gl: 173, pn: 475): 7, 24, 37-38, 41-42, 66, 69, 71-73, 77, 79-80, 84, 91, 96-97, 145, 159-161
exterior cold: 161, 178
exterior exogenous contraction: 70, 153, 160, 178
exterior repletion: 162, 178, 361
exterior resolution: 106, 178, 337, 373, 365, 377, 379
exterior vacuity: 162, 178, 361, 378
extinguishing wind *xī fēng* (gl: 402, pn: 475): 444-445; [liver wind]: 43
extreme cold: 160
extreme heat: 97, 160, 164, 356
exuberance and debilitation *shèng shuāi* (pn: 475)
exuberant fire in the upper body: 236
exuberant heat: 120, 132, 302, 340, 352, 371
exuberant heat in the qi aspect: 366-367
exuberant pathogenic qi: 173
exuberant pulmogastric heat: 351, 366
eyes: 47, 57, 126-127, 239
facial [edema]: 204, 215, 332; [paralysis]: 127, 269, 271, 273
faint: 130; [voice]: 26, 130
faint, fine pulse: 204, 252, 360, 407
faint pulse: 147, 154, 186, 405; [expiry]: 170
false repletion: 372
false signs: 174, 371-372
false-spiritedness: 112
fast, fine pulse: 252
fast, floating pulse: 365
fast, irregularly interrupted pulse: 148
fast, surging, slippery and replete pulse: 182
fatigue: 58, 249, 254; [lack of strength]: 174, 180; [and weakness]: 103, 189, 290

fatigued limbs: 100, 285, 289, 293, 297, 299, 308, 330, 407
fecal incontinence: 86, 437
feeble, fine, and rapid pulse: 282-283
feebleminded withdrawal: 314
fetter *shù* (gl: 141, pn: 476): 266
fever: 6, 53, 87, 97, 99, 105, 121-122, 135, 138, 161, 164-165, 179, 265-268, 279, 282-283, 285, 291-292, 294, 310, 319-320, 324-326, 330, 335, 337-338, 342, 346, 349, 351-352, 354, 356, 360-361, 365-367, 378, 382, 387-388, 391, 398, 400
fever, [general]: 100, 150, 339, 351, 361, 368; [great]: 134, 361; [low]: 134, 290, 325, 377; [moderate]: 314; [non-vigorous surface]: 369; [persistent]: 134, 291, 325, 427, 323, 388; [remittent]: 134, 299, 352, 367, 387; [steady]: 244, 261, 416; [unabating]: 351, 378
fever in the five hearts *wǔ xīn fán rè* (pn: 477): 151, 168, 182, 184, 251
fever in the palms of the hands and soles: 283
fifth-watch diarrhea *wǔ gēng (jīng) xiè* (gl: 44, pn: 477): 262
fine, faint pulse: 165, 343-344, 363; [verging on expiry]: 209
fine, rapid pulse: 182, 184, 208, 251, 261, 328, 344, 356, 363
fine, rough pulse: 195
fine, soft pulse: 189
fine, soggy pulse: 222, 255
fine, weak pulse: 180
fine, weak, rapid pulse: 146
fine pulse: 29, 104, 144, 154, 184, 186, 193, 206, 238, 244, 369, 411
fire *huǒ* (gl: 79, pn: 477): 10, 105, 280, 282; [environmental qi]: 96; [pathogen]: 96, 98-99
fire and kidney vacuity: 139
fire drainage: 97, 340, 382
first-stage construction-aspect: 354
first-stage qi-aspect: 351-352, 366
five forms of taxation damage *wǔ láo suǒ shāng* (pn: 477): 103
five phases: 3, 10-14, 16-17, 114; [in medicine]: 12; [cycles]: 10-11, 13; [organs]: 7-8, 12
flaring nostrils: 127, 212, 349
flatulence: 80, 329
floating *fú* (gl: 218, pn: 477); [fire]: 286-287; [complexion]: 287
floating, tight pulse: 320, 377
floating and rapid pulse: 161, 349
floating pulse: 144, 153, 161, 265-266, 319, 337, 361
flowery vision *mù huā* (gl: 101, pn: 478): 29, 81, 136, 139, 180, 184, 193, 241, 260-261
fluids *jīn yè* (gl: 191, pn: 479): 5, 23-24, 26-27, 31-34, 36-38, 57, 70-71, 73-75, 91-92, 98, 120, 134, 177, 399

flushing *dàng dí* (gl: 440, pn: 479); 367; [cheeks]: 253, 287
foaming at the mouth: 311, 331
food: 30-31, 66, 137, 305; [cold]: 102, 223, 306; [fatty]: 102, 137, 293, 306, 308; [rich, hot, spicy]: 102, 225, 306; [fried]: 306; [raw]: 102, 223, 306; [unclean]: 102
foot-qi disease *jiǎo qì* (gl: 382, pn: 479): 99, 289; [ejection contraindication]: 390
forceless, fine pulse: 251, 322
formation *huà* (gl: 56, pn: 479); [fluids]: 32; [qi and blood]: 42
fostering *yù* (gl: 172, pn: 479): 6, 416
free downflow *tōng jiàng* (gl: 290, pn: 480): 12, 76-77
freeing *tōng* (pn: 480); [and warming the channels]: 405; [strangury]: 326; [connecting channels]: 332
frenetic blood heat *xuè rè wàng xíng* (gl: 115, pn: 480): 197, 281
frenetic movement *wàng xíng* (gl: 107, pn: 480); [blood]: 80, 99, 356, 368, 392
fright inversion *jīng jué* (gl: 488, pn: 480): 314
frigid *lěng* (pn: 480); [extremities]: 279, 314, 414, 416; [limbs]: 87, 169, 179, 186, 190, 204, 209, 212, 215, 250, 262, 394, 408, 447; [excreta]: 98
full pulse: 147
fullness *mǎn* (gl: 400, pn: 480): 46, 70, 138
fullness, infracardiac: 403-404
fullness in the abdomen: 51, 56, 76, 293, 341
fullness in the chest: 42-43, 47, 50, 53, 297, 308, 316
fulminant diarrhea: 166-167, 176
fulminant downpour *bào zhù* (gl: 421, pn: 481): 98
fulminant fluid desertion: 136
fulminant pain in the abdomen: 167
fulminant vomiting: 166-167, 176
gallbladder: 41-42, 46, 50-52, 64-66, 79-80, 125
gallbladder channel: 45-48, 50-51, 56-59, 62-63
gallbladder heat: 341, 401; [fire]: 387; [damp]: 427
gan *gān* (gl: 226, pn: 481); [gan accumulation] *gān jī* (gl: 227, pn: 481): 127, 307
gangrenous lesion *jū* (gl: 228, pn: 481): 105
gaping mouth: 435
gas: 305
gastric heat: 76, 127
gastric disharmony: 76, 218, 227-228
gastric neurosis: 224
gastric qi vacuity cold: 223-224, 255
gastritis: 119, 191, 219, 225
gastrointestinal accumulation: 305-306, 329
gastrointestinal harmonization: 404

gastrointestinal heat-bind: 39, 43, 134, 164, 351, 360, 367, 374
gastrointestinal neurosis: 191
gastrointestinal obstruction: 169
gastrointestinal qi stagnation: 228
gastrointestinal repletion heat: 361
gastrosplenic vacuity cold: 362
gathering *jù* (gl: 409, pn: 481): 104, 148
gingival vacuity edema: 127
gingivitis: 225, 269
girdling vessel: 53
globus hystericus: 101
glomus: 102, 138, 192, 297, 341, 369, 391
glossitis: 120
glossy tongue fur: 122; [black]: 125
governing vessel: 45, 47-51, 53-55, 58-63, 88, 258
great heat *dà rè* (gl: 21, pn: 482): 323, 339, 360, 366
great heat in the qi aspect: 351-352, 366
gynecologic disorders: 56, 122
hair: 126, 263
halitosis: 76, 132, 226, 255, 288, 393
hard stool: 139, 164, 170, 281, 288, 291-293, 302, 342, 352, 386; [bound]: 179, 367, 369; [dry]: 137
hardness *jiān* (gl: 262, pn: 482): [abdomen]: 51; [softeners]: 417
harmonization *hé (fǎ)* (gl: 154, pn: 483): 165, 341, 362, 400
harmonizing construction: 400, 402, 436
headache: 39, 42-43, 47, 49, 52-53, 135, 161, 165, 178, 208, 239, 244, 259, 261, 265-268, 288, 319-320, 337, 350, 365, 379, 393, 426, 445
headache: [lateral]: 58; [recurrent]: 128; [severe]: 135, 236; [wind-cold]: 114
hearing and vision: 139
heart *xīn* (gl: 66, pn: 483): 25, 27-29, 34, 41-42, 47, 49-50, 64-69, 73, 77, 82-83, 90-91, 125, 187
heart, cardiorenal interaction: 69, 87, 107, 139, 203, 208, 252
heart blood: 68-69, 89-90, 139, 156, 193-194
heart blood vacuity: 69, 90, 139, 193, 206-207, 251
heart channel: 43, 46, 50, 59-62
heart disorder: 69, 114-115, 122, 130, 209
heart fire: 13-16, 38, 68-69, 87, 101, 119, 208, 252, 288, 344; [effulgence]: 69, 83, 87
heart governs: 27, 67, 69
heart heat: 114, 252
heart qi: 68, 72, 89, 148, 203, 250
heart qi vacuity: 68, 204-205, 209, 215, 250
heart yang: 7, 14-15, 68, 83, 89, 203-204, 252
heart yang vacuity: 204-205, 210, 250
heart yin: 7, 12, 15, 68, 87, 89, 203-204
heart yin vacuity: 68, 87, 171, 206-207, 251
heartburn: 99

heat *rè* (gl: 424, pn: 483): 29, 69, 78, 98, 102, 113, 132-134, 154, 159, 161, 166, 168-169, 280, 282, 372; [pathogen]: 5, 265; [patterns]: 153, 168
heat clearage: 96, 106, 361, 298, 340, 372-373, 382
heat diseases: 92, 105, 116, 137, 301, 347, 384-385
heat due to insufficiency of yin humor: 168
heat falsely presenting as cold: 170, 372
heat lodging in the triple burner: 367
heat phlegm: 308, 310, 317, 330, 424
heat strangury: 382
heat toxin penetrating the construction aspect: 392
heat-block tetanic inversion *rè bì jìng jué* (gl: 425, pn: 484): 150
heatstroke: 100
heavy bleeding: 176, 199, 442
heavy [head]: 297, 312; [feeling]: 112, 289, 365, 427; [limbs]: 427
heavy micturition *duō niào* (gl: 106, pn: 484): 435
heavy settlers *zhòng zhèn yào* (gl: 198, pn: 484): 444
hemafecia, 197, 219, 222, 255, 345, 441
hematemesis: 236, 322, 390, 441
hematuria *sōu xuè; niào xuè* (gl: 360, pn: 484): 129, 197, 204, 288, 295, 432, 441
hemorrhage: 153, 194, 222, 255, 281, 368, 384; [diseases]: 419; [arrest]: 440
hemorrhoids: 55
hepatic governance of free-coursing: 80; [disruption of]: 80, 192, 403
hepatitis: 115, 151, 174, 191
hepatocystic damp-heat: 129, 138, 232, 293-294, 326
hepatocystic disease, 154, 235, 403
hepatomegaly: 422
hepatorenal essence-blood: 139, 241, 304
hepatorenal yin vacuity: 15, 237, 244, 261
hepatosplenic disharmony: 79, 233, 257, 404
hepatosplenic harmonization: 257, 404
hepatosplenomegaly: 195
hernia: 57
hiccough: 76, 78, 131-132, 228, 256, 346
hidden pulse: 145, 156, 176
high fever: 69, 98, 100, 156, 176, 212, 281, 283, 301, 314, 327, 349, 366, 369, 377, 384, 392, 433, 445
hoarse voice: 72, 130, 253, 303
home *shù* (gl: 477, pn: 484); [connecting relationships between channels and organs]: 41
hot palms: 50, 413
humor *yè* (gl: 276, pn: 485): 31, 76, 92; [depletion]: 31, 34; [desertion]: 31, 33-34, 301
hunger with no desire for food: 346, 364
hyperactivity of the sexual functions: 102, 265, 288

hyperactivity of yang due to yin vacuity: 107
hyperadrenocorticalism: 115
hyperpepsia with rapid hungering: 255
hyperplasia of the connective tissue: 119
hypersomnia: 67
hypertension: 5, 121, 313; [in the elderly]: 416
hyperthyroidism: 121-122, 206, 244
hypertonicity *jŭ* (*jŭ jí, jŭ luán*) (gl: 161, pn: 485): 29, 81-82, 275, 320, 405; [in the limbs]: 113; [elbow and arm]: 50
immediate vomiting [fluids]: 137; [food]: 228
impact trauma: 194
impaired intellect: 247; [memory]: 69, 85, 101, 206, 244, 251, 261
impatience: 233, 236, 259
impeded movement: 270, 405
impotence: 49, 56, 86, 246, 262, 414
inability to assume a recumbent posture: 174, 246
incontinence: 86, 243, 249
incontinent seminal efflux *jīng huá bú jìn* (gl: 162, pn: 485)
increasing appetite: 77, 306, 329
infants: 126-127, 146, 439
infection: 122; [encephalitis B]: 100; [hepatitis]: 6
influenza: 128, 269, 279, 303, 378
ingesta damage: 166, 304-306, 329; [diarrhea]: *shí xiè* (gl: 201, pn: 485); [accumulation]: 304
inhibition *bú lì* (gl: 30, pn: 485); [bending]: 44, 81, 99, 409; [micturition]: 49; [movement of blood]: 204
inhibited sinew-vascular movement: 241, 260
inner body *nèi* (gl: 47, pn: 485): 6, 8, 95
inner-body block *nèi bì* (gl: 49, pn: 485): 156
inner-body yin cold: 155, 170
inner-body heat: 235, 286
inner-body static blood bind: 173, 398
insecurity of construction qi: 134
insecurity of the defensive exterior: 203, 215 216
insomnia: 15, 29, 57, 69, 101, 120, 139, 184, 193, 203, 206, 208, 237, 241, 244, 251-252, 259-261, 282-283, 288, 312, 343-344, 413, 416, 426, 444-445
insufficiency *bù zú* (gl: 31, pn: 486): 29, 58, 376
insufficiency of ancestral qi: 190, 204
insufficiency of blood and fluids: 101
insufficiency of blood and qi, 154-155, 222
insufficiency of blood formation: 192
insufficiency of essence: 30, 243, 416
insufficiency of fluids: 432
insufficiency of form: 416
insufficiency of qi and yin: 154
insufficiency of yang qi: 145, 167, 171, 209-210, 221
insufficiency of yin blood: 112, 206, 233, 237
insufficiency of yin humor: 218, 282
intense heat *chì* (gl: 437, pn: 486): 121, 127, 379, 382-383

interior *lǐ* (gl: 386, pn: 486): 7, 37-38, 41-42, 66, 69, 72-73, 77, 79-80, 84, 87, 91, 114, 145, 153, 159-161
interior cold: 164, 347, 405
interior heat: 164, 347
interiorization *rù lǐ* (gl: 2, pn: 486); [cold]: 406; [heat]: 225
interrupted pulse: 68, 203-204, 250-251
intestine: 32, 42, 64, 71, 218
intestine abscesses: 392
intestine astriction: 437
intestine heat: 129, 352, 367
intestine humor depletion: 231
intestine lubrication: 391, 396, 399
intestine obstruction: 372, 391
intestine parasites: 115, 127
intestinal vacuity efflux desertion *cháng xū huá tuō* (gl: 383, pn: 486): 137, 230
intimidate *líng* (gl: 202, pn: 486); [of the heart by water-qi]: 204
invasion *fàn* (gl: 96, pn: 486): 24; [of exogenous pathogens]: 70, 335; [channels]: 98, 289, 319, 405; [lung]: 211, 217, 265; [the stomach]: 129, 233, 255, 257
inversion *jué* (gl: 302, pn: 487): 115
inversion frigidity of the limbs *sì zhī jué lěng* (pn: 487): 47, 149, 167, 170, 176, 181, 183, 204, 246, 343-344, 346, 363-364
inward fall: 368-369
irascibility: 101, 208, 236-237, 288, 393
iron-band sensation *tóu tòng rú chè* (gl: 444, pn: 487): 239
irregular menses: 56, 141, 233, 244, 246, 258, 398
irregular passage: 358
irritability: 84, 345
issue *chū* (gl: 86, pn: 487): 8, 23, 33
itchy skin: 266, 302
itchy throat: 211, 266, 319
jaundice: 46, 53, 80, 115, 126, 203, 233, 293-294, 326, 340, 386-387, 427
jerking sinews and twitching muscles *jīn tì ròu rùn* (pn: 487): 260
joints: 31, 38, 79
jue yin: 40-42, 46-47, 49-50, 52, 57, 59-64, 91, 135, 342, 345-347
kidney: 23, 26, 30-34, 38, 41-42, 48-49, 53-54, 57, 61, 63-66, 70-71, 73, 76, 82-86, 89, 91-92, 104, 125
kidney channel: 49, 54-55, 57, 60-63
kidney essence: 84, 87, 89, 102
kidney essence vacuity: 244, 247, 416
kidney failing to absorb qi: 73, 174, 447
kidney fire: 13, 288
kidney functions: 32, 66, 73, 83-85
kidney qi: 76, 84-87, 89, 127-128, 136, 243, 249, 259, 263
kidney moistening: 405
kidney supplementation: 73, 263

kidney vacuity: 115, 127, 190, 249, 344
kidney vacuity water flood *shèn xū shuǐ fàn* (pn: 488): 38
kidney yang: 7, 14-15, 17, 35, 78-79, 85, 87-88, 107, 243-245, 308, 375
kidney yang vacuity: 86, 136, 171, 204, 245, 262, 432
kidney yin: 7, 13, 15-16, 83, 87-88, 92, 127, 243, 302, 344, 375, 381, 394
kidney yin vacuity: 13, 206, 208, 244, 261, 416

labored breathing: 316
labored movement: 289
lachrymation: 48-49, 128
lack of strength: 7, 182-183, 254-255, 323
lack of warmth in the extremities: 68, 98, 150, 224, 246, 274, 321, 330
large and vacuous pulse: 283
large appetite with poor digestion: 306
large intestine: 32, 41-43, 64-66, 70, 72-74, 76, 91-92, 339
large intestine channel: 39, 43-44, 58, 60-63, 269, 272
large intestine governs: 32, 76
large intestine qi: 191
large pulse: 144, 147, 155, 173
large, surging pulse: 323, 339, 361, 366
large, surging, rapid pulse: 168
large, weak, rapid pulse: 146
laryngeal patterns: 390
laryngitis: 130
leaden *zhuó* (gl: 385, pn: 488); [obturation]: 289
leprosy: 272
lesion *chuāng (yáng)* (gl: 426, pn: 488): 382; [mouth and tongue]: 288, 393; [serous discharge]: 289
lethargy: 89, 185-186
leukemia: 197
leukorrhagia: 57
limp: [hands]: 435; [knees]: 246, 249, 263; [legs]: 259; [tongue]: 121; [powerless limbs]: 113; [limbs]: 174; [legs]: 416; [lumbar region]: 56
lingering damp-heat: 352
liquid *jīn* (gl: 190, pn: 488): 31, 92, 101; [depletion]: 231; [qi]: 157
little desire for food and drink: 69, 102, 165, 174, 227, 255, 290, 297, 306, 312, 329, 341, 362
liver: 26-28, 30, 38, 41-42, 46, 49, 52-53, 64-66, 78-83, 89-92, 101, 115, 125
liver and spleen failing to store and command blood: 81, 90
liver blood: 81-83, 139, 194, 232, 243
liver blood vacuity: 171, 193, 241, 260
liver channel: 26, 46, 52, 57, 59-63, 296, 387
liver cirrhosis: 6, 114-115, 122, 395
liver fire: 13-14, 38, 82-83, 97, 138-140, 208, 233, 235-236, 239, 259, 288, 387, 391, 393-394
liver functions: 26-27, 78-79, 81-83, 89

liver heat: 138, 379, 389
liver qi: 78-82, 89-90, 101, 191, 129, 223, 232-233, 402-404
liver wind: 42-43, 82, 97, 113, 120, 232, 239, 273, 445
liver yang: 5, 12, 15-16, 81-83, 87, 89, 121, 135-136, 139-140, 146, 203, 232, 237, 239, 259, 266
liver yin: 5, 12, 15, 81-82, 87, 237, 239, 394, 403
liver-calming: 232, 238-240, 260, 279, 312-313, 331
liver-channel qi stagnation: 191-192
liver-clearing: 236, 259, 300, 327, 385
liver-coursing: 232-233, 257, 293, 402
local numbness: 308; [palsy or paralysis]: 269, 319
long micturition with clear urine *xiǎo biàn qīng cháng* (pn: 488): 33, 86, 98, 129, 166, 179, 181, 183, 249, 274
long micturition with copious, clear urine: 246, 414, 439
long pulse: 148, 156
loose teeth: 85, 127, 247, 263
loss of appetite: 100, 289-290, 299, 403, 418
loss of consciousness: 311, 435
loss of hair: 86, 247
loss of hearing: 393
loss of visual acuity: 244
low voice: 112, 171, 180, 183, 186, 211, 213, 216, 253
lower body *xià* (gl: 6, pn: 488); [distress]; [prolapse]: 27; [vacuity]: 175
lower-body cold: 346, 364
lumps: 136, 258; [lump glomus] *pǐ kuài* (gl 325, pn: 488): 46, 53, 80, 417
lung: 23, 26-28, 32-35, 38, 41-44, 46, 49-50, 53, 62, 64-66, 70-74, 77, 83, 91-92, 104, 125, 187
lung abscesses: 128
lung channel: 27, 42-43, 46, 61-63, 72, 91
lung constraining: 436
lung ensures regular flow: 71
lung fire: 288
lung governing qi: 70, 72-73; [diffusion]: 32; [downbearing]: 32; [surface skin and body hair]: 71
lung heat: 13-14, 71-72, 127, 379
lung is the collecting place of phlegm: 73
lung opens at the nose: 65, 71
lung qi: 70-73, 93, 114, 128, 130-131, 203, 213-214, 265, 379
lung qi diffusion: 93, 268, 384
lung qi vacuity: 171, 190, 204, 211, 213, 215-217, 246, 253
lung vacuity: 15, 216, 436
lung yang: 14
lung yin: 15, 87, 131, 213
lung yin vacuity: 87, 211, 216-217, 253, 303

lusterless complexion: 29, 69, 114, 198, 219, 224, 250-251, 254
lusterless conjuctivae: 126
lusterless nails: 241
lusterless skin: 195
lymphadenhypertrophy: 422
macules: 116
maculopapular eruptions *bān zhěn* (gl: 312, pn: 488): 29, 98, 114, 116-117, 198, 281, 286, 322, 348-349, 354, 368, 382, 384, 392
malarial disease *nüè jí* (gl: 403, pn: 489): 45, 52, 55, 134, 383
mania *kuáng* (gl: 144, pn: 489): 98, 195, 281, 332, 339, 354, 444
mania and withdrawal *diān kuáng* (gl: 490, pn: 489): 46, 308, 397
manic agitation *kuáng zào* (gl: 145, pn: 489): 45, 67, 98, 101, 113, 186, 314, 369, 391, 398
marrow vacuity: 85
massive bleeding: 155, 410
massotherapy *tuī ná* (gl: 271, pn: 489): 151
measles: 377
menalgia: 233
menopause: 90
menorrhagia: 81, 83, 90, 197, 236, 141, 442
menorrhalgia: 402, 419
menstruation: 55-56, 83, 89-90, 140-141, 400; [block]: 55-56, 83, 90, 102, 233, 241; [clots]: 198; [delayed]: 141; [discharge]: 141, 398; [disorder]: 90, 102, 195, 402, 419; [prolonged]: 90; [reduced flow]: 90, 141, 241, 260; [short cycle]: 90
mental disorders: 49, 206; [depression]: 233; [distraction]: 180
mental dizziness *yūn* (gl: 355, pn: 489): 193, 198, 265, 312, 411
metrorrhagia *bēng lòu* (gl: 265, pn: 490): 56, 75, 81, 90, 102, 219, 222, 241, 255, 419, 435; [persistent]: 442
middle burner: 27, 30, 91
middle-burner damp obstruction: 297
midstage harmonization: 400
migratory pain: 97, 136, 138, 271
miliaria alba *bái péi* (gl: 98, pn: 490): 116
miliaria crystallina *jīng péi* (gl: 313, pn: 490): 117
miliaria *péi* (gl: 371, pn: 490): 114, 117
ministerial fire *xiàng huǒ* (gl: 193, pn: 490): 88
mirror tongue: 99, 120, 168, 208, 328
miscarriage: 55, 141
mixed gray and white tongue fur: 125
mixed white-and-yellow tongue fur: 352, 354, 366-367
moderate pulse: 144-145, 156, 361
moderate, floating pulse: 162, 178
moderate, soggy pulse: 406
moderate, weak pulse: 362
moist tongue fur: 122

moist white tongue fur: 166-167, 279, 319-320, 330, 377, 394
moistening the intestines: 304, 397
moistening the lung: 304
moxibustion: 187, 191, 198, 223, 405-406
muscular and articular pain: 270, 319, 320
muscular exterior *jī biǎo* (gl: 112, pn: 490): 265
musculocutaneous water swelling: 427
mussitation: 131, 185
myocardiac infarction: 209
myxedema: 119
nasal congestion: 43, 49, 128, 265
nasal polyps: 72
nausea: 6, 27, 46, 76-78, 80, 228, 233, 256-257, 285, 329, 342, 349, 386-388, 400, 418, 423, 427
nausea and vomiting: 49, 100, 104, 291, 294, 305, 308, 323, 331, 400, 426
nephritis: 114, 119, 122, 198, 245, 395, 416
neurasthenia: 245, 416
neurodermatitis: 71
neurologic disorders: 121
neurosis: 204, 206, 233, 244
night blindness: 81-82
night sweating: 134, 182, 184, 206, 216, 251, 253, 261, 322, 412, 435-436
nightmares: 58
nocturia *yè jiān duō niào* (gl: 156, pn: 491): 86, 136, 246, 262
nosebleed: 197, 236, 241, 288, 393
nourish *yǎng* (gl: 428, pn: 491): 24, 31
numbness *má mù* (gl: 296, pn: 491): 270, 272; [limbs]: 184, 315
nurturing yin and subduing yang: 232, 260
nutritional disturbance: 206, 219, 328
obesity: 112
obstruction of qi dynamic: 145
obtundation of the spirit-disposition: 357
obturation *bì* (gl: 372, pn: 491): 113, 138, 273
obturation patterns *bì zhèng* (gl: 373, pn: 491): 270-271, 273, 275, 289, 421
occasional dizziness: 228
ocular rubor *mù chì* (gl: 100, pn: 492): 38, 51, 82-83, 115, 168, 208, 236-237, 259, 269, 281, 288, 379, 383, 393
odors: 132; [malodorous] *chòu* (gl: 248, pn: 455): 129, 132; [putrid]: 132, 305i; [fishy odor]: 128, 132; [foul]: 98, 294, 305, 352
offensive treatment *gōng* (gl: 140, pn: 492): 106, 329, 361, 374-375, 395, 397, 399, 418
oligomenorrhea: 398, 411
oliguria *niào shǎo* (gl: 131, pn: 492): 71, 86, 246, 263, 283, 427, 430
opening: 43, 292, 312, 433
opisthotonos: 82, 113
oppression: 6, 53, 73, 100, 138, 174, 204, 213, 285, 289-290, 297, 299, 312, 349-350, 352, 386-387, 400, 426-427

oral gan *kǒu gān* (gl: 18, pn: 492): 132
orchitis: 56
original qi: 24, 26
osteodystrophy: 247
otogenic vertigo: 313
outer body *wài* (gl: 89, pn: 492): 8
outthrust *tòu* (gl: 287, pn: 492): 286-287, 379, 383
overfloating yang: 170
overuse of diuretic agents: 301
pain: 26, 44, 104, 114, 130, 136, 138, 147, 151, 154, 195, 203, 274, 294, 338-339, 382, 403; [back]: 49, 216, 238, 241, 244, 249, 263, 295, 416; [back of the head and neck]: 135; [cheeks]: 48, 51
pain: [chest]: 38, 47, 52, 58; [chest and lateral costal region]: 6, 52, 80, 84, 101, 203, 303, 316, 342, 402; [corneae]: 126; [ears]: 51; [eyes]: 50; [genitals]: 57; [gums]: 127; [hand and foot]: 345; [hypochondriac region]: 47, 341
pain: [joints]: 161, 362, 378; [knees and lower back]: 203; [lateral aspect of the buttocks]: 52; [lateral aspect of the shoulder]: 48; [lateral gluteal region]: 49; [lumbar region]: 49, 57, 69, 102, 259, 261; [medial aspect of the forearm]: 47; [muscles and joints]: 266
pain: [ocular]: 49; [palms]: 47; [posterior mandibular region]: 46; [posterior thigh]: 49; [precordial region]: 252; [ribs]: 340; [shoulder and upper arm]: 51; [supraclavicular fossa, chest, shoulders and back]: 43; [thigh]: 49, 52; [tongue]: 120; [venter]: 46, 169, 224, 228, 255, 257
pain and distension in the abdomen: 49, 102, 169, 291, 296, 329, 305
pain and distension in the chest: 80, 291
pain and distension in the lateral costal region: 80, 257, 293, 326, 403
pain and distension in the waist: 58
pain and heat in the cardiac region: 346
pain and limpness in the lumbar region and knees: 247
pain and stiffness in the back: 55
pain caused by breathing or coughing: 332
pain experienced when turning over in bed: 316
pain of fixed location: 289
pain or stiffness of the lower lumbar spine: 85
pain penetrating the connecting channels: 420
pain radiating into the testicles: 48
pain soothed by application of heat: 138
pain, burning sensation in the urethra: 431
pain, distention and oppression [chest]: 164, 292, 324, 435; [abdomen]: 292, 374
pain, distention exacerbated by pressure: 305, 367
pain, limp, knees, lumbar region: 262
pain, red tongue with erosion and cracking, 281
pain, sagging of the testicles: 278
pain, scapular region: 47
pain, sinews and bones: 405
pain, soles of the feet: 49

pain, strangury with dark-colored urine: 252
pain, swelling of the gums: 225, 255, 393
pain, swellings and bruises: 419
pain, swollen, red tongue: 119
pain, urination *niào tòng* (gl: 135, pn: 492): 129, 295, 382, 427
pale lips: 127
pale tongue: 120-122, 176, 184, 193, 199, 206, 210, 219, 222, 228, 251, 253-256, 276, 279, 360, 408, 411, 414
pale tongue with white fur: 179, 186, 220, 274, 321
pale white *dàn bái* (gl: 278, pn: 492); [complexion]: 114-115, 184, 193, 206, 411
pale, enlarged tongue: 122, 181, 183, 221, 224, 250, 262-263
palpable heat *zhuó rè* (gl: 143, pn: 492): 281, 382
palpation: 44, 111, 133, 141, 150-151, 176, 391
palpitation *xīn jì* (gl: 69, pn: 493): 15, 29, 35, 50, 67, 69, 72-73, 87, 101, 139, 156, 180, 184, 193, 198, 203-204, 206, 209, 215, 222, 237, 244, 246, 250-251, 259, 261-263, 308, 411, 426, 444
pancreatitis: 391
panting: 131
papules *bān* (gl: 311, pn: 493): 116, 127, 289, 379
paralysis *tān huàn* (gl: 492, pn: 493): 75, 271; [of the limbs]: 273
paranasal sinusitis: 128
parasites: 95, 103, 139, 265, 347
parch *jiāo* (gl: 315, pn: 493); [lips]: 127; [tongue fur]: 124, 354; [mouth]: 44
parotitis: 269
paroxysm: 195, 404
pathogen *xié* (gl: 150, pn: 493): 5, 38, 69, 96, 104, 106, 154, 159, 173, 273, 347, 362, 365, 373; [pathogenic qi] *xié qì* (pn; 493)
pattern *zhèng* (gl: 473, pn: 493): 9, 39-40, 73, 92, 97, 148, 159, 166, 203, 371
peeling tongue: 122-123, 184, 282, 322
penetrating vessel: 53, 55-56, 60, 62, 84, 89-90, 141, 241, 258, 450
pericardium: 41-42, 50-51, 64, 67, 69, 89, 164
pericardium channel: 43, 47, 49-50, 52, 66, 91, 388
pericardium heat: 89, 139, 314, 357, 433
pericardiac patterns: 357, 360, 369
periodontal *gan yá gān* (gl: 81, pn: 494): 132
periodontal *xuan yá xuān* (gl: 80, pn: 494): 393
peritonitis: 125
perverted appetite *shì shí yì wù* (gl: 351, pn: 494): 137
pestilential qi: 95, 101; [wind]: 272
phlegm: 35, 72, 75, 89, 95, 104, 106, 127-128, 131, 139, 153, 161, 173, 233, 265-266, 274, 288, 308, 310, 313-314, 317, 373, 390, 423;

600

phlegm (continued): [white]: 34, 128, 212, 308, 310; [yellow]: 128; [blood in]: 216, 327; [copious]: 128, 330, 434-435; [exuberant]: 174-175
phlegm confounding the cardiac portals: 89, 104, 120, 139, 308, 314, 331, 423, 434
phlegm lodging in the channels: 104, 120, 308, 315, 332
phlegm lodging in the chest: 308 , 316-317, 332
phlegm lodging in the limbs: 308, 315, 332
phlegm lodging in the stomach: 104, 308, 423
phlegm nodules: 308, 315, 332, 417, 422-423
phlegm streaked with blood: 310
phlegm turbidity: 69, 113, 145, 209, 256, 308, 312, 314, 434
phlegm-damp: 69, 210, 213
phlegm-drool *tán xián* (gl: 369.1, pn: 494): 390
phlegm-rheum *tán yǐn* (gl: 370, pn: 494) 33-34, 73-74, 107, 129, 146, 154, 172, 174, 189, 298, 318, 418
physical weakness: 123, 144, 171, 215, 221-222, 230, 328, 400, 406, 410, 443
plum-stone globus *méi hé qì* (gl: 275, pn: 495): 232-233, 258
pneumonia: 130, 269
poisoning: 389
polyuria *niào duō* (gl: 132, pn: 495): 86, 136, 249, 262-263, 439
portal *qiào* (gl: 466, pn: 495); [openers]: 385, 435; [opening]: 357, 369, 435
postpartum disorders: 195, 400; [blood vacuity]: 411; [insufficiency of liquid and blood]: 396
precipitation *xià (fǎ)* (gl: 7, pn: 495): 340, 369, 373-374, 390-391, 418
precipitating qi and downbearing counterflow: 256
precipitation of blood due to intestinal wind: 129
precipitation of depressed upper-body fire: 391, 393
precipitation of gastrointestinal heat-bind: 391
precipitation of heat toxin: 391-392
pregnancy: 141, 145-146, 153, 156, 195, 390, 398, 400
premature ejaculation *zǎo xiè* (gl: 110, pn: 495): 86, 249
premature menstruation: 83, 141
premature senility: 248
pressure in the head: 237, 312, 350
prickles *máng cì* (gl: 148, pn: 495): 120, 391
prolapse: 219, 230; [rectum or uterus]: 221; [rectum]: 77, 410, 437; [uterus]: 56, 410
promoting diffusion: 338, 355, 365, 379
promoting qi perfusion and transforming phlegm: 297
promoting the absorption of qi: 444
promotion of pulmonary depuration: 73
prostatitis: 56
pulmonary abscesses: 382
pulmonary edema: 35
pulmonary emphysema: 131, 246

pulmorenal yin vacuity: 15, 216, 244, 261
pulse: 25, 43, 111, 117-118, 133, 142-143, 145, 147; [children]: 117-118; [combinations]: 144; [depth]: 143-144; [examination]: 141-142; [organ correspondence]: 142; [rate]: 143-144
pungent dissipating lung diffusion: 72
pungent opening and bitter discharge: 325
purgation: 106, 390
purple discharge with clots: 141
purple macules: 195
purple tongue: 68, 122
purple-black blood: 29
purple-black complexion: 115
pustules: 272
putrefaction: 127, 382
qi *qì* (gl: 208, pn: 496): 7, 23-27, 31, 33, 36-39, 53, 57, 68, 70, 76, 80, 84, 117, 163, 173, 199, 286, 370, 395, 412
qi absorption *nà qì* (gl: 242, pn: 497): 73, 87, 215-216, 246, 262
qi and blood: 121, 141, 147
qi ascent *shàng qì* (gl: 5, pn: 497): 27, 131
qi dynamic *qì jī* (gl: 217, pn: 497): 26, 33, 80, 233, 341
qi pain *qì tòng* (gl: 215, pn: 498): 138, 278
qi shortage *qì shǎo* (gl: 210, pn: 498): 73
qi stagnation: 26-27, 29, 80, 98, 139, 189, 191-192, 194-195, 198, 256, 274, 278, 402
qi surging up into the heart: 347
qi thoroughfare *qì jiē* (gl: 214, pn: 498): 25, 45, 52, 55
qi vacuity: 26, 29, 33, 68, 70, 75, 112, 119, 121, 123, 128, 134, 171, 189-190, 194, 205, 219, 278, 380-381, 410
qi, blood relationship: 4, 28; [pattern identification]: 189
qi-aspect: 349, 351-352, 358, 366-367, 384
racing of the heart *zhēng chōng* (gl: 158, pn: 499): 101, 193, 204, 206, 209, 250-251, 347, 444
racing pulse: 146, 156
rapid breathing: 34-35, 43-44, 47, 49, 73, 87, 100, 127, 174, 211, 215-216, 263, 266-267, 310, 316, 349, 351, 366; [at slightest movement]: 183, 250; [while recumbent]: 113
rapid hungering: 46, 77
rapid pulse: 29, 68, 98, 144-146, 153, 156, 168, 173, 179, 186, 197, 206, 208, 281, 291, 295, 314, 343-344, 351, 354, 366-369
rapid, feeble pulse: 99, 200
rapid, fine pulse: 259
rapid, fine, wiry pulse: 193
rapid, floating pulse: 178, 268, 379
rapid, large, surging pulse: 283
rapid, slippery pulse: 310, 212
rapid, surging pulse: 164
rapid, vacuous pulse: 218
rapid, wiry pulse: 259, 326

rashness: 233, 236, 259
rectifying qi *lǐ qì* (gl: 282, pn: 499): 191, 229, 233, 258, 278, 321, 400, 402, 417
red cheeks: 216
red complexion: 50, 115, 168, 179, 236, 259, 281, 314, 349
red speckles: 195
red tongue: 34, 68, 87, 98-99, 120-122, 124, 161, 178, 193, 197-198, 217-218, 238, 244, 251, 255-256, 259, 261, 268, 281, 319, 327, 344, 349, 354, 357, 365, 368, 377, 379; [slightly]: 324
red tongue with dry, yellow fur, 226
red tongue with little fur: 182, 322
red tongue with scant or peeling fur: 413
red tongue with slimy, yellow fur, 170
red tongue with thick, slimy or rough yellow fur: 324
red tongue with yellow fur: 164, 168, 182, 186, 228, 310, 330
red, dry tongue: 301; [furless]: 252
red, mirror tongue: 168, 208, 227, 244, 255, 301
red, swollen lesions: 281
red, swollen tonsils: 268
red and fissured tongue: 282
red or crimson tongue: 179, 184
red-tipped tongue: 208, 252, 292
refloating the grounded ship: 399
regulating the governing and penetrating vessels: 258
reinforcing yang *zhú yáng* (gl: 123, pn: 499): 6
repelling foulness and opening the portals: 433, 435
repelling turbidity: 229
replete pulse: 186
repletion *shí* (gl: 396, pn: 499): 113, 130, 153, 159, 164, 168, 170-173
repletion-cold: 9, 169
repletion-heat: 9, 39, 76, 115, 120, 122, 132, 146, 168-169, 225, 281, 286, 288, 322; [fire]: 99, 286
repletion-heat at blood level: 368
repletion dyspnea: 131, 175
repletion falsely presenting as vacuity: 160
resolution *jiě* (gl: 387, pn: 500); [exterior]: 267, 400; [toxin]: 295, 355
restlessness *xīn fán* (gl: 70, pn: 500): 29, 43, 46-47, 49-50, 67, 99-100, 135, 138, 164-165, 182, 185, 197, 208, 251-252, 281-283, 286, 288, 331, 341, 343-344, 349, 351-352, 354, 361, 363, 366, 368, 393, 413, 416
restoration of hepatic storage of blood and governance: 232
restoring the correct: 176, 343
restoring yang while supporting yin: 416
retching: 46, 48, 227; [nausea]: 293, 308, 312, 403; [blood] *ǒu xuè* (gl: 394, pn: 500): 197
retraction of the scrotum: 345
rhinitis: 71-72

rigid *jiàng zhí* (gl: 267, pn: 500); [limbs]: 266; [neck]: 113, 260, 319; [neck and back]: 269
ringworm patches: 114
rising fire flush: 184
rough breathing: 131, 175, 185-186, 314
rough pulse: 29, 104, 146, 154
rough tongue fur: 34, 122, 259
rough yellow tongue fur: 259
rough, dry skin: 101, 328
running nose: 72, 98, 128
safeguard liquid: 302
salvaging yang: 205, 250, 262, 344, 360, 363, 407
sapor *wèi* (gl: 153, pn: 500): 248
scallion-stalk pulse: 145, 200
scattered pulse: 144, 155
schistosomiasis: 122
scrofula: 52, 128, 308, 315, 332, 417, 422-423
sea of: [blood]: 56 ; [marrow]: 54, 89, 247 ; [qi]: 25 ; [yang channels]: 54 ; [yin channels]: 55
securing *gù* (gl: 155, pn: 501): 249, 263, 408, 442, 447
semiconsciousness: 314, 369
seminal efflux *huá jīng* (gl: 365, pn: 501): 26, 86, 249, 262-263, 435, 438
seminal emission *yí jīng* (gl: 442, pn: 501): 56, 87, 102, 184, 203, 241, 244, 249, 261, 263, 416, 435, 438
seminal loss *shī jīng* (gl: 93, pn: 501): 83, 155, 171
serous discharge: 272, 386
settle *zhèn* (gl: 472, pn: 501): 444
shaking *diào* (gl: 270, pn: 501): 97, 113, 273
shan qi *shàn qì* (gl: 171, pn: 501): 53, 55
shao yang: 40-42, 46-48, 50-52, 56-59, 61-64, 91, 135, 139, 241, 341-342, 347, 360, 362, 400-401
shao yin: 40-42, 46, 48-50, 54-55, 57, 59-64, 139, 344, 347, 363
shivering: 105, 134-135, 371
shock: 114
short micturition: 34-35, 100, 289, 408
short micturition with dark colored urine: 129, 164, 168, 170, 179, 281, 285, 292, 298, 323-325, 386
short micturition with scant urine *xiǎo biàn duǎn shǎo* (pn: 502): 99, 136, 289-291, 324, 352, 367, 432
short pulse: 148, 156
short, rapid breathing: 176, 447
shortness of breath: 49, 68, 70, 73, 87, 180, 183, 185, 199, 204, 209, 215, 217, 222, 250-251, 253, 255, 410
sickly taste in mouth: 290, 292, 325-326
simultaneous dispersion: 306, 329
simultaneous supplementation and attack: 374, 399
sinew-vascular hypertonicity: 81

Concepts Index

sinews *jīn* (gl: 328, pn: 502): 28, 37-38
sinusitis: 128
skin diseases: 70, 117
skipping pulse: 148
slimy tongue fur: 78, 119, 122-123, 174-175, 213, 228, 305, 312, 325-326, 349, 352, 365, 387, 427
slimy white or dry, slightly yellow fur: 324
slimy, glossy tongue fur: 314
slimy, thick tongue fur: 6, 99-100, 125-126, 285, 290, 292, 297, 309, 314, 323, 330, 394, 434
slimy, white tongue fur: 124, 367, 369
slimy, yellow tongue fur: 164, 180, 292, 294, 314, 325, 367, 386
slimy, unclean tongue fur: 329, 331-332
slippery pulse: 144, 146, 173, 186, 213, 226, 291, 313, 315, 330-332, 369
slippery tongue: 309
slippery, rapid pulse: 314, 322, 324
slippery, wiry pulse: 174-175, 236, 314
slow pulse: 68, 87, 145, 153, 156, 166-167, 183, 190, 210, 274, 279
slow interrupted pulse: 148
slow, fine, weak pulse: 250
small intestine: 32, 38, 41-42, 46, 48, 64-67, 69, 73, 75-77, 91-92
small intestine channel: 47, 50-51, 57-60, 62-63
small intestine governs: 32, 76
small pulse: 147
soft, soggy pulse: 174, 199, 219
softening (of hardness) *ruǎn jiān* (gl: 286, pn: 503): 418, 422-423
soggy pulse: 99-100, 147, 154, 183, 186, 221, 224, 254, 285, 290-291, 369, 427
soggy, moderate pulse: 99
soggy, not too rapid pulse: 324
soggy, rapid pulse: 352, 367
somber white complexion: 114-115, 164, 166-167, 179, 183, 185-186, 222, 225, 274, 407-408
somnolence *shì shuì* (gl: 352, pn: 503): 49, 165, 343, 357, 363
soot black *lí hēi* (gl: 429, pn: 503); [complexion]: 29, 195
sore pharynx: 48-49, 170, 265, 268, 319, 350, 365, 379
sore throat: 39, 44, 51, 101, 127, 178, 286, 345, 393
spasm *jìng luán* (gl: 322, pn: 503): 53, 82, 97, 113, 333, 356; [limbs]: 50, 53, 57
speech: 130; [strident]: 131; [deranged]: 112; [faltering]: 130; [feeble]: 215; [impeded]: 183, 239, 260, 423, 425; [incoherent]: 434; [slow]: 112
spermatorrhea: 246, 414
spider nevi: 117, 195
spillage rheum *yì yǐn* (gl: 359, pn: 503): 318
spirit *shén* (gl: 237, pn: 503): 67, 88, 95, 111, 133, 207
spirit-affect *shén qíng* (gl: 239, pn: 504): 22, 176

spirit-disposition *shén zhì* (gl: 240, pn: 504): 22, 67, 104, 112, 331, 354, 433
spiritual fatigue: 6, 68, 102, 165, 171, 183, 209, 217, 220, 222, 262, 406
spleen: 23, 26-28, 30, 32, 34-35, 41-42, 45-46, 57, 61-62, 64-68, 71-78, 83, 85, 87, 90-91, 99, 101-102, 104, 125, 190, 218, 276, 422
spleen and stomach obstructed by the damp pathogen: 289
spleen channel: 45-46, 49, 52, 59-63
spleen fortification: 16, 73, 77-78, 219, 222, 224, 254-255, 313, 331, 428
spleen governs: 27, 35, 65, 73-75
spleen qi: 65, 74, 77-78
spleen qi vacuity: 219, 221, 254
spleen-vacuity qi stagnation: 373
splenic diarrhea *pí xiè* (gl: 337, pn: 504): 14
splenic movement and transformation: 32, 34-35, 69, 102, 192, 218-219, 254, 289, 308, 313
splenic vacuity: 75, 90, 100, 127, 207, 222, 304, 329-330, 342
splenogastric damp: 292-293, 325
splenogastric precipitation: 374
splenogastric qi vacuity: 190
splenogastric transformation failure: 29, 289, 342
splenogastric vacuity: 15, 138, 174, 222, 298, 306, 405-406
splenorenal yang vacuity: 79, 218, 246, 262
stagnant digestate complication: 307
stagnation *zhì* (gl: 398, pn: 504): 7, 26-29, 81, 104, 191, 307, 390
stasis *yū* (gl: 375, pn: 504): 29, 80, 106, 116, 341
stasis macules *yū bān* (gl: 376, pn: 504): 29, 104
stasis speckles *yū diǎn* (gl: 378, pn: 505): 68
stasis-transforming: 196, 252, 418
static blood: 104, 145, 174, 195, 204, 265, 281, 328, 418
steaming bone tidal fever *gǔ zhēng cháo rè* (gl: 254, pn: 505): 134, 168, 244, 283, 288, 322, 388
sterility: 55, 241, 244, 246, 262
stiffness: 58; [neck]: 48-49; [tongue]: 120, 423, 425
stomach: 26-28, 30, 32, 38-39, 41-42, 45-46, 48, 61, 64-67, 73-78, 80, 85, 91, 102, 104, 125, 190, 218, 276, 304, 390
stomach channel: 39, 42-43, 45, 51, 57-63
stomach downbears turbid qi: 65, 78, 403
stomach fire: 226, 288, 375
stomach governs ingestion: 65, 76
stomach harmonization: 78, 228, 423, 426
stomach heat: 129, 132, 137-138, 225-226, 255-256, 298, 348, 358, 369, 383
stomach qi: 65, 76-77, 91, 122-123, 137, 223; [disharmony]: 224; [vacuity]: 219
stomach yin: 225, 227, 255

603

stomachache: 76, 102, 138, 406
stool changes: 100, 136, 322, 398
stool with bright red blood: 129
striations *còu lǐ* (gl: 380, pn: 505): 24, 70-71, 96
strident voice: 175, 186
strong, deep, replete pulse: 339
strong, deep, slippery pulse: 391
strong, full pulse: 395
strong, rapid pulse: 170
strong, rapid, surging pulse: 281
struma: 128, 233, 258, 315, 332, 422-423
subaxillary swelling: 50, 52
subcutaneous hemorrhage: 195
subcutaneous phlegm nodules: 104
subduing yang *qián yáng* (gl: 422, pn: 505): 6, 238-239, 302, 444, 445
summerheat: 96, 100, 105, 108
summerheat diarrhea *shǔ xiè* (gl: 356, pn: 506)
summerheat-damp: 100, 281, 285, 299, 323
summerheat-heat: 100, 281, 283, 323
summerheat-strike (sunstroke): 100, 288
superabundance *yǒu yú* (gl: 111, pn: 506): 58
supplementation *bǔ (fǎ)* (gl: 341, pn: 506): 165, 171, 190, 198, 243, 248, 346, 373-376, 382, 395, 410, 417
supplementation and boosting: 410
supplementation followed by attack, 106, 149, 374
supplementation of blood: 241, 251, 411
supplementation of qi: 6, 410
supplementation of yang: 253, 376, 405, 414
supplementation of yin: 6, 376, 412
supplementing fire: 14
supplementing the center: 222
supporting resistance and outthrusting: 106
surface skin and body hair *pí máo* (gl: 99, pn: 507): 37-38, 65, 70-72
surfeit *piān shèng* (gl: 256, pn: 507): 5, 8-9, 107, 375-376
surging pulse: 100, 147, 154, 173, 186, 383
surging, large pulse: 339
suspended rheum *xuán yǐn* (gl: 474, pn: 507): 318
sweat: 26, 31-32, 71, 87, 105, 164, 176, 178, 339, 349, 360, 405; [retrenchment]: 33
sweating: 68, 71, 96, 134-135, 217, 337-338, 380-381; [absence of]: 100, 178, 266, 268, 283, 323, 361; [cold]: 190, 200, 250, 252, 407; [copious]: 68, 176, 217, 351]; [excessive]: 115, 301; [heavy]: 115; [impeded]: 268, 351; [oily]: 246; [vacuity]: 447
sweating, spontaneous: 134-135, 171, 183, 189, 204, 215, 244, 410, 435-436
sweating: profuse perspiration *dà hàn* (gl: 19, pn: 495): 164, 171, 176, 283, 288, 323, 339, 361, 366
shiver-sweating: 135
sweeping phlegm and opening the portals: 314, 331, 433-434

swelling *zhǒng* (gl: 381, pn: 507): 26, 34, 44, 51, 144, 382; [and distention]: 382; [face]: 265, 316; [lower limbs]: 45, 215; [limbs]: 204; [joints with heaviness]: 427; [throat]: 127; [tonsils]: 390
swill diarrhea *sūn xiè* (gl: 345, pn: 507): 53, 78-79
syncope: 433
tachycardia: 206, 244
tai yang: 40-42, 44-45, 47-48, 50-52, 54, 56-64, 88, 135, 337-338, 341-342, 347, 350, 360, 381
tai yin: 40-43, 46-47, 49-50, 52, 57, 59-64, 342-344, 347, 362
taxation *láo* (gl: 300, pn: 507): 26; taxation strangury *láo lín* (gl: 301, pn: 507); [coughs]: 113; [fatigue]: 95, 103, 219, 265
tenesmus: 27, 137, 294, 306, 326
tension and stiffness in the neck: 239, 337
tetanic disease *jìng bìng* (gl: 320, pn: 507); tetanic inversion *jìng jué* (gl: 321, pn: 507): 164, 260, 266, 283, 301, 354-355, 368-369, 433, 445
tetanus: 271, 273, 319, 333
tetany: 113, 333
thermic disease: 335, 348-349, 353-354
thick tongue fur: 122-124, 291, 305
thick, sticky phlegm: 173, 212
thick, yellow phlegm containing blood or pus: 330
thin stool: 44, 49, 77, 99, 137, 180, 183, 289, 199, 297, 387, 427
thin-stool diarrhea *táng xiè* (gl: 357, pn: 508): 293, 323, 323, 369
thin tongue fur: 122-124, 161, 178, 181, 337, 379
thin, brittle nails: 328
thin, clear phlegm: 128, 253, 330
thin, fast pulse: 413
thin, rapid pulse: 168, 283
thin, slow, weak pulse: 181
thirst: 33-34, 44, 98, 100, 115, 135, 137, 164, 186, 197, 283, 304, 324, 339, 345, 349, 351-352, 361, 366, 379, 383 ; [great thirst] 323, 361, 366
thirst with a desire for warm fluids: 166-167, 170, 176, 179, 186, 394
thirst with desire for cold fluids: 85, 168, 170, 281
thirst with desire for fluids: 281, 287, 301, 324
thirst with no desire for fluids: 47, 137, 292, 297, 324-325, 367
thirst without fluid intake: 291, 352
thoracic glomus: 228, 256, 286, 308
thoracic oppression: 323, 325-326, 329-331, 365, 367
thoracic phlegm turbidity obstruction: 313

thoracic water *xiōng shuǐ; xiōng fù shuǐ* (gl: 244, pn: 508): 395
thrombocytopenic purpura: 197
thyrocele: 422
tidal fever *cháo rè* (gl: 423, pn: 508): 87, 134, 182, 216, 241, 253, 261, 282-283, 322, 339, 341, 361, 369, 388, 391
tidal flushing: 115, 164, 170, 179, 185-186, 217, 322
tight pulse: 147, 155, 161, 166-167, 276-277, 361
tight, floating pulse: 162, 178, 266
tight, wiry pulse: 181, 279
timidity and fear: 58, 138
tingling *má* (gl: 295, pn: 508): 239, 260
tinnitus: 53, 86, 136, 139, 237, 244, 246-247, 261-262, 393, 411; [sudden]: 236, 259
tissue edema: 119
toad-head scourge: 269
tongue: 29, 65, 104, 111, 118-122, 125, 208, 210, 246, 252, 281
toothache: 39, 44, 269, 288, 389
toxin *dú* (gl: 165, pn: 508); toxin-resolving: 372-373
transformation into fire *huà huǒ* (gl: 57, pn: 508): 23, 65, 77
transformation of damp: 290-291, 299, 325, 418, 427
transformation of digestate: 6, 76
transformation of fluids: 73, 221, 298, 308
transformation of phlegm: 229, 256, 309, 311, 331, 367, 391, 418, 423
transformation of static blood: 391, 418-419
transformative action of qi *qì huà* (gl: 209, pn: 509): 26, 34, 91
transforming rheum, expelling phlegm: 317, 332
transforming stasis: 196
transforming turbidity with pungent aromatics: 252
transmutation *biàn* (gl: 485, pn: 509): 23
trauma: 95, 103, 265
trembling; [hands]: 445; [lips and fingers]: 239; [tongue]: 121
tremor: 82, 97, 260, 273
triple burner: 32, 41-43, 64-66, 69, 304, 325, 383
triple burner channel: 43, 50-52, 57-59, 61, 91
trismus: 113, 266, 269, 435
true *zhēn* (gl: 232, pn: 509); true qi *zhēn qì* (gl: 234.1, pn: 509): 70, 73
tuberculosis: 113, 120, 122, 146-147, 213, 244, 388, 390
turbid *zhuó* (gl: 435, pn: 509): 8, 34, 60, 70, 72-73, 76, 78, 130
turbid yellow, foul-smelling mucus: 128
turbid, slimy tongue fur: 123, 256, 369
twitching; [muscles]: 445; [sinews and flesh]: 239
ulcerative diseases: 122, 152, 191, 198, 224-225
unclean *gòu* (gl: 180, pn: 510); [tongue fur]: 122-123, 314, 357
unctuous strangury *gāo lín* (gl: 412, pn: 510): 288

undigested food: 46, 169-170
ungratified desire to vomit: 228, 345, 435
ungratified urge to evacuate: 435
upbearing *shēng* (gl: 60, pn: 510): 8, 12, 23, 27, 33-34, 65, 73, 77-78, 83, 87, 137, 286
upbearing fire: 87, 252, 322, 412
upbearing fire flush *miàn hóng shēng huǒ* (gl: 200, pn: 510): 15, 170, 193, 208, 237, 251, 282-283, 447
upbearing yang and boosting qi: 222, 254
upflow and nausea: 325-326, 350, 352, 365, 367, 387
upper body *shàng* (gl: 3, pn: 511): 175, 308
upper burner: 71, 91
upper ventral vexation *ào nóng* (gl: 433, pn: 511): 351-352
upper-body harrassment by phlegm turbidity: 331
upper-body heat and lower-body cold: 169
upper-body heat: 346, 364
upstirring *shēng dòng* (pn: 511): 12-13, 97
uremia: 125
urethritis: 56
urinary block *niào bì, lóng bì* (gl: 134, pn: 511): 49, 53, 203, 243, 246, 432
urinary calculi: 422
urinary frequency *niào pín* (gl: 136, pn: 511): 51, 249, 262-263, 295, 326, 427
urinary urgency *niào jí* (gl: 133, pn: 511): 129, 295, 431
urination: 26, 31, 86, 129, 136; [burning sensation]: 69; [excessive]: 137, 301; [heavy]: 34; [inhibited]: 35, 46, 71, 341, 345; [red]: 281; [scant]: 33-35, 69, 76, 289; [turbid]: 129; [reduction]: 439; [retention]: 86, 395
urticaria: 272
uterus: 27, 88-90, 398, 450
vacuity: 4, 6-7, 14-15, 26-27, 76, 104, 107, 115-116, 130, 135, 137, 159, 164, 170-171, 337, 343, 347, 376
vacuity and repletion *xū shí* (gl: 338, pn: 512): 7, 173
vacuity cold: 9, 68, 132, 137, 169, 218, 230, 342-343, 363, 397
vacuity desertion *xū tuō* (gl: 340, pn: 512): 134-135, 149, 154, 287, 343, 360, 363, 374, 435
vacuity dyspnea: 131, 174
vacuity edema *xū fú* (gl: 339, pn: 512): 114, 127
vacuity falsely presenting as repletion: 160, 372
vacuity fire: 99, 286
vacuity glomus in the venter: 227, 255
vacuity heat: 68, 115, 122, 169, 282-283, 288, 322, 343-344, 363, 368, 412
vacuity of correct qi: 113, 173-174, 374, 401
vacuity of marrow: 85
vacuity of qi and blood: 122, 199, 145
vacuity of the qi: 26, 130, 344
vacuity of yang: 153

vacuity of yin and hyperactivity of yang: 146
vacuity polyuria in old age: 439
vacuity stirring endogenous wind: 356
vacuous pulse: 288
vacuous, rapid pulse: 147, 344, 407
vacuous, weak pulse: 253
vacuous, wiry pulse: 146-147
vaginal discharge *dài xià* (gl: 266, pn: 512): 99, 102, 289, 296, 435, 443; [checking]: 443
vesicular qi-block: 136
vigorous fever *zhuàng rè* (gl: 130, pn: 512): 168, 182, 186, 322, 383
viral infections: 97, 335
viscera: 24, 26, 28, 31, 35, 38, 40-41, 65-67, 70, 82-83, 101, 189
visceral manifestation theory *zàng xiàng xúe shūo* (pn: 513): 11, 65
visual dizziness *xuàn* (gl: 231, pn: 513): 82, 89, 165, 266, 341-342
vitamin B deficiencies: 120
vomiting *ǒu tù* (gl: 393, pn: 513): 6, 27, 34, 42, 49, 52-53, 76, 78, 80, 98, 100, 129, 137, 145, 164, 169, 203, 224-225, 228, 233, 236, 256-257, 276, 285, 294, 301, 329, 341-343, 345-346, 362, 389, 364, 400, 403-404, 406-407, 418, 423, 426-427
warming: 25, 32, 165, 167, 222, 229, 250, 254-256, 262, 263, 278, 303, 320-321, 330, 346, 358, 362, 364, 405-406, 408-409, 434
warm, bitter damp dryers: 427-428
warm, pungent exterior resolution: 162, 178, 319-320, 361, 377
water *shuǐ* (gl: 73, pn: 513): 10, 84, 144, 399
water amassment: 318, 417
water containment failure: 86
water disinhibition: 106, 373
water expulsion: 395
water qi *shuǐ qì* (gl: 75, pn: 514): 35, 345
water swelling *shuǐ zhǒng* (gl: 76, pn: 514): 5-6, 16, 33-35, 51, 71, 75, 79, 99, 128, 140, 189, 203, 246, 250, 262-263, 289, 405, 408, 430
water-damp *shuǐ shī* (gl: 78, pn: 514): 6, 16, 74, 99, 119, 137, 172, 174, 289, 299, 405, 430
water-rheum *shuǐ yǐn* (gl: 77, pn: 514): 34, 263, 318, 391
weak pulse: 145, 155, 186
weak, deep, fine pulse: 408
weak, faint pulse: 149
weak, moderate pulse: 342-343
weak, rapid pulse: 176
weak, soggy pulse: 262, 410
weak, vacuous pulse: 360
wheezing *xiāo* (gl: 203, pn: 514): 43, 114
wheezing dyspnea *xiāo chuǎn* (gl: 204, pn: 515): 7
white tongue fur: 124, 313, 164, 181, 314-315, 406
white vaginal discharge: 55-56, 289, 443
white, glossy tongue fur: 119, 122, 266, 276, 321

wind: 26, 87, 92, 96-97, 105, 121, 140, 164, 265-268, 270, 272-273, 308, 337-338, 352, 378-379, 425, 446; [barrier]: 117
wind-cold: 114, 161, 266-267, 269, 271, 273-275, 279, 303, 319, 337
wind-cold-damp: 204, 279, 289, 409, 420
wind-extinguishing: 385
wind-fire ocular rubor: 269
wind-fire toothache: 39, 269
wind-heat: 115, 161, 266, 268-269, 271-273, 319, 354
wind-phlegm: 135, 311, 331
wind-strike *zhòng fēng* (gl: 40, pn: 515): 121, 314, 433
wind-thermia: 349-352, 365
wiry pulse: 146, 154, 165, 233, 238, 257, 259, 276-277, 313, 341, 362, 369
withdrawal *diān* (gl: 491, pn: 515): 23, 444
withered yellow *wěi huáng* (pn: 515); [complexion]: 115, 193, 222
wry mouth and eyes: 266, 269, 273, 423, 425; [mouth]: 45, 127; [tongue]: 121
yang channels: 40-41, 58, 135
yang-collapse: 135, 149-150, 175-176, 287, 335, 343-344, 360, 363, 372, 374, 405, 407
yang linking vessel: 53, 58
yang ming: 39, 40-45, 51, 57-64, 120, 135, 269, 339-342, 347, 351-352, 360-361, 388-389, 391, 401
yang motility vessel: 53, 57, 59, 312
yang qi desertion: 121, 145, 156, 175
yang qi vacuity: 8, 114, 122, 190, 405
yang vacuity: 5, 145, 150, 153, 171, 175, 243, 250, 408, 414
yang vacuity water flood *yáng xū shuǐ fàn* (gl: 344, pn: 515): 263
yellow bile: 233
yellow complexion: 29, 103, 115, 306, 411
yellow tongue fur: 98, 124, 173, 212, 281, 295, 305, 313, 322, 325, 339, 351-352, 366, 369, 393; [slight]: 352; [old yellow]: 124, 329, 339, 391
yellow urine: 46, 53, 351, 356-367, 427; [dry] 279
yin and yang: 3-5, 6-7, 9, 16, 37-38, 40, 59, 81, 84, 86-87, 95, 104-107, 133, 159, 166, 175, 375-376
yin channels: 40-41, 59, 90
yin collapse: 175-176
yin humor: 5, 8, 107, 123, 301, 356
yin humor depletion: 120-121, 227, 273
yin linking vessel: 53, 57-58, 388
yin liquid vacuity: 120
yin motility vessel: 53, 56-57, 59, 312
yin vacuity fire effulgence *yin xū huǒ wàng* (gl: 294, pn: 515): 7, 115, 127, 139, 146, 208, 416
yin vacuity: 6, 134, 153, 175, 193, 227, 243, 308, 380, 412